INFLAMMATORY BOWEL DISEASE – ADVANCES IN PATHOGENESIS AND MANAGEMENT

Edited by **Sami Karoui**

Inflammatory Bowel Disease – Advances in Pathogenesis and Management
Edited by Sami Karoui

Published by InTech

Janeza Trdine 9, 51000 Rijeka, Croatia

Publishing Process Manager Bojan Rafaj

Technical Editor Teodora Smiljanic

Cover Designer InTech Design Team

Additional hard copies can be obtained from orders@intechopen.com

Inflammatory Bowel Disease – Advances in Pathogenesis and Management,
Edited by Sami Karoui
p. cm.
ISBN 978-953-307-891-5

For EU product safety concerns:
IN TECH d.o.o., Prolaz Marije Krucifikse Kozulić 3, 51000 Rijeka, Croatia,
info@intechopen.com or visit our website at intechopen.com.

Meet the editor

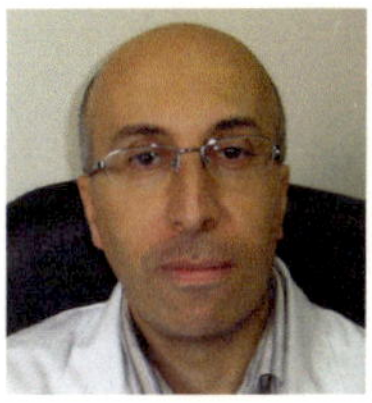

Dr Sami Karoui was born in Tunis in 1968. He studied at the Faculty of Medicine of Tunis and attended Gastroenterology and Hepatology courses at University Hospitals in Tunis. He received the diploma of Gastroenterologist in 1998, and has been working at the Department of Gastroenterology, A. La Rabta Hospital – Tunis, and at the Faculty of Medicine of Tunis since 2000. Dr Karoui also works as a Professor of Gastroenterology and Hepatology since 2008.

Contents

Preface

Inflammatory bowel diseases (IBD), such as ulcerative colitis and Crohn's disease, are chronic and relapsing conditions, characterized by abdominal pain, diarrhea, bleeding and malabsorption. IBD is considered to be a hyper-inflammatory state due to disturbed interactions between the immune system and the commensal bacterial flora of the gut. In recent years, many studies have focused on etiopathogeny of IBD, as well as on advances in diagnosis tools. A better comprehension of mechanisms of the new drugs used for treatment of IBD has enabled new approach strategies in the management of Crohn's disease and ulcerative colitis.

There is accumulating evidence on the importance of microbes in the development and maintenance of both the intestinal and immune systems. No evidence that inflammatory bowel disease is caused by a single agent has been found, whereas a number of microbes have been strongly associated with the presence of disease. The majority of recent studies support a role for the ability of intestinal pathogens to promote chronic inflammation in individuals with genetic susceptibility and/or other environmental factors, which remain to be identified.

The lower gastrointestinal tract houses trillions of microbial cells, representing a large diversity of species in relatively well-defined phylogenetic ratios that are associated with maintenance of key aspects of host physiology and immune homeostasis. It is therefore not surprising that many GI inflammatory diseases, including inflammatory bowel disease, are associated with substantial changes in the composition of these microbial assemblages, either as a cause or consequence of host inflammatory response.

Inflammatory bowel diseases are the consequence of a dysregulated mucosal immune system. The mucosal immune system consists of two arms, innate and adaptive immunity, that have been studied separately for a long time. In the last several years, there has been a huge increase in the discovery of inflammatory bowel disease susceptibility genes. However, similar advances in identifying and defining environmental risk factors associated with IBD have lagged behind.

Treatment of inflammatory bowel disease has changed in recent years. Potential future treatment goals in Crohn's disease include reduction in bowel damage, prevention of complications and maintaining long term remission. Combination therapy with infliximab and azathioprine demonstrated superior rates of sustained clinical remission, when compared to standard therapy. In ulcerative colitis, potential treatment goals include sustained clinical remission, sustained mucosal healing and reduction of rates of colorectal dysplasia and cancer. Although tumor necrosis factor antagonists are effective for the treatment of Crohn's disease and ulcerative colitis, lack and loss of clinical response is a clinical challenge. Accordingly, the use of therapeutic drug monitoring has been proposed as a means to optimize treatment. Several observational studies have demonstrated a relationship between anti-TNF agent serum drug concentrations and/or antidrug antibody presence, and various symptomatic and objective clinical endpoints. However, these relationships are not absolute, and although some algorithms for the use of therapeutic drug monitoring in clinical practice have been proposed, none have yet been validated in a prospective clinical trial.

Dr. Sami Karoui
Department of Gastroenterology A. La Rabta Hospital
Tunis

Part 1

Pathogenesis of Inflammatory Bowel Disease

1

The Role of COX-2 Inhibitors on Experimental Colitis

Ana Paula R. Paiotti[1], RicardoArtigiani-Neto[1], Daniel A. Ribeiro[1,2], Sender J. Miszputen[3] and Marcello Franco[1]
Universidade Federal de São Paulo, Escola Paulista de Medicina
[1]Departament of Pathology
[2]Departament of Biosciences
[3]Division of Gastroenterology
Brasil

1. Introduction

Since the introduction of acetylsalicylic acid (aspirin) as the first nonsteroidal antiinflammatory drug (NSAID) in 1897, NSAIDs have been widely used in the management of pain and inflammation (Botting, 2010; Vane et al., 1990; Wallace, 1997). Today, they are classified as traditional nonsteroidal antiinflammatory drugs (tNSAIDs), characterized by differing degrees of antiinflammatory, analgesic and antipyretic activity. tNSAIDs are among the most widely used medicines in the world. Unfortunately, they are associated with dose-dependent gastrointestinal (GI) adverse events ranging from dyspepsia (10-20%) to symptomatic and complicated ulcers (1-4%) (Scheiman, 2006; Wolfe et al., 1999). The mechanism of tNSAIDs action is attributed to the cyclooxygenase (COX) inhibition (Botting, 2010; Vane, 1971). Cyclooxygenase is a key rate-limiting enzyme that exists in at least two isoforms: COX-1 is observed constitutively expressed in various tissues, whereas COX-2 does not appear to be expressed except at very low levels in most tissues and is rapidly upregulated in response to growth factors and cytokines. More recently, COX-2 has been implicated in several distinct cellular mechanisms, such as angiogenesis, proliferation and the prevention of apoptosis (Dempke et al., 2001). New antiinflammatory drugs have been synthesized, such as selective COX-2 inhibitors (anti-COX-2), however, these drugs may present side effects, such as the ability to modify the epithelial barrier.
Inflammatory bowel disease (IBD) is a common chronic gastrointestinal disorder characterized by alternating periods of remission and active intestinal inflammation. The precise etiology of IBD, including Crohn´s disease (CD) and ulcerative colitis (UC), remains unclear. However, environmental factors, immunological disturbances, genetic influences and the presence of certain chemical mediators (cytokines) have been established as putative participants in the pathogenesis of the disease (Barbieri, 2000; Lashner, 1995; Podolsky, 2002).
In the last few decades, the development of experimental models for studying IBD has greatly contributed to enhance understanding of the immunological mechanisms involved, such as changes in the gut epithelial barrier (Colpaert et al, 2001; Shorter et al, 1972). IBD seems to occur when luminal antigens from the bacterial flora stimulate the immune system

in the gut barrier towards an exacerbated, genetically defined response. Patients present an increase in the amount of intestinal bacterial antigen compared to healthy individuals (Bonen & Cho, 2003). In particular, some human and animal studies have shown the prime importance of gut epithelial barrier integrity and changes that lead to deregulation of the immune system as a result of the loss of intestinal homeostasis (Élson et al., 1995).

A possible association between the use of NSAIDs and the relapse of IBD has been repeatedly suggested. IBD patients seek relief in NSAIDs for non-IBD-related pains (arthralgias, arthritides) and these drugs are also prescribed for the symptons of extraintestinal manifestations of IBD, such as peripheral arthritis, sacroiliitis, ankylosing spondylitis, and osteoporosis-related fractures. NSAIDs are considered to be the first-line treatment for the abnormalities just mentioned (i.e, relieve pain and treat inflammation).

It has been reported that CD is associated with gut barrier dysfunction and that some patients express an instestinal barrier hyperresponsiveness to NSAIDs (Gornet et al., 2002). Thus, clinicians are concerned that the treatment with NSAIDs could increase the risk of disease aggravation relapse in controlled patients. A large number of people suffering from IBD take NSAIDs and COX-2 inhibitors for various reasons, as the efficiency of these drugs in pain control seems to be unquestioned. In some patients, exacerbation disease happens; however it is uncertain whether NSAIDs are implicated in IBD relapse or whether COX-2 inhibitors are safer than NSAIDs.

NSAIDs have been implicated in the onset or the exacerbation of IBD in a number of studies and case reports, whereas in other studies, no relationship has been found between NSAID treatment and an increase in significant disease flares. On the other hand, COX-2 inhibitors have a smaller incidence of toxicity to the small bowel or colon, as recent studies indicate that COX-2 inhibitors are prescribed more often than NSAIDs in patients who are older, sicker, and have risk factors associated with NSAID gastropathy (Bonner et al., 2000; Bonner et al., 2004; Kurahara et al, 2001; Vane et al., 1998). Is the concept that the use of NSAIDs is associated with relapse of IBD is true? For this reason, many studies are conducted with the use of COX-2 in experimental models. So, the objective of this review is to describe the role of COX-2 inhibitors on different experimental models of colitis.

2. COX-1/ COX-2 concept, biochemistry and structural comparisons

Cyclooxygenase (COX) or prostaglandin H2 synthase (PGHs) is the enzyme that catalyzes the first two steps in the biosynthesis of the prostaglandins (PGs) from the substrate arachidonic acid (AA). These are the oxidation of AA to the hydorxyendoperoxide PGH2. The PGH2 is transformed by a range of enzymes and nonenzymic mechanisms into the primary prostanoids, PGD_2, PGE_2, $PGF_{2\alpha}$, PGI_2 and thromboxane A_2 (TXA_2) (DeWitt & Smith , 1988) (**Figure 1**).

COX activity has long been studied in prepraration from sheep seminal visicles, and this enzyme was cloned by three separate groups in 1988 (DeWitt & Smith , 1988; Merlie et al, 1988; Yokoyama et al., 1988;). The discovery of a second form of COX in the early 1990s was the most important event in prostanoid biology in almost 20 years. Induction of this isoform, COX-2, by several stimuli associated with cell activation and inflammation assured the relevance of this finding to inflammatory disease in general. A clear sign of the therapeutic value of this discovery is that in the relatively short time of about five years, several highly effective anti-inflammatory agents and new therapeutic areas have become subjects for investigation (Bakhle & Botting, 1996; Botting, 2010; Herschman, 1996; Jouzeau et al., 1997; Luong et al., 1996).

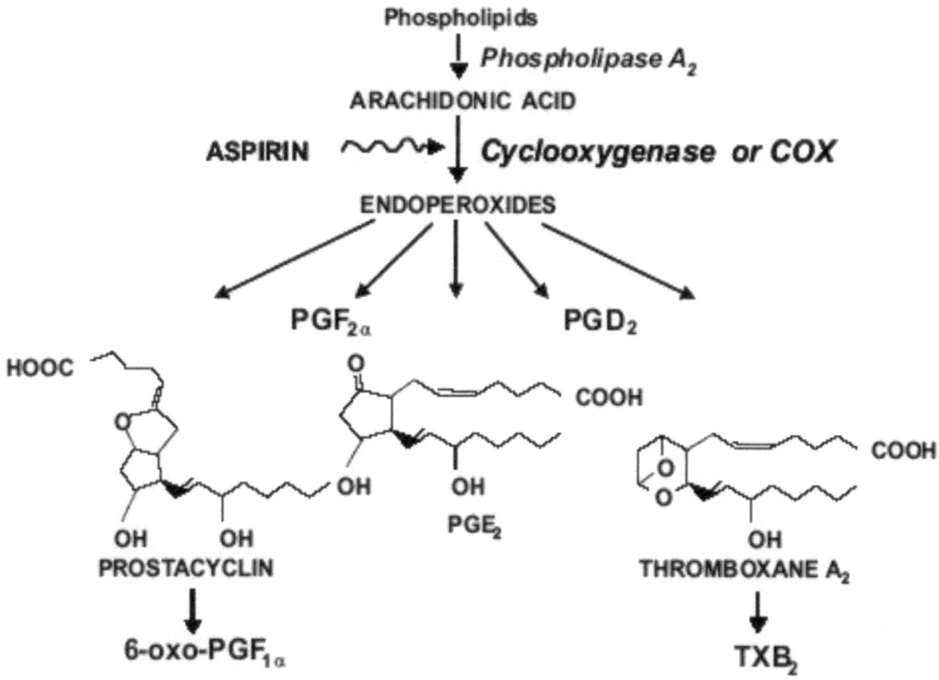

Fig. 1. The arachidonic acid cascade.

The inducible enzyme COX-2 is very similar in structure and catalytic activity to the constitutive COX-1. The biosynthetic activity of both isoforms can be inhibited by aspirin and other NSAIDs (Botting, 2010; Vane, 1971). Both isoforms have a molecular weight of 71 K and are almost identical in length, with just over 600 aminoacids, of which 63% are in an identical sequence. However, the human COX-2 gene at 8.3 kb is a small immediate early gene, whereas human COX-1 originates from a much larger 22-kb gene. The gene products also differ, with the mRNA for the inducible enzyme being approximately 4.5 kb and that of the constitutive enzyme being 2.8 kb (Bakhle & Botting, 1996; Botting, 2010; Jouzeau et al., 1997).

The three-dimensional X-ray crystal structure of human or murine COX-2 (Mancini et al, 1994; Picot etal., 1994) can be superimposed on that COX-1 (Lecomte et al., 1994); the residues that form the substrate binding channel, the catalytic sites, and the residues immediately adjacent are all identical except for two small variations. In these two positions, the same substitutions occur: Ile in COX-1 is exchanged for Val in COX-2 at positions 434 and 523 (the residues in COX-2 are given the same number as their equivalent aminoacids in COX-1).

In spite of this structural identify, there are clear biochemical differences between the isoforms in substrate and inhibitor selectivity. For example, COX-2 will accept a wider

range of fatty acids as substrates than will COX-1 (Bakhle & Botting, 1996; Botting, 2010). Thus, although both enzymes can utilize AA and dihomo-γ-linolenate equally well, COX-2 oxygenates other fatty acid substrates, such as eicosapentaenoic acid, γ-linolenic acid, α-linolenic acid, and linoleic acid more efficiently than does COX-1. Also, COX-2 acetylated by aspirin on Ser 530 will still oxidize AA but to 15-HETE, whereas similarly acetylated COX-1 will not oxidize AA at all (Griswold & Adams, 1996; O'Neill et al., 1994; Wong et al., 1997). In addition (see below), inhibitors will differentiate between COX-2 and COX-1 with over 1000-fold selectivity (Gierse et al., 1996; Luong et al., 1996).
Supporting evidence is strongest from the work on COX-2-selective inhibitors; mutation of Ile 523 to Val in the COX-1 protein allows COX-2-selective inhibitors to bind and inhibit PGH_2 formation without altering the K_m for AA (Guo et al., 1996), and the reverse mutant of COX-2 in which Val 523 is exchanged for Ile shows inhibitor binding and selectivity profiles comparable to those of wild-type COX-1 (Bhattacharyya et al., 1996; Mancini et al., 1995). The structural basis for this has been shown clearly in the crystal analyses of COX-2, which have used either the human or the murine protein, each bound to a nonselective COX-1 or COX-2 inhibitor. The smaller size of Val 523 allows the inhibitor access to a side pocket off the main substrate channel in COX-2-access that is denied sterically by the longer side chain of Ile in COX-1. Selective inhibitors of COX-2 do not bind to Arg 120, which is used by the carboxylic acid ot the substrate AA and by the COX-1-selective or-nonselective NSAIDs, all of which are carboxylic acids (Ren et al., 1995a; Ren et al., 1995b).
Another striking structural difference between the isoforms, but of unknown significance, is the absence of a sequence of 17 amino acids from the N terminus and the insertion of a sequence of 18 amino acids at the C terminus of COX-2 i comparison to COX-1. This accounts for the different numbering for the analogous residues in the two isoforms (e.g. the acetylatable serine is Ser 530 in COX-1 but Ser 516 in COX-2). The C-terminal insert in COX-2 does not alter the last four amino acids residues, which in both proteins form the signal for attachment to the membrane of the endoplasmic reticulum (ER). However, COX-2 is located on the nuclear membrane as well as on the ER, while COX-1 is found attached only to the membranes of the ER. The reason for this selective localization may lie in the different sequence of the C terminus. It is relevant that in the X-ray structural analysis of either isoform, the three-dimensional structures of the last 18 C-terminal residues in COX-1 and the last 30 residues in COX-2 were not resolved, implying a marked flexibility in this region of the proteins even in the crystalline form (Hudson et al., 1993; Mitchell et al., 1993; Morita et al., 1995; Otto & Smith, 1994; Regier et al., 1993). Although emphasis has been placed here on the differences between isorforms, the extensive overall structural and biochemical similarity between COX-1 and COX-2 must be reiterated. Both use the same endogenous substrate, AA, and form the same product by the same catalytic mechanism. Their major difference lies in their pathophysiological functions.

2.1 Physiological and pathological functions of COX-1 and COX-2

Chronic inflammation is an excellent example of a disease that represents a malfunction of normal host defense systems. Thus, rather than classifying PG biosynthesis into physiological and pathological, it may be better to use the classification applied to the COX isoforms: either constitutive or induced. COX-1 activity is constitutive, present in nearly all cell types at a constant level; COX-2 activity is normally absent from cells, and when induced, the protein levels increase and decrease in a matter of hours after a single stimulus (Bakhle & Botting, 1996; Botting, 2010; Jouzeau et al., 1997).

The main reason for labeling COX-1 and COX-2 as physiological and pathological, respectively, is that most of the stimuli known to induce COX-2 are those associated with inflammation, for example, bacterial lipopolysaccharide (LPS) and cytokines such as interleukin (IL)-1, IL-2, and tumor necrosis factor alpha (TNF-α). The anti-inflammatory cytokines, IL-4, IL-10, and IL-13, will decrease induction of COX-2, as will the corticosteroids (Bakhle & Botting, 1996; Luong et al., 1996). The physiological roles of COX-1 have been deduced from the deleterious side effects of NSAIDs, which while inhibiting PG biosynthesis at inflammatory sites, also inhibit constitutive biosynthesis. Thus, COX-1 provides PGs in the stomach and intestine to maintain the integrity of the mucosal epithelium and its inhibition leads to gastric damage, hemorrhage and ulceration.

2.2 Mechanisms of NSAID injury to the gastrointestinal mucosa

For evaluation of the validity of new potentially less toxic NSAIDs it is mandatory to clearly understand the pathogenesis of NSAID induced ulceration (**Figure 2**). Both aspirin and non-aspirin NSAIDs inhibit the COX pathway of prostaglandin synthesis (Botting, 2010; Hudson et al., 1993; Mitchell et al., 1993; Vane, 1971). This represents the basis of anti-inflammatory action but is also responsible for the development of side effects in the gastrointestinal tract and kidney as well as inhibition of platelet aggregation. Inhibition of prostaglandin synthesis can exert injurious actions on the gastric and duodenal mucosa as it abrogates a number of prostaglandin dependent defence mechanisms. Inhibition of COX leads to a decrease in mucus and bicarbonate secretion, reduces mucosal blood flow, and causes vascular injury, leucocyte accumulation, and reduced cell turnover, all factors that contribute to the genesis of mucosal damage. Within this broad spectrum of events, the microvascular damage appears to play a central role. Prostaglandins of the E and I series are potent vasodilators that are continuously produced by the vascular endothelium. Inhibition of their synthesis by an NSAID leads to vasoconstriction (Gana et al., 1987). Furthermore, inhibition of prostaglandin formation results in a rapid and significant increase in the number of neutrophils adhering to the vascular endothelium in both gastric and mesenteric venules (Asako et al., 1992 a;b; Wallace et al., 1993). Adherence is dependent on expression of the â2 integrin (CD11/CD18) on neutrophils and intercellular adhesion molecule on the vascular endothelium (Wallace et al., 1993). Neutrophil adherence in turn causes microvascular stasis and mucosal injury through ischaemia and release of oxygen derived free radicals and proteases (Vaananen et al., 1991).

The severity of experimental NSAID gastropathy was markedly reduced in rats rendered neutropenic by pretreatment with antineutrophil serum or methotrexate (Lee et al., 1992; Wallace et al., 1990) Recently, Wallace et al (2000) provided evidence for an isoenzyme specific role of COX in the homeostasis of the gastrointestinal microcirculation. Thus in rats, the selective COX-1 inhibitor SC-560 decreased gastric mucosal blood flow without affecting leucocyte adherence to mesenteric venules. In contrast, the selective COX-2 inhibitor celecoxib markedly increased leucocyte adherence but did not reduce gastric mucosal blood flow. Only concurrent treatment with the COX-1 and COX-2 inhibitor damaged the gastric mucosa, suggesting that reduction of mucosal blood flow and increase in leucocyte adhesion have to occur simultaneously to interfere with mucosal defence. Inhibition of prostaglandin synthesis thus plays a key role in induction of mucosal injury but does not represent the only pathway by which NSAIDs can damage the gastrointestinal mucosa. NSAIDs can also induce local damage at the site of their contact with the gastrointestinal mucosa. Topical application of NSAIDs increases gastrointestinal permeability allowing luminal aggressive factors access to the mucosa. Aspirin and most non-aspirin NSAIDs are weak organic acids. In the acidic milieu of the stomach, they are converted into more lipid soluble unionised acids that penetrate into the gastric epithelial cells. There, at neutral pH, they are reionised and trapped within the cell causing local injury. Having entered gastric mucosal epithelial cells, NSAIDs uncouple mitochondrial oxidative phosphorylation. This effect is associated with changes in mitochondrial morphology and a decrease in intracellular ATP and therefore a reduced ability to regulate normal cellular functions such as maintenance of intracellular pH. This in turn causes loss of cytoskeletal control over tight junctions and increased mucosal permeability. The ability of NSAIDs to uncouple oxidative phosphorylation stems from the extreme lipid solubility and position of a carboxyl group that acts as a proton translator (Mahmud et al., 1996; Somasundaram et al., 2000). A further mechanism involved in the topical irritant properties of NSAIDs is their ability to decrease the hydrophobicity of the mucus gel layer of the gastric mucosa. NSAIDs can convert the mucus gel from a non-wettable to a wettable state and in experimental animals this effect has been shown to persist for several weeks or months after discontinuation of NSAID administration. Gastric mucosal lesions can also occur in a non-acidic milieu, such as following rectal application. With oral administration, gastric acid however appears to enhance NSAID induced damage. More extensive and deeper erosions occur at low pH and an elevation in gastric pH above 4 is necessary to prevent this acid related component. Prostaglandins do not represent a unique pathway to protect the gastric mucosa. Nitric oxide (NO) has the potential to counteract potentially noxious effects of inhibition of

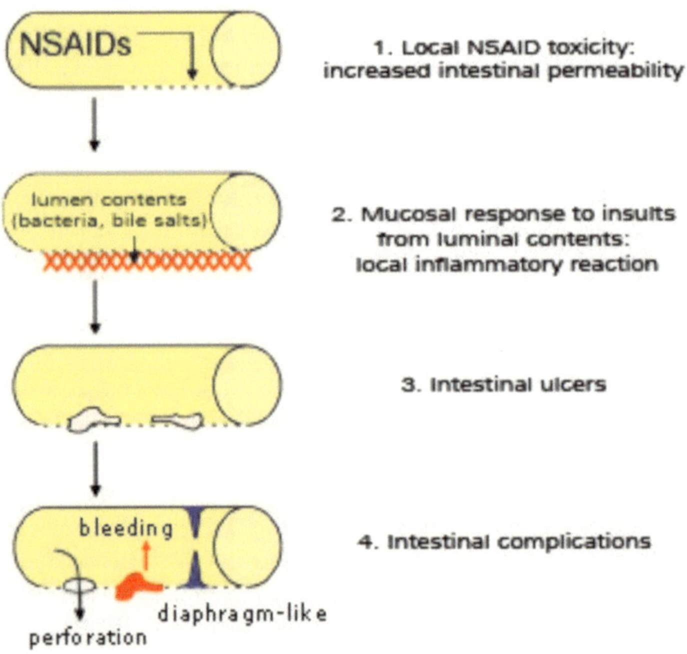

Fig. 2. Pathogenesis of NSAID-induced intestinal lesions (Taken from Thiéfin & Beaugerie, 2005).

prostaglandin synthesis, such as reduced gastric mucosal blood flow and increased adherence of neutrophils to the vascular endothelium of the gastric microcirculation. NO has well characterised inhibitory effects on neutrophil activation/adherence demonstrated in various tissues.

2.3 Chronic inflammatory bowel disease and COX-2

The potential role for prostaglandins in the inflammatory process underlying chronic IBD has been a focus of controversy. Under the hypothesis that prostaglandins may be protective, treatment with exogenous prostaglandins was investigated but found to exacerbate the diarrhea. The possibility that proinflammatory mechanisms might be involved prompted trials of NSAID therapy. However, studies of various NSAIDs in patients with ulcerative colitis showed either no improvement or an exacerbation of the symptoms (Rampton & Sladen, 1981). In keeping with these early findings, some reports suggested a deleterious effect of NSAIDs on the course of IBD (Evans et al., 1997; Felder et al., 2000). The magnitude of the risk, however, remains controversial (Bonner et al., 2002; Nion-Lamurier et al., 2003). The recent review article meets different studies including original papers, case reports, reviews, controlled trials and databases about exacerbation of IBD associated with the use of NSAIDs (Kefalakes et al., 2009). The **Table 1** showed the mechanisms of action of NSAIDs and COX-2 inhibitors in patients with IBD.

2.4 Development of the "COXIBs"

The identification of the COX-2 isoenzyme opened the door to development of NSAIDs which selectivity inhibit COX-2. The main goal of which was to decrease the GI toxicity. The first generation of selective COX-2 inhibitors came from animal models in which compounds were sought that were potent anti-inflammatory agents with minimal side effects on the stomach (Nimesulide, etodolac and meloxicam) (Carvalho et al., 2004). The discovery of the specificity these products was in reality found after the sale, being due, mainly on clinical and experimental observations reduced incidence of gastrointestinal side effects, and subsequently confirmed by *in vitro* studies. The nimesulide is considered an aberrant example of NSAIDs, with good power in vivo inflammatory models, but with weak inhibition in vitro preparations of COX. The nimesulide and display specificity of action on COX-2, has other effects that further enhance their anti-inflammatory activity, as inhibition of neutrophil activation and antioxidant properties. Based on in vitro studies initially suggested that meloxicam selectively inhibited COX-2. However, when tested in *vivo*, in humans, its specificity for COX-2 was only about ten times higher than that for COX-1, with further platelet inhibition (Panara et al., 1999). The molecular modification of these drugs, especially those of nimesulide, in order to increase its COX-2 selectivity, resulted in structures without a carboxylic group and the presence of a sulphonamide or sulphone group, resulting specific inhibitors in the second generation. This group includes celecoxib, rofecoxib, valdecoxib, parecoxib (pro-drug of valdecoxib), APHS [o-(acetoxyphenyl)hept-2-ynyl sulfide] and etoricoxib (Fitzgerald & Patrono, 2001; Kulkarni et al., 2000).

Coxib spare COX-1 and firstly inhibit COX-2 function therefore decrease but do not eliminate NSAIDs associated GI toxicity and are efficacious as tNSAIDs in relieving pain. Data from large GI outcomes studies have characterised the GI effects of coxib. The Celecoxib Longterm Arthritis Safety Study (CLASS Study) that compared high dose Celecoxib (400 mg bid), diclofenac (75 mg bid), and ibuprofen (800 mg 3 times daily) showed that symptomatic ulcers were significantly less common among celecoxib users than tNSAIDs users; however ulcer complication rates were not significantly different (which was probably due to the confounding factor of concomitant low-dose aspirin use which was present in 22% of patients) (Silverstein et al., 2000). However, a recent meta-analysis of available trials of the Cochrane collaboration confirms that celecoxib at any dosewas associated with statistically less GI events (Moore et al., 2005). Moreover, the results of another large outcomes study, celecoxib vs naproxen and diclofenac in osteoarthritis patients (SUCCESS I Study), confirmed the significantly better safety profile of celecoxib compared with tNSAIDs (Singh et al., 2006). The Vioxx Gastrointestinal Safety of Rofecoxib trial (VIGOR Study) concluded that rofecoxib users had 50% fewer GI events compared with naproxen users (Bombardier et al., 2000). Later, in the comparison of lumiracoxib with naproxen and ibuprofen in the Therapeutic Arthritis Research and

Drug	Mechanism of action
Conventional NSAIDs	COX-1 and COX-2 → PGE reduction Surface membrane phospholipid interaction Effect on mitochondrial energy metabolism (oxydase phosphorilation inhibition → ATP deficiency → ↑ mucosal permeability) Escalation of intestinal inflammatory activity Enhancement of enterohepatic circulation Formation of drug enterocyte adducts COX-independent damage to the small intestine Small-bowel enteropathy → blood loss → hypoalbuminemia ↑ TNF-α, IL-1, NO release Lower the thromboxane production
COX-1 inhibitors	Impairs mucosal microcirculatory blood flow Lower the thromboxane production Impairs mucous secretion and acid regulation Impair renal blood flow and platelet aggregation
COX-2 inhibitors	Imunomodulatory and anti-inflammatory role on the GI tract (selective COX-2 inhibition → PGE reduction) Loss of vasodilation Increased of vascular permeability May delay epithelial proliferation Delay wound healing ↑ Oxygen metabolites (LTB4, TNF) ↑ Leukocyte adherence to the vascular endothelium

Table 1. Mechanisms of action of NSAIDs and COX-2 inhibitors in patients with IBD (Taken from Kefalakes et al., 2009).

Gastrointestinal Event Trial (TARGET), showed a 75% decrease in adverse GI events with the coxib (Schnitzer et al., 2004). It is important to emphasise that although the incidence of adverse GI events increased in relation to the presence of GI risk factors, the differences from NSAIDs were maintained in subgroups of patients with and without risk factors (Skelly et al., 2003).

The lumiracoxib is a novel highly selective COX-2 inhibitor. Lumiracoxib differs structurally from others drugs in the class of selective COX-2 inhibitors (**Figure 3**) (Brune & Hinz 2004; Mangold et al., 2004). Differently, the lumiracoxib is a phenyl acetic acid derivative. It has the highest selectivity (selective for COX-2 compared with COX-1 in the human whole blood assay with a ratio of 515:1 in healthy subjects and a fairly short plasm half-life (3-6 hours) compared with other COX-2 selective inhibitors (Esser et al., 2005). In endoscopic studies, lumiracoxib has been associated with a rate of acute gastric injury and chronic ulcer formation that does not differ form placebo (Rordorf et al., 2003) and which was significantly lower than with the NSAID ibuprofen and with celecoxib (Hawkey et al., 2004; Kivitz et al 2004).

Notwithstanding, it is important to note that 3 of the above commented outcome studies (CLASS, TARGET and SUCCESS studies) (Schnitzer et al., 2004; Silverstein et al., 2000; Singh et al., 2006), one endoscopy study (Solomon et al., 2005) and several epidemiological studies (Lanas et al., 2005) have shown that the concomitant use of low-dose aspirin and coxib or tNSAIDs increases further the risk of upper GI bleeding in NSAIDs users and attenuates the GI advantage of a coxib over an tNSAID.A recent meta-analysis of RCTs has shown that coxib plus low-dose ASA use was associated with a lower risk of upper GI complications when compared to non-selective NSAID plus low-dose ASA (Rostom et al., 2009). These gastrointestinal benefits have to be balanced against the known cardiovascular risks, particularly with long-term use. The VIGOR and Adenomatous Polyp Prevention on Vioxx Trial Investigators (APPROVe) studies showed that rofecoxib were associated with increased risk of cardiovascular events after 12 and 36 months of treatment when compared to naproxen (VIGOR) or placebo (APPROVe) (Bombardier et al., 2000; Bresalier et al., 2005). Other outcome studies have shown also that celecoxib at doses of 400 mgbid or 200 mgbid (Laine et al., 2004), but not 400 mg once a day (Arber et al., 2006) is associated with increased risk of cardiovascular events. Observational studies have shown, however, that celecoxib at 200 mg/day dose was not associated with increased risk of cardiovascular events (Bombardier et al., 2000; Silverstein et al., 2000). Recent observational studies have shown that also most NSAIDs (including nonselective) may be associated with increased cardiovascular risk and this may be different for the different compounds, dose and length of treatment (Chan et al., 2006; Lanas et al., 2005; McHippisley-Cox & Coupland, 2005). Of all traditional NSAIDs, diclofenac have been found to be the one increasing the CV risk the most (Mc Gettigan & Henry, 2006). In the MEDAL program etoricoxib at the dose of 60–90 mg/day was found to be not different to diclofenac in the incidence of CV events (Cannon et al., 2006). The study also showed no differences in the incidence of upper GI complications between these 2 compounds, although the total number of events (symptomatic ulcers and complications) was statistically lower in etoricoxib users (Laine et al, 2007). Lastly, both tNSAIDs and coxib may also increase blood pressure and reduce kidney function. Following, we describe the effects of these COX-2 inhibitors on differents studies on experimental colitis models.

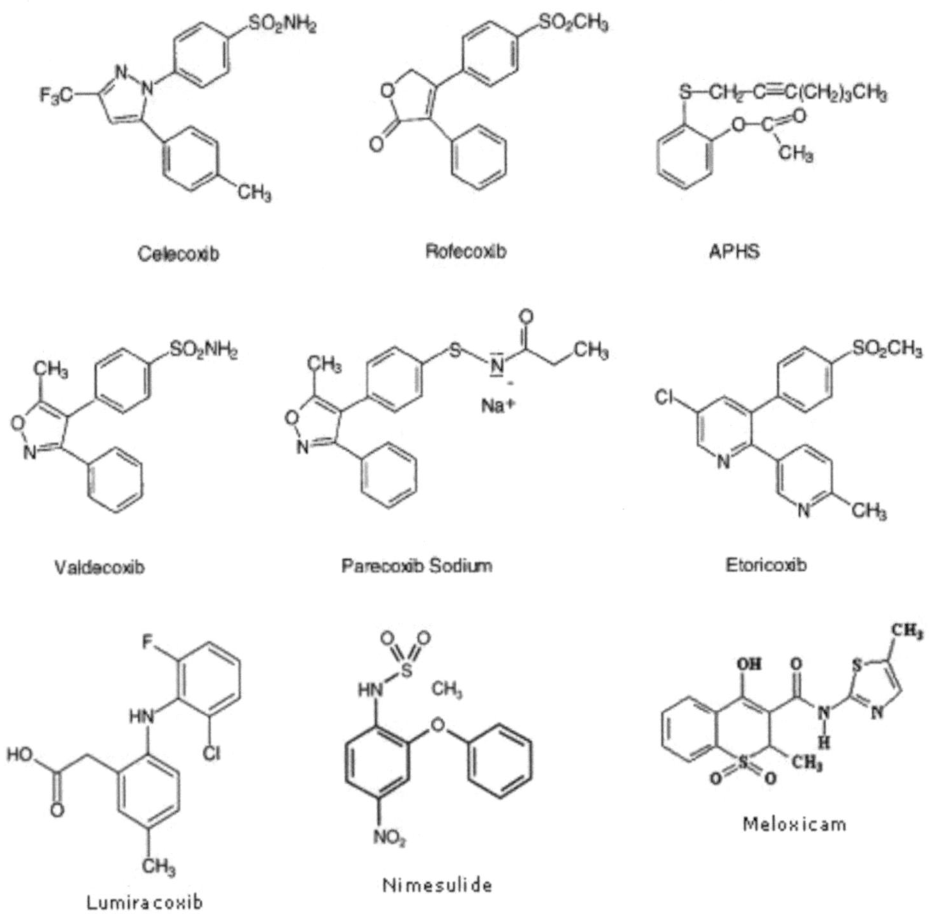

Fig. 3. The chemical structures of some COX-2 inhibitors.

2.5 COX-2 inhibitors on experimental colitis models

The role of selective inhibition of COX-2 for the inflammatory process and the course of experimental and human colitis is controversially discussed, even though increased levels of prostaglandins (PGE_2 and PGI_2) and other eicosanoids were detected in both colitis models and patients with chronic inflammatory bowel disease, which correlates well with the disease activity. PGE_2 is produced by mononuclear cells in the lamina propria and is dependent on COX-2 expresion. It modulates the intestinal immune response, including the differentiation of T cells and the production and release of proinflammatory cytokines. During the course of inflammatory bowel disease and experimental colitis, some prostanoids are released and subsequently modulate the course of the disease.

Animal models are used extensively to study the pathogenesis and pathophysiology of IBD and to evaluate therapies. The more extensively used models were: acetic acid colitis, dextran sodium sulphate (DSS) and 2,4,6′-trinitrobenzene sulphonic acid (TNBS). Acetic-acid-induced colitis in rats resembles human ulcerative colitis in histology, eicosanoid production and excessive oxygen-derived free radicals release by inflamed mucosa (Millar et al., 1996). DSS-induced ulcerative colitis is accompanied by erosion and ulceration as well as inflammatory cell infiltration, characteristics resembling those of human ulcerative colitis (Okayama et al., 2007). TNBS-induced colitis is accompanied by marked thickening of the colonic wall, infiltration of polymorphonuclear leukocytes and ulceration, resembling the human Crohn´s disease (Morris et al., 1989). A number of animal studies have reported the positive effect of COX-2 inhibition, others exacerbation of colitis (**Table 2**).

Study	Model of colitis	Drug	Results
Reuter et al. (1996)	TNBS	diclofenac (10mg/kg) naproxen (5mg/kg) etodolac (10 or 50mg/kg) nabumetone (25 or 75mg/kg) L745,337 (1 or 5mg/kg)	unfavorable
Lesch et al. (1999)	TNBS	NS-398* SC-58125* PD-138387* *dose of 100mg/kg	unfavorable
Karmeli et al. (2000)	Acetic-acid or iodoacetamide	nimesulide (10mg/kg) SC-236 (6mg/kg)	favorable
Cuzzocrea et al. (2001)	DNBS	celecoxib (5mg/kg)	favorable
Martin et al. (2003)	TNBS	rofecoxib	favorable
Martin et al. (2005)	DSS	Rofecoxib (2.5-10mg/kg)	favorable
Singh et al. (2003)	Acetic-acid; LTB4-induced IBD)	nimesulide (9 and 18mg/kg)	favorable
Zhang et al. (2004)	TNBS	celecoxib (1.25mg/kg)	unfavorable
El-Medany et al. (2005)	Acetic-acid	celecoxib (5mg/kg) rofecoxib (2.5mg/kg)	favorable
Kruschewski et al. (2006)	TNBS	NS-398 (10mg/kg)	favorable
Tsubouchi et al. (2006)	DSS	rofecoxib	unfavorable
Dudhgaonkar et al. (2007)	TNBS	rofecoxib (10mg/kg)	favorable
Okayama et al. (2007)	DSS	celecoxib (3mg/kg)	unfavorable
Paiotti et al. (2009)	TNBS	lumiracoxib (6mg/kg)	unfavorable

Table 2. COX-2 inhibitors on experimental colitis.

Karmeli et al. (2000) reported that nimesulide, ameliorates the extent of tissue damage in acetic acid and iodoacetamide-treated rats. The decrease in the extent of colitis induced by nimesulide was accompanied by a significant decrease in mucosal MPO and nitric oxide synthase (NOS) activities.

There is good evidence that an enhanced formation of reactive oxygen species contributes to the pathophysiology of IBD (Guo et al., 1999; Kruidenier & Verspaget, 2002). Quantitatively, the principal free radical in tissues is superoxide anion (O_2^-), which is converted to H_2O2 by superoxide dismutase. Superoxide anion (O_2^-) can be produced by activated neutrophils through NADPH oxidase, which reduces molecular oxygen to the O_2^- radical through the enzyme myeloperoxidase. Nitric oxide (NO), a reactive free radical gas, is generated enzymatically in a variety of cells from the L-arginine pathway by three isoforms of NO synthetase (Yue et al., 2001). In the GI tract, NO can be either protective or damaging to tissues, depending on what type of NOS is involved in the pathological condition. In experimental colitis, NO derived from iNOS, together with other free radicals, contribute significantly to the inflammatory response in the colon. The mechanism for this inflammatory response is likely explained by the interaction of NO with superoxide to produce peroxynitrite, which is a strong oxidizing agent that initiates lipid peroxidation (El-Medany et al., 2005). Combination of rofecoxib and aminoguanidine hydrochloride has protective effect on colonic injury by TNBS which is probably, via mechanism of local inhibition of iNOS and COX-2 activity in colonic mucosa (Dudhgaonkar et al., 2007).

Cuzzocrea et al. (2001) have provided evidence for the potential protective effect of celecoxib in reducing the severity of colonic injury induced by dinitrobenzene sulfonic acid (DNBS). They observed reduction of the degree of colonic injury, the MPO activity, hemorrhagic diarrhoea and the weight loss. Martin et al. (2003; 2005) have demonstrated that rofecoxib seems to have beneficial effects in TNBS-induced colitis in rats and in acute DSS-induced colitis in mice; probably by the initial diminishing the initial stage of inflammation by a mechanism related to inhibition of PGE_2 by the COX-2 pathway as well by reducing neutrophil infiltration and inhibiting up-regulation of IL-1β. The use of nimesulide in two different models (acetic acid -and LTB4-induced IBD) significantly prevented development of inflammatory changes, decreased MPO activity, and also restored the altered contractility response of the isolated colon segment (Singh et al., 2003). In addition, El-Medany et al. (2005) showed that treatment with the celecoxib and rofecoxib reduced the inflammation and subsequent tissue damage to the colon induced by acetic acid, as verified by macroscopic, histological and biochemical findings. They demonstrated that these drugs exert a significant attenuation of the extent and severity of the histological signs of cell damage, significant reduction in tissue PGE_2 production, as well reduction in NOS activity.

The acute phase of TNBS colitis is characterized by a significant reduction of capillary blood flow, capillary density, diuresis, and weight and a significant increase in capillary permeability, leukocyte sticking, and hematocrit (Kruschewski et al., 2006). Kruschewski et al. (2006) demonstrated that the selective COX-2 inhibitor NS-398 leads to a significant improvement of all microcirculatory parameters and clinical findings compared to the (untreated) colitis.

On the other hand, Reuter et al. (1996) reported that administration of three types of COX-2 inhibitors with moderate to high selectivity significantly exacerbated the severity of colonic damage in experimental colitis. Continued twice-daily administration of these compounds for one week resulted in perforation of the colon, leading to death in a substancial number of the animals. Lesch et al. (1999) evaluated three highly selective COX-2 inhibitors (NS-398, SC-58125 and PD-138387) on TNBS-induced colitis and observed that these three compounds do not seem to have any beneficial effect in this model. Zhang et al. (2004) showed that celecoxib resulted in exacerbation of inflammation-associated with colonic damage and even led to perforation, megacolon and death of the rats, with the mortality rate reaching 50%. Tsubouch et al. (2006) demonstrated that daily administration of indomethacin and rofecoxib significantly delayed the healing of colitis with deleterious influences on histological restitu as well as mucosal inflammation. Okayama et al. (2007) showed that celecoxib aggravated the severity of colonic ulceration and inflammation, as represented by the gross injury and the shortening of colon length as well as the myeloperoxidase activity (MPO) on dextran sulfate sodium (DSS) induced colitis.

Although lumiracoxib interacts with the COX-2 enzyme via mechanisms different from other COX-2 selective inhibitors and is associated with improved gastrointestinal tolerability, Paiotti et al. (2009) showed this did not reduce inflammation-associated colonic injury in TNBS-induced colitis. They demonstrated that macroscopic and the histopathological assessment on the TNBS nontreated induced-colitis and lumiracoxib-treated induced-colitis were similar.

3. Conclusion

The ability of selective COX-2 inhibitors to significantly exacerbate colonic injury in differents models of colitis suggests that prostaglandins derived from COX-2 are beneficial in the setting of colonic inflammation. There is a strong body of evidence to suggest that prostaglandins do exert anti-inflammatory and mucosal protective effects in experimental colitis. It is known that PGE_2 inhibits inflammatory cytokines and stimulates mucus secretion in the GI mucosa through activation of EP4 receptors (Kabashima et al., 2002; Nitta et al., 2002). Nitta et al reported that a selective EP4 agonist decreased the levels of IL-1β and cytokine-induced neutrophil chemoattractant in the colorectal mucosa with marked downregulation of the corresponding cytokine mRNA expression. They also found that the IL-10 concentration was higher following administration of the EP4 agonist. These findings may suggest that endogenous PGE_2 ameliorates the severity of dextran sodium sulphate colitis (DSS), presumably by suppressing the induction of proinflammatory cytokines. Prostaglandins are capable of reducing the production of reactive oxygen metabolites and a number of inflammatory mediators suggested to contribute to the pathogenesis of human and experimental colitis, included leukotriene B_4 and TNF-α. In addition prostaglandins increase the secretion of water and electrolytes into the intestinal tract and in the acute stage of UC and CD, activated monocytes promote the increased concentration of PG in the enteric mucosa, which in turn suppresses the effect of the Na^+, Ka^+-ATP enzyme and prevents the reabsorption of Na^+, resulting in diarrhea. Some studies demonstrated that pretreatment with intraluminal PGE analogs (e.g. 16,16′-dimethyl PGE_2) caused a reduction in the severity of injury induced by TNBS and acetic acid (Feng et al., 1993; Nitta et al., 2002; Sasaki et al., 2000 Tso et al., 1995).

In conclusion, the relative role of COX-2 selective inhibitors on human and experimental colitis to be explored. Thus, the use of COX-2 inhibitors in IBD should be considered with caution.

4. References

Arber N, Eagle CJ, Spicak J, et al. (2006). Pre-SAP Trial Investigators. Celecoxib for de prevention of colorectal adenomatous polyps. *N Engl J Med*, Aug; 355(9):885-95. ISSN 1533-4406.

Asako H, Kubes P,Wallace JL, et al. (1992). Indomethacin-induced leukocyte adhesion in mesenteric venules: role of lipoxygenase products. *Am J Physiol*, 262:G903-8; a. ISSN 0363-6119.

Asako H,Kubes P,Wallace JL, et al. (1992). Modulation of leukocyte adhesion in rat mesenteric venules by aspirin and salicylate. *Gastroenterology*, Jul; 103(1):146-52;b. ISSN 1440-1746.

Bakhle YS, Botting RM. (1996). Cyclooxygenase-2 and its regulation in inflammation. *Mediat Inflamm*, Oct; 5(5):305-23. ISSN 0962-9351.

Barbieri D. (2000). Inflammatory bowel diseases. *J Pediatr (Rio J)*, Jul; 76(suppl 1):S173-S180. ISSN 0021-7557.

Bhattacharyya DK, Lecomte M, Rieke CJ, et al. (1996). Involvement of arginine 120, glutamate 524 and tyrosine 355 in the binding of arachidonate and 2-phenylpropionic acid inhibitors to the cyclooxygenase active site of ovine prostaglandin endoperoxide H synthase-1. *J Biol Chem*, Jan; 271(4):2179-84. ISSN 0021-9258.

Bombardier C, Laine L, Reicin A, et al. (2000). Comparison of upper gastrointestinal toxicity of rofecoxib and naproxen in patients with rheumatoid arthritis. VIGOR Study Group. *N Engl J Méd*, Nov; 343(21):1520-8. ISSN 1533-4406.

Bonen DK, Cho JH. (2003). The genetics of inflammatory bowel disease. *Gastroenterology*, Feb; 124(2):521-536. ISSN 1440-1746.

Bonner GF, Fakhri A, Vennamaneni SR. (2004). A long-term cohort study of nonsteroidal anti-inflammatory drug use and disease activity in outpatients with inflammatory bowel disease. *Inflamm Bowel Dis*, Nov; 10(6):751-757. ISSN 1078-0998.

Bonner GF, Walczak M, Kitchen L, et al. (2000). Tolerance of nonsteroidal antiinflammatory drugs in patients with inflammatory bowel disease. *Am J Gastroenterol*, Aug; 95(8):1946-1948. ISSN 0002-9270.

Botting RM. (2010). Vane's discovery of the mechanism of action of aspirin changed our understanding of its clinical pharmacology. *Pharmacol Reports*, 62:518-25. ISSN 1734-1140.

Bresalier RS, Sandler RS, Quan H, et al. (2005). Adenomatous polyp prevention on Vioxx (APPROVe) trial investigators. Cardiovascular events associated with rofecoxib in a colorectal adenoma chemoprevention trial. *N Engl J Med*, Marc; 352(11):1092-102. ISSN 1533-4406.

Brune K, Hinz B (2004). Selective cyclooxygenase-2 inhibitors: similarities and differences. *Scand J Rheumatol*, 33(1):1-6. ISSN 03009742.

Cannon CP, Curtis SP, FitzGerald GA, et al. (2006). MEDAL Steering Committee. Cardiovascular outcomes with etoricoxib and diclofenac in patients with osteoarthritis and rheumatoid arthritis in the Multinational Etoricoxib and Diclofenac Arthritis Long-term (MEDAL) programme: A randomized comparison. *Lancet*, Nov 18; 368(9549):1771-81. ISSN 0140-6736.

Carvalho WA, Carvalho RDS, Rios-Santos F. (2004). Specific cyclooxygenase-2 inhibitor analgesics: Therapeutic advances. *Rev Bras Anestesiol*, Aug; 54(4):448-64. ISSN 0034-7094.

Chan AT, Manson JE, Albert CM, et al. (2006). Nonsteroidal antiinflammatory drugs, acetaminophen, and the risk of cardiovascular events. *Circulation* 2006 Mar; 113(12):1578-87. ISSN 0009-7322.

Colpaert S, Liu Z, De Greef B, et al. (2001). Effects of anti-tumour necrosis factor, interleukin-10 and antibiotic therapy in the indometacin-induced bowel inflammation rat model. *Aliment Pharmacol Ther*, Nov; 15(11):1827-1836. ISSN 0269-2813.

Cuzzocrea S, Mazzon E, Serraino I, et al. (2001). Celecoxib , a selective cyclooxygenase-2 inhibitor reduces the severity of experimental colitis induced by dinitrobenzene sulphonic acid in rats. *Eur J Pharmacol*, Nov; 431(1):91-102. ISSN 0014-2999.

Dempke W, Rie C, Grothey A, et al. (2001). Cyclooxygenase-2: a novel target for cancer chemotherapy? *J Cancer Res Clin Oncol*, Jul; 127(7):411-417. ISSN 0171-5216.

DeWitt DL, Smith WL. (1988). Primary structure of prostaglandin G/H synthase from sheep vesicular gland determined from the complementary DNA sequence. *Proc Natl Acad Sci USA*, Marc; 85(5):1412-1416. ISSN 0027-8424.

Dudhgaonkar SP, Tandan SK, Kumar D, et al. (2007). Influence of simultaneous inhibition of cyclooxygenase-2 and inducible nitric oxide synthase in experimental colitis in rats. *Inflammopharmacology*, Oct 15(5):188-95. ISSN 09254692.

El-Medany Azza, Mahgoub Afaf, Mustafa ali, et al. (2005). The effects of selective cyclooxygenase-2 inhibitors, celecoxib and rofecoxib, on experimental colitis induced by acetic acid in rats. *Eur J Pharmacol*, Jan; 507(1-3):291-299. ISSN 0014-2999.

Élson CO, Sartor RB, Tennyson GS, et al. (1995). Experimental models of inflammatory bowel disease. *Gastroenterology*, Oct; 109(4):1344-1367. ISSN 1440-1746.

Esser Ronald, Berry Carol, Du Zhengming , et al. (2005). Preclinical pharmacology of lumiracoxib: a novel selective inhibitor of cyclooxygenase-2. *Br J Pharmacol*, Feb; 144(4):538-550. ISSN 0007-1188.

Evans JM, McMahon AD, Murray FE, et al. (1997). Non-steroidal anti-inflammatory drugs are associated with emergency admission to hospital for colitis due to inflammatory bowel disease. *Gut* , May; 40(5):619-22. ISSN 0017-5749.

Felder JB, Korelitz BI, Rajapakse R, et al. (2000). Effects of nonsteroidal antiinflammatory drugs on inflammatory bowel disease: a case-control study. *Am J Gastroenterol*, Aug; 95(8):1949-54. ISSN 0002-9270.

Feng L, Sun W, Xia Y, et al. (1993). Cloning two isoforms of rat cyclooxygenase: Differential regulation of their expression. *Arch Biochem Biophys*, Dec; 307(2):361-8. ISSN 00039861.

Fitzgerald GA, Patrono C. (2001). The coxibs, selective inhibitors of cyclooxigenase-2. *N Engl J Med*, Aug; 345(6):433-442. ISSN 1533-4406.

Gana TJ, Huhlewych R, Koo J (1987). Focal gastric mucosal blood flow in aspirininduced ulceration. *Ann Surg*, Apr; 205(4):399-403. ISSN 0003-4932.

Gierse JK, McDonald JJ, Hauser SD, et al. (1996). A single amino acid difference between cyclooxygenase-1 and -2 reverses the selectivity of COX-2 specific inhibitors. *J Biol Chem*, Jun; 271(26):15810-14. ISSN 0021-9258.

Gornet JM, Hassani Z, Modiglian R, et al. (2002). Exacerbation of Crohn's colitis with severe colonic hemorrhage in a patient on rofecoxib. *Am J Gastroenterol*, Dec; 97(12):3209-3210. ISSN 0002-9270.

Griswold DE, Adams JL. (1996). Constitutive cyclooxygenase (COX-1 and inducible cyclooxygenase (COX-2): rationale for selective inhibition and progress to date. *Med Res Rev*, Mar; 16(6):181-206. ISSN 1077-5587.

Guo Q, Wang L, Ruan K, et al. (1996). Role of Val509 in time-dependent inhibition of human prostaglandin H synthase-2 cyclooxygenase activity by isoform-selective agents. *J Biol Chem*, Aug; 271(32):19134-39. ISSN 0021-9258.

Guo X, Wang WP, Ko JK, et al. (1999). Involvement of neutrophils and free radicals in the potentiating effects of passive cigarette smoking on inflammatory bowel disease in rats. *Gastroenterology*, Oct; 117(4):884-92. ISSN 1440-1746.

Hawkey CJ, Svoboda P, Fiedorowicz-Fabrycy IF, et al. (2004). Gastroduodenal safety and tolerability of lumiracoxib compared with ibuprofen and celecoxib in patients with osteoarthritis. *J Rheum*, Sep; 31(9):1804-1810. ISSN 0315-162X.

Herschman HR. (1996). Prostaglandin synthase 2. *Biochim Biophys Acta*, Jan; 1299(1):125-40. ISSN 0006-3002.

Hudson N, Balsitis M, Everitt S, et al. (1993). Enhanced gastric leukotriene B4 synthesis in patients taking non-steroidal anti-inflammatory drugs. *Gut*, Jun; 34(6):742-7. ISSN 0017-5749.

Jouzeau J-Y, Terlain B, Abid A, et al. (1997). Cyclooxygenase isoenzymes. How recent findings affect thinking about nonsteroidal anti-inflammatory drugs. *Drugs*, Apr; 53(4):563-82. ISSN 0012-6667.

Kabashima K, Saji T, Murata T, et al. (2002). The prostaglandin receptor EP4 suppresses colitis, mucosal damage and CD4 cell activation in the gut. *J Clin Invest*, Apr; 109(7):883-93. ISSN 0021-9738.

Kafalakes H, Stylianides TJ, Amanakis G, et al. (2009). Exacerbation of inflammatory bowel diseases associated with the use of nonsteroidal anti-inflammatpry drugs: myth or reality. *Eur J Clin Pharmacol*, Oct; 65(10):963-70. ISSN 0031-6970.

Karmeli F, Cohen P, Rachmilewitz D. (2000). Cyclo-oxygenase-2 inhibitors ameliorate the severity of experimental colitis in rats. *Eur J Gastroenterol Hepatol*, Feb 12(2):223-31. ISSN 0954-691X.

Kivitz AJ, Nayiager S, Schimansky T, et al. (2004). Reduced incidence of gastroduodenal ulcers associated with lumiracoxib compared with ibuprofen in patients with rheumatoid arthritis. *Aliment Pharmacol Ther*, Jun; 19(11):1189-1198. ISSN 0269-2813.

Kruidenier L, Verspaget HW. (2002). Oxidative stress as a pathogenic factor in inflammatory bowel disease-radicals or ridiculous? *Aliment Pharmacol Ther*, Dec; 16(12):1997-2015. ISSN 0269-2813.

Kruschewski M, Anderson T, Burhr HJ, et al. (2006). Selective COX-2 inhibition reduces leukocyte sticking and improves the microcirculation in TNBS colitis. *Dig Dis Sci*, Apr 51 (4):662-70. ISSN 0002-9211.

Kulkarni SK, Jain NK, Singh A. (2000). Cyclooxygenase isoenzymes and newer therapeutic potential for selective COX-2 inhibitors. *Methods Find Exp Clin Pharmacol*, Jun; 22(5):291-298. ISSN 0379-0355.

Kurahara K, Matsumoto T, Iida M, et al. (2001). Clinical and endoscopic features of nonsteroidal antiinflammatory drug-induced colonic ulcerations. *Am J Gastroenterol*, Feb; 96(2):473-480. ISSN 0002-9270.

Kurumbail RG, Stevens AM, Gierse JK, eta l. (1996). Structural basis for selective inhibition of cyclooxygenase-2 by anti-inflammatory agents. *Nature*, Dec; 384(6610):644-48. ISSN 0028-0836.

Laine L, Curtis SP, Cryer B, et al (2007). MEDAL Steering Committee. Assessment of upper gastrointestinal safety of etoricoxib and diclofenac in patients with osteoarthritis and rheumatoid arthritis in the Multinational Etoricoxib and Diclofenac Arthritis Long-term (MEDAL) programme: A randomized comparison. *Lancet*, Feb 10;369(9560): 465-73. ISSN 0140-6736.

Laine L, Maller ES, Yu C, et al. (2004). Ulcer formation with low-dose enteric-coated aspirin and the effect of COX-2 selective inhibition: a double-blind trial. *Gastroenterology*, Aug; 127(2):395-402. ISSN 1440-1746.

Lanas A, Garcia-Rodriguez LA, Arroyo MA, et al. (2005). Coxibs, NSAIDs, aspirin, PPIs and the risks of upper GI bleeding in common clinical practice. *Gastroenterology*, 128:629. ISSN 1440-1746.

Lashner BA. (1995). Epidemiology of inflammatory bowel disease. *Gastroenterol Clin North Am*, Sep; 24(3):467-474. ISSN 0889-8553.

Lecomte M, Laneuville O, Ji C, et al. (1994). Acetylation of human prostaglandin endoperoxide synthase-2 (cyclooxygenase-2) by aspirin. *J Biol Chem*, May; 269(18):13207-15. ISSN 0021-9258.

Lee M, Aldred K, Lee E, et al. (1992). Aspirin-induced acute gastric mucosal injury is a neutrophil-dependent process in rats. *Am J Physiol*, Dec; 263(6PT1):G920-6. ISSN 0363-6135.

Lesch CA, Kraus ER, Sanchez B, et al. (1999). Lack of beneficial of COX-2 inhibitors in an experimental model of colitis. *Methods Find Exp Clin Pharmacol*, Marc 21(2):99-104. ISSN 0379-0355.

Luong C, Miller A, Barnett J, et al. (1996). Flexibility of the NSAID binding site in the structure of human cyclooxygenase-2. *Nat Struct Biol*, Nov; 3(11):927-933. ISSN 1072-8368.

Mancini JA, O'Neill GP, Bayly C, et al. (1994). Mutation of serine-516 in human prostaglandin G/H synthase-2 to methionine or aspirin cetylation of this residue stimulates 15-R-HETE synthesis. *FEBS Lett*, Mar; 342(1):33-37. ISSN 0014-5793.

Mancini JA, Riendeau D, Falgueyret JP, et al. (1995). Arginini 120 of prostaglandin G/H synthase-1 is required for the inhibition by nonsteroidal anti-inflammatory drugs containing a carboxylic acid moiety. *J Biol Chem*, Dec; 270(49):29372-77. ISSN 0021-9258.

Mangold JB, Gu H, Rodriguez LC, et al. (2004). Pharmacokinetics and metabolism of lumiracoxib in healthy male subjects. *Drug Metab Dispos*, May; 32(5):566-571. ISSN 0090-9556.

Martin AR, Villegas I, La-Casa C, et al. (2003). The cyclooxygenase-2 inhibitor , rofecoxib, attenuates mucosal damage due to colitis induced by trinitrobenzene sulphonic acid in rats. *Eur J Pharmacol*, Nov; 481(2-3):1-10. ISSN 0014-2999.

Martin AR, Villegas I, Alarcon de la Lastra C. (2005). The COX-2 inhibitor, rofecoxib, ameliorates dextran sulphate sodium induced colitis in mice. *Inflamm Res*, Apr 54(4):145-51. ISSN 1023-3830.

Mc Gettigan P, Henry D. (2006). Cardiovascular risk and inhibition of cyclooxygenase: a systematic review of the observational studies of selective and non selective inhibitors of cyclooxygenase 2. *J Am Med Assoc*, Oct;296(13):1633-44. ISSN 0002-9955.

McHippisley-Cox J, Coupland C. (2005). Risk of myocardial infarction in patients taking cyclo-oxygenase-2 inhibitors or conventional non-steroidal anti-inflammatory drugs: population based nested case-control analysis. *BMJ*, Jun; 330(7504):1366. ISSN 09598138.

Merlie JP, Fagan D, Mudd J, et al. (1988). Isolation and characterization of the complementary DNA for sheep seminal vesicle prostaglandin endoperoxidase synthase (cyclooxygenase). *J Biol Chem*, Mar; 263(8):3550-53. ISSN 0021-9258.

Millar AD, Rampton DS, Chander CL, et al. (1996). Evaluating the antioxidant potential of new treatments for inflammatory bowel disease using a mouse model of colitis. *Gut*, Sep; 39(3):407-15. ISSN 0017-5749.

Mitchell JA, Akarasereenont P, Thiemermann C, et al. (1993). Selectivity of nonsteroidal antiinflammatory drugs as inhibitors of constitutive and inducible cyclooxygenase. *Proc Natl Acad Sci USA*, Dec; 90(24):11693-7. ISSN 0027-8424.

Moore RA, Derry S, Makinson GT, et al. (2005). Tolerability and adverse events in clinical trials of celecoxib in osteoarthritis and rheumatoid arthritis: systematic review and meta-analysis of information from company clinical trial reports. *Arthritis Res Ther*, Mar; 7(3):R644-65. ISSN 1478-6354.

Morita I, Schindler MS, Regier MK, et al. (1995). Different intracellular locations for prostaglandin endoperoxide H synthase 1 and 2. *J Biol Chem*, May; 270(18):10902-8. ISSN 0021-9258.

Morris GP, Beck PL, Herridge MS, et al. (1989). Hapten-induced model of chronic inflammation and ulceration in the rat colon. *Gastroenterology*, Mar; 96(3):795-803. ISSN 1440-1746.

Nitta M, Hirata I, Toshina K, et al. (2002). Expression of the EP4 prostaglandin E2 receptor subtype with rat dextran sodium sulphate colitis: colitis suppression by a selective agonist, ONO-AE1-329. *Scand J Immunol*, Jul; 56:66-75. ISSN 0300-9475.

Okayama M, Hayashi S, Aoi Y, et al. (2007). Aggravation by selective COX-1 and COX-2 inhibitors of dextran sulfate sodium (DSS)-induced colon lesions in rats. *Dig Dis Sci*, Sep; 52(9):2095-2103. ISSN 0163-216.

O'Neill GP, Mancini JA, Kargman S, et al. (1994). Overexpression of human prostaglandin G/H synthase-1 and -2 by recombinant vacinia virus: inhibition by nonsteroidal anti-inflammatory drugs and biosynthesis of 15-hydroxyeicosatetraenoic acid. *Mol Pharmacol*, Feb; 45(2):245-54. ISSN 0026-895X.

Otto JC, Smith WL. (1994). The orientation of prostaglandin endoperoxide synthases 1 and 2 in the endoplasmic reticulum. *J Biol Chem*, Aug; 269(31):19868-75. ISSN 0021-9258.

Paiotti APR, Miszputen SJ, Oshima CTF, et al. (2009). Effect of COX-2 inhibitor after TNBS-induced colitis in wistar rats. *J Mol Hist*, Aug; 40(4):317-24. ISSN 1567-2379.

Panara MR, Renda G, Sciulli MG, et al. (1999). Dose-dependent inhibition of platelet cyclooxygenase-1 and monocyte cyclooxygenase-2 by meloxicam in healthy subjects. *J Pharmacol Exp Ther*, Jul; 290(1):276-280. ISSN 00223565.

Picot D, Loll PJ, Garavito RM. (1994). The X-ray crystal structure of the membrane protein prostaglandin H2 synthase-1. *Nature*, Jan; 367(6460):243-49. ISSN 0028-0836.

Podolsky DK. (2002). Inflammatory bowel disease. *N Engl J Med*, Aug; 347(6):417-429. ISSN 1533-4406.

Rampton DS, Sladen GE. (1981). Prostaglandin synthesis inhibitors in ulcerative colitis: flurbiprofen compared with conventional treatment. *Prostaglandins*, Mar; 21(3):417-25. ISSN 1098-8823.

Regier MK, DeWitt DL, Schindler MS, et al. (1993). Subcellular localization of prostaglandin endoperoxide synthase-2 in murine 3T3 cells. *Arch Biochem Biophys*, Mar; 301(2):439-44. ISSN 0003-9861.

Ren Y, Loose-Mitchell DS, Kulmacz RJ. (1995). Prostaglandin H synthase-1: evaluation of C-terminus function. *Arch Biochem Biophys*, Feb; 316(2):751-57. ISSN 0003-9861.

Ren Y, Walker C, Loose-Mitchell DS, et al. (1995). Topology of prostaglandin H synthase-1 in the endoplasmic reticulum membrane. *Arch Biochem Biophys*, Oct; 323(1):205-14. ISSN 0003-9861.

Reuter BK, Asfaha S, Buret, et al. (1996). Exacerbation of inflammatory associated colonic injury in rat through inhibition of cyclooxygenase-2. *J Clin Invest*, Nov; 98(9):2076-2085. ISSN 0210-573X.

Rordorf C, Kellett N, Mair S, et al. (2003). Gastroduodenal tolerability of lumiracoxib vs placebo and naproxen: a pilot endoscopic study in healthy male subjects. *Aliment Pharmacol Ther*, Sep; 18(5):533-541. ISSN 0269-2813.

Rostom A, Muir K, Dube C, et al. (2009). Prevention of NSAID-related upper gastrointestinal toxicity: a meta-analysis of traditional NSAIDs with gastroprotection and COX-2 inhibitors. *Drug Healthc Patient Saf*, Oct; 1:1-25. ISSN 1179-1365.

Sasaki S, Hirata I, Maemura K, et al. (2000). Prostaglandin E2 inhibits lesion formation in dextran sodium sulphate-induced colitis in rats and reduces the levels of mucosal inflammatory cytokines. *Scand J Immunol*, Jan; 51:23-28. ISSN 0300-9475.

Scheiman JM. (2006). Unmet needs in non-steroidal antiinflammatory drug-induced upper gastrointestinal diseases. *Drugs*, 66 (Suppl 1):15-21, discussion 29-33. ISSN 0012-6667.

Schnitzer TJ, Burmester GR, Mysler E, et al. (2004). Comparison of lumiracoxib with naproxen and ibuprofen in the Therapeutic Arthritis Research and Gastrointestinal Event Trial (TARGET), reduction in ulcer complications: randomised controlled trial. *Lancet*, Aug; 364(9435):665-74. ISSN 0140-6736.

Shorter RG, Huizenga KA, Spencer RJ, et al. (1972). Inflammatory bowel disease. The role of lymphotoxin in the cytotoxicity of lymphocytes for colonic epithelial cells. *Am J Dig Dis*, Aug; 17(8):689-696. ISSN 0002-9211.

Silverstein FE, Faich G, Goldstein JL, et al. (2000). Gastrointestinal toxicity with celecoxib vs nonsteroidal anti-inflammatory drugs for osteoarthritis and rheumatoid arthritis: the CLASS study: a randomized controlled trial.

Celecoxib Long-term Arthritis Safety Study. *J Am Med Assoc*, Sep; 284(10):1247-55. ISSN 0002-9955.

Singh G, Fort JG, Goldstein JL, et al. (2006). Celecoxib versus naproxen and diclofenac in osteoarthritis patients: SUCCESS-I Study. *Am J Med*, Mar; 119(3):255-66. ISSN 0002-9343.

Singh VP, Patil CS, Jain NK, et al. (2003). Effect of nimesulide on acetic acid- and leukotriene-induced inflammatpry bowel disease in rats. *Prostaglandins Other Lipid Mediat*, Jul; 71(3-4):163-75. ISSN 1098-8823.

Skelly MM, Hawkey CJ. (2003). Dual COX inhibition and upper gastrointestinal damage. *Curr Pharm Des*, 9(27):2191-5. ISSN 1381-6128.

Solomon SD, Mc Murray JJ, Pfeffer MA, et al. (2005). Adenoma Prevention with Celecoxib (APC) study Investigators. Cardiovascular risk associated with celecoxib in a clinical trial for colorectal adenoma prevention. *N Engl J Med*, Mar; 352(11):1071-80. ISSN . ISSN 1533-4406.

Suenaert P, Bulteel V, Vermeire S, et al. (2005). Hyperresponsiveness of the mucosal barrier in Crohn´s disease is not tumor necrosis factor-dependent. *Inflamm Bowel Dis*, Jul; 11(7):667-673. ISSN 1078-0998.

Thiéfin G, Beaugerie L. (2005). Review: Toxic effects of nonsteroidal antiinflammatory drugs on the small bowel, colon and rectum. *Joint Bone Spine*, Jul; 72(4):286-94. ISSN 1297-319X.

Tso JY, Sun X-H, Kao T-H, et al. (1995). Isolation and characterization of rat and human glyceraldehyde-3-phosphate dehydrogenase cDNAs: Genomic complexity and molecular evolution of the gene. *Nuclei Acids Res*, Apr; 13(7):2485-2502. ISSN 0305-1048.

Tsubouch R, Hayashi S, Aoi Y, et al. (2006). Healing impairment effect of cyclooxygenase inhibitors on dextran sulfate sodium-induced colitis in rats. *Digestion*, Dec 74(2):91-100. ISSN 0012-2823.

Vaananen PM, Meddings JB, Wallace JL. (1991). Role of oxygen-derived free radicals in indomethacin-induced gastric injury. *Am J Physiol*, Sep; 261(3 Pt 1):G470-5. ISSN 0002-9513.

Vane JR, Bakhle YS, Botting RM (1998). Cyclooxygenases 1 and 2. *Annu Rev Pharmacol Toxicol*, 38:97-120. ISSN 0362-1642.

Vane JR, Flower RJ, Botting RM. (1990). History of aspirin and its mechanism of action. *Stroke*, Dec; (Suppl 12):IV12-IV23. ISSN 00392499.

Vane JR. (1971). Inhibition of prostaglandin synthesis as a mechanism of action for aspirine-like drugs. *Nat New Biol*, Jun; 231(25):232-235. ISSN 0090-0028.

Wallace JL, Keenan CM, Granger DN. (1990). Gastric ulceration induced by nonsteroidal anti-inflammatory drugs is a neutrophil-dependent process. *Am Jphysiol*, Sep; 259(3 Pt 1):G462-7. ISSN 0002-9513.

Wallace JL, McKnight W, Miyasaka M, et al. (1993). Role of endothelial adhesion molecules in NSAID-induced gastric mucosal injury. *Am J Physiol*, Nov; 265(5 Pt 1):G993-8. ISSN 0002-9513.

Wallace JL,McKnight W, Reuter BK, et al. (2000). NSAID-induced gastric damage in rats: requirement for inhibition of both cyclooxygenase 1 and 2. *Gastroenterology*, Sep; 119(3):706-14. ISSN 1440-1746.

Wallace JL. (1997). Nonsteroidal anti-inflammatory drugs and gastroenteropathy: the second hundred years. *Gastroenterology*, Mar; 112(3):1000-1016. ISSN 1440-1746.

Wolfe MM, Lichtenstein DR, Singh G. (1999). Gastrointestinal toxicity of nonsteroidal antiinflammatory drugs. *N Engl J Med*, Jun; 340(24):1888-1899. ISSN 1533-4406.

Wong E, Bayly C, Waterman HL, et al. (1997). Conversion of prostaglandin G/H synthase-1 into an enzyme sensitive to PGHS-2 selective inhibitors by a double His513 to Arg and Ile523 to Val mutation. *J Biol Chem*, Apr; 272(14):9280-86. ISSN 0021-9258.

Yokoyama C, Takai T, Tanabe T. (1988). Primary structure of sheep prostaglandin endoperoxidase synthase deduced from cDNA sequence. *FEBS Lett*, Apr; 231(2):347-51. ISSN 0014-5793.

Yue G, Pi-Shiang L, Kingsley Y, et al. (2001). Colon epithelial cell death in 2,4,6 trinitrobenzene sulfonic acid induced colitis is associated with increased inducible nitric-oxide synthase expression and peroxynitrite production. J *Pharmacol Exp Ther*, Jun; 297(3):915-25. ISSN 0022-3565.

Zhang L, Lu YM, Dong XY. (2004). Effects and mechanism of the selective COX-2 inhibitor, celecoxib, on rat colitis induced by trinitrobenzene sulfonic acid. *Chin J Dig Dis*, 5(3):110-114. ISSN 1443-9611.

2

Intestinal Barrier Dysfunction: The Primary Driver of IBD?

Pieter Hindryckx and Debby Laukens
Ghent University
Belgium

1. Introduction

The healthy gastrointestinal tract is functionally maintained by an epithelial barrier, a monocellular layer that acts as a critical interface between the "outside" lumen and host tissues. This selectively permeable barrier controls the equilibrium between tolerance and immunity to microbes and non-self antigens. It is physically composed of epithelial cells linked through tight junctions, and it is reinforced by a mucus layer and the secretion of antimicrobial peptides such as defensins, cathelicidins and lysozymes. Intestinal epithelial cells are also responsible for the transport of water and nutrients while simultaneously preventing the uptake of noxious agents and luminal flora. Pathogens are selectively eradicated and should therefore be distinguished from the commensal flora to elicit a balanced inflammatory response. This capacity is tightly governed by pathogen recognition receptors, such as NOD proteins and the Toll-like receptors (TLRs). To avoid immunologic hyper-responsiveness against harmless intra-luminal food and bacterial antigens, the selective transport of small quantities of these antigens takes place by dendritic cells and M cells in Peyer's patches, leading to oral tolerance.

Several defects related to intestinal barrier function have been found in patients with inflammatory bowel disease (IBD), but for many, it remains to be clarified whether these are primary defects or secondary bystander effects of the inflammatory state. Nevertheless, evidence suggests that a "leaky gut" is an early and possibly primary defect in IBD pathogenesis. It has been demonstrated that increased intestinal epithelial permeability in Crohn's disease (CD) may indeed precede clinical relapse by as much as 1 year and that unaffected first-degree relatives of CD patients may also have barrier dysfunction. In addition, it is well known that mucosal barrier-breaking substances, such as non-steroidal anti-inflammatory drugs (NSAIDs), may cause flare-ups in IBD patients. Finally, transgenic animal models have clearly demonstrated that a unique defect in the intestinal epithelial barrier is a sufficient trigger of the development of chronic gut inflammation. The recent advances in genotyping technology have greatly improved the knowledge base regarding genetic susceptibility for IBD and have revealed several IBD-associated single nucleotide polymorphisms (SNPs) in genes involved in intestinal barrier function.

In this chapter, we first describe the components of the normal intestinal barrier. Next, we focus on the different barrier anomalies found in IBD both at the genetic and molecular level. The current evidence for a role of these barrier disturbances in the inflammatory process is extensively discussed. As a final point, the different therapeutic strategies for protecting or restoring the barrier function of the gut during IBD are discussed.

2. Components of the normal intestinal barrier

2.1 The physical barrier is composed of a tightly linked intestinal epithelial cell layer and a mucus shield

The surface lining of the intestine is composed of a single cell layer of tightly linked columnar epithelial cells. Intestinal epithelial cells are polarised, possessing an apical surface facing the lumen and a basolateral surface that is in direct contact with the immune compartment of the underlying lamina propria. The cells are tightly sealed by intercellular protein complexes consisting of tight junctions, adherens junctions and desmosomes (see 2.1.2), thus creating two physical compartments that separate the outside lumen from the inner host immune system. As such, these epithelial cells serve as a physical line of defence against harmful components passing the lumen, including foreign antigens, bacteria and the toxins they produce. Simultaneously, this barrier acts as a selective filter that permits the passage of essential dietary nutrients, electrolytes and water across the epithelial layer.

Selective transport through the intestinal epithelial membrane is accomplished in three ways: via the transcellular route, via the paracellular route and through microfold (M) cells (figure 1). The transcellular passage of amino acids, ions, sugars and short-chain fatty acids is performed by specific pumps and channels embedded in the cell membrane. This process is called transcytosis, and it involves the uptake of entities and their subsequent endosomal degradation. As such, the transport of intact proteins is limited, as they are degraded by the lysosomal system. The transcellular transport of bacteria and toxins is usually linked with mucosal inflammation. Paracellular transport refers to the passage of luminal materials through the space between the epithelial cells that is controlled by the intercellular junctional complexes. These complexes permit the diffusion of ions and solutes through the pores created by the protein structures and prevent the flux of larger entities such as microbes. Both the junctional pore size and the presence and activity of membrane pumps are highly regulated by such factors as cytokines and hormones, and these factors largely determine the passage and "leakiness" of the intestine. A final route of epithelial transport is mediated by M cells, which are typically located in overlying lymphoid aggregates called Peyer's patches. Unlike other epithelial cells, M cells lack microvilli and a mucus coat and represent a "guarded gateway" for the entry of microbes that are quickly recognised by the underlying lymphoid tissue.

2.1.1 Specialised epithelial cells

The epithelial lining of the gastrointestinal tract is composed of self-renewing epithelial cells that are arranged as crypts and villus projections. Stem cells within the crypts give rise to different types of specialised epithelial cells that migrate to the tip of the villus, where they undergo programmed cell death. Paneth cells represent one exception because they remain in the crypts. In addition to its role in antigen trafficking, the intestinal epithelial lining represents an anatomic barrier (see 2.1.2). Moreover, epithelial cells play an active role in barrier protection; they produce mucus, regulate the composition of the mucus layer (see 2.1.3) and serve as antigen-presenting cells for the immune cells residing in the lamina propria (see 2.2). Several different types of specialised epithelial cells can be distinguished, each of which participates in specific barrier functions (Table 1).

Cell type	Characteristics	Role in barrier function
Goblet cells	Production and release of mucus and trefoil factors (see 2.1.3)	Formation of a semi-permeable mucus layer preventing direct contact and adhesion between microflora and epithelial cells. Increase in repair mechanisms and tight junctions by trefoil factors.
Paneth cells	Production and release of antimicrobial peptides	Direct bactericidal or bacteriostatic effects elicited by defensins, lysosyme and phospholypase A2. Some enveloped viruses and fungi can be specifically lysed by these antimicrobial peptides.
Enteroendocrine cells	Production and release of serotonin	Release of serotonin into the lamina propria activates nerve fibres resulting in the stimulation of mucin secretion from goblet cells and passive water efflux.
M cells	Selective uptake of bacteria and antigens from the lumen via endocytosis or phagocytosis	Controlled stimulation of the gut-associated immune system.

Table 1. Main characteristics of the different epithelial cell types found in the gut and their role in intestinal barrier protection.

2.1.2 Intercellular junction complexes

Intestinal epithelial cells are sealed together by dynamic protein complexes composed of transmembrane proteins linked to the actin cytoskeleton through adaptor proteins. The intestinal epithelial cell lining in the gut is permanently self-renewing through the continuous migration of cells from the bottom of the crypt to the villus tip. To maintain the integrity of the epithelial barrier, intercellular complexes are rapidly assembled and disassembled without any dysfunction of the barrier function.

At the ultrastructural level, contacts between cells can be classified as tight junctions, adherens junctions or desmosomes. On the apical side of the epithelial monolayer, cells are attached to each other by means of tight junctions. These can be easily identified by electron microscopy because they leave no free space between two cells, in contrast to other junctional complexes in which cells are separated by 15 to 20 nm. Tight junctions consist of three types of proteins: occludins, claudins and junctional adhesion molecules. These molecules are linked to the cytoskeleton by members of the zonula occludens (ZO) family. Below the tight junctions, cells are attached by adherens junctions composed of E-cadherin

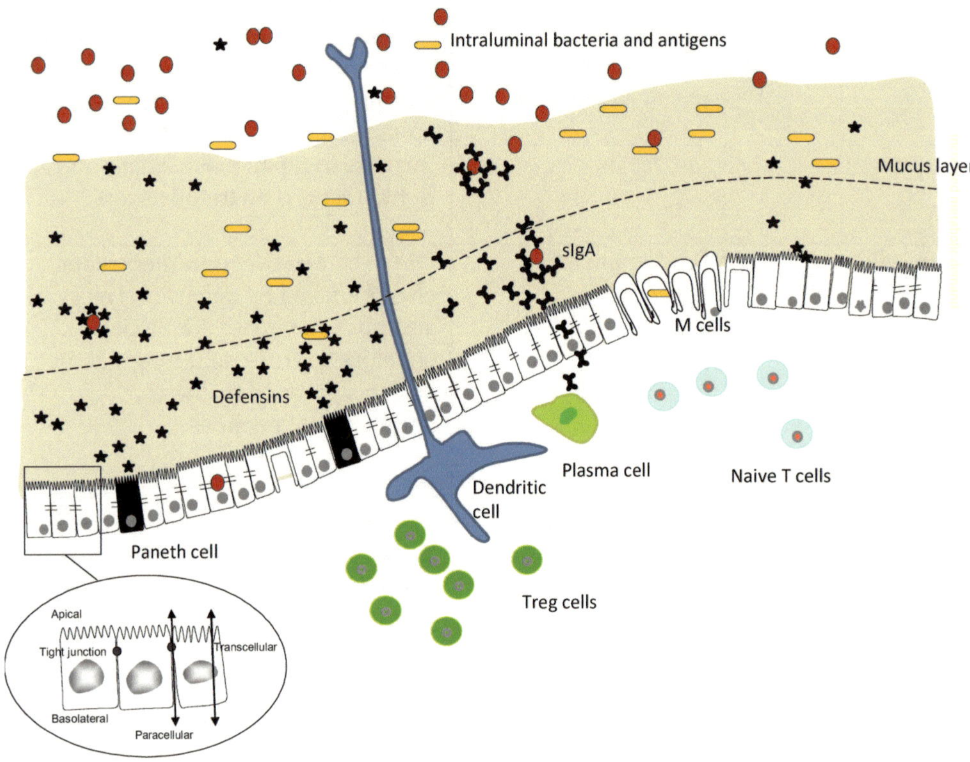

Fig. 1. Components of the normal intestinal barrier. Polarized intestinal epithelial cells provide a physical barrier between the outer luminal surfaces (apical) from the inner host immune tissues (basolateral). Highly selective transport across this barrier is accomplished by transcellular and paracellular routes and through M cells. A thick glycoprotein layer prevents direct contact between luminal bacteria and the epithelial cells. Further overgrowth of bacteria is prevented by the secretion of Paneth cell-derived antimicrobial peptides such as defensins and secreted IgA molecules (sIgA) produced by plasma cells. Tolerance within the gut is mediated by the large number of tolerogenic dendritic cells that are able to sense the lumen for bacterial antigens, resulting in the development of regulatory T (Treg) cells.

molecules that are connected via catenin proteins. Finally, desmosomes reside at the basal part of the epithelial cell and provide anchoring points for keratin filaments that are attached to intracellular desmoplakin, which connects the cytoskeleton to proteins belonging to the cadherin family.

2.1.3 The extracellular mucus shield

Throughout the gastrointestinal tract, intestinal epithelial cells are covered on the apical side with a viscous glycoprotein layer, although the sites of M cells are an exception. This layer acts as a lubricant for the propulsion of gut contents and prevents direct contact between bacteria and epithelial cells, thus preventing inappropriate immune reactions. The mucus layer is porous, permitting the diffusion of macromolecules required for gastrointestinal absorption and digestion while impeding the invasion of bacterial-sized particles.

Four major components can be found in the complex mixture of the mucus barrier: secreted mucins and trefoil peptides (produced by goblet cells), antimicrobial peptides (produced by Paneth cells) and immunoglobulin A (IgA) molecules (produced by B cells residing in the lamina propria).

The mucus barrier consists of two layers: a thin, sterile inner layer and a bulkier outer mucus layer that contains bacteria. The outer mucus layer physically protects the underlying cells from luminal bacteria. However, another important function is that it represents a niche that houses the commensal bacteria colonising the gut, thereby maintaining a balanced microflora that facilitates digestion. This outer layer is a dynamic compartment that is continuously degraded by luminal flora and replaced by the underlying cells. The differentiation of goblet cells and the release of mucins and antimicrobial peptides are directly regulated by the microbial flora. In addition, pathogen recognition by innate mechanisms (see 2.2) leads to the production of cytokines, which consequently stimulate mucin release. High concentrations of antimicrobial peptides and secretory IgA, which exert immune pressure on luminal bacteria, are found in the inner layer of the mucus barrier. Bile salts, which are produced mainly in the small intestine, greatly contribute to the suppression of bacterial growth in the mucus coat.

The mucus layer in the colon is thicker than that of the ileum. Furthermore, bile salt concentrations are much lower in the colon, whereas bacterial load and dwell time are higher.

2.2 The innate defence system: Sensing microbe-associated molecular patterns

When bacteria are able to break through the mucus barrier, either because of active pathogenic mechanisms or because the mucus layer is compromised, they reach the surface of epithelial cells. This triggers a rapid innate immune reaction mediated by TLRs and NOD-like receptors on the cell surface and inside epithelial cells, respectively. Rather than recognising specific antigens, these receptors discriminate self from non-self entities by recognising highly conserved molecular structures, the so-called microbe-associated molecular patterns. Examples include lipopolysaccharide (LPS), bacterial DNA, flagellin and peptidoglycan. Upon the binding of these ligands to their receptors, they recruit adaptor proteins, such as MyD88, inducing a signalling cascade that ends in the activation of nuclear factor kappa B (NFκB) and subsequent chemokine and pro-inflammatory cytokine expression, including tumour necrosis factor alpha (TNFα, see 4.1).

At least 11 TLR homologues have been identified, each of which has the unique capacity to recognise a specific microbial pattern. The best-studied apical TLR is TLR4, which recognises LPS, a cell-wall constituent of Gram-negative bacteria. In contrast, TLR5 can bind bacterial flagella, and it is located on the basolateral side of epithelial cells, suggesting its involvement in the eradication of invading bacteria.

The NOD-like receptors are expressed exclusively within the cell. NOD1 and NOD2 have been widely studied, and each binds to a specific moiety of peptidoglycan, the main constituent of the bacterial cell wall of both Gram-negative and Gram-positive bacteria. After ligand binding, these receptors recruit the Rip2 protein, which in turn also leads to the activation of NFκB.

The final outcome of innate signalling is the induction of pro-inflammatory cytokines and subsequent recruitment of phagocytes, which present bacterial antigens, leading to the activation of adaptive immune responses and clearance of the infection. Surprisingly, the deletion of *TLR4* or *MyD88* in mice leads to increased susceptibility to chemically induced colitis. Antibiotic therapy or germ-free cultivation of mice also results in a higher sensitivity to colitis. In addition, TLR4 signalling increases transepithelial resistance, indicating increased gut barrier function. It is clear that TLR and NOD signalling is important in maintaining a physiological state of immune activation to preserve intestinal homeostasis (see 2.3), and these signalling pathways are actively involved in repair mechanisms.

2.3 The immunological barrier characterised by oral tolerance

Once antigens invade the epithelial barrier, they are sensed by antigen-presenting cells (dendritic cells and resident macrophages), which prime naïve T cells *in situ* or after they migrate to the mesenteric lymph nodes. Activated T cells then differentiate into T helper type 1 (Th1), Th2, Th17 or regulatory T (Treg) cells and up-regulate specific gut-homing receptors ($\alpha 4\beta 7$ integrin and CCR9) to exert their functions at the site of infection. Whereas invasive pathogens can actively intrude on gut epithelial cells or induce their own phagocytosis via M cells, non-invasive bacteria can enter dendritic cells because of their frequent sampling. In the gut, dendritic cells can access the lumen by opening the intercellular space through the expression of tight junction proteins without compromising epithelial barrier function.

The balance between responsiveness towards foreign antigens and unresponsiveness towards self-antigens is critical because any breakdown of these mechanisms can lead to autoimmunity or an inability to respond to harmful infections. An intriguing question, therefore, is how the gut, which contains an enormous amount of food components and bacteria and houses an elaborate network of lymphoid tissue, is not in a state of massive inflammation as a result of the constant triggering of innate immune responses, both from epithelial cells and the underlying lymphoid cells. The control of such responses is called oral tolerance, and this control precisely defines a healthy mucosal barrier. Immune homeostasis in the gut utilises innate signalling triggered mainly by the commensal microflora and provides an environment rich in Treg cells, which produce anti-inflammatory cytokines such as interleukin 10 (IL10).

Oral tolerance is defined as the absence of a systemic immune response towards an antigen that has previously been encountered by the host. Thus, tolerance is an antigen-specific event. Together with anergy and apoptosis of antigen-specific T cells in the gut, the induction of antigen-specific Treg cells represents a method of actively inhibiting unnecessary inflammation. The key players in maintaining oral tolerance are the gut-resident antigen-presenting cells, which produce regulatory and immunosuppressive cytokines and present antigens to naïve T cells. In particular, dendritic cells exert the greatest stimulatory effect on T cells, as they express high levels of MHC class II and co-stimulatory molecules. Emerging evidence suggests that dendritic cells in the gut are conditioned to a tolerogenic state, mediated by transforming growth factor beta 1 (TGFβ), thymic stromal lymphopoietin (TSLP) and retinoic acid.

An important role exists for TGFβ, a well-known immunosuppressive cytokine that is expressed abundantly in the gut. TGFβ inhibits the expression of the transcription factors T-bet and GATA-3, which are necessary for the differentiation of Th1 and Th2 cells, respectively. In addition, TGFβ stimulates cells to differentiate into Treg cells that express the transcription factor Foxp3, which in turn inhibits the expression of IL2 and results in reduced T cell proliferation. Finally, TGFβ induces Th17 cells that express the transcription factor RORγT and produce inflammatory cytokines IL17A, IL17F and IL22. Although these cells play an important role during infection, an excess of Th17 cells has been associated with tissue injury and chronic inflammation. The expansion of established Th17 cell populations is accomplished by IL23, a cytokine that alters intestinal homeostasis and that has been linked with susceptibility to IBD (see 3.2.5).

2.4 Commensal bacteria

Commensal bacteria are by definition non-pathogenic microbes (bacteria or yeast) that can colonise the intestinal environment and confer benefit to the host. Typically, these bacteria are known to play a role during food digestion. However, they also elicit considerable protective effects related to barrier function. A very important role of commensal bacteria relates to immunomodulation by promoting tolerogenic dendritic cell and Treg cell populations and inhibiting pro-inflammatory cytokine production as described above. For example, commensal bacteria can induce TSLP and TGFβ expression from epithelial cells. Some *Lactobacillus* species can increase mucus, IgA and defensin secretion, and several *Bifidobacteria* strains can directly inhibit adherence or invasion of specific pathogens into epithelial cells or inhibit their growth and destroy them. Finally, some commensals can strengthen epithelial junctional complexes by inducing the expression of host proteins in these complexes.

3. Intestinal barrier dysfunction in IBD

IBD is characterised by loss of controlled ion and water transport, which is a direct consequence of intestinal barrier dysfunction. Increased permeability in IBD is largely determined by tight junction deregulation and apoptosis of epithelial cells. Functionally, barrier loss is associated with uncontrolled immune responses because of increased bacterial translocation and high expression of inflammatory cytokines such as TNFα and IFNγ (in CD) and IL13 (in the case of ulcerative colitis (UC)). In addition, recent advances in metagenomic sequencing have greatly aided in the characterisation and understanding of the composition of microflora, which was found to be significantly altered in IBD (see 4.2.2). Although barrier dysfunction has indisputably been recognised as a component of IBD pathogenesis, the question whether these defects are a primary cause or a consequence of the chronic disease process remains unanswered. Over the last decade, evidence has mounted that intestinal barrier impairment may be the primary driver of IBD.

3.1 Clinical data

The first clue that an intestinal mucosal barrier defect could be an early pathogenic event in IBD came from studies of first-degree healthy relatives of patients with CD. It was found that these relatives exhibit increased intestinal permeability compared to that in unrelated control subjects despite the absence of inflammation.

Complete mucosal healing appears to become the goal of future treatment for IBD. Preliminary data indicate that patients with complete mucosal healing have long-lasting and deep remission. Interestingly, CD patients in remission with a persistent increase in intestinal permeability appear to have a greater risk of disease relapse.

NSAID use, stress and smoking are known risk factors for IBD relapse. All of these factors are known to cause intestinal barrier dysfunction. NSAIDs inhibit the synthesis of mucosa-protective prostaglandins, potentially leading to ulcerations and barrier breakdown. Prolonged psychological stress can induce ultrastructural epithelial abnormalities, increased bacterial translocation and low-grade inflammation. Finally, smoking is associated with an increase in apoptotic cell death of the intestinal epithelium, leading to conductive leaks in the gut barrier.

3.2 Genetic and molecular evidence for intestinal barrier dysfunction in IBD

Evidence suggests that increased gut permeability tends to be familial and is most likely genetically determined. Up to 40% of healthy first-degree relatives of patients with CD have been reported to exhibit increased intestinal permeability, compared to 5% in the control population.

Epidemiological evidence clearly indicates that CD and UC are related polygenic diseases, and this has been supported by results from genetic association studies. In 2009, the International IBD Genetics Consortium (www.ibdgenetics.org), a network of researchers investigating the genetics of IBD, was established. At present, 20,000 CD and a similar number of UC cases have been collected, together with equivalent numbers of population-based healthy controls, from several countries in Europe, North America and Australia. This collaboration has resulted in three large-scale genome-wide association studies for CD and UC in which multiple risk loci have been identified (Anderson et al., 2011; Barrett et al., 2008; Imielinski et al., 2009). At the end of 2010, 99 replicated loci were found, and the genes within these loci have led to the discovery of new pathways involved in chronic gut inflammation. Many of these pathways involve intestinal barrier dysfunction, particular for UC (Barrett et al., 2009). Although the genome-wide scans have greatly improved our understanding of IBD pathogenesis, only an estimated 25% of the total genetic susceptibility can be explained by the currently identified disease-associated SNPs. In addition, due to linkage disequilibrium, the exact causative mutations remain to be identified. In the next section, the best-studied genetic associations involved in barrier function are discussed.

3.2.1 Paneth cell dysfunction

Paneth cells, which secrete antimicrobial factors, are found in the base of the crypts of the ileum. Many of the risk factors identified for IBD converge on Paneth cells and their function, including *XBP1*, *NOD2*, *TCF4* and *ATG16L1*. The most intriguing finding of Paneth cell dysfunction was found in the intestinal epithelial-specific knockout of *XBP1*, a central regulator of endoplasmic reticulum (ER) stress. These mice spontaneously develop small bowel inflammation that markedly resembles some features observed in human IBD, such as crypt abscesses, leucocyte infiltration and ulcerations (Kaser et al., 2008). Among several identified abnormalities, including goblet cell depletion and accelerated cell renewal, Paneth cells were completely lost in these mice. These data demonstrate that XBP1 function, or ER stress in general, is critical for proper intestinal epithelial cell functioning. Obviously, cells with the highest protein synthesis burden (Paneth cells and goblet cells) suffer most from a deletion of ER stress mediators. In human IBD, increased ER stress can be detected in inflamed areas of the intestine (Bogaert et al., 2011). However, it remains to be investigated whether this is a primary dysfunction or secondary to inflammation. One of the arguments that ER stress abnormalities are a primary event in IBD arises from genetic studies. Linkage of the region that is in close proximity to *XBP1* has been established previously, and deep sequencing of this gene resulted in the identification of polymorphisms associated with both CD and UC. Rare *XBP1* variants can be found to a much higher degree in IBD patients than in healthy controls. In particular, four non-synonymous mutations are present only in IBD patients. Interestingly, these mutations have been linked with hampered ER stress responses *in vitro*.

Another well-characterised risk gene specifically for ileal CD is the innate immune receptor *NOD2* (see 3.2.4). The finding that NOD2 is highly expressed in Paneth cells is particularly of interest because these cells provide host defence against microbes in the ileum, whereas they are not present in the normal colon. Lysozyme is an enzyme that breaks down bacterial cell wall components into muramyl dipeptide (MDP, GlcNAc-MurNAc), which is recognised by NOD2. Ileal expression of defensins was diminished in active regions in patients with *NOD2* mutations, although this was not observed in the diseased colon. NOD2 acts as an inducer of defensins, an effect that is lost in patients carrying a homozygous mutation in *NOD2*. Rather, these patients exhibit defective epithelial defence, proliferation of bacteria and the potential loss of epithelial barrier function. Similarly, variants in *TCF4* have been associated with ileal CD. TCF4 is a Wnt signalling transcription factor that plays a crucial role in Paneth cell development and directly activates defensin expression.

Finally, a coding variant in *ATG16L1*, a gene involved in autophagy, was identified in CD. Mice with only a partial loss of this gene and CD patients carrying the causal *ATG16L1* variant exhibit structural defects in Paneth cell granules, the "protein storage" compartment of the cell (Cadwell et al., 2008). Proteins that are normally found within granules were visible in the cytoplasm. In addition, an altered transcriptional profile was found specifically in Paneth cells, consistent with a pro-inflammatory state. However, Atg16l1-deficient mice do not develop spontaneous intestinal inflammation. Unexpectedly, NOD2 with MDP activation has recently been reported to induce autophagy via an ATG16L1-dependent pathway, and monocytes isolated from patients carrying a CD-associated *NOD2* variant fail to induce autophagy in response to MDP and bacterial infection.

Taken together, the apparently divergent genetic findings point to a central impairment in Paneth cell function that is associated with IBD. Although the risk genes act at different levels, this can be explained by the fact that innate sensing, ER stress and autophagy are interconnected.

3.2.2 Junctional complex genes

A locus containing *CDH1*, which encodes E-cadherin, a component of adherens junctions, was found to be associated with UC and possibly with CD. With this finding, the first genetic link between colorectal carcinoma and chronic colonic inflammation was established, with routine colonoscopic surveillance recommended for those at greatest risk. Some mutations have been associated with reduced levels of E-cadherin at the plasma membrane and an accumulation of cytoplasmic cadherin. Another interesting genetic candidate gene for UC is *hepatocyte nuclear factor 4 alpha* (*HNF4A*), a transcription factor involved in the regulation of genes that comprise cell-cell contacts that is aberrantly expressed in human IBD. The full knockout of this gene is lethal, with embryological anomalies in the intestine including reduced epithelial cell proliferation, loss of crypt formation and defective goblet cell maturation. The conditional knockout of *HNF4A* in the

intestinal epithelium results in mice that develop increased epithelial permeability and alterations in mucin-associated genes. A strong association was found, specifically for UC, in a region containing *laminin beta 1* (*LAMB1*), which encodes a subunit of the laminin family of proteins. Laminins are extracellular matrix glycoproteins that serve as major constituents of the basement membranes and play a key role in anchoring epithelial cells. Again, strongly reduced expression of laminins has been demonstrated in UC.
The inflammatory cytokines TNFα and *interferon gamma* (*IFNγ*), both of which are highly expressed during active CD, significantly influence tight junction reorganisation, but the exact mode of action is incompletely understood. The pore-forming claudins (claudin 1, 3, 4, 5 and 8), which can form size- and charge-specific paracellular pores, are up-regulated in CD, whereas occludin expression is reduced. Most likely, these changes occur as a consequence of inflammation, as they are not apparent during inactive disease. Nevertheless, determining how cytokines can modulate tight junction organisation is of great importance, as drugs targeting these cytokines have proven clinical efficacy in IBD.

3.2.3 Genes involved in the constitution of the mucus shield

A decrease of the number of goblet cells in IBD is associated with the reduced expression of mucins and a thinning of the mucus layer. Clinically, mucus diarrhoea is observed in UC, most likely because of the poor quality of the secreted mucus. Conversely, goblet cell dystrophy has been observed in CD with an increase in mucus production and decreases in antimicrobial peptides and tissue-regenerating trefoil factors. Moreover, colonic glycoprotein composition appears to be genetically determined, as it is more similar between monozygotic twins than between unrelated individuals.
In human intestinal tissue isolated from patients with IBD, disturbed expression of several mucin genes has been reported, and allelic variants in *MUC2*, *MUC3A*, *MUC4* and *MUC13* have been associated with IBD.
Striking evidence for a role of mucus secretion in the development of colitis arise from mice that carry mutations in *muc2*. Aberrant mucus biosynthesis in these mice results in the spontaneous development of colitis with striking resemblance to some aspects of human UC. Targeted mutations in *muc2* lead to misfolding of the mucin 2 protein in goblet cells followed by massive ER stress induction accompanied by increased intestinal permeability and enhanced production of pro-inflammatory cytokines in the distal colon.

3.2.4 Genes involved in innate immunity

The IBD1 locus, originally mapped in 1996, represents the best-replicated region exhibiting linkage specifically to CD and not to UC. In 2001, two groups simultaneously identified *NOD2* as the first susceptibility gene for CD (Hugot et al., 2001; Ogura et al., 2001). Hugot and colleagues employed the positional cloning strategy, whereas Ogura and co-workers identified *NOD2* by the positional candidate gene approach.
The NOD2 protein belongs to the NOD1/Apaf-1 family, which comprises cytosolic proteins composed of an N-terminal caspase recruitment domain, a centrally located nucleotide-binding domain, and a C-terminal leucine-rich regulatory (LRR) domain. Three common SNPs in *NOD2* were independently associated with CD: two missense mutations [R702W (c.2104C>T, SNP8) and G908R (c.2722G>C), SNP12], and one frameshift mutation [1007fs (c.3020insC, SNP13)] that truncates the protein by 30 amino acids. All three variants alter the C-terminal domain of the protein, and they are located within or close to the LRR domain, which is involved in ligand recognition. The heterozygous carrier frequency of these

variants in CD ranges from 30 to 50%, compared to frequencies of 3–15% for homozygous or compound heterozygote. By comparison, 8–15% of healthy controls are heterozygous, and 0–1% of individuals carry a homozygous variant. The relative risk of developing CD if one of these variants is carried increases by a factor of 1.5 to 3 for heterozygous carriers, but the risk increases by a factor of 20 to 40 in homozygous or compound heterozygous individuals. Although this relative risk appears high, it must be stated that the absolute risk for developing CD is no more than 1 in 25 for homozygous carriers. This reduced penetrance can undoubtedly be explained by the requisite of environmental risk factors and/or additional genetic determinants. Clinically, 40% of healthy relatives of IBD patients who carry one of these SNPs have increased intestinal permeability.

The Nod1/Apaf-1 family of proteins displays striking similarity to a class of disease resistance (R) proteins found in plants. Following specific recognition of pathogen products, these R proteins mediate a defence response associated with metabolic alterations and localised cell death at the site of pathogen invasion. The LRR domains of R proteins are highly diverse and appear to be involved in the recognition of a wide array of pathogen components. Similar to the R proteins, NOD2 appears to play an important role in innate and acquired immunity as a sensor of bacterial components. Specifically, NOD2 participates in the signalling events triggered by host recognition of specific bacterial motifs and subsequently activates NFκB, the key mediator in the production of pro-inflammatory mediators. Naturally occurring peptidoglycan fragments were identified as the microbial motifs sensed by NOD2, specifically MDP, which is found in Gram-negative and Gram-positive bacterial peptidoglycans.

The expression of NOD2 was first thought to be restricted to myeloid lineage cells, primarily monocytes. Moreover, its expression is enhanced by pro-inflammatory cytokines and bacterial components via NFκB, a mechanism that may contribute to the amplification of the innate immune response. Consistent with this observation, elevated NOD2 expression has been detected in inflamed areas of colonic tissue of CD patients.

Although the function of NOD2 in bacterial sensing is widely accepted, its physiological function is less well understood. Consequently, the implications of the CD-associated mutations in disease onset and progression remain unclear. Several hypotheses have been postulated that involve both loss-of-function and gain-of-function mutations in *NOD2*, although the gain-of-function hypotheses have received criticism. The gain-of-function hypotheses evolved from *NOD2* knockout and transgenic mice, but they are not consistent with the observations in humans. It is important to note that these hypotheses are not mutually exclusive and may be physiologically relevant in combination.

In vitro and *ex vivo* experiments have indicated that the three CD-associated polymorphisms actually decreased the activation of NFκB and pro-inflammatory cytokine production, which are inconsistent with the observation that NFκB is up-regulated in patients. However, this might reflect a lack of primary innate immune triggering in response to bacterial invasion. As the three CD-associated variants of *NOD2* are located in or near the LRR, it was suggested that bacterial sensing is impaired, thereby explaining the susceptibility to disease. Consequently, the clearing of bacterial products is inefficient, which may lead to a secondary, compensatory activation of NFκB independent of NOD2. Notably, peripheral blood mononuclear cells from individuals homozygous for the major disease-associated SNP13 mutation did not respond to synthetic MDP. These cells also exhibit defective pro-inflammatory cytokine release after stimulation with MDP. Mononuclear cells isolated from CD patients carrying *NOD2* polymorphisms produced significantly less IL1β, IL6 and IL10 after stimulation with adherent-invasive *E. coli* LF82 in a gene-dose effect. This was the first study in which aberrations were found in heterozygous carriers of SNP8 and SNP12 *NOD2* mutations, which represent the largest group of patients.

In human monocyte-derived dendritic cell cultures, NOD2 agonists synergistically induce IL12 production in combination with TLR3, TLR4 and TLR9 agonists to induce Th1-lineage immune responses. This synergistic effect was lost in patients carrying a mutant NOD2 protein. The inflammatory phenotype of CD is difficult to reconcile with decreases in TNFα and IL12 levels. However, it was recently demonstrated that the synergistic induction of IL10 in response to MDP and TLR stimuli was lost in NOD2 mutant monocyte-derived dendritic cells. IL10 is crucially involved in the down-regulation of the inflammatory process. It was thus postulated that IL10-mediated immune suppression is impaired, and the counter-effect for pro-inflammatory cytokines is lost, thereby contributing to chronic inflammation in CD.

Incubation of normal murine macrophages with MDP was demonstrated to suppress IL12 secretion induced by stimulation with TLR2 ligands. This suppression did not occur in cells lacking NOD2 or in cells expressing a mutant form of NOD2 during transfection experiments. Once secreted, IL12 promotes IFNγ production and the growth and differentiation of Th1 cells. A major concern, however, is the reproducibility of these results. Furthermore, NOD2 and TLR2 stimulation of human mononuclear cells isolated from patients with the 1007fs mutation led to a loss of the synergistic induction of pro-inflammatory cytokines, which is also inconsistent with a TLR2 inhibitory function of NOD2.

LPS, a cell wall component of Gram-negative bacteria, is a major inducer of inflammation, and its signalling is mediated through the cell-surface receptor TLR4. During intestinal inflammation, TLR4 is up-regulated on epithelial cells, macrophages and dendritic cells, thus providing a first line of defence against enteric Gram-negative bacteria. An association between a polymorphism in the LRR region of *TLR4* has been reported within a Dutch CD and UC cohort. Allele frequencies of 11% were found in CD patients, versus 5% in healthy controls. The association was replicated twice but could not be reproduced in three other studies. This mutation was previously linked to decreased bronchial responsiveness to LPS and impaired LPS signalling. However, no functional defect, e.g., cytokine release or LPS recognition, has been attributed to heterozygous carriers among CD patients. However, TLR4 is generally up-regulated on intestinal epithelial cells of patients with IBD, contributing to prolonged and increased responsiveness to normal luminal bacteria.

3.2.5 Genes involved in oral tolerance

IBDs are characterised by a loss of tolerance towards commensal bacterial flora. Animal models of enteritis, such as the *IL10* knockout model, do not develop disease when they are housed in a germ-free environment. Likewise, diversion of the faecal stream in IBD patients can stop the disease until the faecal stream is restored.

Anti-inflammatory cytokines, such as IL10, play a crucial role in maintaining tolerance. Deletion of the gene encoding *IL10* or its receptor (*IL10R*) in mice results in spontaneous small intestinal inflammation. IL10R mutations have been found in CD. These mutations lead to inefficient immunosuppression via IL10.

Treg cells are important for the maintenance of intestinal self-tolerance. Concentrations of TSLP, a major inducer of Treg development, are reduced in patients with IBD. Although Treg numbers increase during active IBD, they are significantly lower when compared to

non-IBD inflammatory conditions, such as diverticulitis. The addition of Treg cells in established colitis in mice results in complete remission of intestinal inflammation.
The first large genome-scan for CD resulted in the identification of multiple genes involved in IL23/Th17 signalling (Barrett et al., 2008), with CD-associated SNPs in *CCR6, STAT3, JAK2, IL23R* and *IL12B*.

3.3 Animal data

Additional evidence that barrier dysfunction may be the *primum movens* in IBD can be derived from animal studies. One of the earliest histological signs of dextran sodium sulphate (DSS)-induced colitis, a commonly used mouse model of UC, is increased apoptosis in colonocytes. This finding occurs before any histological sign of inflammation, such as an influx of polymorphonuclear cells in the colonic mucosa. A similar finding has been observed in the SAMP1/Yit and *IL10* gene-deficient mouse models of CD. These mice both exhibit a disturbance of the intestinal epithelial integrity prior to the onset of inflammation.
Some genetically engineered mice with a primary defect in a component of the normal intestinal mucosal barrier (*Muc2, Hnf4a* gene-knockout mice) spontaneously develop chronic intestinal inflammation, suggesting that intestinal barrier disruption may be a primary and sufficient trigger of IBD.

4. Strategies to defend or restore the gut barrier in IBD

4.1 Currently used therapies

Little is known about the barrier-protective actions of the currently used drugs in IBD treatment.
Preparations *of 5-aminosalicylic acid (5-ASA)* are mainly used in the treatment of mild to moderate UC. The exact mechanism of action of 5-ASA is incompletely known. In the DSS-induced colitis model, mesalazine both reduces colonic inflammation and permeability. It has been claimed that part of the mode of action of 5-ASA might rely on a reduction of IFNγ-induced epithelial barrier dysfunction during inflammation.
Although sometimes used for maintenance of remission in patients with CD, *methotrexate* appears instead to promote barrier dysfunction by promoting the production of reactive oxygen species and by altering ZO-1. Hence, it can be speculated that the anti-inflammatory actions of methotrexate overrule its negative effects on intestinal barrier function in patients with CD.
The introduction of *anti-TNF agents* was a breakthrough in the management of IBD. These biologics can rapidly induce remission and mucosal healing in both CD and UC patients. Anti-TNF agents share the ability to rapidly restore intestinal mucosal barrier function (within 2 weeks after a single infusion), which has been attributed to their strong anti-apoptotic effect on the gut epithelium rather than an effect on tight junction proteins.

4.2 Experimental therapies

Compounds with strong protective effects on the gut barrier often have spectacular efficacy in experimental gut inflammation, making them attractive candidates for the treatment of IBD. In this part, we give an overview of the most promising barrier-protecting molecules that might enter clinical practice in the future.

4.2.1 Prolyl hydroxylase-inhibiting compounds

Active inflammation is associated with low levels of oxygen and nutrients. Severe intestinal mucosal hypoxia has been clearly demonstrated in both experimental colitis and human IBD. The intestinal epithelial cells lining the gut lumen are particularly prone to these decreased oxygen levels during inflammation because of their anatomic position, which is relatively far from the richly vascularised sub-epithelial mucosa (figure 2). Mucosal hypoxia will lead to epithelial inflammation and barrier dysfunction by stimulating the release of pro-inflammatory cytokines. Animals exposed to full-body hypoxia display increased colonic permeability and an increase in myeloperoxidase levels, which is a marker for neutrophil accumulation.

The inhibition of cellular PHDs during hypoxia is an endogeneous adaptive system of the enterocytes aimed at protecting against hypoxia-induced cell death. As a result of PHD inactivation, both *hypoxia-inducible factor 1* (HIF-1) and NFκB are activated. HIF-1 is a transcription factor of many genes involved in angiogenesis, metabolism and barrier preservation. Mice with a conditional knockout of *HIF-1* in the intestinal epithelium are more susceptible to chemically induced colitis. NFκB is considered a pro-inflammatory transcription factor. However, it has recently been recognised that NFκB also has strong anti-apoptotic effects on the gut epithelium. Mice lacking NEMO, an important and essential positive regulator of NFκB, exhibit severe spontaneous colitis.

PHD-inhibiting compounds have a very strong protective action in murine models of colitis and in a murine model of Crohn's ileitis. A strong inhibitory effect on intestinal epithelial apoptosis appears to be an important mode of action. Future studies must address the feasibility and safety of these molecules for human use (Hindryckx et al., 2011a)

4.2.2 Probiotics

The normal intestinal microflora plays an important role in maintaining intestinal health. These microflora protect against pathogens and maintain epithelial barrier integrity. A microbial imbalance in the gut (termed "dysbiosis"), with a relatively low proportion of beneficial flora and a relatively high proportion of potentially harmful flora, has been associated with IBD. For example, some patients with CD have remarkably reduced levels of *Faecalibacterium prausnitzii*, a butyrate-producing commensal bacterium of the gut. Low ileal levels of this bacterial species are associated with a higher risk of postoperative recurrence of ileal CD. In addition, oral administration of *Faecalibacterium prausnitzii* or its supernatant appears to correct the dysbiosis in experimental colitis and strongly reduces the severity of inflammation. Butyrate functions as a potent anti-inflammatory factor through the inhibition of NFκB activation and the increased production of mucins, antimicrobial peptides and tight junction proteins. Therefore, the selection of probiotic strains from the *Clostridium* IV cluster of bacteria that can locally produce butyrate is under investigation (Van Immerseel et al., 2010)

Preliminary data on the use of probiotics in IBD patients to induce and maintain remission are promising, although the results appear to depend on the exact type of probiotic employed. For example, the addition of *Saccharomyces boulardii* to baseline therapy in patients with CD in remission may reduce the intestinal permeability and reduce the risk of relapse, although this was not observed for *Lactobacillus casei GG*.

Several probiotics have been successfully tested in the preclinical IBD setting, but they remain to be examined in human disease. For example, *Lactobacillus plantarum* has been demonstrated to ameliorate colonic epithelial barrier dysfunction and prevent colitis in *IL10* knockout mice.

A careful selection of probiotic agents, combined with more convincing efficacy in large clinical trials, will determine whether some probiotics can be used to treat IBD in clinical practice.

4.2.3 Flavonoids

Flavonoids, a class of plant secondary metabolites, have long been recognised to exhibit some anti-inflammatory properties that may have potential applicability in IBD. For example, the flavonoid quercetin ameliorates experimental colitis in rats. *In vitro* studies have demonstrated that quercetin improves the barrier function of the gut by changing the expression and distribution of several tight junction proteins.

Curcumin, a flavonoid extract from the spice turmeric, has been demonstrated to protect the mucosal barrier during rat enteritis. In a double-blind, multicentre trial of UC patients, the combination of curcumin and 5-ASA was superior in the prevention of disease relapse to 5-ASA alone.

Although evidence for a beneficial role in human IBD is still scarce, the available data on flavonoids suggest that it could be an effective and safe supplement to conventional IBD treatments.

4.2.4 Phosphatidylcholine

Phosphatidylcholine is a major phospholipid component of cell membranes. Insufficient phosphatidylcholine in the colonic mucus may lead to impaired phospholipid barrier function in UC, resulting in exposure to colonic commensal bacteria and mucosal inflammation. Exogenously administered phosphatidylcholine has anti-inflammatory properties in murine models of colitis.

Phase IIa/b clinical trials have demonstrated that delayed-release phosphatidylcholine can induce clinical improvement and even remission in UC patients.

4.2.5 Oxygenated perfluorodecalin

PFD is a member of the perfluorochemical (PFC) family of chemicals, which are high-density inert liquids with a remarkable capacity to dissolve high amounts of oxygen. These molecules can be used as powerful oxygen carriers and releasers into ischemic tissues. Topical administration of oxygenated PFCs has already been successfully used to treat difficult-to-treat chronic wounds, such as burns and diabetic ulcers. Intrarectal administration of oxygenated PFD both prevents and cures experimental colitis (Hindryckx et al., 2011b). The mechanism of action largely relies on a protective effect on colonic epithelial barrier function during inflammation. Due to its high density, PFD covers the colonic mucosa with an impermeable film, thereby preventing the influx of luminal antigens through the damaged colonic mucosa. In addition, the oxygen released by oxygenated PFD prevents apoptosis and stimulates proliferation of the colonocytes during inflammatory hypoxia (figure 2).

No study on the use of oxygenated PFCs in human IBD has been conducted thus far. However, intrarectal administration of oxygenated PFCs is a typical example of a barrier-promoting treatment that could be a very attractive strategy to heal therapy-resistant distal IBD or pouchitis.

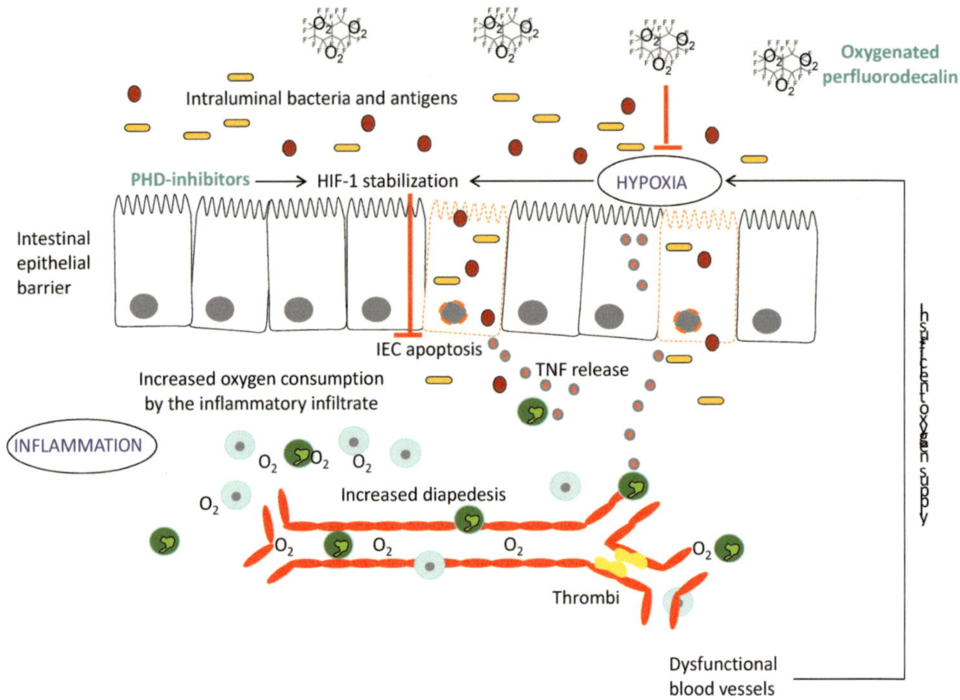

Fig. 2. Targeting inflammatory hypoxia in IBD to protect the gut barrier during inflammation. IBD is characterized by dysfunctional blood increased oxygen consumption by the active inflammatory infiltratea disturbed barrier function of the gut. Severe mucosal hypoxia during active IBD may lead to IEC death and further disruption of the gut barrier. Moreover, both hypoxia and inflammation stimulate the release of TNF-α, which also has a pro-apoptotic action on the gut epithelium. Prolyl hydroxylase- (PHD-) inhibiting compounds mimick hypoxia and stabilize hypoxia-inducible factor-1 (HIF-1), which is a major transcription factor for cell survival and barrier-protection. Intra-luminal administration of oxygenated perfluorodecalin (O_2-PFD) directly delivers O_2 to the intestinal epithelium and suppresses inflammatory cytokines such as TNF-α.
Both PHD-inhibitors and O_2-PFD have been succesfully used in animal models of IBD.

4.2.6 Growth factors

Several observations have suggested that therapeutic growth factor administration attenuates the mucosal barrier function defect in CD.

Epidermal growth factor (EGF) plays a key role in the healing response of the gut. In a small but randomised placebo-controlled trial, EGF enemas were superior to placebo in inducing remission at week 2 in mesalazine-treated patients with distal UC.

Keratinocyte growth factor administration improved mucosal healing in murine colitis models but failed in a placebo-controlled trial in patients with active UC.

In addition to improving the microbicidal activity of phagocytic cells, *granulocyte-macrophage colony-stimulating factor* (GM-CSF) also stimulates the proliferation of colonic epithelial cells. In a multicentre, randomised, controlled clinical trial using patients with active CD, sargramostim (a recombinant version of GM-CSF) was superior to placebo in terms of disease remission and quality of life improvement.

Transforming growth factors (TGFα, TGFβ) play an important role in mucosal defence and repair. Both TGF subtypes have been demonstrated to be crucially protective in murine colitis. Preliminary maintenance studies with a polymeric diet rich in TGFβ have been performed in both paediatric and adult CD patients with satisfactory results.

Although the supplementation of some growth factors appears promising for treating IBD, concern exists regarding potential carcinogenic action, which should be addressed.

4.2.7 Stem cells

Stem cells (SCs) have pluripotent potential and can differentiate into every type of cell, including intestinal epithelial cells. This unique capacity may allow SCs to restore the intestinal epithelium as well as the immune balance in IBD. Currently, both haematopoietic SC transplantation and mesenchymal SC transplantation in IBD patients are under evaluation in phase III clinical trials.

5. Conclusions

IBDs are chronic, relapsing inflammatory conditions of the digestive tract, with an incompletely known multifactorial aetiology. Clinical, experimental and genetic data suggest that intestinal mucosal barrier dysfunction is a hallmark of IBD. The occurrence of increased permeability in healthy first-degree relatives of IBD patients and its predictive value of clinical relapse suggests that these events are of primary origin or are at least very early events in the pathogenesis of IBD. Therefore, restoration of the barrier integrity may be a highly effective treatment strategy to promote the recovery of the barrier function and help to alleviate inflammation.

6. References

Anderson C. A., Boucher G., Lees C. W., Franke A. et al. (2011). Meta-analysis identifies 29 additional ulcerative colitis risk loci, increasing the number of confirmed associations to 47. *Nat Genet*, Vol.43, No.3, pp. 246-52, ISSN 1546-1718

Barrett J. C., Hansoul S., Nicolae D. L., Cho J. H. et al. (2008). Genome-wide association defines more than 30 distinct susceptibility loci for Crohn's disease. *Nat Genet*, Vol.40, No.8, pp. 955-62, ISSN 1546-1718

Barrett J. C., Lee J. C., Lees C. W., Prescott N. J. et al. (2009). Genome-wide association study of ulcerative colitis identifies three new susceptibility loci, including the HNF4A region. *Nat Genet*, Vol.41, No.12, pp. 1330-4, ISSN 1546-1718

Bogaert S., De Vos M. Olievier K., Peeters H. et al. (2011). Involvement of endoplasmic reticulum stress in inflammatory bowel disease: A different implication for colonic and ileal disease? *PloS One*, E25589. ISSN 1932-6203

Cadwell K., Liu J. Y., Brown S. L., Miyoshi H. et al. (2008). A key role for autophagy and the autophagy gene Atg16l1 in mouse and human intestinal Paneth cells. *Nature*, Vol.456, No.7219, pp. 259-63, ISSN 1476-4687

Hindryckx P., Laukens D. & De Vos M. (2011a). Boosting the hypoxia-induced adaptive response in inflammatory bowel disease: A novel concept of treatment. *Inflamm Bowel Dis*, Vol.17, No.9, pp. 2019-22. ISSN 1536-4844

Hindryckx P., Devisscher L., Laukens D., Venken K. et al. (2011b). Intrarectal administration of oxygenated perfluorodecalin promotes healing of murine colitis by targeting inflammatory hypoxia. *Lab Invest*, Vol.91, No.9, pp. 1266-76 ISSN 1530-0307

Hugot J. P., Chamaillard M., Zouali H., Lesage S. et al. (2001). Association of NOD2 leucine-rich repeat variants with susceptibility to Crohn's disease. *Nature*, Vol.411, No.6837, pp. 599-603, ISSN 0028-0836

Imielinski M., Baldassano R. N., Griffiths A., Russell R. K. et al. (2009). Common variants at five new loci associated with early-onset inflammatory bowel disease. *Nat Genet*, Vol.41, No.12, pp. 1335-40, ISSN 1546-1718

Kaser A., Lee A. H., Franke A., Glickman J. N. et al. (2008). XBP1 links ER stress to intestinal inflammation and confers genetic risk for human inflammatory bowel disease. *Cell*, Vol.134, No.5, pp. 743-56, ISSN 1097-4172

Ogura Y., Bonen D. K., Inohara N., Nicolae D. L. et al. (2001). A frameshift mutation in NOD2 associated with susceptibility to Crohn's disease. *Nature*, Vol.411, No.6837, pp. 603-6, ISSN 0028-0836

Van Immerseel F., Ducatelle R., De Vos M., Boon N. et al. (2010) Butyric acid-producing anaerobic bacteria as a novel probiotic treatment approach for inflammatory bowel disease. *J Med Microbiol*, Vol.59, No.2, pp. 141-3, ISSN 1473-5644

3

Adenosine Receptors: New Targets to Protect Against Tissue Damage in Inflammatory Bowel Symptoms

Sebastian Michael[1,3], H.-W. Rauwald[1], Haba Abdel-Aziz[2], Dieter Weiser[2], Christa E. Müller[4], Olaf Kelber[2] and Karen Nieber[1]

[1]University of Leipzig, Institute of Pharmacy
[2]Scientific Department, Steigerwald Arzneimittelwerk GmbH, Darmstadt
[3]Loewen-Apotheke, Waldheim, Germany, [4]PharmaCenter Bonn, Pharmaceutical Institute,Pharmaceutical Chemistry I, University of Bonn
Germany

1. Introduction

Irritable bowel syndrome (IBS) is a disease in which, typically, alterations in intestinal motility and visceral hypersensitivity appear to exist, apparently without any organic alteration (Thompson, 1991). Several pathogenic factors responsible for IBS have been suggested. It seems that there are cell factors, which give reason to believe that there is a low-grade intestinal inflammation in this pathology (Ortiz-Lucas et al., 2010). Several cytokines, such as tumour necrosis factor α (TNFα), interleukin 1, and interleukin 6, contribute to the pathogenesis (Ardizzone and Bianchi Porro, 2005; Pizarro et al., 2006). Macrophages are the major producers of TNFα, and, interestingly, they are also highly responsive to TNFα. TNFα has been shown to play a pivotal role in activating the cytokine cascade in many inflammatory diseases and it has been proposed as a therapeutic target for a number of diseases. Consequently, recent strategies for the treatment of intestinal inflammation have primarily targeted the immunopathogenic processes that mediate intestinal inflammation at the cytokine level (Bamias et al., 2003; Sandborm and Targan, 2002). At present, pharmacotherapy represents the mainstay of inflammatory bowel disease management (Stein and Hanauer, 1999). Some anti-inflammatory or immuno-modulating drugs, including salicylates and methotrexate, are able to decrease intracellular adenosine 5′-triphosphate concentrations and raise extracellular adenosine levels. It has been proposed that such properties can significantly contribute to the drugs' pharmacological actions in inflammatory diseases (Cronstein et al., 1999).

Several lines of evidence suggest that adenosine regulates immunity and inflammation (Amann and Peskar, 2002; Montesinos et al., 2007). The wide distribution of adenosine receptors (AR) as well as enzymes for purine metabolism in different gut regions suggests a complex role for this mediator in the regulation of gastrointestinal functions (Antonioli et al., 2008). Adenosine binds to four different types of G protein-coupled cell surface receptors referred to as A_1R, $A_{2A}R$, $A_{2B}R$, and A_3R, each having a unique pharmacological profile, tissue distribution and signalling pathway (Jacobson and Gao, 2006). All known ARs contribute to the modulation of inflammation, as demonstrated by many *in vitro* and *in vivo* pharmacological studies (Hasko and Cronstein, 2004; Montesinos and Constein, 2001). The involvement of adenosine pathways in the anti-inflammatory and immunomodulating effects becomes evident. These observations have stimulated the research of novel drugs suitable for treatment of intestinal inflammatory disorders through the pharmacological modulation of adenosine pathways (Cavalcante et al., 2006; Guzman et al., 2006; Odashima et al., 2005).

One medication which is successfully used in functional dyspepsia and IBS is the fixed herbal combination product STW 5 (Iberogast®; Madisch et al., 2004; Perez and Youssef, 2007; Raedsch et al., 2007; Schmulson, 2008). There is growing evidence that STW 5 besides being effective in functional dyspepsia, also improves IBS symptoms (Madisch et al., 2004; Krueger et al., 2009). STW 5 and its fresh plant component *Iberis amara* (STW 6) show a powerful reduction of morphological and contractile damages observed after experimental inflammation within the small intestine, and may thus have a promising therapeutic value as anti-inflammatory drug (Michael et al., 2009).

We therefore investigated the effect of STW 5 and its main component STW 6 on experimentally induced inflammation in rat ileum/jejunum preparations and the mechanisms of action. Using RT-PCR the expression of the ARs mRNA was determined and an interaction between the receptors and STW 5 as well as STW 6 was characterized. The results were confirmed by receptor binding experiments and pharmacological use of selective receptor antagonists.

2. Materials and methods

2.1 Animals

All procedures used throughout this study were conducted according to the German Guidelines for Animal Care and approved by the Institutional Review Board of Animal Care Committee.

Adult male Wistar rats (8-10 weeks old, 150-220 g body weight) were obtained from the Biomedical Centre, Medical Faculty, University of Leipzig, and were maintained at room temperature in a light (12 h light/12 h dark) controlled environment with food and water ad libitum. The rats were anaesthetized with CO_2 and killed by decapitation. The abdomen was immediately opened; intestinal segments (ileum and distal part of the jejunum) of about 15 cm were rapidly removed and placed in a dish containing aerated modified Krebs solution at 37 °C.

2.2 Materials

STW 5 contains *Iberis amara* totalis (STW 6) fresh plant extract and eight dried plants as drug extracts (Table 1).

STW 5 and STW 6 were kindly provided by Steigerwald Arzneimittelwerk GmbH, Darmstadt, Germany, in form of ethanol-free lyophilisates (58.0 mg resp. 18.2 mg corresponding to 1 ml of the fluid extract). STW 5 and STW 6 were dissolved in water. The concentrations of STW 5 were used as described before (Hohenester et al., 2004). STW 6 was used in equivalent concentrations to its proportion in STW 5.

ACh (1 M) was prepared as fresh 1:10 dilution from a 10 M stock solution. The final concentration in the organ baths was 1 mM. ACh (1 mM) was used as positive control. PSB-1115 (1-propyl-8-*p*-sulfophenylxanthine) was synthesized at the PharmaCenter Bonn,

Department of Pharmaceutical Chemistry I, University of Bonn, Germany, according to previously described procedures (Kirfel et al., 1997; Müller et al., 1993; Yan and Müller, 2004), and purified by preparative HPLC to obtain a purity of >98 %.

Plant extract	Drug-extract ratio	ml/100ml
Iberis amara totalis (STW 6)	1:1.5-2.5	15
Menthae piperitae folium	1:2.5-3.5	5
Matricariae flos	1:2.0-4.0	20
Liquiritiae radix	1:2.5-3.5	10
Angelicae radix	1:2.5-3.5	10
Carvi fructus	1:2.5-3.5	10
Silybi mariani fructus	1:2.5-3.5	10
Melissae folium	1:2.5-3.5	10
Chelidonii herba	1:2.5-3.5	10

Table 1. Constituents of STW 5

The modified Krebs solution contained (mM): NaCl (130.5), KCl (4.86), $MgCl_2$ (1.2), NaH_2PO_4 (1.97), Na_2HPO_4 (4.63), $CaCl_2$ (2.4) and glucose (11.4). The pH value was adjusted to 7.3. The reverse transcription (RT)-buffer contained 250 mM tris-HCl (pH 8.3 at 25 °C), 250 mM KCl, 20 mM $MgCl_2$ and 50 mM DTT. Phosphate buffered saline (PBS) contained (mM): NaCl (15.0), NaH_2PO_4 (4.0), Na_2HPO_4 (1.0) adjusted to a pH of 7.4. Tris-HCl was obtained from Carl Roth GmbH & Co KG, Karlsruhe, Germany.

The RNA preparation kit was from Qiagen GmbH. Primers were from Invitrogen. Enzymes used for reverse transcription were from Fermentas GmbH. The PCR reaction kit was from Bio-Rad Laboratories GmbH, Munich, Germany. All other substances were purchased from Sigma-Aldrich Chemie GmbH, Steinheim, Germany.

2.3 Radioligand binding assays

The radioligand binding assays were performed according to methods established by Klotz and Muller (Klotz et al., 1989; Muller, 2000; Muller et al., 2002). All studies were carried out as competition assays.

A_1R was taken from rat cortical tissue homogenates. Boards with 48 or 96 cavities were used. Each cavity carried 30 µg proteins in 200 µl final volume. 2-Chloro-N^6-[^{3}H]cyclopentyladenosine ([^{3}H]CCPA, specific activity 42.6 Ci/mmol, K_D 0.2 nM) was used as standard A_1R agonist in a final concentration of 1 nM. Tris-HCl was used as medium. Unspecific binding was determined with complete displacement by adenosine deaminase resistant adenosine analogue 2-chloroadenosine (CADO 10 µM). The extracts were dissolved in water. Incubation of boards took place at room temperature for 1.5 h. After that all samples were filtered on a cell harvester (Brandel) with ice-cold tris-HCl and filled into scintillation tubes. After addition of 40 µl ultima gold cocktail (Perkin Elmer) for the amplification of [^{3}H] signal the radiation intensity was measured in a LS counter (Packard).

$A_{2A}R$ was taken from rat brain striatal tissue homogenates. Boards with 48 or 96 cavities were used. Each cavity carried 50 µg protein in 200 µl final volume. [^{3}H]CGS 21680 (specific activity 41 Ci/mmol, K_D 15.5 nM) was used as standard $A_{2A}R$ agonist in a final concentration of 5 nM. Tris-HCl was used as medium. Unspecific binding was determined with complete displacement by broad spectrum AR agonist 5'-N-ethylcarboxamidoadenosine (NECA 50 µM).

The extracts were dissolved in water. Incubation of boards took place at room temperature for 1.5 h. The final procedure was the same as for A_1R preparations.
The results were analyzed and displayed with GraphPad PRISM®.

2.4 Induction of inflammation and drug application

Inflammation was induced as previously described (Michael et al., 2009). In brief, an ileum/jejunum preparation approximately 10 cm long was prepared, cleaned and divided into four segments. One end of each segment was tied up with a thread and in the other end a canula was inserted through which TNBS (0.01 M) and/or test substances were instilled. Thereafter the canula was removed, and the end was closed with a thread. The preparation was suspended for 30 min in a 10 ml incubation chamber containing aerated modified Krebs solution. After preincubation the threads were removed and the preparation was rinsed with modified Krebs solution. Sections of 1.5 cm in length were prepared for the experiments.
Four preparations per animal were used to test the effects of STW 5 and STW 6 in the same experiment. All experiments were repeated using at least three animals. Modified Krebs solution (control), TNBS (0.01 M) alone, or TNBS together with STW 5 (512 µg/ml) and STW 6 (24.1 µg/ml) respectively were instilled and incubated for 30 min.

2.5 Recording of mechanical activity

The preparations were suspended in 20 ml organ baths containing oxygenated (95 % O_2, 5 % CO_2) modified Krebs solution maintained at 37 °C. Then they were attached to fixed pins in the bath and to isometric transducers (TSE Systems, Bad Homburg) using polyester threads. The preparations were allowed to equilibrate for 40 min under a tension of 10 mN interrupted by a wash out before starting the experiment. ACh (1 mM) was applied at the beginning of each experiment to test the sensitivity of the preparations. Thereafter ACh was applied into the organ bath every 20 min. A washout and equilibration period followed after registration of the maximum contraction.
The ACh-evoked contraction was defined as difference between the basal tone and the first maximum contraction after drug application. For each experiment an untreated preparations (control 100%) and TNBS-treated preparation were used from the same animal. The TNBS-induced alterations of ACh-induced contractions differed strongly between several experimental series. To evaluate the experimental series the damage was calculated as an internal standardisation of the TNBS-induced alterations of the ACh-contractions. 100% damage represents the effect of TNBS on ACh-contractions under control conditions.

2.6 Van Gieson staining and morphometric analysis

The middle part (0.5 cm) of each preparation was fixed in phosphate buffered paraformaldehyde (4 %), washed with PBS, dehydrated in sequential ethanol baths with increasing concentrations of ethanol (50 % to 99.8 %) and embedded in paraffin wax. Slices of 7 µm were cut with a Jung Biocut microtome (Leica). The slices were dewaxed with xylene and rehydrated in three sequential ethanol baths with decreasing concentrations that ranged from 99.8 % to 70 % ethanol. For histological studies, the sections were stained with haemalaun solution (Mayer, cell nuclei) and van Gieson solution (picric acid with sour fuchsine) according to the method of Romeis (Mikroskopische Technik, 1989). The slides were examined qualitatively under a light microscope at 20x magnification. For analysing of the histological photographs the method of calibrated ocular micrometer gauge was used. Largest and smallest diameters of the tissue layers were determined to calculate the area of mucosa as well as muscularis (longitudinal and circular muscle layers). Three positions were implemented in the calculation. Ten objects from at least three animals were used for statistics.

2.7 RNA isolation and reverse transcription

Following the manufacturers protocol total RNA from ileum/jejunum segments was extracted after preincubation for 3 h using the RNeasy Mini kit® (Qiagen). 10 µl of the RNA eluates were activated with 1 µl of oligo-dT (20) 500 µg primers in a 5 min incubation step at 70 °C in the Crocodile III cycler. Reverse transcription was performed with 200 units of RevertAID (Fermentas) and dNTP (1 mM) in the Crocodile III cycler in the RT-buffer. The final volume was 20 µl. The reaction was stopped by heating at 70 °C for 10 min.

2.8 Real-time fluorescence PCR

AR mRNA expression as well as the expression of TNFα and IL-10 mRNA were measured quantitatively by a ready-to-use real-time fluorescence polymerase chain reaction (PCR) assay. SYBR Green® Mix reaction (BioRad) was used in a MyIQ® cycler (BioRad) according to manufacturers protocol. β-actine was used as a housekeeping gene. The primers for β-actin and the adenosine A_1R were self-designed, whereas the primers for the $A_{2A}R$, TNFα and IL-10 were found in literature (Chen et al. 2004). Table 2 summarizes the sequences of the primers.

primer	sequence	origin
ß-Actin sense	5′-TGTCACCAACTGGGACGATA-3′	designed by the authors
ß-Actin antisense	5′-GGGGTGTTGAAGGTCTCAAA-3′	
A_1 sense	5′- CTGCTCCTCATGGTCCTCAT-3′	designed by the authors
A_1 antisense	5′- GGGCAGAAGAGGGTGATACA-3′	
A_{2A} sense	5′- CTCACGCAGAGTTCCATCTT-3′	Chen, 2004
A_{2A} antisense	5′- TCCATCTGCTTCAGCTGTCT-3′	
TNFα sense	5′-TCAGCCTCTTCTCATTCCTG-3′	designed by the authors
TNFα antisense	5′-GGCTACGGGCTTGTCACTCG-3′	
IL-10 sense	5′- TTTAAGGGTTACTTGGGTTGC-3′	Klingenberg, 2006
IL-10 antisense	5′- GCTCCACTGCCTTGCTTTTA-3′	

Table 2. Primers for RT-PCR.

Each sample contained 10 µl of the SYBR Green® SuperMix, 1 µl sense primer, 1 µl antisense primer, 1 µl complementary DNA and 7 µl sterile water in a volume of 20 µl. The results were analyzed using the $\Delta\Delta c_t$-method (Pfaffl et al., 2002) and expressed as relative gene expression.

2.9 Maceration

STW 6 (24.2 µg/ml) was extracted three times each with hexane, chloroform and ethyl acetate (water saturated). Emulsions were centrifuged. The solvent phase was siphoned off. The solvent phases of the three extractions of each solvent were combined and vacuum evaporated. The fractions as well as the remaining aqueous fraction were lyophilised. The lyophylisates were analysed qualitatively by thin layer chromatography using standard protocols (Wagner, 1996) and quantitatively by high pressure liquid chromatography (HPLC, Kroll, 2006). The results of HPLC are shown in table 3.

fraction	Cucurbitacin E	Cucurbitacin I	mass percentage
STW 6	44.4 µg/ml	31.6 µg/ml	100 %
STW 6-$CHCl_3$	31.4 µg/ml	14.9 µg/ml	3.2 %
STW 6-EA	1.2 µg/ml	0.65 µg/ml	2.1 %
STW 6-H_2O	n.d.	n.d.	93.5 %

Table 3. Quantitative results of the fraction chromatography (n.d. not detected).

2.10 Statistics

Experimental data are presented as the means±SEM of the number (n) of experiments. Multiple comparisons with a control value were performed by one-way analysis of variance followed by Student´s *t-test.* A probability level of 0.05 or less was considered statistically significant. K_i values were calculated by nonlinear correlation.

3. Results

3.1 Effects of STW 5 and STW 6 on ACh-contractions in inflamed preparations

The ileum/jejunum preparations were pre-incubated with TNBS for 30 min. During this time a marked inflammation developed, manifested by a constant inhibition of the ACh-induced contractions. As shown previously TNBS (1 mM - 1 M) resulted in a concentration-dependent inhibition of ACh-induced contractions (damage) with an IC_{50} value of 63 mM. 100 mM TNBS reduced the ACh-induced contraction to approximately 35 % in comparison to intact preparation of the same animal (Michael et al., 2010). The combined preincubation of the ileum/jejunum preparation with TNBS (0.01 M, 30 min) and STW 5 (64-512 µg/ml) or STW 6 in equivalent concentrations (3-24.1 µg/ml) diminished concentration-dependently the TNBS-induced damage of the ACh-contraction. STW 5 (128-512 µg/ml) prevented up to 30 % of the TNBS-induced damage, whereas STW 6 at the highest concentration of 24.1 µg/ml had even a stronger effect of 56.8±6.6 % (Fig. 1A).

To study whether the TNBS-induced damage is linked with morphological alterations van Gieson staining was done followed by detailed morphometric analysis. Histological assessment revealed tissue damages in preparations pre-incubated with TNBS. As seen in Fig. 1 B, the mucosal area of control preparations was 22,150±100 μm^2. It was reduced to 16,080±810 μm^2 by TNBS (0.1 M). The combined pre-incubation with TNBS and STW 5 (29,980±2,150 μm^2) or STW 6 (20,690±1,010 μm^2) preserved the mucosa. The gradual reduction of the muscularis area (longitudinal and circular muscle layers) was even greater after TNBS incubation. The decrease was from 5,770±300 μm^2 to 2,750±140 μm^2. STW 5 and STW 6 also prevented this TNBS-induced morphological disturbance (5,530±450 μm^2 and 5590±360 μm^2, Fig. 1C).

3.2 Effects of STW 5 and STW 6 on the gene expression of TNFα and IL-10

Human monocyte is an established model to study the inflammatory or anti-inflammatory drugs (Linden, 2006; Sitkovsky et al., 2004). In previous studies we have shown that treatment of monocytes with STW 5 (128 µg/ml) or STW 6 (6.0 µg/ml) had no effect on the

TNFα release whereas LPS, a well described inflammatory mediator, stimulated the release of TNFα from 0.007±0.007 ng/ml to 1.4±0.1 ng/ml. STW 5 prevented the LPS-induced TNFα release by depressing the release to 0.4±0.2 ng/ml. No inhibitory effect was found with STW 6 (Michael et al., 2009).

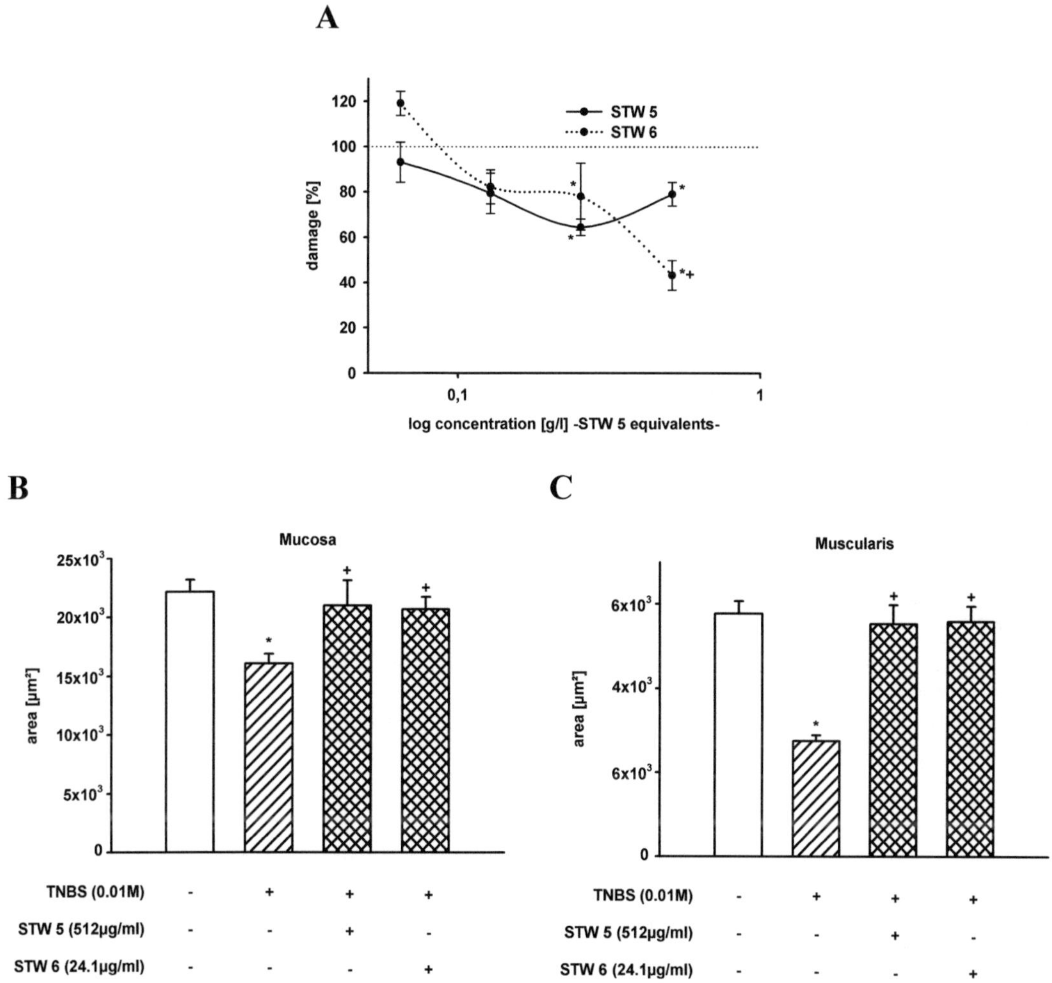

Fig. 1. Effects of STW 5 and STW 6 on TNBS-induced damage of ACh-induced contractions in ileum/jejunum preparations. (A) Concentration response curves of the effect of STW 5 (64-512 µg/ml) and STW 6 in equivalent concentrations (3-24 µg/ml) after coincubation with TNBS (0.01 M, 30 min). STW 5 and STW 6 prevented concentration dependently the TNBS-induced damage. STW 6 at maximum concentration mediated a <20 % stronger effect than STW 5. Mean±SEM of nine experiments, *p<0.05, significant vs. control; $^{+}$p<0.05 significant vs. previous value. Morphometric analysis of the effects of STW 5 and STW 6 on mucosa (B) and muscularis (C). STW 5 (512 µg/ml) and STW 6 (24.1 µg/ml) prevented the TNBS-induced effects. Mean±SEM of 30 measurements (B and C), *p<0.05, significant vs. control; $^{+}$p<0.05 significant vs. TNBS.

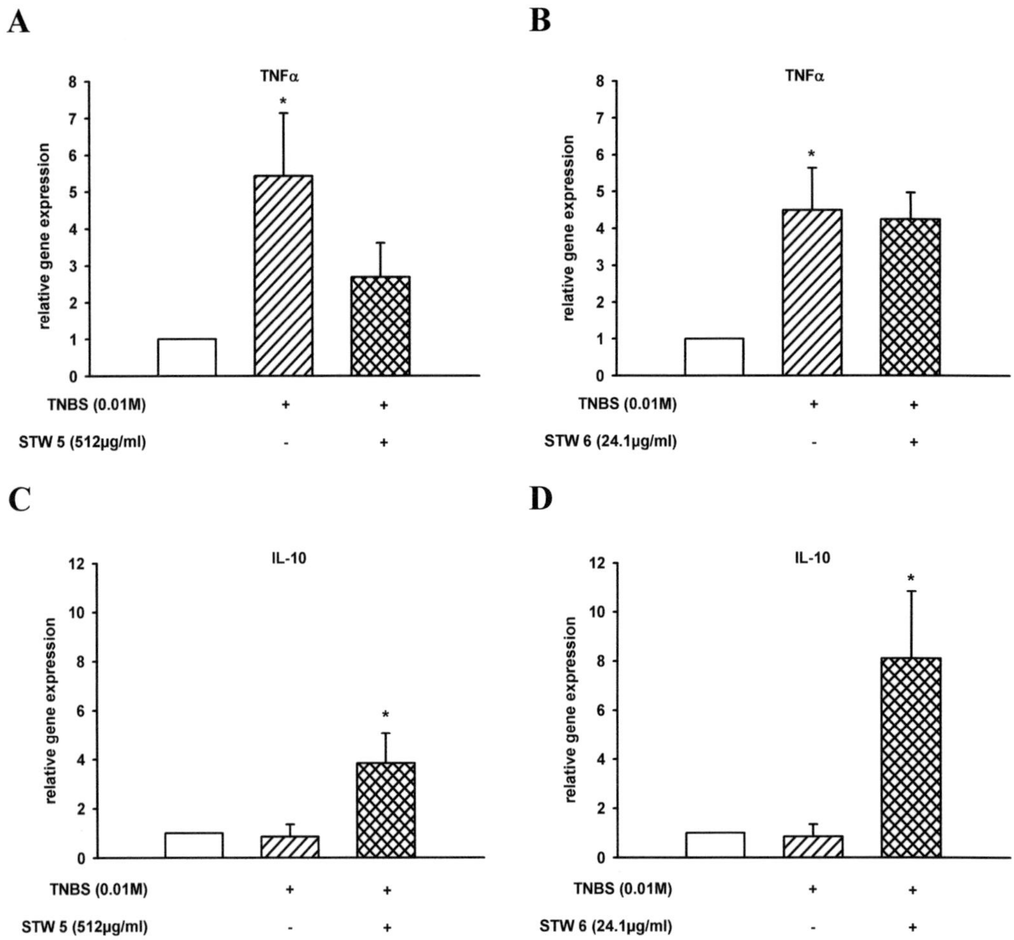

Fig. 2. Effects of TNBS alone and after coincubation of TNBS with STW 5 or STW 6 on TNFα and IL-10 gene expression in ileum/jejunum preparations. TNBS (0.01 M) increased significantly the TNFα gene expression. STW 5 (512 µg/ml, A) but not STW 6 (24.1 µg/ml, B) prevented the gene activation. The IL-10 gene expression was not affected significantly by TNBS (0.01 M). It was increased by coincubation of TNBS and STW 5 (512 µg/ml, C) and this effect was more pronounced with STW 6 (24.1 µg/ml, D). Mean±SEM of five experiments, * $p<0.05$ significant vs. control (blank column).

Here, we investigated the gene expression of TNFα and additionally the gene expression of the anti-inflammatory cytokine IL-10. Preincubation of ileum/jejunum preparations with TNBS (0.01 M) resulted in a significant increase of the relative gene expression of TNFα by factor 5.4±1.7 (Fig. 2A) and 4.5±1.1 (Fig. 2B) compared to the gene expression in control preparations. The combined preincubation with TNBS and STW 5 (512 µg/ml) reduced this factor to 2.7±0.9 (Fig. 2A), whereas STW 6 had no significant effect (4.2±0.7) on the TNBS-increased gene expression (Fig. 2B). In contrast, TNBS did not influence the relative gene expression of IL-10 (factor 0.86±0.50). After combined preincubation with STW 5 (512 µg/ml), the relative gene expression was significantly increased by factor 3.85±1.21 compared to the gene expression in control preparations (Fig. 2C). The increase was even more pronounced after combined preincubation with STW 6 (24.1 µg/ml, factor 8.10±2.73, Fig. 2D).

3.3 Gene expression and functionality of adenosine receptors

RT-PCR was used to study the expression of receptor mRNA for A_1R and $A_{2A}R$ in intact and TNBS-treated ileum/jejunum preparations.

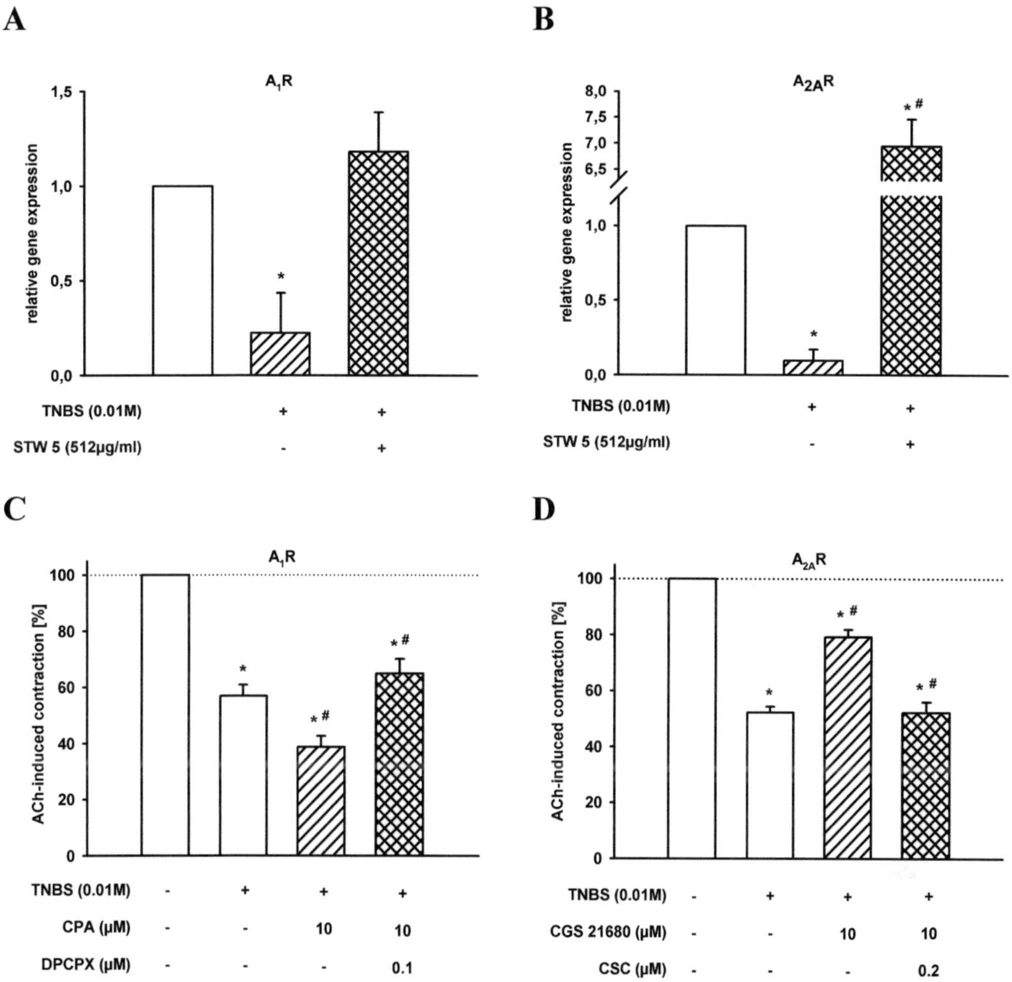

Fig. 3. Gene expression of A_1R and $A_{2A}R$ as well as their alteration after incubation with TNBS and STW 5 (A and B). AR-mRNA expression was measured quantitatively by a ready-to-use real-time fluorescence polymerase chain reaction (PCR) assay and expressed as relative gene expression using the $\Delta\Delta c_t$-method. Effect of the A_1R agonist CPA (10 µM) and the A_1R antagonist DPCPX (0.1 µM) on the TNBS-induced decrease of the ACh (1 mM) -induced contractions (C). Effect of the $A_{2A}R$ agonist CGS 21680 (10 µM) and the $A_{2A}R$ antagonist CSC (0.2 µM) on TNBS-induced decrease of the ACh (1 mM) contractions (D). Mean±SEM of 12 experiments, *$p<0,05$ vs. control (open column), #$p<0.05$ vs. previous column.

A_1R and $A_{2A}R$ mRNA were identified in intact preparations. Incubation of the preparations with TNBS (10 mM,) resulted in a significant suppression of the mRNA expression. STW 5 (512 µg/ml) coincubated with TNBS (10 mM) protected from TNBS-induced suppression of the A_1R (Fig. 3A). The gene expression remained at control levels. For $A_{2A}R$ mRNA even a significant induction by factor 6.9±0.5 was detectable (Fig. 3B).
The functionality of the adenosine A_1R and $A_{2A}R$ was tested pharmacologically. Ileum/jejunum preparations were incubated with TNBS together with specific receptor agonists and antagonists for 30 min. After that ACh (1 mM)-induced contractions were recorded. TNBS (10 mM) decreased the ACh-induced contraction to 57.9±3.9 % ($p<0.05$ vs. control, n=12). After preincubation together with the A_1R agonist CPA (10 µM), the decrease to 38.8±3.26 % (n=12, $p<0.05$ vs. control). DPCPX (0.1 µM), described as inverse agonist on A_1R, enhanced slightly the TNBS-reduced contractions but prevented the CPA-induced inhibition (65.0±5.1 %, $p<0.05$ vs. CPA, n=12, Fig. 3C). The activation of $A_{2A}R$ by CGS 21680 (10 µM) enhanced the TNBS-reduced contraction by 27 % (79.3±2.6 % vs. 52.3±2.1 %, $p<0.05$, n=9). The $A_{2A}R$ antagonist CSC (0.2 µM) had negligible effect on the TNBS-reduced contraction (52.3±2.6 % vs. 46.4±6.6 %, $p>0.05$, n=9), but it abolished completely the agonist-induced enhanced contraction (52.3±3.7 %, $p<0.05$ vs. CGS 21680, n=9, Fig. 3D).

A

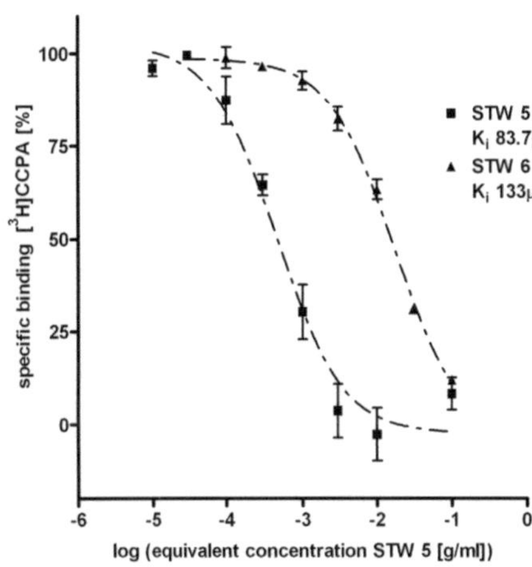

B

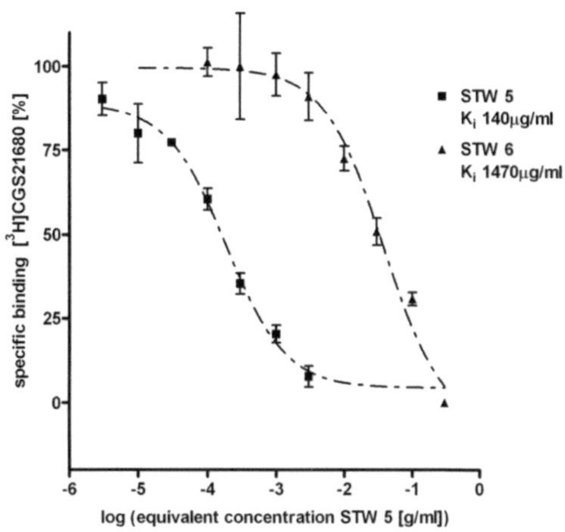

Fig. 4. Competition curves of STW 5 and STW 6 at the A_1R and the $A_{2A}R$. Displacement of (A) the radioactive labelled A_1R agonist [^{3}H]CCPA and (B) the radioactive labelled $A_{2A}R$ agonist [^{3}H]CGS 21680. Half logarithmic line graphs of mean ± SEM of specific binding of [^{3}H]CCPA and [^{3}H]CGS 21680 from 3 independent experiments, respectively. A decreased binding of the radioactive labelled agonist represents competitive displacement by STW 5 or STW 6. The concentrations of STW 6 were calculated as equivalent to STW 5. Mean±SEM of three independent experiments.

3.4 Receptor binding assays

To evaluate an interaction between STW 5 and STW 6 and A_1R and $A_{2A}R$, receptor binding studies were designed. STW 5 and STW 6 were able to displace the radioactive labelled A_1R

agonist [^{3}H]CCPA (Fig. 4A) as well as radioactive labelled $A_{2A}R$ agonist [^{3}H]CGS 21680 (Fig. 4B) from these receptors in a concentration dependent manner. The shift of the displacement curve of STW 6 to the right indicates a very weak binding of this extract, which may be due to nonspecific interactions.

3.5 Interaction of STW 5 and $A_{2A}R$ in inflamed preparations

According to data from gene expression in further experiments the role of A_1R and $A_{2A}R$ in STW 5 responses is indicative for an anti-inflammatory action and was therefore investigated in TNBS-treated ileum/jejunum preparations. STW 5 (512 µg/ml) was able to prevent the TNBS-induced damage of the ACh-contraction by 19.0 % ($p<0.05$ vs. control, n=18) in ileum/jejunum preparations. The $A_{2A}R$ antagonist CSC (0.2 µM) was significantly effective in blocking the effect of STW 5 ($p<0.05$, n=18, Fig. 5). The experiments were repeated in the presence of A_1R antagonist DPCPX. The additional preincubation with DPCPX (0.1 µM) enhanced the damage of the ACh-induced contractions but did not affect the effective blockade by CSC (Fig. 5).The experiments indicate that the protective effect of STW 5 in TNBS-inflamed preparations is mediated primarily by activation of $A_{2A}R$.

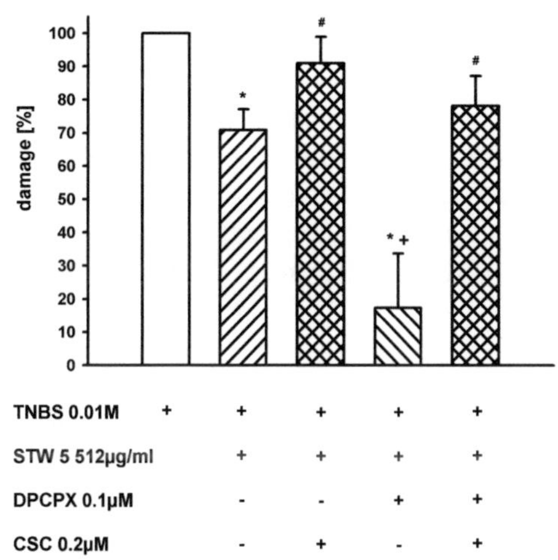

Fig. 5. Impact of $A_{2A}R$ antagonist CSC and A_1R antagonist DPCPX on the STW 5 mediated effect on the TNBS-induced damage of the ACh contraction. STW 5 (512 µg/ml) was incubated together with TNBS (0.01 M), CSC (0.2 µM) and DPCPX (0.1 µM,) or the combination of the antagonists. Means±SEM from 12 to 18 experiments. *$p<0.05$ vs. TNBS (open column), $^{\#}$ $p<0.05$ vs. previous column, $^{+}$ $p<0.05$ vs. STW 5.

3.6 Mechanism of action of STW 6 in inflamed preparations

The experiments described above clearly indicate that the protective effect of STW 6 was not mediated by activation of $A_{2A}R$ or interaction with TNFα pathway rather than by activation of IL-10 pathway. Therefore, the next set of experiments was designed to study the mechanisms involved in the action of STW 6. Bio-guided isolation of active ingredients within STW 6 was performed using solvents of different polarities. The hexane fraction had only a marginal mass portion (1.3 %) and was, therefore, excluded from further experiments. The chlorophorm, ethyl acetate and water fractions were concentrated to the equivalent concentration of STW 6 (24.1 µg/ml), respectively, and used for simultaneous incubation of ileum/jejunum preparations with TNBS. The chloroform (37.9±12.8%, $p<0.05$, n=9) and ethyl acetate fraction (29.7±9.9%, $p<0.05$, n=9), which contained the cucurtacines E and I (Fig. 6A), prevented the TNBS inhibition of the ACh-induced contractionsrespectively. The water fraction, devoid of cucurbitacins, was without effect. This observation was further supported by the fact that purified cucurbitacin E and I could antagonize the TNBS-induced damage of ACh- stimulated contraction with EC_{50} of 0.12 µM and 0.04 µM, respectively (Fig. 6B). Additionally, cucurbitacins were able to stimulate the IL-10 gene expression. TNBS was without effect on the relative IL-10 gene expression. Cucurbitacin E (10 mM) coincubated with TNBS (10 mM, 30 min) significantly induced IL-10 mRNA by the factor 7.0±2.8 ($p<0.05$ vs. control, n=3, Fig. 6C).

4. Discussion

Gastrointestinal inflammation is accompanied by structural and functional changes of the gut, leading to gastrointestinal motility disturbances during both acute and chronic inflammation (Collins, 1996). Motility disturbance may persist in the period following an episode of gastrointestinal inflammation, resulting in the development of IBS or functional dyspepsia, which are suggested to be part of a single syndrome (Holtmann et al., 1997). Both IBS and functional dyspepsia are associated with disturbed gastric motor function and decreased gastric emptying (Caballero-Plasencia et al., 1999). It is well established that inflammatory bowel diseases are chronic immune-mediated intestinal disorders. Both subtypes, Crohn's disease (CD) and ulcerative colitis (UC), are considered to arise as a consequence of an aberrant intestinal immune response in genetically predisposed individuals (Xavier and Podolsky, 2007). In inflamed segments of the bowel, persistent overproduction of pro-inflammatory cytokines, such as TNFα and IL-6 and impaired production of anti-inflammatory cytokines are characteristic features (Strober and Fuss, 2006). Furthermore, gut inflammation is associated with extensive structural and functional alterations of the enteric nervous system and dysregulation in neuroimmune interactions (Bischoff and Gebhardt, 2006). Different experimental animal models are used to address these clinical findings.

In this study, using an *in vitro* inflammation model (Michael et al., 2009), we demonstrated that the action of STW 5 resulted in a reduction of TNBS-induced disturbance of contractions possibly by attenuation of the TNBS-induced morphological damages. The mechanism of action of STW 5 is based at least on two distinctive mechanisms. STW 5 inhibited the pro-inflammatory TNFα pathway by activation of $A_{2A}R$ and STW 6, the fresh plant component of STW 5, stimulated the anti-inflammatory IL-10 pathway. It seems that cucurbitacins are involved in influencing this pathway. Both pathways effectively contribute to the overall effect of STW 5. It is known from numerous studies carried out with plant extracts that the whole extract has in most cases a better efficacy than a single substance isolated from the extract (Wegener and Wagner, 2006). Our findings are in accordance with other pharmacological studies showing different effects of a single

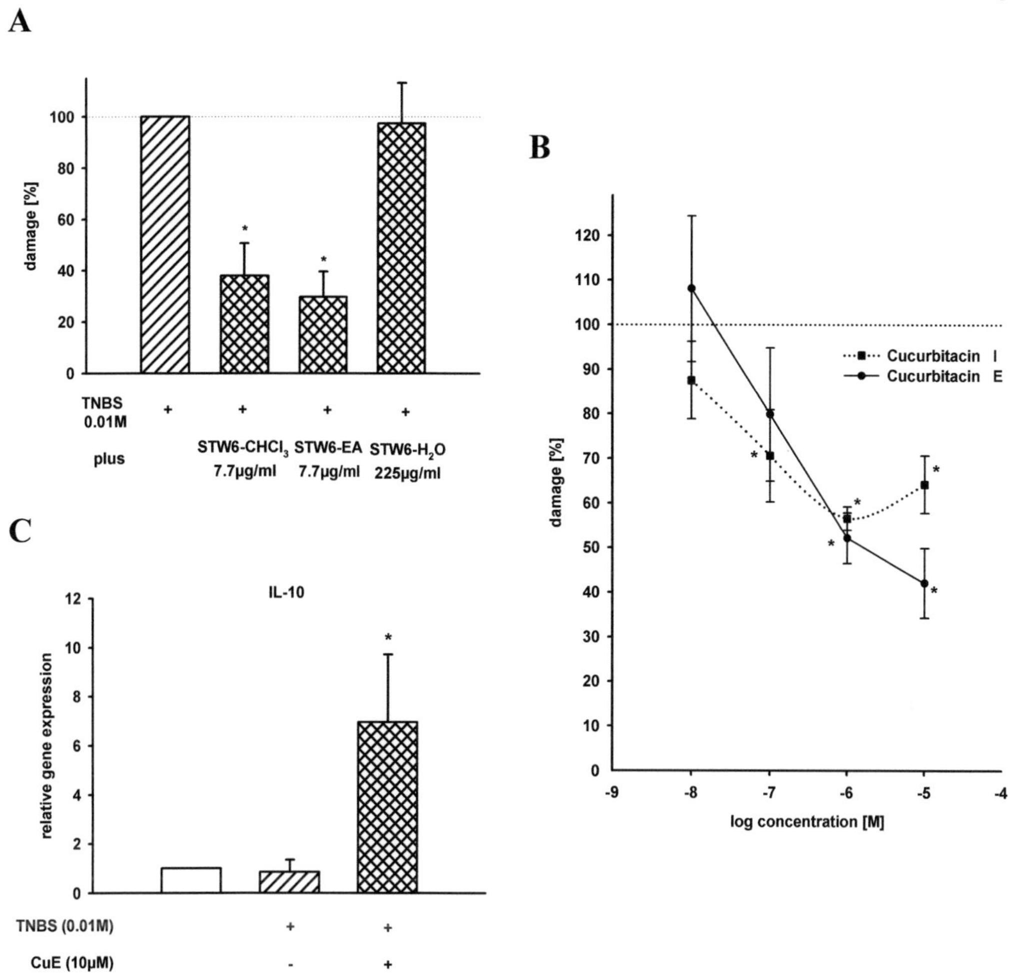

Fig. 6. Effects of the fractions of STW 6 and the cucurbitacins E and I on the TNBS-induced damage and the influence of cucurbitacin E on IL-10 gene expression. (A) The chloroform and ethyl acetate fractions containing the cucurbitacins E and I but not the water faction without cucurbitacins antagonized the damage of the ACh-contraction. (B) cucurbitacin E and I coincubated wit TNBS reduced concentration dependently the TNBS-induced damage of the ACh contraction. (C) Cucurbitacine E coincubated with TNBS enhanced the IL-10 gene expression. Means±SEM from 9 (A), 9 (B) and 3 (C) experiments. *$p<0.05$ significant vs. control.

constituent of STW 5 on mechanisms which are discussed as underlying the manifestation of IBS (Heinle et al., 2006, Ammon et al., 2006). At present it is not understood in detail how this multi-target principle of STW 5 arises (Wagner, 2006; Wagner and Ulrich-Merzenich, 2009). TNFα is a pro-apoptotic cytokine, which is produced by a wide variety of cell types in response to various inflammatory stimuli. It promotes the pathogenesis of several health disorders, in particular those related to ulcerative colitis and Crohn's disease. In both diseases there is an increased synthesis of pro-inflammatory cytokines, including TNFα and an influx of nonspecific inflammatory cells into the mucosa. The cytokines contribute to tissue damage either directly or indirectly (Heuschkel, 2000; Pallone and Monteleone, 2001). The main sources of TNFα *in vivo* are stimulated monocytes, fibroblasts, and endothelial cells. The signals triggering the TNFα secretion are not completely understood. LPS, the endotoxin of Gram-negative bacteria, stimulates *in vitro* these cells including cells of the monocytic lineage (Rietschel et al., 1996). Human monocytes are characterised by their high level production of TNFα and by their propensity to preferentially develop into potent dendritic cells. Therefore, the effect of STW 5 was not only determined on the gene expression in TNBS-pretreated tissue but also on the TNFα release from untreated and LPS-stimulated human monocytes. Our data clearly show that TNBS increased the TNFα gene expression in rat intestinal tissue, which was reduced by STW 5. Additionally, STW 5 inhibited the increased TNFα release in LPS-stimulated monocytes (Michael et al., 2009). These results point out that those inflammatory processes contribute to the damaged morphology and to the reduced contractility and provide evidence that the protective effect of STW 5 in TNBS-pretreated preparations is largely related to inflammatory processes. Interestingly, STW 6, the fresh plant component of STW 5, neither stimulated the gene expression nor the release of TNFα (Michael et al., 2011). On the other hand, STW 6 enhanced drastically the gene expression of the anti-inflammatory cytokine IL-10 whereas STW 5 did it moderately. These results suggest that at least two different processes contribute to the protective effects of STW 5 in the gastrointestinal inflammation, and therefore, we focused to the mechanisms underlying the regulation of TNFα and IL-10.

The purine nucleoside adenosine has been recognized for its regulatory functions in situations of cellular stress like ischemia, hypoxia and inflammation. The importance of agonists or antagonists of AR as modulators in the immune system is of great interest of the field of gastrointestinal inflammation (Estrela and Abraham, 2011). RT-PCR and immunohistochemical analysis demonstrated a wide distribution of AR in the neuromuscular compartment and mucosal/submucosal layers of both small and large intestine (Christofi et al., 2001; Puffinbarger et al., 1995). The protective effect of STW 5 against inflammation in ileum/jejunum preparations is mainly mediated by activation of $A_{2A}R$. Activation of $A_{2A}R$ by a selective agonist protects against TNBS-induced damage of the ACh-induced contractions and the results of binding studies clearly show an affinity of STW 5 to $A_{2A}R$. In accordance with the present experiments the $A_{2A}R$ antagonist CSC was shown recently to be effective in blocking the STW 5-induced enhanced ACh contraction in inflamed rat small intestinal preparation (Michael et al., 2011). Although, STW 5 enhanced the gene expression of by A_1R. The contribution of this receptor subtype could be excluded. STW 5 did not bind significantly to A_1R and the activation of A_1R by the selective agonist CPA enhanced the damage induced by TNBS.

We found that both STW 5 and STW 6 protected from TNBS-induced damage but STW 6 did not interact with $A_{2A}R$ and therefore it did not inhibit the TNFα pathway. Others than this pathway must be involved. Based on recently published results we focused on the anti-inflammatory cytokine IL-10. IL-10 was first identified as a cytokine, secreted by $CD4^+$Th2-cells, which inhibit cytokine production in antigen-presenting cells (Fiorentino et al., 1989). Its main function within the gastrointestinal tract is limitation and ultimately termination of immune responses. It acts as a key mediator for maintaining gut homeostasis (Paul et al., 2011). IL-10 has long been known for its substantial role in regulating gut immunity, but its contribution to inflammatory gut diseases was somewhat elusive. A recent study identified mutations in either IL-10 receptor subunits that are associated with early-onset enterocolitis, a severe phenotype of IBD. Other than genetic variants of IL-10 receptors, IL-10 and STAT3 genes are also associated with IBD, emphasizing the involvement of the IL-10 signalling cascade in the pathogenesis of CD and UC. Interestingly, cucurbitacin E and I are inhibitors of STAT3. Cucurbitacin E inhibits tumor angiogenesis through VEGFR2-mediated Jak2-STAT3 signaling pathway (Dong et al., 2010). Cucurbitacin I potently induces apoptosis in leukemia cell lines and in primary chronic lymphocytic leukemia cells and was associated with a reduction in serine 727 phosphorylation of STAT3 (Ishdorj et al., 2010). In our experiment the fractions of STW 6 containing cucurbitacin E and I prevented significantly the TNBS-mediated disturbance of the ACh-induced contraction. The involvement of the cucurbitacins was confirmed by coincubation of cucurbitacins with TNBS. Under these conditions the cucurbitacins reduced the TNBS-induced disturbance of the ACh-induced contractions in a concentration-dependent manner. Additionally, they increased significantly IL-10 mRNA. Therefore, it appears, that the induction of the anti-inflammatory cytokine IL-10 by cucurbitacins is a second mechanism underlying the protective action of STW 5 in our *in vitro* inflammation model.

In conclusion, STW 5 exhibits significant anti-inflammatory properties which contribute to the reduction of TNBS-induced morphological and contractile changes. Its mode of action seems to be twofold: inhibition of the TNFα pathway by activation of $A_{2A}R$ and activation of the IL-10 pathway. These anti-inflammatory mechanisms appear to be involved in the multi-target action of STW 5 as a new therapeutic approach in IBS.

5. References

Amann R, Peskar BA. Anti-inflammatory effects of aspirin and sodium salicylate. Eur J Pharmacol 2002;447:1-9

Ammon HPT, Kelber O, Okpanyi SN. Spasmolytic and tonic effect of Iberogast (STW 5) in intestinal smooth muscle. Phytomedicine 2006;13 Suppl 5:67-74

Antonioli L, Fornai M, Colucci R, et al. Regulation of enteric functions by adenosine: pathophysiological and pharmacological implications. Pharmacol Ther 2008;120:233-253

Ardizzone S, Bianchi Porro G. Biologic therapy for inflammatory bowel disease. Drugs 2005;65:2253-2286

Bamias G, Sugawara K, Pagnini C, Cominelli F. The Th1 immune pathway as a therapeutic target in Crohn's disease. Curr Opin Investig Drugs 2003;4:1279-1286

Bischoff SC, Gebhardt T. Role of mast cells and eosinophils in neuroimmune interactions regulating mucosal inflammation in inflammatory bowel disease. Adv Exp Med Biol 2006;579:177-208

Caballero-Plasencia AM, Valenzuela-Barranco M, Herrerias-Gutierrez JM, Esteban-Carretero JM. Altered gastric emptying in patients with irritable bowel syndrome. Eur J Nucl Med 1999;26:404-409

Cavalcante IC, Castro MV, Barreto AR, et al. Effect of novel A2A adenosine receptor agonist ATL 313 on Clostridium difficile toxin A-induced murine ileal enteritis. Infect Immun 2006;74:2606-2612

Chen Y, Epperson S, Makhsudova L, et al. Functional effects of enhancing or silencing adenosine A2b receptors in cardiac fibroblasts. Am J Physiol Heart Circ Physiol 2004;287:H2478-2486

Christofi FL, Zhang H, Yu JG, et al. Differential gene expression of adenosine A1, A2a, A2b, and A3 receptors in the human enteric nervous system. J Comp Neurol 2001;439:46-64

Collins SM. The immunomodulation of enteric neuromuscular function: implications for motility and inflammatory disorders. Gastroenterology 1996;111:1683-1699

Cronstein BN, Montesinos MC, Weissmann G. Salicylates and sulfasalazine, but not glucocorticoids, inhibit leukocyte accumulation by an adenosine-dependent mechanism that is independent of inhibition of prostaglandin synthesis and p105 of NFkappaB. Proc Natl Acad Sci U S A 1999;96:6377-6381

Dong Y, Lu B, Zhang X, et al. Cucurbitacin E, a tetracyclic triterpenes compound from Chinese medicine, inhibits tumor angiogenesis through VEGFR2-mediated Jak2-STAT3 signaling pathway. Carcinogenesis;31:2097-2104

Estrela AB, Abraham WR. Adenosine in the inflamed gut: a janus faced compound. Curr Med Chem;18:2791-2815

Fiorentino DF, Bond MW, Mosmann TR. Two types of mouse T helper cell. IV. Th2 clones secrete a factor that inhibits cytokine production by Th1 clones. J Exp Med 1989;170:2081-2095

Guzman J, Yu JG, Suntres Z, et al. ADOA3R as a therapeutic target in experimental colitis: proof by validated high-density oligonucleotide microarray analysis. Inflamm Bowel Dis 2006;12:766-789

Hasko G, Cronstein BN. Adenosine: an endogenous regulator of innate immunity. Trends Immunol 2004;25:33-39

Heinle H, Hagelauer D, Pascht U, Kelber O, Weiser D. Intestinal spasmolytic effects of STW 5 (Iberogast) and its components. Phytomedicine 2006;13 Suppl 5:75-79

Heuschkel RB. New immunologic treatments for inflammatory bowel disease. Curr Opin Gastroenterol 2000;16:565-570

Hohenester B, Ruhl A, Kelber O, Schemann M. The herbal preparation STW5 (Iberogast) has potent and region-specific effects on gastric motility. Neurogastroenterol Motil 2004;16:765-773

Holtmann G, Goebell H, Talley NJ. Functional dyspepsia and irritable bowel syndrome: is there a common pathophysiological basis? Am J Gastroenterol 1997;92:954-959

Ishdorj G, Johnston JB, Gibson SB. Inhibition of constitutive activation of STAT3 by curcurbitacin-I (JSI-124) sensitized human B-leukemia cells to apoptosis. Mol Cancer Ther;9:3302-3314

Jacobson KA, Gao ZG. Adenosine receptors as therapeutic targets. Nat Rev Drug Discov 2006;5:247-264

Kirfel A, Schwalbenlander F, Müller CE. Crystal structure of 1-propyl-8-(4-sulfophenyl)-7H-imidazol[4,5-d]pyrimidin-2,6(1H,3H)-dione dihydrate, $C_{14}H_{14}N_4O_5S$ x $2H_2O$. Z.Kristallographie-New Cryst Struct 1997; 3:447-448.

Klotz KN, Lohse MJ, Schwabe U, et al. 2-Chloro-N^6-[^{3}H]cyclopentyladenosine ([^{3}H]CCPA)--a high affinity agonist radioligand for A1 adenosine receptors. Naunyn Schmiedebergs Arch Pharmacol 1989;340:679-683

Kroll U, Cordes C. Pharmaceutical prerequisites for a multi-target therapy. Phytomedicine 2006;13 Suppl 5:12-19

Krueger D, Gruber L, Buhner S, et al. The multi-herbal drug STW 5 (Iberogast) has prosecretory action in the human intestine. Neurogastroenterol Motil 2009;21:1203-e1110

Linden J. New insights into the regulation of inflammation by adenosine. J Clin Invest 2006;116:1835-1837

Madisch A, Holtmann G, Plein K, Hotz J. Treatment of irritable bowel syndrome with herbal preparations: results of a double-blind, randomized, placebo-controlled, multi-centre trial. Aliment Pharmacol Ther 2004;19:271-279

Michael S, Kelber O, Hauschildt S, Spanel-Borowski K, Nieber K. Inhibition of inflammation-induced alterations in rat small intestine by the herbal preparations STW 5 and STW 6. Phytomedicine 2009;16:161-171

Michael S, Warstat C, Michel F, et al. Adenosine A(2A) agonist and A(2B) antagonist mediate an inhibition of inflammation-induced contractile disturbance of a rat gastrointestinal preparation. Purinergic Signal 2010;6:117-124

Michael S, Voss U, Weiser D, Kelber O, Nieber K: The plant extracts STW 5 and STW 6 interact differently with adenosine receptors in inflamed rat gastric preparations. Gastroenterology Research and Practice 2011 (submitted)

Montesinos M and Cronstein BN, Role of P1 receptors in inflammation : In Handbook of Experimental Pharmacology, Purinergic and Pyrimidinergic Signalling II Cardiovascular, Respiratory, Immue, Metabolic and Gastrointestial Tract Function Volume 151/II. Edited by: MP Abbrachio and M.Billiams. Berlin. Springer-Verlag, 2001: 303-321.

Montesinos MC, Takedachi M, Thompson LF, et al. The antiinflammatory mechanism of methotrexate depends on extracellular conversion of adenine nucleotides to adenosine by ecto-5'-nucleotidase: findings in a study of ecto-5'-nucleotidase gene-deficient mice. Arthritis Rheum 2007;56:1440-1445

Müller CE. Adenosine receptor ligands-recent developments part I. Agonists. Curr Med Chem 2000;7:1269-1288

Müller CE, Shi D, Manning M, Jr., Daly JW. Synthesis of paraxanthine analogs (1,7-disubstituted xanthines) and other xanthines unsubstituted at the 3-position: structure-activity relationships at adenosine receptors. J Med Chem 1993;36:3341-3349

Müller CE, Thorand M, Qurishi R, et al. Imidazo[2,1-i]purin-5-ones and related tricyclic water-soluble purine derivatives: potent A(2A)- and A(3)-adenosine receptor antagonists. J Med Chem 2002;45:3440-3450

Odashima M, Bamias G, Rivera-Nieves J, et al. Activation of A2A adenosine receptor attenuates intestinal inflammation in animal models of inflammatory bowel disease. Gastroenterology 2005;129:26-33

Ortiz-Lucas M, Saz-Peiro P, Sebastian-Domingo JJ. Irritable bowel syndrome immune hypothesis. Part one: the role of lymphocytes and mast cells. Rev Esp Enferm Dig;102:637-647

Pallone F, Monteleone G. Mechanisms of tissue damage in inflammatory bowel disease. Curr Opin Gastroenterol 2001;17:307-312

Paul G, Khare V, Gasche C. Inflamed gut mucosa: downstream of interleukin-10. Eur J Clin Invest

Perez ME, Youssef NN. Dyspepsia in childhood and adolescence: insights and treatment considerations. Curr Gastroenterol Rep 2007;9:447-455

Pfaffl MW, Horgan GW, Dempfle L. Relative expression software tool (REST) for group-wise comparison and statistical analysis of relative expression results in real-time PCR. Nucleic Acids Res 2002;30:e36

Pizarro TT, De La Rue SA, Cominelli F. Role of interleukin 6 in a murine model of Crohn's ileitis: are cytokine/anticytokine strategies the future for IBD therapies? Gut 2006;55:1226-1227

Puffinbarger NK, Hansen KR, Resta R, et al. Production and characterization of multiple antigenic peptide antibodies to the adenosine A2b receptor. Mol Pharmacol 1995;47:1126-1132

Raedsch R, Hanisch J, Bock P, et al. [Assessment of the efficacy and safety of the phytopharmacon STW 5 versus metoclopramide in functional dyspepsia--a retrolective cohort study]. Z Gastroenterol 2007;45:1041-1048

Rietschel ET, Brade H, Holst O, et al. Bacterial endotoxin: Chemical constitution, biological recognition, host response, and immunological detoxification. Curr Top Microbiol Immunol 1996;216:39-81

Romeis B. Mikroskopische Technik. München: Urban&Schwarzenberg Verlag; 1989

Sandborn WJ, Targan SR. Biologic therapy of inflammatory bowel disease. Gastroenterology 2002;122:1592-1608

Schmulson, MJ. How safe and effective is the herbal drug STW 5 for patients with functional dyspepsia? Nature clinical practice gastroenterology & hepatology 2008; 5:136-137

Sitkovsky MV, Lukashev D, Apasov S, et al. Physiological control of immune response and inflammatory tissue damage by hypoxia-inducible factors and adenosine A2A receptors. Annu Rev Immunol 2004;22:657-682

Stein RB, Hanauer SB. Medical therapy for inflammatory bowel disease. Gastroenterol Clin North Am 1999;28:297-321

Strober W, Fuss I, Mannon P. The fundamental basis of inflammatory bowel disease. J Clin Invest 2007;117:514-521

Thompson WG. Symptomatic presentations of the irritable bowel syndrome. Gastroenterol Clin North Am 1991;20:235-247

Wagner H: Multitarget therapy - the future of treatment for more than just functional dyspepsia. Phytomedicine 2006;13:122-129.

Wagner H, Ulrich-Merzenich G: Synergy research: approaching a new generation of phytopharmaceuticals. Phytomedicine 2009;16:97-110.

Wagner HB, S. Plant drug analysis. A Thin Layer Chromatography Atlas english ed: Springer-Verlag GmbH; 1996:384

Wegener T, Wagner H. The active components and the pharmacological multi-target principle of STW 5 (Iberogast). Phytomedicine 2006;13 Suppl 5:20-35

Xavier RJ, Podolsky DK. Unravelling the pathogenesis of inflammatory bowel disease. Nature 2007;448:427-434

Yan L, Müller CE. Preparation, properties, reactions, and adenosine receptor affinities of sulfophenylxanthine nitrophenyl esters: toward the development of sulfonic acid prodrugs with peroral bioavailability. J Med Chem 2004;47:1031-1043

4

Role of Dipeptidyl Peptidase IV/CD26 in Inflammatory Bowel Disease

Dijana Detel[1], Lara Batičić Pučar[1], Ester Pernjak Pugel[2],
Natalia Kučić[3], Sunčica Buljević[1], Brankica Mijandrušić Sinčić[4],
Mladen Peršić[5] and Jadranka Varljen[1*]
School of Medicine, University of Rijeka
Croatia

1. Introduction

Inflammatory bowel disease (IBD) comprises two main chronic pathologies of the gastrointestinal tract: ulcerative colitis (UC) and Crohn's disease (CD), both characterized by alternating phases of active inflammation and clinical remission with different complications and extraintestinal manifestations (Colletti, 2004; Hanauer & Hommes, 2010). The ethiopathogenesis of IBD has still not been elucidated, but it has been suggested that inflammatory processes emerge in genetically susceptible individuals as a result of an irregular, over-expressed immunological reaction to some undefined food antigens or some other agents of microbial origin (Baumgart et al., 2011).
Given the complexity of etiological factors in human IBD, a lot of current knowledge regarding IBD pathogenesis has arisen from the study of various animal models. Although no ideal model of IBD has been accomplished so far, they resemble different important clinical, histopathological and immunological aspects of human IBD (Mizoguchi & Mizoguchi, 2010). Chemically induced murine models by oral administration of dextran sulfate sodium (DSS) and intrarectal application of 2,4,6-trinitrobenzene sulfonic acid (TNBS) are the most commonly used ones, due to their onset and duration of colonic inflammation which is immediate, reproducible and shares a lot of similarities with human IBD. TNBS-induced colitis is one of the most accepted and used Crohn-like disease while the DSS-model is clinically and histologically similar to human ulcerative colitis (Wirtz & Neurath, 2007). These models, together with other animal models of IBD, have given insight in different processes at the molecular level and have revealed the importance of different molecules involved in IBD etiology, representing therefore essential tools in investigating different mechanisms underlying acute or chronic inflammation in the IBD (Uhlig & Powrie, 2009).

* Corresponding Author
[1]*Department of Chemistry and Biochemistry,*
[2]*Department of Histology and Embryology,*
[3]*Department of Physiology and Immunology,*
[4]*Department of Internal Medicine,*
[5]*Department of Pediatrics*

Growing body of knowledge proposes proteases as key factors in the occurrence of inflammatory processes due to their ability to metabolize different biologically active molecules implicated in maintaining the integrity of mucosal barrier (Ravi et al., 2007). Dipeptidyl peptidase IV, known also as CD26 molecule (DPP IV/CD26) is one of them (Gorrell et al., 2001). DPP IV/CD26 is also T-cell differentiation antigen, expressed on various cell types, having numerous functions in a variety of biological processes, as well as immunological mechanisms (Fleischer, 1994). It is also present in a soluble form circulating in body fluids in living organisms with specific peptidase function having unique features in substrate processing: it cleaves dipeptides from the N terminus of polypeptides having proline or alanin at the penultimate position. Since Xaa-Pro peptides are not easily metabolized by other proteases, the action of DPP IV/CD26 is an essential step in the degradation of many polypeptides (Gorrell et al., 2001). Numerous biologically important cytokines, chemokines and neuropeptides with potential and/or confirmed role in IBD ethiopathogenesis are effective DPP IV/CD26 substrates (Mentlein, 2004).
Previous studies proposed a role of DPP IV/CD26 in the pathogenesis of IBD, given its involvement in immune regulations via its expression on immune cells and capability to cleave biologically active molecules (Hildebrandt et al., 2001; Varljen et al., 2005). Additionally, DPP IV/CD26 inhibitors have been pointed out as therapeutic agents in ameliorating inflammatory processes in immunologically mediated diseases such as IBD (Yazbeck et al., 2009; Yazbeck et al., 2008).
The aim of this study was to review our previously published results regarding correlation between disease severity and serum DPP IV/CD26 activity in young and adult patients affected with IBD. Furthermore, our aim was to investigate and review does it and in which manner DPP IV/CD26 affect the immune homeostasis during development, progression and resolution of inflammatory events in two animal models of IBD.

2. Dipeptidyl peptidase IV/CD26 molecule

The exoprotease dipeptidyl peptidase IV (DPP IV, EC 3.4.14.5), also known as surface antigen CD26, is a transmembrane glycoprotein with molecular mass of 220-240 kDa, expressed constitutively on a variety of cell types (Lambeir et al., 2003). It is also present in a soluble form in serum, saliva, urine and other biological fluids. So far, the role of this molecule has been investigated in different fields of biochemistry, immunology, endocrinology, oncology, pharmacology, physiology and pathophysiology.

Structural and molecular characteristics

According to the current biochemical and structural data, DPP IV/CD26 is a type II transmembrane, homodimeric glycoprotein. Each monomer consists of a large extracellular part (739 amino acids), a hydrophobic transmembrane segment of 23 amino acids and a short cytoplasmic N-terminal tail. The primary sequence of DPP IV/CD26 is composed of 766 amino acids and it was found to be conserved in different species (85% similarities between rat and human and 92% similarities between rat and mouse), mostly in the C-terminal protease segment (Lambeir et al., 2003). DPP IV/CD26 is a member of the POP (prolyl oligopeptidase) gene family with an α/β hydrolase domain and a N-terminal β-propeller domain that enclose the large cavity (30-40 Å) which contains a small pocket with the active site. The catalytic site, as a part of extracellular domain of the molecule, contains Ser-630, His-740 and Asp-708, which is not common for classical serine-type peptidases, but is characteristic for the previously mentioned α/β hydrolase fold (Gorrell et al., 2006).

Based on structural and biochemical features, DPP IV/CD26 is a member of a family of DPP IV activity and/or structure homologue (DASH) proteins, which also includes quiescent cell proline dipeptidase (QPP), DPP8, DPP9, fibroblast activation protein (FAP), attractin and DPP IV-β (Sedo & Malik, 2001). Since it is well known that most DASH proteins have protease activity, having the possibility to modify the activity of biologically active peptides, it could be suggested that they are important regulatory molecules (Gorrell, 2005). However, further research is necessary in order to clarify their biological role.

Distribution and expression

DPP IV/CD26 is widely distributed in mammalian tissues, mainly on epithelial and endothelial cell surfaces, as well as on fibroblasts and lymphocytes (Boonacker & Van Noorden, 2003). The expression of DPP IV/CD26 on hematopoietic cells is well regulated according to the activation status. In humans, it is expressed on a fraction of resting lymphocytes at low density, but is strongly up-regulated following T-cell activation (Fleischer, 1987). In resting peripheral blood mononuclear cells, a small subpopulation of T cells expresses CD26 at high density on the surface (CD26-bright cells), which belongs to the CD45RO+ population of T cells (memory cells) (De Meester et al., 1999; Ishii et al., 2001). Moreover, CD26 expression on T cells may correlate with T-helper subsets. High expression is found on Th1 and Th0 cells, whereas Th2 cells display lower CD26 expression (Willheim et al., 1997).

Soluble DPP IV/CD26

Soluble DPP IV/CD26 activity was firstly discovered in the serum in 1968 by Nagatsu et al. (Nagatsu et al., 1968). Later, DPP IV/CD26 activity has been shown in other body fluids including plasma, serum, cerebrospinal and synovial fluids, semen and urine. Although soluble DPP IV/CD26 lacks the transmembrane domain and intracellular tail, due to glycosylations processes, its molecular weight is similar to the transmembrane form. The origin of the soluble DPP IV/CD26 is still not elucidated, but it was suggested that it could be released from the surface of all CD26 expressing cells in contact with blood by proteolytic cleavage (Gorrell et al., 2001). The physiological role of soluble DPP IV/CD26 in biological fluids with respect to the transmembrane DPP IV/CD26 remains poorly understood, but according to previous findings it has been proposed that, as an enzyme, it is involved in the regulation of many processes in human body (Aytac & Dang, 2004; Mentlein, 1999).

Functions in immune regulations

Immune regulation is a complex and important process in which DPP IV/CD26 as a costimulatory molecule in T-cell activation and a regulator of the functional effect of selected biological factors through its enzyme activity, certainly has an important function (Boonacker & Van Noorden, 2003). Furthermore, biochemical and immune studies provide evidence that CD26 interacts with many biologically important molecules including CD45, adenosine deaminase protein, chemokine receptor CXCR4 on the surface of human peripheral blood lymphocytes (Herrera et al., 2001) and the mannose-6-phosphate/insulin-like growth factor II receptor (Ikushima et al., 2000). The costimulatory properties of DPP IV/CD26 have been studied extensively, although different experimental settings sometimes provide conflicting results. It is generally accepted that several distinct anti-CD26 mAbs have costimulatory activities in anti-CD3-driven activation of pure T-cell subsets (either $CD4^+$ or $CD8^+$ T cells), and that the extent and kinetics of the response differs between mAbs, recognizing different epitopes. High CD26 surface expression is correlated with the production of Th1-type cytokines such as IFN-γ (Reinhold et al., 1997b).

Furthermore, $CD26^+$ $CD4^+$ T cells support differentiation of B cells into antibody-producing plasma cells (Dang et al., 1990).
The question whether the DPP IV/CD26 enzyme activity is involved in T cell activation is still controversial (Lambeir et al., 2003; Schon et al., 1985). Upon CD26-mediated costimulation, IL-2 production is higher in cells expressing wild-type CD26, suggesting that the DPP IV enzymatic activity of CD26 might contribute to, but is not essential for signal transduction. On the other hand, studies with inhibitors of DPP IV/CD26 activity have demonstrated that DPP IV/CD26 plays a key role in T cell activation (Munoz et al., 1992). It was shown that antigen-specific T cell proliferation and IL-2 production *in vitro* could be inhibited by application of the chemical inhibitor Pro-boro-Pro (Flentke et al., 1991). In addition, Lys(Z(NO_2))-thiazolidide, Lys(Z(NO_2))-piperidide, and Lys(Z(NO_2))-pyrrolidide, all synthetic competitive DPP IV/CD26 inhibitors, significantly inhibit DNA synthesis and the production of IL-2, IL-10, IL-12 and IFN-γ in pokeweed mitogen-stimulated purified T lymphocytes (Hildebrandt et al., 2000; Thompson et al., 2007). On the other hand, the presence of these inhibitors enhance the secretion of the immune-inhibitory cytokine TGF-β1, suggesting that TGF-β1 helps regulate DPP IV/CD26 effect on T cell function (Reinhold et al., 1997a).

DPP IV/CD26 substrates

Neuropeptides	**Glucose regulators**
Neuropeptide Y	Glucagon
Vasoactive intestinal peptide	Glucagon-like peptide 1 (GLP-1)
Peptide YY	Glucagon-like peptide 2 (GLP-2)
Endomorfin 1 and 2	Gastrin-releasing peptide
Beta-casomorphine	
Substance P	
Mediators of inflammation	**Other bioactive peptides**
Stromal cell derived factor- 1α and 1β (SDF-1α and 1β)	Bradykinin Growth hormone-releasing factor
RANTES (regulated on activation, normal T-cell expressed and secreted)	Prolactin Enterostatin Alpha-1-microglobulin
Interleukines: IL-1, IL-2, IL-6, IL-10	Monomeric fibrin (α chain)
Tumor necrosis factor α (TNF-α)	Melanostatin
Macrophage-derived chemokine	Tripsinogen
Interferon-inducible protein 10 (IP-10)	
Eotaxin	

Table 1. Selected DPP IV/CD26 biologically important substrates (Gorrel et al, 2006)

Firstly, DPP IV/CD26 was considered to cut off distinctively after a proline or an alanine on the second position from the N-terminal end of a polypeptide chain. Meanwhile, the list of DPP IV/CD26 substrates has been enlarged as it has been shown that a DPP IV/CD26

substrate could also have a serine, glycine, valine, threonine, leucine, or hydroxyproline at the penultimate position (Lambeir et al., 2001). However, DPP IV/CD26 is unable to hydrolyze substrates with proline, hydroxyproline or N-methyl glycine on the third position from the N-terminus (Puschel et al., 1982) and therefore, these peptides are DPP IV inhibitors.
A large number of various biologically important peptides have been shown to be substrates of DPP IV/CD26. Some of the most important DPP IV/CD26 substrates are presented in Table 1.

3. Inflammatory bowel disease and DPP IV/CD26

During the past 50 years, IBD affected millions of people worldwide and therefore has become one of the major gastroenterological problems, especially in the Westernized world. It is a disorder of multiple etiologies, with generally accepted definition that occurs in genetically susceptible individuals, under influence of environmental and microbiological factors, as an overexpressed immunological response to antigens of unknown origin, characterized by chronic uncontrolled inflammation of intestinal mucosa, resulting in its destruction and lost of its function (Colletti, 2004). IBD comprises two main chronic inflammatory diseases of humans, namely ulcerative colitis and Crohn's disease, both characterized by alternating phases of active inflammation and clinical remission with diverse complications and extraintestinal manifestations (Hanauer & Hommes, 2010).
Although the scientific knowledge increases exponentially, there are still many unanswered questions in several fundamental aspects of the IBD. The most stimulating field of IBD research is the interaction among the three major factors of the pathophysiology, including genetic predisposition, environmental bacteria and immune deregulation. The early inductive phases of these diseases are particularly difficult to study in humans because patients usually come to clinic only after their symptoms have been established (Hanauer, 2006).

3.1 Clinical relevance of serum DPP IV/CD26 activity in adult patients and children with IBD

Many investigations and reviews have discussed the role of DPP IV/CD26 activity in inflammation and the potential usefulness of this protein in therapeutics and diagnostics purpose (Hildebrandt et al., 2001; Varljen et al., 2005). However, its exact role still remains unclear. In clinical practice, the differential diagnosis of CD and UC is often difficult. Different biochemical, clinical, endoscopic, pathological and histological features should be combined in order to allocate the appropriate diagnosis. However, a precise diagnosis is not possible in about 10% of patients with chronic colitis, which results in the designation »indeterminate colitis« (Geboes et al., 2008).
Given the role of DPP IV/CD26 in the modulation of the immune response, we hypothesized that DPP IV/CD26 is altered in patients with CD and UC and that changes in DPP IV/CD26 serum activity could be related to the disease activity together with other inflammatory parameters. Therefore, the aim of this study was to evaluate the clinical relevance of changes in serum DPP IV activity in adult patients IBD (CD and UC). Furthermore, given the different immune background in patients with CD and UC as well as different expression of DPP IV/CD26 on Th1 and Th2 cells, we wanted to evaluate if DPP IV/CD26 serum activity could be used as differentiating marker in the diagnosis of these diseases.

3.2 Material and methods

Adult patients

The study was performed on 62 patients, 38 with CD (mean age ± SD: 42.7±14.4; 19 males, 19 females), and 24 with UC (mean age ± SD: 45.6±17.6; 13 males, 11 females). All patients were admitted to the Department of Gastroenterology, Clinical Hospital Centre Rijeka. Diagnoses of CD or UC were established on the basis of clinical history, laboratory, endoscopic and histological data. The control group included 65 healthy donors (mean age ± SD: 41.6±12.1; 32 males, 33 females). The CD activity was evaluated using the Crohn's Disease Activity Index (CDAI), while the UC activity was evaluated according to the Truelove and Witts' (TW) classification (Truelove & Witts, 1955). The localization of the disease was determined according to the Wienna classification for CD while UC was divided into proctosigmoiditis, left-side colitis and pancolitis. Blood samples were obtained after all patients and controls signed informed consents under the protocols approved by the Ethics Committee.

Children

The study involved also young patients, 31 children with IBD. Diagnoses of CD or UC were established on the basis of clinical history, laboratory, endoscopic and histological data. CD activity was evaluated by using the Paediatric Crohn´s Disease Activity Index (PCDAI) (Hyams et al., 1991). Blood samples were obtained after all children's parents gave their signed informed consent under the protocols approved by the Ethics Committee. The study group comprised 24 patients with CD (12 with (PCDAI)≥15 and 12 with (PCDAI)<15) and 7 with UC. Their mean ± SD age at diagnosis was 13.84±1.72 years. The control group included 46 healthy children (mean age ± SD: 13.80±2.83 years; 22 males and 24 females).

3.2.1 DPP IV/CD26 assay

Sera were separated from fasting blood samples and stored at –80°C until thawed for enzyme activities. Determination of serum DPP IV/CD26 activities was performed as described by Kreisel et al (Kreisel et al., 1982). DPP IV/CD26 activities were determined by measuring the release of 4-nitroaniline from an assay mixture containing 0.1 mol Tris-HCl (pH 8.0), 2 mmol Gly-Pro *p*-nitroanilide (Sigma Chemical, Steinheim, Germany) as the substrate and serum in a total volume of 0.20 mL. After 30 minutes of incubation at 37°C, the reaction was stopped by the addition of 800 µL of 1 mol sodium acetate buffer (pH 4.5). The absorbance at 405 nm was measured by use of a Varian Cary UV/VIS spectrophotometer (Cary, NC). All of the reactions were performed in duplicate. Enzyme activities in serum were expressed as µmol of hydrolyzed substrate in a volume of 1 dm^3 per minute under the assay conditions.

3.3 Results and discussion

Here reviewed results for adult patients were previously published in *Croatica chemica acta,* (Varljen et al., 2005), while results of investigations that included children were previously published in *Pediatric Gastroenterology* - Reports from the 2nd World Congress of Pediatric Gastroenterology, Hepatology and Nutrition (Varljen et al., 2004).

Adult patients

Results of serum DPP IV/CD26 activity in adult patients with CD and UC compared to the control group are presented on Fig. 1. It could be seen that both serum DPP IV/CD26 activities in CD as well as UC are statistically significantly ($P < 0.05$) reduced compared to healthy controls.

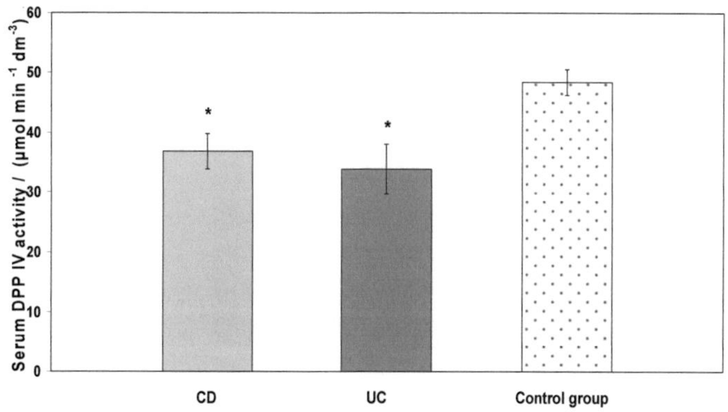

*, statistically significantly different compared to control group ($P < 0.001$)

Fig. 1. Serum DPP IV/CD26 activity in patients affected with Crohn's disease (CD) and ulcerative colitis (UC) compared to healthy controls.

When analyzing the correlation between serum DPP IV/CD26 activity in patients with CD and UC, it was noticed that patients affected with CD, having CDAI>250 had statistically significantly lower serum DPP IV/CD26 activity compared to patients having CDAI<150 (Fig. 2).

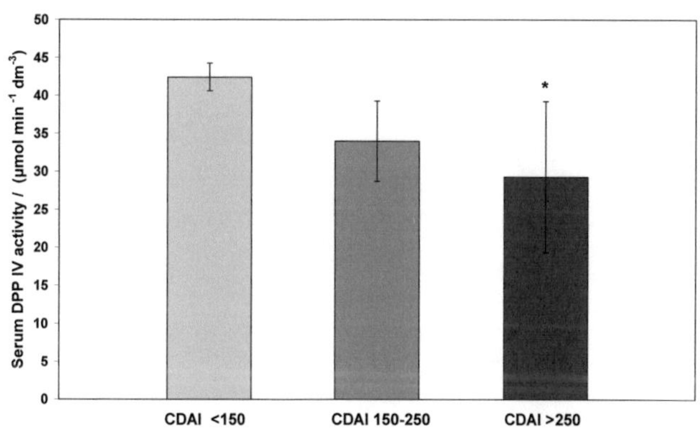

*, statistically significantly different compared to CDAI<150 ($P = 0.023$).
CDAI - Crohn's Disease Activity Index
CDAI ≤ 150 – remission
CDAI >150 – active disease

Fig. 2. Serum DPP IV/CD26 activity in three groups of patients with Crohn's disease.

Likewise, an inverse correlation between serum DPP IV/CD26 activity and disease severity was found in patients affected with UC (Fig. 3). It could be seen that patients with severe UC had statistically significantly ($P < 0.05$) lower DPP IV/CD26 activity compared to patients having mild UC.

Children

In young patients affected with IBD, DPP IV/CD26 activity in serum was also reduced compared to the levels in healthy controls, likewise in adult patients. The serum DPP

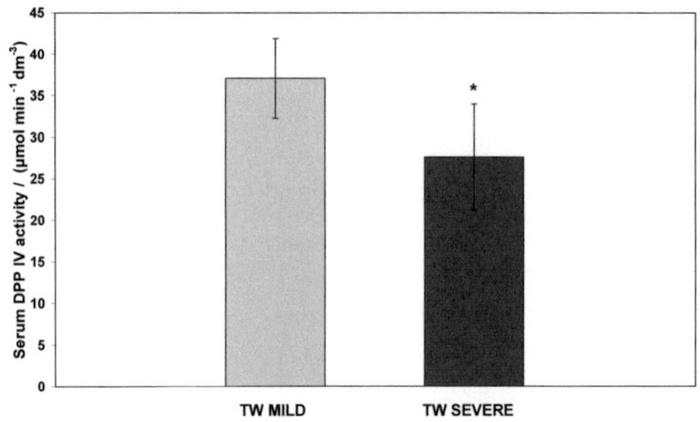

TW-mild and TW-severe - Truelove and Witts' classification (Truelove & Witts, 1955)
*, statistically significantly different compared to TW-mild (P=0.035)

Fig. 3. Serum DPP IV/CD26 activity in two groups of patients with ulcerative colitis.

IV/CD26 activity in children with CD was statistically significantly (P < 0.05) decreased compared to the levels in healthy controls. The DPP IV/CD26 activity in children with UC was also decreased but not statistically significantly when compared to controls (Fig. 4).

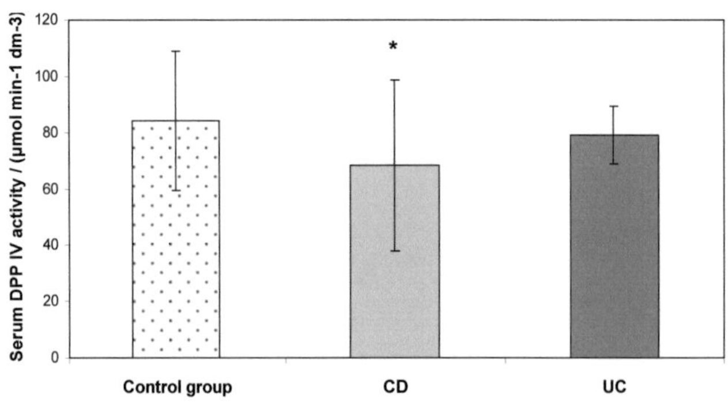

*, statistically significantly different compared to control group (P < 0.05)

Fig. 4. Serum DPP IV/CD26 activity in children affected with Crohn's disease (CD) and ulcerative colitis (UC)

The serum DPP IV/CD26 activity in children with active CD was statistically significantly decreased (P < 0.05) compared with the levels in healthy controls, while in patients with inactive CD it was also found to be decreased, but not statistically significantly (Fig. 5).
Based on obtained results, it could be concluded that soluble DPP IV/CD26 in serum seems to be involved in the pathophysiology of IBD and appears to be useful as an available non-invasive marker in the diagnosis of disease activity. Changes of DPP IV/CD26 expression and serum activity were found to occur in several clinical and experimental situations of altered immune function (Gorrell et al, 2006). Results of our study accord with previous investigation which confirmed lower serm DPP IV/CD26 activity in patients affected with IBD (Hildebrandt et al., 2001; Rose et al., 2003). Obtained data, together with previously published results, suggest that the persisted immune dysbalance could have a significant

impact on the pathogenesis of IBD. Our results can suggest a functional compartmentalization of DPP IV/CD26, which can be interpreted as an adaptive systemic immune response to a local inflammatory reaction. Meanwhile, the obtained results do not corroborate the hypothesis that the serum DPP IV/CD26 enzymatic activity differs between patients with CD and patients with UC, thus reflecting the concept of different cytokine patterns in one or the other subtype of IBD. Consequently, it seems that the serum DPP IV/CD26 activity could not be used as a specific differential diagnostic marker between CD and UC, and further investigations are necessary in order to establish a new parameter for differentiation of CD from UC.

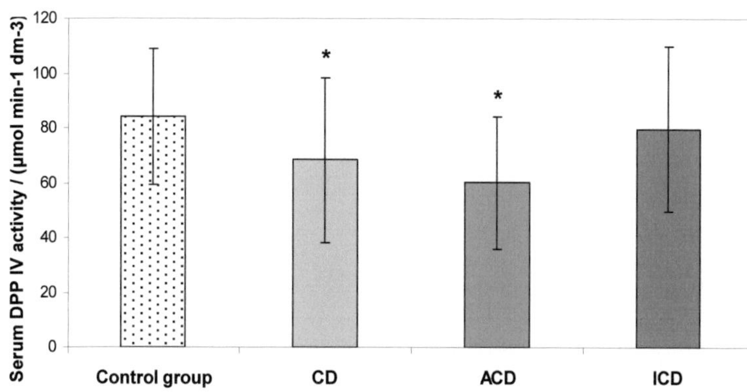

(ACD-Active Crohn's disease, ICD-Inactive Crohn's disease)
*, statistically significantly different compared to control group ($P<0.05$)

Fig. 5. Serum DPP IV/CD26 activity in children affected Crohn's disease (CD),

4. Animal models of IBD

Throughout the last decade, several experimental animal models of IBD have been developed in order to define different components of the pathophysiological processes that characterize these disorders (Mizoguchi & Mizoguchi, 2010; Strober et al., 1998; Wirtz & Neurath, 2007). Experimental animal models have a number of advantages which include allowing the study of specific pathophysiological events occurring before symptoms onset. Furthermore, investigators can perform genetic and immunologic manipulations of relevant mouse genes, possibly involved in disease pathogenesis (Bhan et al., 1999).
Although no ideal model of IBD has been accomplished so far, they resemble different important clinical, histopathological and immunological aspects of human IBD. The value of the animal models is the insight they allow into the complex, multifaceted processes and mechanisms that can result in acute or chronic intestinal inflammation. Animal models of IBD have given insight in different processes at the molecular level and have revealed the importance of different molecules involved in IBD etiology, representing therefore essential tools in investigating different mechanisms underlying acute or chronic inflammation in IBD. In recent years quite a number of new experimental models of intestinal inflammation have been described (Table 2).

Animal model	Disease type
Spontaneous	
C3H-HeJBir	Colitis, superficial, acute-resolving, Th1
SAMP1/Yit	Ileitis, chronic, transmural, granulomatous, Th1
SAMP1/YitFc	Perianal disease, early onset of disease
Genetically engineered	
IL-2 knockout	Spontaneous colitis, Th1
IL-10 knockout	Colitis, acute, chronic, transmural, Th1 (early)/Th2 (late)
T-cell receptor α mutant mice	Colitis, chronic, Th2
TNF-3' UTR knockout mice	Colitis
STAT-4 transgenic mice	Colitis, acute, chronic, transmural, Th1
IL-7 transgenic mice	Colitis, acute, chronic, Th1
HLA B27 transgenic	Spontaneous, entire colon, Th1
Chemically induced	
Trinitrobenzene sulfonic acid-induced colitis	Colitis, acute, chronic, transmural, Th1
Oxazolone colitis	Colitis, Th2
Dextran sulfate sodium colitis	Colitis, superficial, Th1 (acute), Th1/Th2 (chronic)
Peptidoglycan-polysaccharide colitis	Enterocolitis, transmural
Adoptive transfer	
CD4/CD45RB^{high} T-cell transfer colitis	Colitis, chronic transmural, Th1
Transfer of hsp60-specific CD8 T cells	Colitis, Th1

TNF, Tumor necrosis factor; UTR, untranslated region; STAT, signal transducer and activating transcription; hsp, heat shock protein

Table 2. Selected animal models of IBD (Mizoguchi & Mizoguchi, 2010)

4.1 DSS-induced colitis (ulcerative-like model of colitis)

Ulcerative colitis (UC) is a chronic inflammatory condition of the colon that may affect individuals of any age. It generally begins in the anus and extends at a variable length from the rectum in a continuous fashion. Patients usually present with a constellation of symptoms including diarrhea, lower abdominal cramping and tenesmus (Shah & Feller, 2009). The dextran sulfate sodium (DSS) model of induced colitis is an excellent preclinical animal model that exhibits numerous phenotypic features with human ulcerative colitis. It was originally described by Ohkusa et al. (Ohkusa, 1985) as a hamster model and was adapted to mice subsequently by Okayasu and its coworkers (Okayasu et al., 1990).

DSS is a polyanionic derivate of dextrane produced by esterification with chlorosulphonic acid. The exact mechanism through which DSS initiates colitis is unknown but according to previously published data, it is supposed that DSS alternates the gut permeability. It was shown that administration of DSS reduces the expression of tight junction proteins like zona occludens-1, leading to increased gut permeability. Another suggested mechanism involves direct cytotoxic action of DSS on the colonic mucosa, which leads to the alteration of integrin-α4 and M290 subunit levels on epithelial cells. Through these effects, DSS induces mucosal injury with consequent activation of immune response, leading to the development of acute or chronic colitis (Dieleman et al., 1998). Inflammation induced by DSS is most frequent and severe in the distal part of the colon (Okayasu et al., 1990) and its severity depends on the concentration and molecular weight of DSS (Kitajima et al., 2000). Concentrations described in literature range between 1% and 7%, while the most commonly used molecular weight ranges between 30 kDa and 50 kDa.

4.1.1 Induction of DSS-colitis in mice

This study was performed using pathogen-free, male, 8-10-week-old (weighting 20±2 g) wild type (C57BL/6) mice and mice with inactivated gene for DPP IV/CD26 molecule ($CD26^{-/-}$) generated on a C57BL/6 genetic background, as described previously (Marguet et al., 2000). $CD26^{-/-}$ mice were kindly provided by Dr. Didier Marguet, Centre d'Immunologie Marseille-Luminy, France. Animals were housed and bred under standard conditions at the Central Animal Facility of the School of Medicine, University of Rijeka.

Colitis was induced in both mice strains using 3% (w/v) sodium dextran sulfate sodium (DSS; MW 50 kDa; MP Biomedicals, USA) during seven days in drinking water *ad libitum* (Wirtz & Neurath, 2007). Control mice received regular drinking water throughout the experiment (days 1-15).

Handling with animals, experimental procedures and anesthesia were performed in accordance with the general principles contained in the Guide for the Care and Use of Laboratory Animals (National Academic Press). The Ethical Committee at the School of Medicine, University of Rijeka approved all of the experiments.

Experimental design

Animals included in the study were randomly divided into four groups as follows: C57BL/6 and $CD26^{-/-}$ mice treated with the 3% DSS solution for 7 days and control C57BL/6 and $CD26^{-/-}$ group treated with tap water. At day 7, in order to compare the colitis severity, treated and control animal of each genotype were anesthetized by intraperitoneal administration of ketamine (2.5 mg/mice) and sacrificed by cervical dislocation. The remaining animals were given normal drinking water until day 15 when they were sacrificed in order to compare the strain difference during colitis resolution. At each time point, 6-8 animals of each group were sacrificed. During the entire experiment, body mass was measured daily and clinical symptoms were assessed using the disease activity score. The colon segments from the ileocecal valve to the anus were excised *post mortem,* washed with ice-cold phosphate-buffered saline (PBS) and their length and weight were measured, as indirect markers of inflammation. After colon length and weight measurements, tissue samples were opened longitudinally, washed in PBS and proceeded for histology, morphometry and biochemical analysis. *Morphometrical measurements* included evaluation of crypt number, crypt depth and crypt width on hematoxilin - eosin stained tissue samples. Analyses were performed using software Issa (VAMS, Zagreb, Croatia), Pulmix camera (TMC 76S, Japan) and Olympus BX 40 microscope.

The *clinical score* was assessed as described previously (Howarth et al. 2000; Murthy et al. 1993). Briefly, weight loss of >5% was scored as 0 points, weight loss of 5 to 10% as 1 point, 10 to 15% as 2 points, 15 to 20% as 3 points, and more than 20% as 4 points. For stool consistency, 0 points were given for well formed pellets, 2 points for pasty and semiformed stools that did not stick to the anus, and 4 points for liquid stools that remained adhesive to the anus. Bleeding was scored 0 points for no presence of rectal bleeding and 4 points for gross bleeding from the rectum. These scores were added and divided by three, resulting in a total clinical score ranging from 0 (healthy) to 4 (maximal activity of colitis).

Mucosa fractions isolation from duodenum, jejunum, ileum and colon segments were prepared from mucosal scrapings according to Ahnen et al. (Ahnen et al., 1982).

4.1.2 Establishment and validation of the DSS-induced colitis at systemic and local level

Oral administration of DSS in rodents induces a colonic inflammation with many similarities to human IBD. Consistent with previous studies, as disease progressed, clinical symptoms, including loss of body mass, changes of stool consistency and appearance of rectal bleeding, were aggravated. Until day 3, no clinical symptoms of colitis were seen. From day 3 and later, both mice strain showed blood in their feces and diarrhea. From the results presented in Table 3, it could be concluded that body mass of healthy animals, control group, CD26-/- mice, in comparison to the control C57BL/6 mice is lower which is in agreement with previously published data (Marguet et al., 2000). Administration of the DSS solution caused a statistically significant decrease ($P < 0.05$) of body mass on day 3 in C57BL/6 mice, while in CD26-/- mice, extensive body mass loss began one day after, with a maximum fall on the ninth day. As the inflammation progressed, the disease activity index (DAI) in each group, increased gradually and reached its maximum on day 7 in both mice strains. Body weight increased gradually in both control groups. Variations in clinical symptoms and body mass during colitis development, established in C57BL/6 and CD26-/- mice, are shown in Table 3.

Mice strain	Day of experiment	Body mass (g)	DAI[a]	Diarrhea[b]	Gross bleeding[b]	Colon length (cm)[a]
C57BL/6	0	24.17 ± 1.97	0	0/6	0/6	8.5 ± 0.1
	7	19.19 ± 3.62	4.00 ± 0.20	6/6	6/6	7.3 ± 0.4
	15	23.35 ± 2.79	0	0/6	0/6	8.0 ± 0.2
CD26-/-	0	23.63 ± 1.73	0	0/6	0/6	8.5 ± 0.1
	7	19.35 ± 2.16	3.66 ± 0.25	6/6	5/6	7.7 ± 0.2
	15	21.57 ± 1.55	0.33 ± 0.05	0/6	0/6	8.0 ± 0.3

[a]Data are presented as mean ± SD
[b]Number of mice with diarrhea or gross bleeding/total number of mice in each group
DSS: dextran sulfat sodium; DAI: Disease activity index

Table 3. Changes of clinical variables during DSS-induced colitis development and resolution in C57BL/6 and CD26-/- mice.

In order to assess the degree of inflammation at the local level, length and weight of each colon sample was measured. Statistically significant shortening of the colon was observed on day 7 of the experiment in both CD26-/- and C57BL/6 mice. Together with colon shortening, statistically significant increase of colon weight was observed on day 7 and 15 in CD26-/- and C57BL/6 mice. It is known that during colitis development, DSS induces colon tissue obliteration, but recent studies in rats showed that changes through the small intestine are also present (Geier et al., 2009; Ohtsuka & Sanderson, 2003). Therefore, in order to provide further evidence, we isolated small intestinal and colonic mucosa and measured the *changes of mucosa weight* during colitis development. A significant decrease of colonic mucosa weight was observed in C57BL/6 mice, while in CD26-/- mice the statistically significant decrease of ileum and colon mucosa weight was observed (Fig. 6). Our results and results of previously published studies showed that DSS-induced damage could extend to the small intestine and therefore, further studies are necessary to validate physiological impact of this damage.

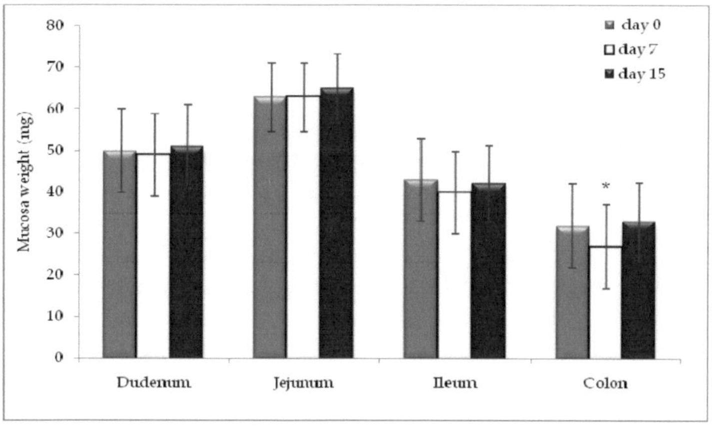

A

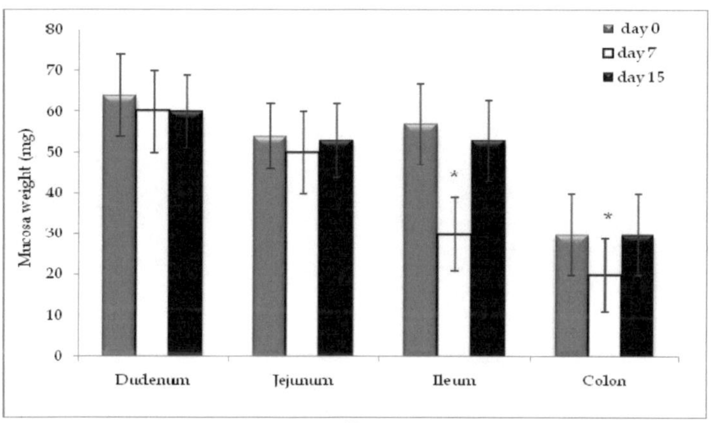

B

Data are presented as mean ± SD
*$P < 0.05$, statistically significantly different compared to day 0

Fig. 6. Influence of DSS-induce damage on small intestine and colon mucosa weight during colitis development and resolution in C57BL/6 (A) and CD26$^{-/-}$ (B) animals.

In compliance with our results, it could be concluded that administration of DSS in drinking water for seven days resulted in a prominent colon inflammation and gastrointestinal dysfunction, followed by regeneration of the colonic epithelium in C57BL/6 and CD26$^{-/-}$ mouse strains. Shortening of the colon and increase of colon weight, as macroscopic measures for the degree of inflammation, correlates with changes of mucosa weight and pathological changes (Okayasu et al., 1990). Given the fact that the symptoms of inflammation were the most prominent between the seventh and tenth day following DSS administration, this period was classified as acute phase, which is in accordance with previously reported findings. Furthermore, our findings suggest and confirm that the DSS model of colitis, because of similarities to human IBD, represents a good model to study the molecular and immune mechanisms activated during colitis development and resolution.

In accordance with previously published histological data regarding colonic inflammation present in DSS model of colitis, inflammatory changes are superficial, mainly affecting the mucosa, but may extend to the submucosa and the muscularis mucosa as well. The inflammation is characterized by superficial ulcers, mucosal oedema, crypt distortion and mucosal inflammatory cell infiltration with large numbers of neutrophils, macrophages and lymphocytes (Cooper et al., 1993). *Pathohistological* and *morphometrical analyses* of colon tissue sections confirmed the presence of inflammatory changes in both mice strains. During colitis development, a statistically significant decrease in number of crypts of Lieberkühn per milimetar of mucosa followed by its shortening was recorded in both mice strains along with the infiltration of inflammatory cells in lamina propria (Fig. 7). In the acute phase (day 7), crypt architectural distortion reached its maximum and during this phase, typical sign of disease, patches of totally destroyed epithelial sheet with deep ulcerations, can be seen. The resolution of inflammation and regeneration of crypts started during the second week and finished on the day 15 (Fig. 7D). In this period, mononuclear types of inflammatory cells were predominant.

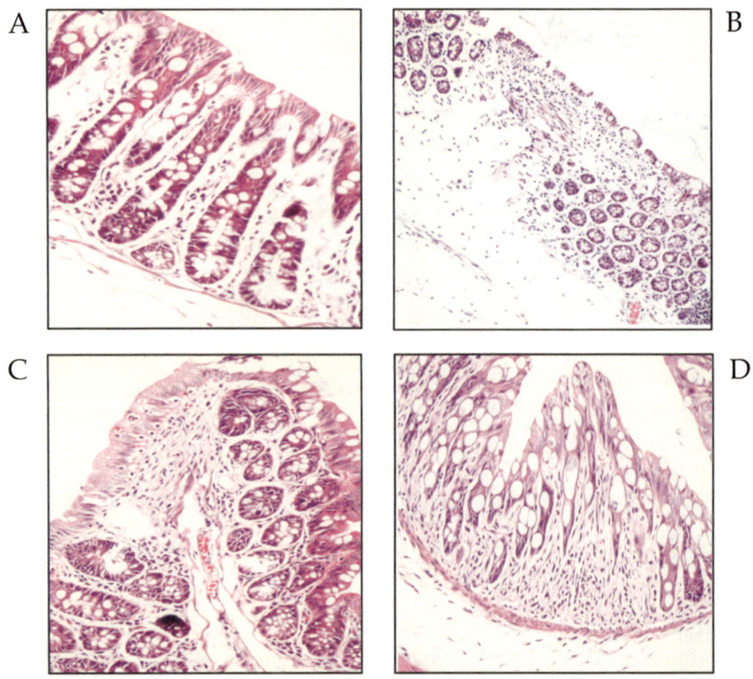

Fig. 7. Histological changes in colon tissues during dextran sulfate sodium-induced (DSS) colitis development and resolution in CD26$^{-/-}$ animals. Normal colon (A), acute phase of colitis (B) and process of tissue damage resolution (C, D). Colon sections (2 µm) were stained with hematoxylin and eosin and examined for histological properties. Magnification: 20x (A, C, D); 10x (B).

There is evidence that susceptibility to DSS varies with the animal species and mice strain. Guinea pig is the most susceptible, with inflammation usually fully established in less than 72 h (Iwanaga et al., 1994). In mice, some strains such as C3H/HeJ and C3H/HeJ Bir were found to be highly susceptible, while others such as NON/LtJ were quite resistant to DSS colitis (Mahler et al., 1998). Our results are in agreement with previously published study regarding the intensity of clinical symptoms between C57BL/6 and CD26$^{-/-}$ mice. Given the fact that there is no statistically significant difference in the intensity of clinical symptoms between mice strains it could be suggested that CD26 deficiency does not increase resistance to the development of DSS-induced experimental colitis (Geier et al., 2005).

4.1.3 DPP IV/CD26 and DPP IV/CD26-like activity in DSS-colitis

Functional studies have demonstrated that inhibition of DPP IV/CD26 enzyme activity may lead to changes in chemokine regulation and a subsequent immunological effect, while *in vitro* studies using activated T lymphocytes have shown that inhibition of DPP IV/CD26 activity can result in a decreased secretion of proinflammatory cytokines, including TNF-α and IFN-γ as well as an increase in the anti-inflammatory cytokine TGF-β. This evidence suggests that DPP IV/CD26 enzyme activity plays an essential role in the immune response and therefore, its enzymatic role is being extensively investigated. In our study, a statistically significant decrease in serum DPP IV/CD26 activity was observed in the acute phase in serum of C57BL/6 mice. The results regarding serum DPP IV/CD26 activity established in a DSS mouse model of colitis are consistent with our previous work in patients with IBD (Varljen et al., 2005). Furthermore, a decrease in DSS colitis disease activity was observed in wild type mice treated with inhibitors but on the other hand the inhibitors were not effective in CD26$^{-/-}$ animals (Yazbeck et al., 2010). Concurrently, during colitis development, an increased expression of DPP8 in wild type and CD26$^{-/-}$ animals and DPP2 mRNA expression in wild type animals was observed.

Considering that DPP IV/CD26 is a member of a large S9b family of structurally homologous serine proteases that possess a unique catalytic activity, and since two recent studies have demonstrated a broad tissue distribution of DPP IV-like enzyme activity in both wild type and CD26$^{-/-}$, a possible explanation of results obtained in our study could be that other DPP IV-like protease are involved in the activation of the inflammatory response in animal model of colitis (Ansorge et al., 2009; Yu et al., 2009). Furthermore, it was recently demonstrated by Yazbeck and its coworkers (Yazbeck et al., 2008) that inhibition of DPP-like activity ameliorates the severity of inflammation in experimental colitis in mice. However, further studies are required to characterize the role of DPP IV-like proteins in the initiation and activation of immune mechanisms leading to intestinal inflammation and development of IBD.

4.2 TNBS-induced colitis (Crohn-like model of colitis)

One of the most widely used and accepted Crohn-like colitis in scientific research is the TNBS-induced colitis. The TNBS-colitis resembles human Crohn's disease in different aspects, from the clinical manifestation, histological appearance and immunological features. TNBS-colitis is induced in experimental animals by rectal application of TNBS in an adequate, experimentally determined dilution of ethanol, usually 30 to 50%. Ethanol serves as a barrier-breaker which allows TNBS molecules, a contact-sensitizing agent, to enter in deeper layers of the colonic mucosa. The mechanism of TNBS-induced inflammation involves reaction of TNBS, which is a hapten, with tissue host proteins. TNBS is a covalently reactive compound that attachs to autologous proteins and stimulates a delayed-type hypersensitivity response (Camoglio et al., 2000). This generates a variety of new antigens in situ, as well as stimulates the production of proinflammatory molecules and free radicals which initiate a whole cascade of complex immunological interactions (Grisham et al., 1991). The colonic administration of a single dose of TNBS/ethanol solution induces in mice and rats a granulomatous, transmural inflammation with tissue destruction, mainly localized in the distal part of the colon (Scheiffele & Fuss, 2002).

4.2.1 Induction of TNBS-colitis in mice

Two mice strains were used in our study: wild type mice strain C57BL/6 and mice with inactivated gene for molecule CD26 (C57BL/6 Jbom-ob, CD26$^{-/-}$), generated on a C57BL/6 genetic background. CD26$^{-/-}$ mice were kindly provided by Dr. Didier Marguet, Centre d'Immunologie Marseille-Luminy, France. Generation of CD26$^{-/-}$ mice has been described previously (Marguet et al., 2000). Male, 8-10-week-old mice were used in the study. Animals were housed and bred under standard conditions at the Central Animal Facility of the School of Medicine, University of Rijeka. Laboratory animals were housed in plastic cages, fed with standard pellet food (MK, Complete Diet for Laboratory Rats and Mice, Slovenia), given tap water *ad libitum* and maintained under a 12/12 hours dark/light cycle at constant temperature (20±1)°C and humidity (50±5)%. Each study group comprised 8-10 experimental animals. Handling with animals, experimental procedure and anesthesia were performed in accordance with the general principles contained in the Guide for the Care and Use of Laboratory Animals (National Academic Press). The Ethical Committee of the School of Medicine, University of Rijeka, approved all experimental procedures.

TNBS-colitis was induced by rectal administration of 5% (w/v) TNBS (Sigma-Aldrich, Germany) dissolved in 50% ethanol (Kemika, Croatia). Each animal received 0.1 mL of TNBS-ethanol solution, using a vinyl catheter that was positioned 4 cm from the anus, according to the protocol of (Scheiffele & Fuss, 2002). Two control groups of mice were used for each mice strain. Control mice underwent identical procedures, but were instilled equal volumes of saline (NaCl 0.9%) or ethanol solution. Mice were anesthetized with ketamine/xylazine while receiving TNBS, saline or ethanol solution.

4.2.2 Analytical methods

Experimental animals were sacrificed by cervical dislocation after 2, 7, 15 and 30 days upon administration of TNBS, saline or ethanol solution. Peripheral blood samples were taken and serum samples were collected by centrifugation at 3000 rpm for 10 minutes. Livers and spleens were isolated and their weights were noted. Colons were freed from adhering tissue and macroscopic changes were noted. The colon lumen was carefully washed with ice-cold saline, its weight and length was measured after which underwent homogenization procedure. Brains were separated immediately after sacrifice, washed in ice-cold saline and then homogenized on ice. Colon and brain homogenates were centrifuged at 14000 rpm for 20 minutes at +4°C. Resulting supernatants were measured for total protein concentrations according to the method of Bradford (Bradford, 1976).

Colon tissues for *histological and histomorphometrical analyses* were collected and fixed in 4% formalin for 24 h. Samples were processed and embedded in paraffin wax. Two-micrometer sections were stained with hematoxylin and eosin. An experienced pathologist blinded to

treatment allocation scored microscopical changes, which included overall severity of mucosal damage, number of crypts of Lieberkühn and their depth and width.
The DPP IV/CD26 (in C57BL/6) and DPP IV/CD26-like *enzymatic activities* (in CD26$^{-/-}$ mice) in mice serum, brain and colon homogenates were measured according to the protocol of (Kreisel et al., 1982), as described in section 3.2.1.
Brain and colon samples for *Western blot analyses* of CD26 molecule expression were homogenized on ice using RIPA lysis buffer including inhibitors of proteases and phosphatases. After that, homogenates were centrifuged at 14000 rpm for 20 minutes at +4°C and resulting supernatants were measured for total protein concentrations according to the method of Bradford (Bradford, 1976). Equal amounts of total proteins were separated by SDS-PAGE (sodium dodecyl sulphate-polyacrylamide gel electrophoresis). Proteins were transferred from the gels to polyvinylidenedifluoride membranes by semi-dry electroblotting. Membranes were incubated overnight with primary anti-CD26 (Santa Cruz Biotechnology Inc., CA), followed by 45 min incubation with secondary antibody, horseradish peroxidase-conjugated mouse-anti-rabbit IgG (Santa Cruz Biotechnology Inc., CA). Membranes were incubated with chemiluminescent Amersham ECL-plus Western blotting detection reagents (Amersham, Little Chalfont, UK) and bands revealing protein expression of the CD26 molecule were visualized after exposure to photosensitive films (AGFA Ortho CP-G plus). Equal total protein loading was ensured with use of the primary mouse ß-actin antibody (Chemicon International, USA), and secondary horseradish peroxidase-conjugated goat-anti-mouse IgG (Santa Cruz Biotechnology Inc., CA).

4.2.3 Evaluation of TNBS-colitis assessment

All groups of experimental mice were monitored daily for their body weights, stool consistence and presence of blood, eventual occurrence of rectal bleeding and general clinical state. Characteristic findings associated with intrarectal administration of TNBS solution in mice included their poor clinical state, body weight loss up to 15% and a mortality rate of approximately 11% in both CD26$^{-/-}$ and C57BL/6 mice. Disease symptoms were mostly pronounced in the first five days of experiment.
Body mass of individual experimental animals of all groups of both investigated mice strains were determined each day at about the same time, starting from the day of application of TNBS-ethanol solution, ethanol solution or saline, until the day of sacrifice (the second, seventh, fifteenth and thirtieth day). It has been noticed that body weights of CD26$^{-/-}$ animals, as compared to C57BL/6 strain of animals of the same age and gender, are statistically significantly different ($P < 0.05$) and amount (25.29±2.23)g for C57BL/6 and (23.41±2.51)g for CD26$^{-/-}$ animals. Lower body mass of CD26$^{-/-}$ animals in comparison with their genetic background (C57BL/6) mice as well as enhanced insulin secretion and improved glucose tolerance in mice lacking CD26 was reported before (Marguet et al., 2000).
The weights of the brain, liver and spleen were measured analytically for each experimental animal and presented in Table 4.
It was noticed that weights of livers and spleens were slightly higher in CD26$^{-/-}$ animals as compared to the corresponding groups of C57BL/6 animals, nevertheless their lower body mass. The trend of reduction in weight of liver and spleen on the second day of induction of colitis was observed in both strains of experimental animals. The hepatosomatic index (relative ratio of liver weight and body mass) and the relative ratio of spleen weight and body mass of animals were calculated for all animals. It was found that CD26$^{-/-}$ mice have statistically significantly higher ($P < 0.05$) values of the hepatosomatic index compared to

Mice strain	Experimental group	Day of experiment	Brain mass (g)	Liver mass (g)	Spleen mass (g)
C57BL/6	physiological	0	0.44776 ± 0.02273	1.32092 ± 0.11335	0.07822 ± 0.00951
	colitis	2	0.44733 ± 0.02117	0.89232 ± 0.14574	0.07596 ± 0.01806
	colitis	7	0.44019 ± 0.01498	1.12842 ± 0.19671	0.08650 ± 0.02623
	colitis	15	0.44037 ± 0.03687	1.24861 ± 0.12537	0.08424 ± 0.02037
	colitis	30	0.44113 ± 0.02342	1.36642 ± 0.14692	0.07707 ± 0.01311
C57BL/6	physiological	0	0.44776 ± 0.02273	1.32092 ± 0.11335	0.07822 ± 0.00951
	control	2	0.44716 ± 0.01527	1.27890 ± 0.15756	0.07680 ± 0.01630
	control	7	0.44488 ± 0.00435	1.23160 ± 0.05487	0.07462 ± 0.00938
	control	15	0.44838 ± 0.25067	1.26048 ± 0.05868	0.07630 ± 0.01327
	control	30	0.43701 ± 0.03043	1.35711 ± 0.17414	0.07728 ± 0.00697
CD26$^{-/-}$	physiological	0	0.41532 ± 0.02409	1.43343 ± 0.12470	0.08170 ± 0.01447
	colitis	2	0.41836 ± 0.02203	1.08765 ± 0.12792	0.06012 ± 0.01982
	colitis	7	0.42448 ± 0.02631	1.53770 ± 0.07895	0.11080 ± 0.04752
	colitis	15	0.42556 ± 0.01740	1.47498 ± 0.18033	0.11300 ± 0.01758
	colitis	30	0.41040 ± 0.01315	1.36693 ± 0.10567	0.09158 ± 0.02720
CD26$^{-/-}$	physiological	0	0.41532 ± 0.02409	1.43343 ± 0.12470	0.08170 ± 0.01447
	control	2	0.40117 ± 0.02964	1.33858 ± 0.22979	0.08222 ± 0.03727
	control	7	0.41232 ± 0.02331	1.38604 ± 0.07852	0.08058 ± 0.00259
	control	15	0.41924 ± 0.03450	1.24388 ± 0.08975	0.08260 ± 0.00995
	control	30	0.42334 ± 0.02402	1.34925 ± 0.24189	0.08338 ± 0.01257

Table 4. Average brain, liver and spleen weights (g) for different groups of experimental animals at scheduled days of experiment.

C57BL/6 animals. Hepatosomatic index decreased the second day of colitis induction in both strains of experimental animals, as a result of reduction in liver weight, despite of body weight loss. On the other hand, analyzed mice strains did not differ statistically significantly in the relative values of the ratio of spleen weight and body weight in physiological conditions, as well as in the control group treated with ethanol solution. Regardless of the reduction of the weight of the spleen on the second day of induction of colitis in both strains of experimental animals, due to a reduction in body weights no statistically significant reduction in their relative ratios was observed. Statistically significant increase in the relative ratio of spleen weight and body mass was recorded in the group of CD26-/- animals on the fifteenth day of the induction of colitis, compared to the corresponding control group and compared to C57BL/6 animals sacrificed on the same day.

Macroscopic examination of the distal part of the colon discovered localized inflammation with several ulcerations, mucosal erosions and bowel obstruction with enhanced edematous changes. Colon shortening and thickening with marked colonic edema, accompanied by increased colon weight and presence of hemorrhagic changes was most prominent two days following TNBS administration (Fig. 8). Therefore, day 2 of experiment was classified as acute phase of colitis, which is in accordance with previously reported findings (Scheiffele & Fuss, 2002).

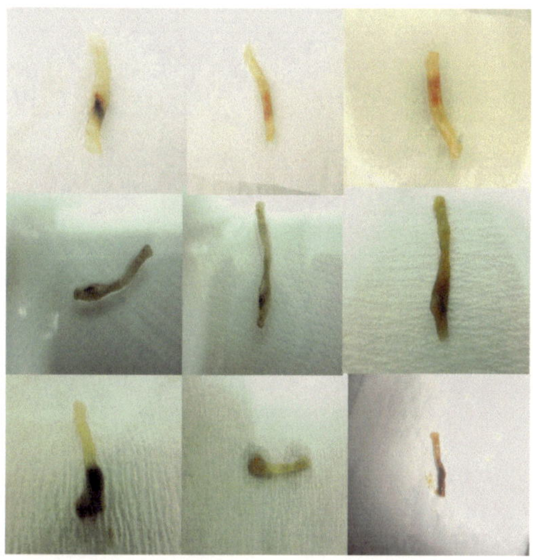

Fig. 8. Macroscopic appearance of the distal part of mice colons in the acute phase of colitis, two days after administration of TNBS-ethanol solution.

Results of our histopathological analyses of colon tissue sections in wild type and CD26-/- mice that received TNBS-ethanol solution confirmed the presence of inflammatory processes and accomplishment of colitis induction. *Microscopic changes*, as well as macroscopic, were most conspicuous in the acute phase of colitis. *Pathohistological analyses* confirmed the presence of inflammatory changes very similar to those seen in human Crohn's disease and revealed that under physiological conditions no differences in histological architecture was observed between analyzed mice strains (Fig. 9).

Pathohistological analyses of a wider number of colonic section samples discovered some differences in the manifestation of inflammatory processes between CD26-/- and wild type mice: in CD26-/- mice, ulcerations were mainly localized in one part of the mucosal surface, and inflammatory changes did not overtake the entire mucosa. In most analyzed colon samples from CD26-/- mice, a part of the colonic mucosa was preserved with physiological appearance of crypts, but a transmural inflammation was observed in a number of mice (Fig. 10A). On the other hand, no transmural inflammatory changes were observed in wild type animals, but in a number of experimental animals, inflammatory processes affected the entire colonic circumference with very little or no areas of preserved mucosa (Fig. 10B).

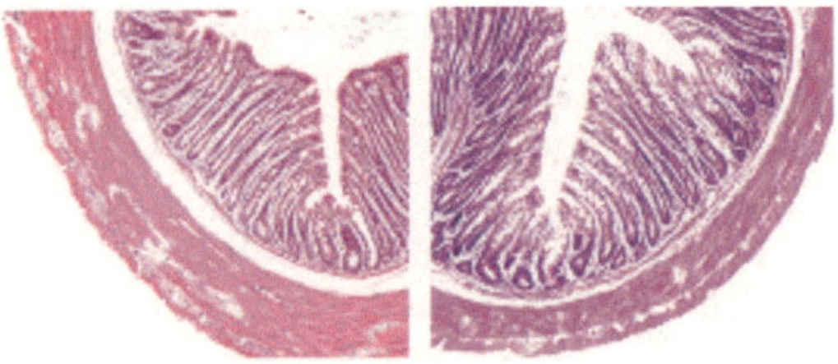

A B

Fig. 9. Histological appearance of colonic tissue sections of CD26-/- (A) and wild type mice (B) two days after application of saline solution. Colon sections (2 µm) were stained with hematoxylin and eosin and examined for histological properties. Magnification: 10x.

CD26-/- C57BL/6

A B C D

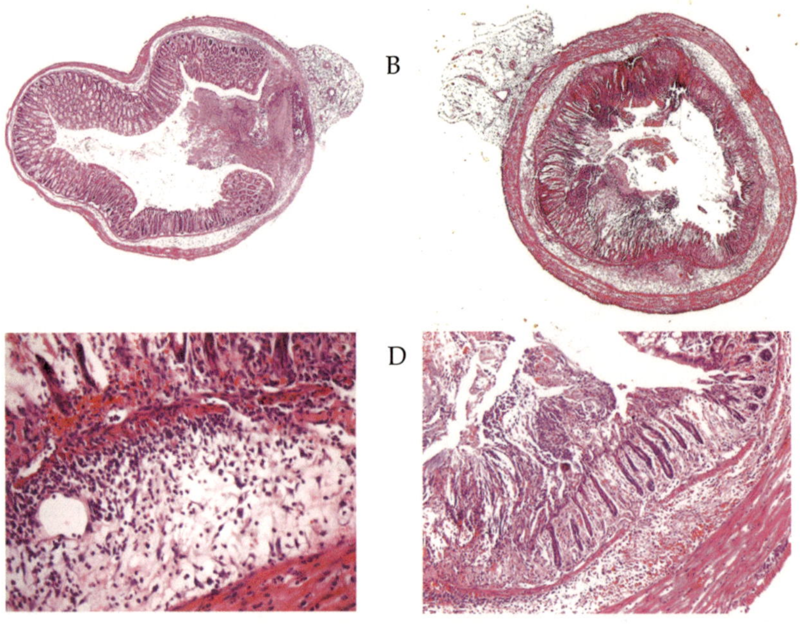

Fig. 10. Pathohistological appearance of colonic tissue sections of CD26-/- (A, C) and wild type mice (B, D) in the acute phase of colitis, two days after application of TNBS-ethanol solution. Colon sections (2 µm) were stained with hematoxylin and eosin and examined for histological properties. Magnification: 4x (A, B), 10x (D) and 20x (C).

Results of *histomorphometrical analyses* also confirmed the presence of inflammatory changes in both mice strains that received TNBS-ethanol solution. Number of crypts of Lieberkühn per mm of mucosa, and their depth and width for different groups of both mice strains at given days of experiment were measured (data not shown). Statistical analyses of obtained results among both control groups of animals did not reveal statistically significant changes in observed parameters, nor at different days of sacrifice. In both mice strains with induced colitis, a statistically significant ($P < 0.05$) decrease in number of crypts of Lieberkühn per mm of mucosa was observed in the acute phase of colitis. Changes persisted even during tissue healing in $CD26^{-/-}$ mice. The width of crypts of Lieberkühn was increased in the acute phase of colitis in both mice strains, but it took longer to achieve physiological values in wild type mice. Furthermore, the depth of crypts of Lieberkühn was decreased in acute colitis in both mice strains. All those changes represent consequences of inflammatory processes in the colon which include mucosa thickening and formation of edema due to TNBS-ethanol-induced tissue damage.

4.2.4 DPP IV/CD26 and DPP IV/CD26-like activity in TNBS-colitis

Measurements of DPP IV/CD26 activity and protein expression in wild type mice were performed at systemic and local levels, in the serum and within the gut-brain axis respectively. Furthermore, in order to evaluate whether in conditions of DPP IV/CD26 deficiency other DPP IV/CD26-like enzymes could partially undertake its enzymatic function, DPP IV/CD26-like systemic and local activities were determined in $CD26^{-/-}$ mice. Results of investigations concerning DPP IV/CD26 and DPP IV/CD26-like molecules in TNBS-induced colitis in mice reviewed here are accepted for publication in *Croatica Chemica Acta* (*in press*, vol.no.4, 2011). Fig. 11 shows results of serum DPP IV/CD26 activity in wild type mice with induced colitis compared to control groups.

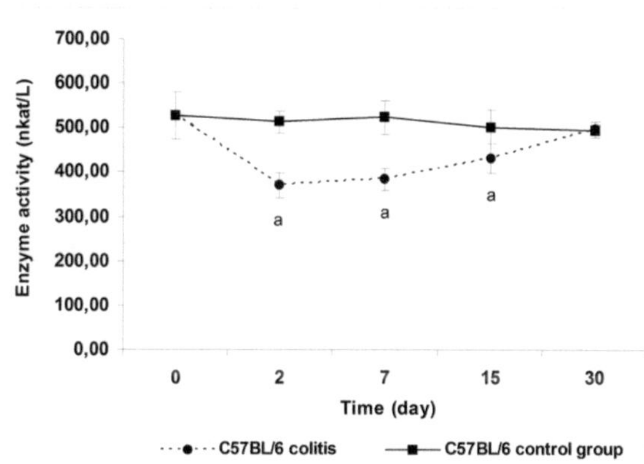

[a], statistically significantly different compared to control group ($P < 0.05$)
0 - control group, physiological condition; 2, 7, 15, 30 - days after administration of TNBS-ethanol solution (colitis group) or ethanol solution (control group).

Fig. 11. Serum DPP IV/CD26 activity in C57BL/6 mice during colitis development and resolution compared to control group.

A statistically significant decrease ($P < 0.05$) in serum DPP IV/CD26 activity, starting in the acute phase of colitis and achieving physiological values after disease healing could be seen. Our results accord with previously published results that included determination of serum DPP IV/CD26 activity in patients with IBD, as described before in this chapter. Furthermore, our results are in accordance with the observation that serum DPP IV/CD26 activity correlates inversely with disease severity in patients with IBD (Varljen et al., 2005), since the lowest DPP IV/CD26 activity in mice was found in the acute phase of disease.

Furthermore, we wanted to evaluate possible changes in serum DPP IV/CD26-like activities during colitis development and healing as well. Therefore, CD26-/- mice with induced colitis as well as their control groups were analyzed. Obtained results showed that CD26-/- mice express approximately 10% of total serum DPP IV/CD26 activity detected in wild type mice. Fig. 12 shows results of serum DPP IV/CD26-like activity in CD26-/- mice with induced colitis compared to their control groups.

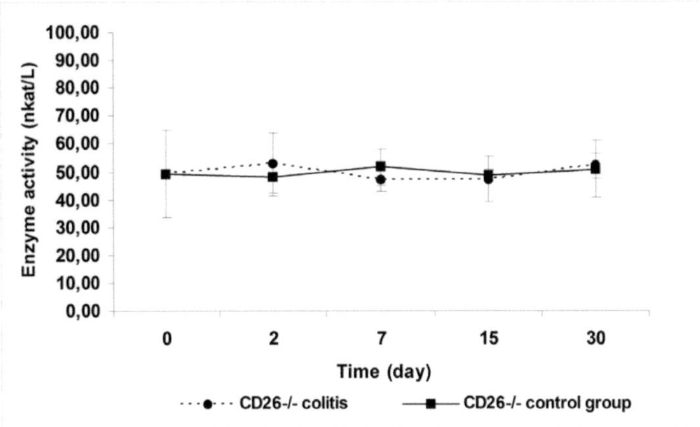

0 – control group, physiological condition; 2, 7, 15, 30 – days after administration of TNBS-ethanol solution (colitis group) or ethanol solution (control group).

Fig. 12. Serum DPP IV/CD26-like activity in CD26-/- mice during colitis development and resolution compared to control group.

Our results indicated that there are no statistically significant differences in serum DPP IV/CD26-like activity between groups of CD26-/- animals with colitis and their control groups. Therefore, the significance of DPP IV/CD26 over DPP IV/CD26-like serum activity is proposed.

4.2.5 DPP IV/CD26, IBD and the gut-brain axis

Growing scientific evidence emphasizes neuroimmunomodulation as an important factor in the occurrence of inflammatory and autoimmune processes, as described in different investigations in the last few years (Ohman and Simren, 2010). The complex causal connection between central and enteric nervous system caused the introduction of the term **gut-brain axis** (Romijn et al., 2008). DPP IV/CD26 has previously been shown to play a key role in the metabolism of important bioactive neuro- and immunopeptides, as well as in the activation of the immune response (Vanderheyden et al., 2009). Due to its localization on the cell surface of the nervous and digestive system, likewise on the surface of important immune cells (Matteucci & Giampietro, 2009), we aimed to investigate possible changes in DPP IV/CD26 activity and protein expression at sight of inflammation, in the colon, and in which way those changes reflect on examined parameters in the brain.

Results of our research showed an accentuated decrease in DPP IV/CD26 activity at site of inflammation, in the inflamed colon in wild type animals compared to their control groups

(Fig. 13A). On the other hand, an increased CD26 protein expression in the acute phase of disease was revealed by Western blotting technique (Fig. 13B).

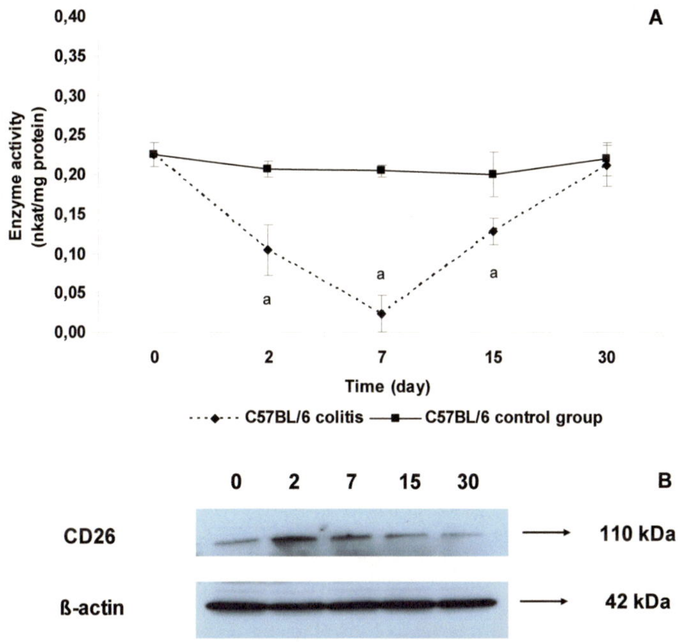

[a], statistically significantly different compared to control group ($P < 0.05$).
0 - control group, physiological condition; 2, 7, 15, 30 - days after administration of TNBS-ethanol solution (colitis group) or ethanol solution (control group).

Fig. 13. DPP IV/CD26 activity (A) and protein expression (B) in colon of C57BL/6 mice during colitis development and resolution.

Besides a regulatory system at the enzymatic level, this observed fact could also be partly explained as a compensatory mechanism, considering that a part of the decreased DPP IV/CD26 activity in the colon of wild type mice is indeed a consequence of severe mucosal damage induced by TNBS-ethanol solution. Consequently, increased CD26 protein expression in the acute phase of disease could represent an effort to realize a compensatory mechanism. Since damaged DPP IV/CD26 conformation is present in inflamed tissue, with the consequence of an improper enzyme activity, enhanced DPP IV/CD26 protein expression could represent a mechanism of feed-back. Our results are in agreement with previously reported observations regarding enhanced CD26 mRNA production in inflamed tissue (Nemoto et al., 1999).
We have determined that, in physiological conditions, CD26$^{-/-}$ mice express less than 2% of total DPP IV/CD26 activity detected in the colon of wild type mice. This enzyme activity was defined as DPP IV/CD26-like activity in the colon and was investigated during colitis development and resolution, as well. Our results showed statistically significantly ($P < 0.05$) decreased DPP IV/CD26-like activity in inflamed colon homogenates in CD26$^{-/-}$ mice, compared to their controls (Fig. 14).

Nevertheless, this observation could not entirely be explained as a consequence of an intrinsic regulatory mechanism which downregulates the activity of DPP IV/CD26-like enzymes in inflammatory processes, but could also partially be attributable to tissue damage induced by TNBS/ethanol solution.

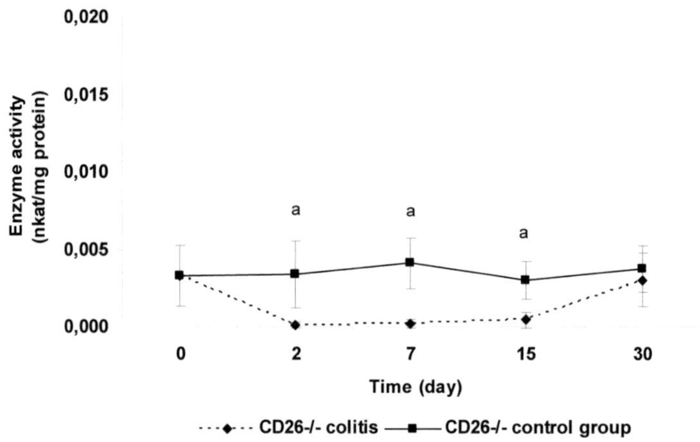

[a], statistically significantly different compared to control group ($P < 0.05$).
0 – control group, physiological condition; 2, 7, 15, 30 – days after administration of TNBS-ethanol solution (colitis group) or ethanol solution (control group).

Fig. 14. DPP IV/CD26-like activity in colon of $CD26^{-/-}$ mice during colitis development and resolution compared to control group.

DPP IV/CD26 and DPP IV/CD26-like activities were also analyzed in brain homogenates during colitis development and resolution in wild type and $CD26^{-/-}$ mice. Our results showed that DPP IV/CD26 activity in brain is statistically significantly decreased ($P < 0.05$) in the acute phase of colitis compared to control groups (Fig. 15A). On the other hand, CD26 protein expression, as confirmed by Western blotting (Fig. 15B) remains constant. Furthermore, the activity of DPP IV/CD26-like enzymes was found to remain unchanged (Fig. 15C).
It could be seen that changes in DPP IV/CD26 activity in the colon during inflammatory events, reflect on its activity in the central nervous system, which accentuates the importance of the gut-brain axis in IBD pathogenesis. Therefore, a decreased DPP IV/CD26 activity in the brain is most probably causally connected with its accentuated changes in the colon. Furthermore, a regulatory mechanism which regulates DPP IV/CD26 activity in brain, independently of its protein expression is proposed.
This study reveals new data about DPP IV/CD26 activity and protein expression in a model of Crohn-like colitis in mice. Likewise, due to very little available results of colitis investigation under conditions of CD26 deficiency, our study gives new insights in inflammatory manifestations induced by TNBS-ethanol administration in CD26 $^{-/-}$ mice.

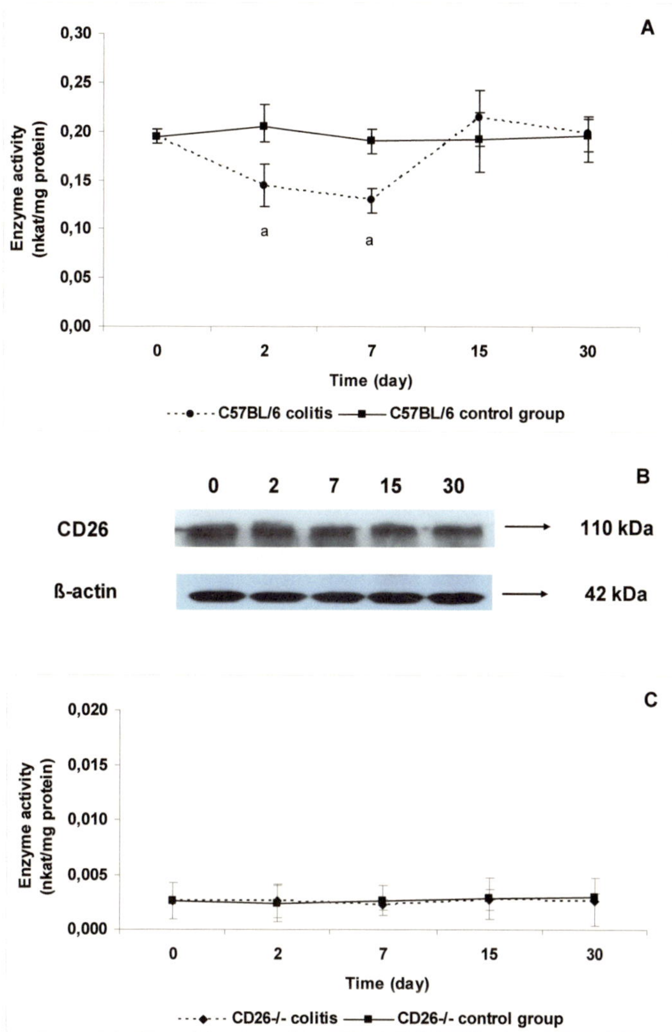

[a], statistically significantly different compared to control group ($P < 0.05$).
0 - control group, physiological condition; 2, 7, 15, 30 - days after administration of TNBS-ethanol solution (colitis group) or ethanol solution (control group).

Fig. 15. Brain DPP IV/CD26 activity and protein expression in C57BL/6 mice (A, B), DPP IV/CD26-like activity in CD26-/- mice (C) during colitis development and resolution.

5. Conclusions

Results of our studies show that DPP IV/CD26 is involved in the pathogenesis of IBD. In patients, its activity seems to be a good marker of disease activity, given its inverse correlation with disease severity. Given the potential role of DPP IV/CD26 in IBD, animal models of UC and CD have been established in CD26-/- and wild type mice. Our results showed that CD26-/- mice are not protected from two chemically induced colitis (DSS and TNBS colitis), but show specificity in histological damage compared to wild type mice, as well as differences in the time course of the disease. When analyzing targeted immunobiochemical parameters, it was noticed that changes occurring during inflammatory processes in the colon reflect on investigated parameters in the central nervous system. Therefore, our results indicate and confirm the importance of the gut-brain axis in the pathogenesis of IBD.

6. Acknowledgements

This study was supported by the Croatian Ministry of Science, Education and Sports (grant No. 062-0061245-0213). We gratefully acknowledge Dr. Didier Marguet (Centre d'Immunologie Marseille-Luminy, France), for providing us CD26$^{-/-}$ mice. Many thanks to professor Siniša Volarević, PhD, head of the department of Molecular Medicine and Biotechnology and professor Stipan Jonjić, PhD, head of the department of Histology and Embryology, School of Medicine, University of Rijeka, for allowing us to complete a part of experiments using the equipment at their departments.

7. References

Ahnen, D.J.; Santiago, N.A.; Cezard, J.P. & Gray G.M. (1982). Intestinal aminooligopeptidase. In vivo synthesis on intracellular membranes of rat jejunum. *J Biol Chem* 257:12129-35. ISSN: 0021-9258

Ansorge, S.; Bank, U.; Heimburg, A.; Helmuth, M.; Koch, G.; Tadje, J.; Lendeckel, U.; Wolke, C.; Neubert, K.; Faust, J.; Fuchs, P.; Reinhold, D.; Thielitz, A. & Tager, M. (2009). Recent insights into the role of dipeptidyl aminopeptidase IV (DPIV) and aminopeptidase N (APN) families in immune functions. *Clin Chem Lab Med* 47:253-61. ISSN: 1434-6621

Aytac, U. & Dang, N.H. (2004). CD26/dipeptidyl peptidase IV: a regulator of immune function and a potential molecular target for therapy. *Curr Drug Targets Immune Endocr Metabol Disord* 4:11-8. ISSN: 1568-0088

Baumgart, D.C.; Bernstein, C.N.; Abbas, Z.; Colombel, J.F.; Day, A.S.; D'Haens, G.; Dotan, I.; Goh, K.L.; Hibi, T.; Kozarek, R.A.; Quigley, E.M.; Reinisch, W.; Sands, B.E.; Sollano, J.D.; Steinhart, A.H.; Steinwurz, F.; Vatn, M.H. & Yamamoto-Furusho, J.K. (2011). IBD Around the world: Comparing the epidemiology, diagnosis, and treatment: Proceedings of the World Digestive Health Day 2010 - Inflammatory bowel disease task force meeting. *Inflamm Bowel Dis.* Feb;17(2):639-44. ISSN: 1536-4844

Bhan, A.K.; Mizoguchi, E.; Smith, R.N. & Mizoguchi, A. (1999). Colitis in transgenic and knockout animals as models of human inflammatory bowel disease. *Immunol Rev* 169:195-207. ISSN: 0105-2896

Boonacker, E. & Van Noorden, C.J. (2003). The multifunctional or moonlighting protein CD26/DPPIV. *Eur J Cell Biol* 82:53-73. ISSN: 0171-9335

Bradford, M.M. (1976). A rapid and sensitive method for the quantitation of microgram quantities of protein utilizing the principle of protein-dye binding. *Anal Biochem* 72:248-54. ISSN: 0003-2697

Camoglio, L.; te Velde, A.A.; de Boer, A.; ten Kate, F.J.; Kopf, M. & van Deventer, S.J. (2000). Hapten-induced colitis associated with maintained Th1 and inflammatory responses in IFN-gamma receptor-deficient mice. *Eur J Immunol* 30:1486-95. ISSN: 0014-2980

Colletti, T. (2004). IBD--recognition, diagnosis, therapeutics. *Jaapa* 17:16-8, 21-4. ISSN 1547-1896

Cooper, H.S.; Murthy, S.N.; Shah, R.S. & Sedergran, D.J. (1993). Clinicopathologic study of dextran sulfate sodium experimental murine colitis. *Lab Invest* 69:238-49. ISSN: 0023-6837

Dang, N.H.; Torimoto, Y.; Sugita, K.; Daley, J.F.; Schow, P.; Prado, C., Schlossman, S.F. & Morimoto, C. (1990). Cell surface modulation of CD26 by anti-1F7 monoclonal antibody. Analysis of surface expression and human T cell activation. *J Immunol* 145:3963-71. ISSN: 0022-1767

De Meester, I.; Korom, S.; Van Damme, J. & Scharpe, S. (1999). CD26, let it cut or cut it down. *Immunol Today* 20:367-75. ISSN: 0167-5699

Dieleman, L.A.; Palmen, M.J.; Akol, H.; Bloemena, E.; Pena, A.S.; Meuwissen, S.G. & Van Rees, E.P. (1998). Chronic experimental colitis induced by dextran sulphate sodium (DSS) is characterized by Th1 and Th2 cytokines. *Clin Exp Immunol* 114:385-91. ISSN: 0009-9104

Fleischer, B. (1987). A novel pathway of human T cell activation via a 103 kD T cell activation antigen. *J Immunol* 138:1346-50. ISSN: 0022-1767

Fleischer, B. (1994). CD26: a surface protease involved in T-cell activation. *Immunol Today* 15:180-4. ISSN: 0167-5699

Flentke, G.R.; Munoz, E.; Huber, B.T.; Plaut, A.G.; Kettner, C.A. & Bachovchin, W.W. (1991). Inhibition of dipeptidyl aminopeptidase IV (DP-IV) by Xaa-boroPro dipeptides and use of these inhibitors to examine the role of DP-IV in T-cell function. *Proc Natl Acad Sci U S A* 88:1556-9. ISSN: 0027-8424

Geboes, K.; Colombel, J.F.; Greenstein, A.; Jewell, D.P.; Sandborn, W.J.; Vatn, M.H.; Warren, B. & Riddell, R.H. (2008). Indeterminate colitis: a review of the concept--what's in a name? *Inflamm Bowel Dis* 14:850-7. ISSN: 1536-4844

Geier, M.S.; Smith, C.L.; Butler, R.N. & Howarth, G.S. (2009). Small-intestinal manifestations of dextran sulfate sodium consumption in rats and assessment of the effects of Lactobacillus fermentum BR11. *Dig Dis Sci* 54:1222-8. ISSN: 1573-2568

Geier, M.S.; Tenikoff, D.; Yazbeck, R.; McCaughan, G.W.; Abbott, C.A. & Howarth, G.S. (2005). Development and resolution of experimental colitis in mice with targeted deletion of dipeptidyl peptidase IV. *J Cell Physiol* 204:687-92. ISSN: 0021-9541

Gorrell, M.D. (2005). Dipeptidyl peptidase IV and related enzymes in cell biology and liver disorders. *Clin Sci (Lond)* 108:277-92. ISSN: 0143-5221

Gorrell, M.D.; Gysbers, V. & McCaughan, G.W. (2001). CD26: a multifunctional integral membrane and secreted protein of activated lymphocytes. *Scand J Immunol* 54:249-64. ISSN: 0300-9475

Gorrell, M.D.; Wang, X.M.; Park, J.; Ajami, K.; Yu, D.M.; Knott, H.; Seth, D. & McCaughan, G.W. (2006). Structure and function in dipeptidyl peptidase IV and related proteins. *Adv Exp Med Biol* 575:45-54. ISSN: 0065-2598

Grisham, M.B.; Volkmer, C.; Tso, P. & Yamada, T. (1991). Metabolism of trinitrobenzene sulfonic acid by the rat colon produces reactive oxygen species. *Gastroenterology* 101:540-7. ISSN: 0016-5085

Hanauer, S.B. (2006). Inflammatory bowel disease: epidemiology, pathogenesis, and therapeutic opportunities. *Inflamm Bowel Dis* 12 Suppl 1:S3-9. ISSN: 1536-4844

Hanauer, S.B. & Hommes, D.W. (2010): Inflammatory bowel disease. *Expert Rev Clin Immunol* 6:499-500. ISSN: 1744-8409.

Herrera, C.; Morimoto, C.; Blanco, J.; Mallol, J.; Arenzana, F.; Lluis, C. & Franco, R. (2001). Comodulation of CXCR4 and CD26 in human lymphocytes. *J Biol Chem* 276:19532-9. ISSN: 0021-9258

Hildebrandt, M.; Reutter, W.; Arck, P.; Rose, M. & Klapp, B.F. (2000). A guardian angel: the involvement of dipeptidyl peptidase IV in psychoneuroendocrine function, nutrition and immune defence. *Clin Sci (Lond)* 99:93-104. ISSN: 0143-5221

Hildebrandt, M.; Rose, M.; Ruter, J.; Salama, A.; Monnikes, H. & Klapp, B.F. (2001). Dipeptidyl peptidase IV (DP IV, CD26) in patients with inflammatory bowel disease. *Scand J Gastroenterol* 36:1067-72. ISSN: 0036-5521

Howarth, G.S.; Xian, C.J. & Read, L.C. (2000). Predisposition to colonic dysplasia is unaffected by continuous administration of insulin-like growth factor-I for twenty weeks in a rat model of chronic inflammatory bowel disease. *Growth Factors* 18(2):119-33. ISSN: 0897-7194

Hyams, J.S.; Ferry, G.D.; Mandel, F.S.; Gryboski, J.D.; Kibort, P.M.; Kirschner, B.S.; Griffiths, A.M.; Katz, A.J.; Grand, R.J.; Boyle, J.T. et al. (1991). Development and validation of a pediatric Crohn's disease activity index. *J Pediatr Gastroenterol Nutr* 12:439-47. ISSN: 0277-2116

Ikushima, H.; Munakata, Y.; Ishii, T.; Iwata, S.; Terashima, M.; Tanaka, H.; Schlossman, S.F. & Morimoto, C. (2000). Internalization of CD26 by mannose 6-phosphate/insulin-like growth factor II receptor contributes to T cell activation. *Proc Natl Acad Sci U S A* 97:8439-44. ISSN: 0027-8424

Ishii, T.; Ohnuma, K.; Murakami, A.; Takasawa, N.; Kobayashi, S.; Dang, N.H.; Schlossman, S.F. & Morimoto, C. (2001). CD26-mediated signaling for T cell activation occurs in lipid rafts through its association with CD45RO. *Proc Natl Acad Sci U S A* 98:12138-43. ISSN: 0027-8424

Iwanaga, T.; Hoshi, O.; Han, H. & Fujita, T. (1994). Morphological analysis of acute ulcerative colitis experimentally induced by dextran sulfate sodium in the guinea pig: some possible mechanisms of cecal ulceration. *J Gastroenterol* 29:430-8. ISSN: 0944-1174

Kitajima, S.; Takuma, S. & Morimoto, M. (2000). Histological analysis of murine colitis induced by dextran sulfate sodium of different molecular weights. *Exp Anim* 49:9-15. ISSN: 1341-1357

Kreisel, W.; Heussner, R.; Volk, B.; Buchsel, R.; Reutter, W. & Gerok, W. (1982). Identification of the 110000 Mr glycoprotein isolated from rat liver plasma membrane as dipeptidylaminopeptidase IV. *FEBS Lett* 147:85-8. ISSN: 0014-5793

Lambeir, A.M.; Durinx, C.; Proost, P.; Van Damme, J.; Scharpe, S. & De Meester, I. (2001). Kinetic study of the processing by dipeptidyl-peptidase IV/CD26 of neuropeptides involved in pancreatic insulin secretion. *FEBS Lett* 507:327-30. ISSN: 0014-5793

Lambeir, A.M.; Durinx, C.; Scharpe, S. & De Meester, I. (2003). Dipeptidyl-peptidase IV from bench to bedside: an update on structural properties, functions, and clinical aspects of the enzyme DPP IV. *Crit Rev Clin Lab Sci* 40:209-94. ISSN: 1040-8363

Mahler, M.; Bristol, I.J.; Leiter, E.H.; Workman, A.E.; Birkenmeier, E.H.; Elson, C.O. & Sundberg, J.P. (1998). Differential susceptibility of inbred mouse strains to dextran sulfate sodium-induced colitis. *Am J Physiol* 274:G544-51. ISSN: 0002-9513

Marguet, D.; Baggio, L.; Kobayashi, T.; Bernard, A.M.; Pierres, M.; Nielsen, P.F.; Ribel, U.; Watanabe, T.; Drucker, D.J. & Wagtmann, N. (2000). Enhanced insulin secretion and improved glucose tolerance in mice lacking CD26. *Proc Natl Acad Sci U S A* 97:6874-9. ISSN: 0027-8424

Matteucci, E. & Giampietro, O. (2009). Dipeptidyl Peptidase-4 (CD26): Knowing the Function before Inhibiting the Enzyme. *Curr Med Chem* 16:2943-51. ISSN: 0929-8673

Mentlein, R. (1999). Dipeptidyl-peptidase IV (CD26)--role in the inactivation of regulatory peptides. *Regul Pept* 85:9-24. ISSN: 0167-0115

Mentlein, R. (2004). Cell-surface peptidases. *Int Rev Cytol* 235:165-213. ISSN: 0074-7696

Mizoguchi, A. & Mizoguchi, E. (2010). Animal models of IBD: linkage to human disease. *Curr Opin Pharmacol* 10:578-87. ISSN: 1471-4973

Munoz, E.; Blazquez, M.V.; Madueno, J.A.; Rubio, G. & Pena, J. (1992). CD26 induces T-cell proliferation by tyrosine protein phosphorylation. *Immunology* 77:43-50. ISSN: 0019-2805

Murthy, S.N.; Cooper, H.S.; Shim, H.; Shah, R.S.; Ibrahim, S.A. & Sedergran, D.J. (1993). Treatment of dextran sulfate sodium-induced murine colitis by intracolonic cyclosporin. *Dig Dis Sci.* 38(9):1722-34. ISSN: 0163-2116

Nagatsu, I.; Nagatsu, T. & Yamamoto, T. (1968). Hydrolysis of amino acid beta-naphthylamides by aminopeptidases in human parotid salva and human serum. *Experientia* 24:347-8. ISSN: 0014-4754

Nemoto, E.; Sugawara, S.; Takada, H.; Shoji, S. & Horiuch, H. (1999). Increase of CD26/dipeptidyl peptidase IV expression on human gingival fibroblasts upon stimulation with cytokines and bacterial components. *Infect Immun* 67:6225-33. ISSN: 0019-9567

Ohkusa, T. (1985). (Production of experimental ulcerative colitis in hamsters by dextran sulfate sodium and changes in intestinal microflora). *Nippon Shokakibyo Gakkai Zasshi* (*The Japanese journal of gastro-enterology*) 82:1327-36. ISSN: 0446-6586

Ohman, L. & Simren, M. (2010). Pathogenesis of IBS: role of inflammation, immunity and neuroimmune interactions. *Nat Rev Gastroenterol Hepatol* 7:163-73. ISSN: 1759-5053

Ohtsuka, Y. & Sanderson, I.R. (2003). Dextran sulfate sodium-induced inflammation is enhanced by intestinal epithelial cell chemokine expression in mice. *Pediatr Res* 53:143-7. ISSN: 0031-3998

Okayasu, I.; Hatakeyama, S.; Yamada, M.; Ohkusa, T.; Inagaki, Y. & Nakaya, R. (1990). A novel method in the induction of reliable experimental acute and chronic ulcerative colitis in mice. *Gastroenterology* 98:694-702. ISSN: 0016-5085

Puschel, G.; Mentlein, R. & Heymann, E. (1982). Isolation and characterization of dipeptidyl peptidase IV from human placenta. *Eur J Biochem* 126:359-65. ISSN: 0014-2956

Ravi, A.; Garg, P. & Sitaraman, S.V. (2007). Matrix metalloproteinases in inflammatory bowel disease: boon or a bane? *Inflamm Bowel Dis* 13:97-107. ISSN: 1536-4844

Reinhold , D.; Bank, U.; Buhling, F.; Tager, M.; Born, I.; Faust, J.; Neubert, K. & Ansorge, S. (1997a). Inhibitors of dipeptidyl peptidase IV (DP IV, CD26) induces secretion of transforming growth factor-beta 1 (TGF-beta 1) in stimulated mouse splenocytes and thymocytes. *Immunol Lett* 58:29-35. ISSN: 0165-2478

Reinhold, D.; Kahne, T.; Tager, M.; Lendeckel, U.; Buhling, F.; Bank, U.; Wrenger, S.; Faust, J.; Neubert, K.; & Ansorge, S. (1997b). The effect of anti-CD26 antibodies on DNA synthesis and cytokine production (IL-2, IL-10 and IFN-gamma) depends on enzymatic activity of DP IV/CD26. *Adv Exp Med Biol* 421:149-55. ISSN: 0065-2598

Romijn, J.A.; Corssmit, E.P.; Havekes, L.M. & Pijl, H. (2008). Gut-brain axis. *Curr Opin Clin Nutr Metab Care* 11:518-21. ISSN: 1363-1950

Rose, M.; Walter, O.B.; Fliege, H.; Hildebrandt, M.; Monnikes, H. & Klapp, B.F. (2003). DPP IV and mental depression in Crohn's disease. *Adv Exp Med Biol* 524:321-31. ISSN: 0065-2598

Scheiffele, F. & Fuss, I.J. (2002). Induction of TNBS colitis in mice. *Curr Protoc Immunol* Chapter 15:Unit 15 19. ISSN: 1934-368X

Schon, E.; Mansfeld, H.W.; Demuth, H.U.; Barth, A. & Ansorge, S. (1985). The dipeptidyl peptidase IV, a membrane enzyme involved in the proliferation of T lymphocytes. *Biomed Biochim Acta* 44:K9-15. ISSN: 0232-766X

Sedo, A. & Malik, R. (2001). Dipeptidyl peptidase IV-like molecules: homologous proteins or homologous activities? *Biochim Biophys Acta* 1550:107-16. ISSN: 0006-3002

Shah, S.A. & Feller, E.R. (2009). Inflammatory bowel disease. *Med Health R I* 92:72. ISSN: 1086-5462

Strober, W.; Fuss, I.J.; Ehrhardt, R.O.; Neurath, M.; Boirivant, M. & Ludviksson, B.R. (1998) Mucosal immunoregulation and inflammatory bowel disease: new insights from murine models of inflammation. *Scand J Immunol* 48:453-8. ISSN: 0300-9475

Thompson, M.A.; Ohnuma, K.; Abe, M.; Morimoto, C. & Dang, N.H. (2007). CD26/dipeptidyl peptidase IV as a novel therapeutic target for cancer and immune disorders. *Mini Rev Med Chem* 7:253-73. ISSN: 1389-5575

Truelove, S.C. & Witts, L.J. (1955). Cortisone in ulcerative colitis; final report on a therapeutic trial. *Br Med J* 2:1041-8. ISSN: 0007-1447

Uhlig, H.H. & Powrie, F. (2009). Mouse models of intestinal inflammation as tools to understand the pathogenesis of inflammatory bowel disease. *Eur J Immunol* 39:2021-6. ISSN: 1521-4141

Vanderheyden, M.; Bartunek, J.; Goethals, M.; Verstreken, S.; Lambeir, A.M.; De Meester, I. & Scharpe, S. (2009). Dipeptidyl-peptidase IV and B-type natriuretic peptide. From bench to bedside. *Clin Chem Lab Med* 47:248-52. ISSN: 1434-6621

Varljen, J., Sincic, B.M.; Baticic, L.; Varljen, N.; Detel, D. & Lekic, A. (2005). Clinical relevance of the serum dipeptidyl peptidase IV (DPP IV/CD26) activity in adult patients with Crohn's disease and ulcerative colitis. *Croatica Chemica Acta* 78:427-432. ISSN: 0011-1643

Varljen, J.; Detel, D.; Lupis, T. & Peršić, M. (2004). Serum Dipeptidyl Peptidase IV (DPP IV/CD26) Activity in Children with Inflammatory Bowel Disease. Pediatric Gastroenterology 2004 - Reports from the 2nd World Congress of Pediatric Gastroenterology, Hepatology and Nutrition. Medimont S.r.l., 559-563. ISBN 88-7587-106-X

Willheim, M.; Ebner, C.; Baier, K.; Kern, W.; Schrattbauer, K.; Thien, R.; Kraft, D.; Breiteneder, H.; Reinisch, W. & Scheiner, O. (1997). Cell surface characterization of T lymphocytes and allergen-specific T cell clones: correlation of CD26 expression with T(H1) subsets. *J Allergy Clin Immunol* 100:348-55. ISSN: 0091-6749

Wirtz, S. & Neurath, M.F. (2007). Mouse models of inflammatory bowel disease. *Adv Drug Deliv Rev* 59:1073-83. ISSN: 0169-409X

Yazbeck, R.; Howarth, G.S. & Abbott, C.A. (2009). Dipeptidyl peptidase inhibitors, an emerging drug class for inflammatory disease? *Trends Pharmacol Sci* 30:600-7. ISSN: 1873-3735

Yazbeck, R.; Howarth, G.S.; Geier, M.S.; Demuth, H.U. & Abbott, C.A. (2008). Inhibiting dipeptidyl peptidase activity partially ameliorates colitis in mice. *Front Biosci* 13:6850-8. ISSN: 1093-4715

Yazbeck, R.; Sulda, M.L.; Howarth, G.S.; Bleich, A.; Raber, K.; von Horsten, S.; Holst, J.J. & Abbott, C.A. (2010). Dipeptidyl peptidase expression during experimental colitis in mice. *Inflamm Bowel Dis* 16:1340-51. ISSN: 1536-4844

Yu, D.M.; Ajami, K.; Gall, M.G.; Park, J.; Lee, C.S.; Evans, K.A.; McLaughlin, E.A.; Pitman M.R.; Abbott, C.A.; McCaughan, G.W. & Gorrell, M.D. (2009). The in vivo expression of dipeptidyl peptidases 8 and 9. *J Histochem Cytochem* 57:1025-40. ISSN: 1551-5044

5

The Roles of Interleukin-17 and T Helper 17 Cells in Intestinal Barrier Function

Elizabeth Trusevych, Leanne Mortimer and Kris Chadee
University of Calgary
Canada

1. Introduction

Inflammatory bowel diseases (IBD) are caused by chronic inflammation of the gastrointestinal tract, affecting as many as 1.4 million persons in the United States, and 2.2 million persons in Europe (Loftus, 2004). Crohn's disease (CD) and ulcerative colitis (UC), the two major forms of IBD, affect different regions of the intestinal tract and have distinct cytokine profiles. In CD, transmural inflammation can occur over the entire length of the gastrointestinal tract, whereas UC inflammation is restricted to the mucosa of the colon. The T helper (T_h) paradigm was established by Mosmann et al (1986) who observed distinct cytokine patterns were produced by two types of fully differentiated effector T cells which they termed termed T_h1 and T_h2 cells. The initial cytokine profiles observed in IBD helped to classify CD as a T_h1 disease, due to the increased production of the main T_h1 effector cytokine, interferon-gamma (IFN-γ). UC was slightly more difficult to classify because levels of a central T_h2 effector cytokine, IL-4, are not increased; however, other T_h2 effector cytokines, such as IL-5 and IL-13 are produced at higher levels (Fuss et al, 1996). Therefore, UC is not considered fully T_h2, but rather a T_h2-like disease (Fuss et al, 2004).

Conventional IBD therapies, including corticosteroids and anti-tumor necrosis factor-alpha (TNF-α) therapy, are aimed at reducing nonspecific inflammation. TNF-α is a central pro-inflammatory cytokine that contributes to the pathology of many autoimmune disorders. Anti-TNF-α was the first biological therapy introduced for patients with IBD in the late 1990s, and corticosteroid-refractory or fistulizing CD and refractory UC generally respond very well to anti-TNF-α treatment (Hoentjen & van Bodegraven, 2009; Rutgeerts et al., 2006). The initial identification of disease-specific inflammatory mediators in CD and UC, T_h1 and T_h2-associated cytokines respectively, lead to the development of more specific anti-inflammatory treatment options, and the efficacies of these new biological agents have in turn helped evolve our understanding of IBD pathogenesis. Using mouse models of intestinal inflammation that resemble CD, and targeting the main cytokine that drives T_h1 cellular development, IL-12, with an antibody to the IL-12p40 subunit either prevented the development of colitis, or completely cured established colitis (Liu et al., 2001; Neurath et al, 1995). These observations further supported the link between CD and T_h1 responses, in addition to warranting the development of an anti-IL-12p40 antibody for human patients with CD. In clinical trials, anti-IL-12p40 therapy induced clinical responses and remissions in patients with active CD (Mannon et al., 2005; Sandborn et al., 2008), which lead to its acceptance as a new therapy for CD.

Around the same time as anti-IL-12p40 therapy was being tested, discrepancies within the T_h1/T_h2 paradigm observed over the previous two decades were beginning to be resolved (Steinman, 2007). Two models in particular provided the first inconsistencies with the T_h1/T_h2 hypothesis: experimental autoimmune encephalomyelitis (EAE) and collagen-induced arthritis (CIA). EAE is a mouse model of human multiple sclerosis, caused by cell-mediated tissue damage that results in delayed-type hypersensitivity (DTH). DTH reactions are cell-mediated immune reactions to a challenge antigen, leading to swelling, induration, and redness appearing 24 to 72 hours after antigen exposure. Initially, DTH was believed to be mediated by a T_h1 response (Cher & Mosmann, 1987). Therefore, it was hypothesized that EAE would worsen with the addition of the T_h1 effector cytokine, IFN-γ. Interestingly, the results were just the opposite and IFN-γ administration ameliorated EAE damage (Billiau et al., 1988; Voorthuis et al., 1990). Similarly, CIA as a second model of autoimmune tissue destruction was also predicted to worsen with the administration of IFN-γ. Although the disease did worsen when IFN-γ was given before the administration of the adjuvant, it was ameliorated when IFN-γ was given after the adjuvant (Jacob et al., 1989; Nakajima et al., 1991). These puzzling inverse relationships between disease states thought to be controlled by T_h1 responses and the presence of IFN-γ, eventually lead to the discovery of IL-23 and it's role as a master regulator of a new T_h cell subset. IL-23, like IL-12, is a heterodimeric cytokine comprised of two subunits: a unique p19 subunit and a p40 subunit that is also shared by IL-12 (Oppmann et al., 2000). After it was discovered that IL-12 and IL-23 share a common subunit, divergent functions of these cytokines were unraveled, and the autoimmune inflammation in both EAE and CIA was found to result from the actions of IL-23, and not the T_h1 associated cytokine IL-12 (Cua et al., 2003; Murphy et al., 2003). In the same regard, when models of innate and adaptive chronic intestinal inflammation were re-evaluated, IL-23 was found to play a greater role than IL-12 in the induction of inflammation (Hue et al., 2006; Kullberg et al., 2006).

Around the time that IL-23 was found to be a central mediator of autoimmune inflammation, it was also discovered as a master regulator of an emerging T_h cell subset, T_h17 (Aggarwal et al., 2003). This was a significant event, as it shifted the long-standing T_h1/T_h2 paradigm of inflammation to include a novel subset of adaptive T_h cells. Consequently, all inflammatory conditions involving the adaptive immune response have needed re-evaluation. T_h17 cells have high expression of the transcription factors RORα and ROR-γt, produce the cytokines IL-17A, IL-17F and IL-22, have high surface expression of the IL-23R as well as the chemokine receptor CCR6, and can also secrete the CCR6 ligand, CCL20 (O'Connor et al., 2010). Importantly, the CCL20-CCR6 ligand-receptor pair plays an important chemoattractant role at mucosal surfaces (Schutyser et al., 2003). In addition to T_h17 cells, CCR6 is also expressed on T regulatory (T_{reg}) cells that function to maintain homeostatic conditions (Lim et al., 2008). By producing CCL20, T_h17 cells are able to promote the migration of additional T_h17 cells as well as T_{reg} cells (Yamazaki et al., 2008), and both cell types are enriched at mucosal surfaces.

Since their characterization, T_h17 cells have been shown to play an important protective role in infectious immunity where they promote the clearance of extracellular pathogens by enhancing neutrophil recruitment and promoting the expression of antimicrobial factors. Additionally, T_h17 cells have been associated with many autoimmune diseases, such as rheumatoid arthritis, dermatitis, psoriasis, asthma, multiple sclerosis, as well as IBD (Hemdan et al., 2010). Studies of human IBD have shown that the T_h17 effector cytokines IL-17A and IL-17F are both increased in the affected mucosa and sera of CD and UC patients

(Fujino et al., 2003; Rovedatti et al., 2009). Furthermore, polymorphisms in the *IL-17A* and *IL-17F* genes have been linked to UC and animal models indicate that they are fundamentally involved in the etiology of IBD (Arisawa et al., 2008). However, their precise roles in pathogenesis are not entirely clear. This chapter will focus on the cytokines IL-17A and IL-17F, and review what is known about their contributions to mucosal barrier function in the gastrointestinal tract with special emphasis on IBD.

2. The intestinal mucosal barrier

The gastrointestinal tract forms the largest surface in contact with the external environment. The intestinal mucosal barrier separates the internal intestinal tissues from an estimated 10^{14} organisms (Savage, 1977), and is composed of a physical barrier as well as specialized immune cells, primed to react if the physical barrier is breached.

2.1 Anatomy and function of the physical barrier

The physical barrier is comprised of an outer mucus layer less than a millimeter thick, and a single layer of epithelial cells joined together by tight junctions (Figure 1). The main structural component of the outer mucus layer is the heavily O-glycosylated glycoprotein MUC2, which is produced by goblet cells and gives mucus its viscous properties. The outer mucus layer was recently discovered to contain within it two distinct layers: an outer loose mucus layer with high numbers of commensal bacteria, and a dense inner layer that is sterile, containing high concentrations of antimicrobial molecules including nonspecific antimicrobial peptides and specific antimicrobial immunoglobulins (IgA) (Johansson et al., 2008). Commensal bacteria contribute to the function of the mucosal barrier by inducing the production of IgA, recruiting intraepithelial lymphocytes, and providing a physical blockade to prevent the colonization of pathogens (Umesaki et al., 1999).

The second component of the physical mucosal barrier is the single layer of epithelial cells supporting the outer mucus layer. The majority of epithelial cells are transporting enterocytes, but specialized epithelial cell types contribute to mucosal barrier integrity by producing the main constituents of the mucus layer, which minimizes microbial contact with the epithelium. Additionally, epithelial cells have a dense glycocalyx overlaying microvillar projections that prevent microbial attachment (Linden et al., 2008; L. Shen & Turner, 2006). The epithelial barrier needs to be selective to allow the absorption of essential nutrients while preventing the entry of potentially noxious compounds. As depicted in Figure 1, tight junctions that connect the epithelial cells allow the cellular barrier to respond to changes in the environment by regulating the tight junction protein composition, which leads to general or ion-selective changes in paracellular permeability (Arrieta et al., 2006).

In both animal models of IBD and the clinical disease in humans, changes in the physical mucosal barrier have been observed. In patients suffering from UC, MUC2 protein levels are significantly decreased during active phases of the disease, resulting in a thinner protective mucus layer (Hinoda et al., 1998; Tytgat et al., 1996). In animal models of chronic intestinal inflammatory conditions that cycle between active and quiescent phases, paracellular permeability remains increased regardless of the inflammatory state, whereas transcellular permeability is only increased during active inflammation (Porras et al., 2006). Similar observations have been made in humans, where patients with quiescent CD have significantly increased intestinal permeability when compared to controls (Wyatt et al.,

1993). It is believed that the sustained increase in paracellular permeability, indicative of epithelial cell layer dysfunction, contributes to the chronic nature of the disease.

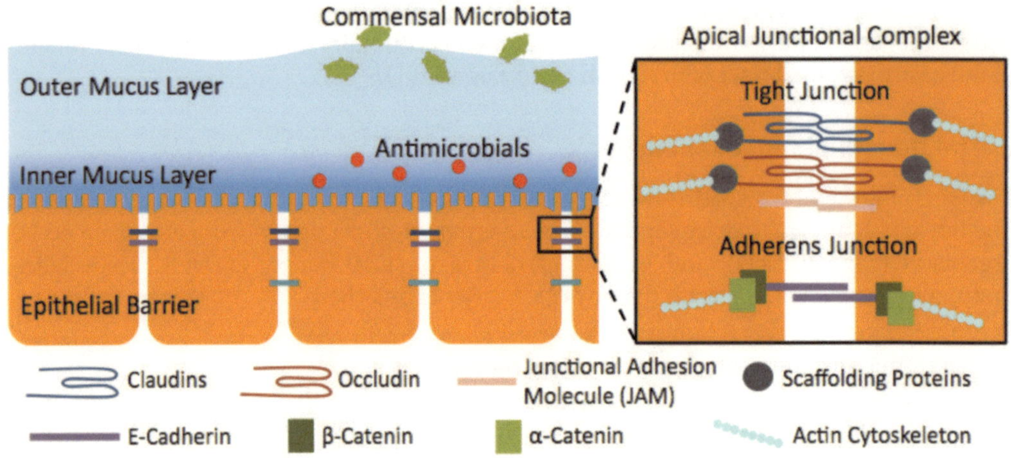

Fig. 1. The physical intestinal mucosal barrier. A single layer of epithelial cells linked together at the apical junctional complex (AJC) and an overlying mucus layer form the physical mucosal barrier. AJCs are comprised of tight junctions and adherens junctions. The protein composition of the tight junction is dynamic, and different claudin-family proteins as well as varying levels of occludin and the junctional adhesion molecule (JAM) allow for specific alterations of paracellular permeability. The foundation of the adherens junction is formed by contacts between epithelial cadherin (E-cadherin)-catenin complexes, which functions to connect neighboring epithelial cells and maintain cell polarity.

2.2 Immune cells of the mucosal barrier: Surveillance and tolerance

In addition to the physical boundary, there are immune cells and gut associated lymphoid tissues (GALT) situated within and below the epithelium. In a healthy intestine these cells and tissues strike a balance between immunity and tolerance, and maintain barrier function. The intestinal tract harbors vast populations of leukocytes. Innate immune cells typically mediate the first line of host defense, and in the intestine these include dendritic cells, macrophages, natural killer (NK) cells, γδ T cells, NKT cells and polymorphonuclear cells (Meresse & Cerf-Bensussan, 2009). Innate immunity evolved to recognize molecular signatures within the products of microbes that are essential to microbial survival. The innate immune system is comprised of pathogen recognition receptors (PRRs), such as toll-like receptors (TLR) and nucleotide-binding and oligomerization domain-like receptors (NLR), which recognize pathogen-associated molecular patterns (PAMPs). Binding of PAMPs to their cognate PRR activates signaling pathways that in turn activate host defense mechanisms. Different cell types have distinct immune functions; they express different combinations and levels of PRRs, and the downstream targets of PRR signaling are cell specific (Wells et al., 2010). Consequently, PAMP-PRR signaling mediates cell specific responses that enable the surrounding tissue to adapt to the dynamic intestinal environment.

Additionally, intestinal tissues are unique in that they harbor large numbers of adaptive immune cells expressing effector or memory phenotypes (Mowat, 2003). These include IgA and IgG secreting plasma B cells and canonical αβ T cells located in the lamina propria.

Adaptive immune responses are antigen specific and typically facilitate expeditious removal of pathogens. In the gut however, adaptive immune tolerance is crucial for maintaining quiescent relationships with the microbial flora and food antigens. In this regard, the intestine is a prime inductive site for large numbers of adaptive T_{reg} cells that home back to the intestinal mucosa, where they help to maintain intestinal tolerance (Belkaid & Oldenhove, 2008; Coombes et al., 2007). Thus, innate and adaptive immune cells in the gut are primed for action so that they can maintain a tolerant immune environment, while still being able to rapidly respond to invading pathogens.

3. Interleukin-17

IL-17 is a central pro-inflammatory cytokine at mucosal surfaces, with important functions in innate and adaptive immunity, as well as host defense against extracellular pathogens. Originally named cytotoxic T-lymphocyte antigen (CTLA)-8, IL-17 was first described in the mid 1990s (prior to the identification of T_h17 cells) as a cytokine produced by activated $CD4^+$ T cells that acts on stromal cells to up regulate inflammatory and hematopoietic processes (Fossiez et al., 1996; Rouvier et al., 1993; Yao et al., 1995a). IL-17 is now best known as the signature cytokine secreted from the recently characterized T_h17 cells, however numerous innate cells can also produce IL-17, including innate-like γδ intraepithelial lymphocytes (IEL), natural killer (NK) T cells, lymphoid tissue inducer (LTi)-like cells, Paneth cells, and neutrophils, as well as other unidentified cell types (Buonocore et al., 2010; Cua & Tato, 2010; Doisne et al., 2011; L. Li et al., 2010; Maele et al., 2010; Michel et al., 2007; Shibata et al., 2007; Takahashi et al., 2006; Takatori et al., 2008). In the context of the intestinal mucosa, γδ IELs are currently the best-characterized innate sources of IL-17. γδ IELs reside at the intestinal mucosal surface between epithelial cells on the basolateral side of tight junctions. They play an essential role in the restitution of epithelial cells following mucosal injury through the production of growth factors, a distinct ability that does not occur in other mucosal T cell populations (Y. Chen et al, 2002). Additionally, γδ IELs play an essential role in controlling bacterial penetration across injured mucosal surfaces, and recruiting neutrophils following *Escherichia coli* infection by acting as the major source of early IL-17 (Ismail et al., 2009; Shibata et al., 2007).

Importantly, since the discovery of IL-17 additional IL-17 family members have been identified. The IL-17 cytokine family consists of six members in mammals: IL-17A (also called IL-17), IL-17B, IL-17C, IL-17D, IL-17E (also called IL-25), and IL-17F (X. Zhang et al., 2011). IL-17F shares 50% sequence homology with IL-17A, is also produced by T_h17 cells, binds the same receptor as IL-17A and in turn shares certain biological activities (Hymowitz et al., 2001). IL-17A and IL-17F are either produced as homodimeric cytokines or as heterodimers composed of IL-17A/F (Wright et al., 2007). When acting on fibroblasts, endothelial cells, or epithelial cells, both IL-17A and IL-17F induce the production of pro-inflammatory cytokines (notably IL-6 and IL-8), chemokines, antimicrobial peptides, and matrix metalloproteinases (Iwakura et al., 2011; Starners et al., 2001). Despite their similar pro-inflammatory actions, IL-17A and IL-17F appear to have distinct roles in mediating inflammatory processes and autoimmune diseases (*discussed later*). IL-17B, IL-17C, and IL-17D are the least well-characterized members of the IL-17 family. IL-17B and IL-17C have 27% homology with IL-17A, but are not produced by activated T cells and do not induce the same pro-inflammatory cytokines as IL-17A and IL-17F (H. Li et al., 2000). IL-17D, which is most similar to IL-17B with 27% sequence identity, is highly expressed in skeletal muscle,

brain, adipose, heart, and lung tissue, but poorly expressed in activated T cells. However, similar to IL-17A and IL-17F, IL-17D can induce the expression of IL-6 and IL-8 from endothelial cells (Starnes et al. 2002). Lastly, IL-17E has the most divergent primary sequence compared to IL-17A with 16% homology, and plays a role in pro-allergic type 2 immune responses (Angkasekwinai et al., 2007; Lee et al., 2001; Pan et al., 2001).
Despite the varying degrees of sequence homology and varying functions, the C-terminal region of each IL-17 family member is quite conserved, containing 4 cysteine and 2 serine residues. Three IL-17 crystal structures have been resolved thus far: IL-17A with its neutralizing antibody, IL-17F, and IL-17F with its receptor IL-17RA. These structures have demonstrated the 6 conserved residues adopt a cysteine knot fold, which differs from the canonical cysteine knot found in TGF-β and neurotrophin proteins due to the absence of two cysteine residues (Ely et al., 2009; Gerhardt et al., 2009; Hymowitz et al, 2001).

3.1 IL-17 receptor and signaling

Cytokine receptors are generally classified into six main categories: IL-1 receptors, class I cytokine receptors, class II cytokine receptors, TNF receptors, tyrosine kinase receptors and chemokine receptors (Wang et al., 2009). The IL-17 receptors do not belong to any of these categories based on their unique structure and cytokine interaction (X. Zhang et al., 2011).
The IL-17 receptor family contains 5 members: IL-17RA (or IL-17R), IL-17RB, IL-17RC, IL-17RD, and IL-17RE. IL-17B is known to signal through IL-17RB, IL-17C through IL-17RE, and IL-17E through IL-17RA/IL-17RB (Iwakura et al., 2011; Wright et al., 2008). The receptor for IL-17D remains unknown. IL-17RA and IL-17RC are normally required for IL-17A, IL-17F, and IL-17A/F signaling (Iwakura et al., 2011). However, the IL-17RA is highly expressed on mouse T cells, while IL-17RC is undetectable, and only IL-17A but not IL-17F can induce signaling (Ishigame et al., 2009). Thus, it appears in some cell types IL-17RC is dispensable for IL-17RA signaling. This has lead to the hypotheses that IL-17RA forms either a homodimeric signaling complex or that other subunits can pair with IL-17RA in some cell types that do not express IL-17RC (Gaffen, 2009). Clarification of the receptor complexes for IL-17A and IL-17F is important for understanding how a cell or tissue responds to IL-17A versus IL-17F and will undoubtedly reveal crucial aspects of tissue specific T_h17 responses.
Signaling through IL-17 receptors triggers pathways that are usually associated with innate immune signaling (F. Shen et al., 2005; Park et al., 2005). Classical T_h1 and T_h2 cytokines activate JAK/STAT signaling, however IL-17A and IL-17F mediate signaling through nuclear factor (NF)-κB, NF-κB activator 1 (Act1) and tumor necrosis factor (TNF) receptor associated factor 6 (TRAF6) (Chang et al., 2006; Schwandner et al., 2000; Yao et al., 1995b). This mode of signaling is similar to those used by TLRs and the IL-1 receptor family, which function in innate immunity. Furthermore, IL-17A and IL-17F generally induce events that are typical of early inflammation (Gaffen, 2009). Upon receptor binding, IL-17A and IL-17F induce expression of many pro-inflammatory genes including: the cytokines TNF, IL-1, IL-6, granulocye-colony stimulating factor (G-CSF) and granulocyte-macrophage (GM)-CSF; the chemokines CXCL1, CXCL5, IL-8, CCL2, and CCL7; antimicrobial defensins, and S100 proteins; as well as matrix metalloproteinases (MMP)-1, -3, and -13 (Iwakura et al., 2011). In this regard, signaling by IL-17A and IL-17F through an IL-17 receptor complex is considered to mediate innate-like inflammatory events.

3.2 Interleukin-17 and the mucosal barrier

Although the majority of the defined roles played by IL-17 in mucosal barrier function are related to innate and adaptive immune functions, IL-17 has also been found to directly regulate components of the physical mucosal barrier. In colonic epithelial monolayers IL-17A enhances tight junction formation by increasing claudins 1 and 2 association with the membrane (Kinugasa et al., 2000). Direct application of IL-17A to T84 monolayers increased transepithelial resistance and decreased manitol flux through monolayers. Thus, IL-17A may have an important role in maintaining tight junctions and epithelial restitution during repair processes. In airway epithelial cells IL-17A induces mucin gene expression, and it may have similar inductive effects in the intestine on goblet cells (Chen et al., 2003). IL-17A also induces expression of β-defensins in the colon (Ishigame et al., 2009). Furthermore, in subepithelial myofibroblasts, which sit just below the epithelium, IL-17A reduced TNF-α-induced secretion of pro-inflammatory cytokines, demonstrating that IL-17 is not implicitly a pro-inflammatory cytokine. Additionally, IL-17 receptor-deficient mice show increased dissemination of *S. typhimurium* from the gut (Raffatellu et al., 2008). Taken together, it appears IL-17 can dynamically regulate components of the physical intestinal epithelial barrier, and the barrier is dysfunctional when IL-17 signaling is impaired.

4. Adaptive immunity and T_h17 cell development

4.1 Induction of adaptive immunity

There are numerous locations in the gut where adaptive immune responses are initiated. These include organized lymphoid tissue such as Peyer's patches and isolated lymphoid follicles (ILF) that are embedded directly in the epithelial wall, and mesenteric lymph nodes (MLN), which are connected to the intestinal mucosa by draining lymphatic vessels (Figure 2, Mowat, 2003). Furthermore, there is evidence that adaptive responses occur directly in the lamina propria via dendritic cell and epithelial cell signaling (He et al., 2007).

Under homeostatic conditions, intestinal luminal contents are constitutively sampled and processed by professional antigen presenting cells (pAPC). pAPC present processed antigen to the naive T cell population, which has an infinite repertoire of antigen-specific receptors. Upon presentation of antigen to a T cell bearing a cognate receptor, the pAPC drives an antigen specific T cell response. Depending on the accompanying signals from the pAPC and surrounding environment, the T cell may become activated into an effector cell, anergic (unresponsive to antigen) or apoptotic. Classically there are three types of cells that act as pAPC: B cells, macrophages and dendritic cells. Arguably, antigen acquisition by dendritic cells is most critical for priming adaptive immune responses, as dendritic cells are the most efficient class of pAPC.

In Peyer's patches and ILF, antigen is transported from the lumen by microfold (M) cells to dendritic cells located in the follicle associated epithelium or the underlying subepithelial dome. From there, dendritic cells move into local T cell/follicular areas or drain to the MLN to initiate adaptive responses (Artis, 2008; Kelsall, 2008; Mowat, 2003). The other site for antigen entry is the non-follicular associated epithelium overlying the lamina propria. Under normal conditions antigen is moved across the non-follicular associated epithelium by receptor-mediated transport (Kelsall, 2008) and by dendritic cells located in the lamina propria, which project dendrites through the tight junctions into the lumen (Figure 2, Chieppa et al., 2006; Rescigno et al., 2001). When the epithelium is damaged, as occurs in IBD and pathogenic infections, antigens also enter directly.

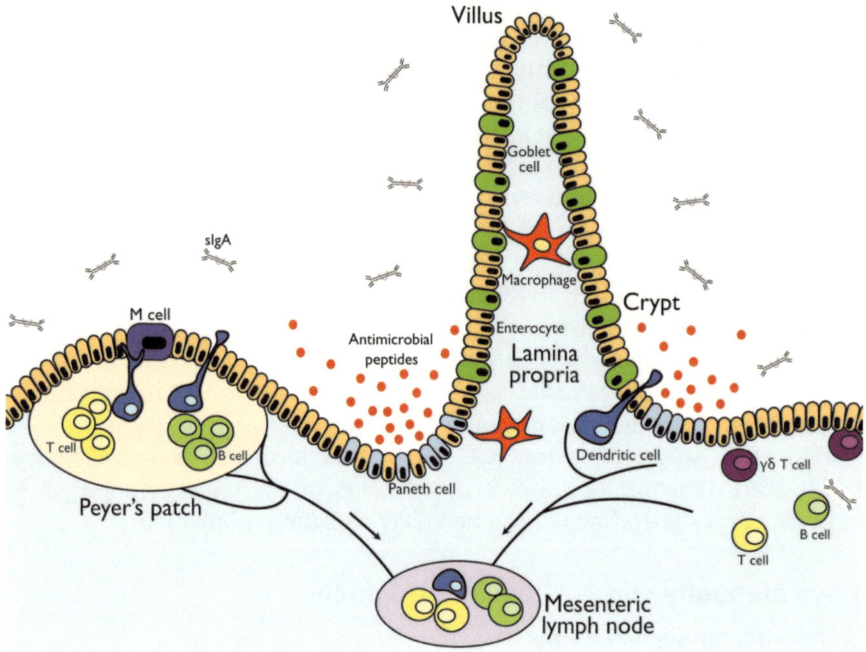

Fig. 2. Schematic of organized gastrointestinal lymphoid tissues. Antigens can be transported from the lumen to antigen presenting cells, such as dendritic cells (DC), by the specialized M cells of Peyer's patches where adaptive immune responses can be generated. Additionally, DCs are able to directly sample luminal antigens by projecting dendrites through the intestinal barrier. DCs can then migrate to local T cell areas, or drain to mesenteric lymph nodes (MLN) through lymphatic vessels. Other immune cells in the lamina propria include: mucosal macrophages, γδ T cells, αβ T cells and IgA-secreting B cells.

Dendritic cells are equipped to recognize microbial products with an array of PRR and in doing so, undergo a process of maturation in order to become proficient antigen presenters for naive T cells. In addition to down-regulating their phagocytic machinery and up-regulating antigen processing pathways, dendritic cells secrete an array of immuno-modulatory cytokines. At first, they express a mixed cytokine profile. However, a dominant cytokine profile emerges and this dictates the type of adaptive immunity that develops (Wilson et al., 2009). The specific constellation of PRRs that are engaged on a dendritic cell is what determines their cytokine profile.

4.2 Adaptive immune cells

The defining feature of an adaptive immune system is antigen-specific immunity. The first encounter with antigen leads to clonal expansion of a few antigen-specific lymphocytes, which target immune responses towards their cognate antigens. Some of these cells become long-lived memory cells and they enable the immune system to remember antigen that has already been encountered, so that upon re-exposure a tailored immune response is quickly recalled. The cells of the adaptive immune system are T and B-lymphocytes. Each lymphocyte bears a surface receptor of a single specificity that binds antigen in a highly specific manner. T and B cell development generates an infinitely diverse repertoire of T and B cell receptors, so that in theory any possible antigen can be recognized. Classical naive T cells express an αβ T cell receptor and a co-receptor, which comes in two flavors: CD4 or CD8. Accordingly, CD4 expressing T cells are called $CD4^+$ T cells and CD8 expressing T cells are called $CD8^+$ T cells. $CD4^+$ T cells are also called T helper cells because following establishment of the adaptive phase by innate defenses, $CD4^+$ T cells become the central coordinators of the adaptive immune response. The primary effector function of $CD4^+$ T cells is to help and regulate other immune cells. Upon encountering their cognate antigen on mature pAPCs, $CD4^+$ T cells proliferate and differentiate into antigen-specific effector cells.

4.2.1 T Helper cell differentiation

There are currently four well characterized lineages of T_h cells: T_h1, T_h2, T_{reg}, and T_h17 (Figure 3). Naïve $CD4^+$ T cells differentiate into T_h1 cells in the presence of IFNγ and IL-12, which enhances the expression of the principal T_h1 transcription factors, T-box family of transcription factors (T-bet) and the signal transducers and activators of transcription protein 4 (STAT4). Effector cytokines produced by T_h1 cells include IFNγ, TNFα and IL-2, which help to clear intracellular pathogens. T_h2 cells differentiate in the presence of IL-4, which activates STAT6 and leads to the expression of the transcription factor GATA binding protein 3 (GATA3). T_h2-derived cytokines, including IL-4, IL-5 and IL-13, are important in mediating asthma and allergic responses (Zhu & Paul, 2010).

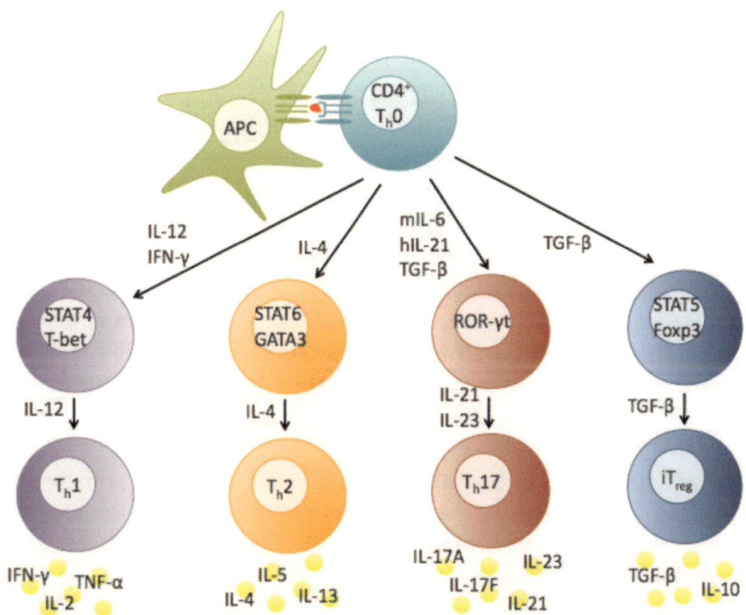

Fig. 3. T helper cell differentiation. After encountering an antigen-presenting cell (APC) within the periphery, naïve T helper (T_h0) cells are able to differentiate into one of four T_h subsets based on the cytokine milieu present. In the presence of interleukin (IL)-12, the activation of transcription factors STAT4 and T-bet lead to T_h1 development, whereas IL-4 results in the activation of STAT6 and GATA3, leading to T_h2 development. In the presence of TGF-β, T_h0 cells will differentiate into inducible T regulatory (iT_{reg}) cells following transcription of STAT5 and Foxp3, unless IL-6 (in mouse) or IL-21 (in human) is present in addition to TGF-β, in which case T_h17 cells will develop following ROR-γt transcription.

Most T_{reg} cells, termed natural T_{reg} (nT_{reg}) cells, are fully differentiated before leaving the thymus, upon TCR stimulation and encountering IL-2 or IL-15. This results in the activation of STAT5 and leads to forkhead box (Fox)p3 expression, the characteristic transcription factor of T_{reg} cells (Burchill et al., 2008). Once these cells leave the thymus, they can home to mucosal surfaces, including the GI tract where the presence of TGF-β helps them to maintain their regulatory phenotype (Barnes & Powrie, 2009). TGF-β is also able to induce the expression of Foxp3 in naïve T cells within the periphery, resulting in inducible T_{reg} (iT_{reg}) cells. Primarily through the production of IL-10, nT_{reg} and iT_{reg} cells share the same suppressive phenotype and function to maintain peripheral tolerance and prevent autoimmunity (Maloy et al., 2003; Read et al., 2000; Zheng & Rudensky, 2007).

T_h17 cellular differentiation also depends on TGF-β, however with the additional presence of IL-6 in mice (Veldhoen et al., 2006), or IL-21 in humans (L. Yang et al., 2008), Foxp3 expression is inhibited and STAT3 activation leads to expression of the transcriptional regulator retinoic acid receptor-related orphan receptor-γt (RORγt), which drives T_h17 differentiation (Ivanov et al., 2006). Once differentiated, T_h17 cells are highly responsive to IL-21 and IL-23, cytokines that function to maintain the T_h17 phenotype. The principle effector cytokines produced by T_h17 cells include IL-17A, IL-17F, IL-21, and IL-22.

5. Role of IL-17 in enteric infections

Several murine models of infectious disease highlight the presence and importance of IL-17 in intestinal inflammation: *Helicobacter hepaticus, Salmonella enterica* serotype *typhimurium*, and *Citrobacter rodentium*. In *H. hepaticus*-induced typhlocolitis, a model of T-cell independent innate inflammation, local increases in IL-23 induced the secretion of IL-17 from non-T cell sources (Hue et al., 2006). A similar study using the same *H. hepaticus* model of bacteria-driven innate colitis confirmed the IL-23-dependent increases in IL-17, and went on to characterize the IL-17-producing cells. This led to the identification of a novel innate lymphoid cell population that accumulates in the inflamed colon, and is able to mediate acute and chronic innate colitis in response to IL-23 stimulation (Buonocore et al., 2010).

In the second infectious model with *S. typhimurium*, initial inflammatory responses are important to contain the infection as localized gastroenteritis, and prevent the systemic spread of bacteria. Macrophages and dendritic cells infected with *S. typhimurium* are a major source of IL-23, and five hours post- *S. typhimurium* infection, IL-17 expression is markedly up regulated (Raffetulla et al., 2008, 2009). The increased IL-17 production resulted in IL-17-dependent intestinal epithelial induction of antimicrobial peptides (Raffatellu et al. 2009). In IL-23p19-deficient mice, the increased expression of IL-17 during *S. typhimurim* infection was abrogated. Although αβ T cells were found to be the predominant cell type expressing the IL-23R, there was a marked increase in γδ T cells expressing the IL-23R during *S. typimurium* infection. γδ T cell-deficient mice demonstrated a blunted expression of IL-17, suggesting that γδ T cells are a significant source, but not the only source of IL-17 during an acute bacterial infection (Godinez et al., 2009).

Lastly, *C. rodentium* is a non-invasive bacterium that transiently colonizes the large intestine of mice. In addition to serving as a model for attaching/effacing bacteria, *C. rodentium* infection can be used a model of IBD, as the infection-associated pathology shares many features with IBD (Mundy et al., 2005). The first evidence of IL-17 involvement in *C. rodentium* infection implicated its importance during the peak and late stages of infection, demonstrating a role for adaptive T_h17 cells in clearing the infection (Symonds et al., 2009;

Zheng et al., 2008). More recent evidence also suggests there is an early T_h17-like response during *C. rodentium* infection that is dependent on the activation of the innate immune receptors Nod1 and Nod2 (Geddes et al., 2011). Whether or not this will directly relate to the *NOD2* coding variants identified as risk factors for IBD (Hugot & Cho, 2002) remains to be explored.

6. Role of IL-17 in IBD pathogenesis

Since the discovery of IL-23 as a critical regulator of T_h17 responses and that there are increased numbers of T_h17 cells in IBD patients (Kleinschek et al., 2009), the importance of T_h17 cells and their effector cytokines has been an active area of IBD research. To help elucidate the precise role of the T_h17 subset, three principle animal models of intestinal inflammation resembling CD have been employed: T cell transfer models of colitis, trinitobenzene sulfonic acid (TNBS)-induced colitis, and dextran sulfate sodium (DSS)-induced colitis. With the T cell-transfer model, the initiation of colitis via an adaptive immune response is modeled through the transfer of naïve $CD4^+$ T cells ($CD45RB^{high}$) to immune-deficient mice that lack T cells and B cells, such as recombination activating gene (RAG)-deficient mice, or severe combined immune-deficient (SCID) mice. The naïve cells introduced develop into pro-inflammatory effector T cells in the absence of a mature immune cell population ($CD45RB^{low}$) containing T_{reg} cells, and spontaneous intestinal inflammation develops (Powrie et al., 1994a). TNBS-induced colitis is also dependent on the adaptive immune system, where mucosal inflammation following the administration of the haptenizing agent TNBS is mediated by T_h1 and T_h17 responses (Alex et al, 2009). In contrast to the latter two models, DSS-induced colitis does not require T cells to initiate inflammation. DSS is thought to disrupt the epithelial barrier, resulting in the activation of lamina propria cells by the normal microflora. In the acute DSS model both T_h1 and T_h17 cells accumulate; however, if the DSS is given in several cycles to establish chronic inflammation, the cytokine profile shifts towards T_h2 (Alex et al., 2009). Therefore, acute DSS can be used as a model for CD whereas chronic DSS is more representative of UC.

6.1 The IL-23/T_h17 axis and IBD

IL-23 has been found to critically mediate intestinal inflammation through both adaptive and innate immune pathways. Interestingly, an uncommon coding variant of the *IL23R* gene, which encodes a subunit of the IL-23 receptor, was found to confer strong protection against both CD and UC (Duerr et al., 2006). T cell transfer models show that IL-23 is required for spontaneous development of colitis by activated $CD4^+$ T cells (Elson et al., 2007; Hue et al., 2006). Similarly, RAG deficient mice that are also IL-23p19 or IL-12p40 deficient (do not produce IL-23) do not develop spontaneous intestinal inflammation, whereas RAG deficient mice that lack IL-12p35 (do not produce IL-12) still develop colitis (Hue et al., 2006). In these experimental systems IL-23 and not IL-12 drives intestinal inflammation. Interestingly, though IL-23p19 deficient mice fail to develop intestinal inflammation, they still develop a systemic inflammatory response (Hue et al., 2006). This demonstrates that IL-23 driven inflammation by $CD4^+$ T cells is localized to the gut. A transfer model with bacteria-reactive $CD4^+$ T cells showed that neutralization of IL-23p19 with a monoclonal antibody attenuates intestinal inflammation and that individually, bacteria-reactive T_h17 cells induce more inflammation than bacteria-reactive T_h1 cells (Elson et al., 2007). The latter study also highlights that T_h1 and T_h17 cells have an overlapping ability to promote pathologic responses. Although IL-12 as a T_h1 inducing cytokine is dispensable for initiating colitis, T_h1 responses should not be considered insignificant in inflammatory bowel disease. Previous studies have shown that neutralization of IFN-γ (signature T_h1 cytokine) prevents intestinal inflammation and severe wasting, and transfer of IFN-γ deficient T cells into RAG deficient mice fails to induce colitis (Ito & Fathman, 1997; O'Connor et al., 2009; Powrie et al., 1994b). Taken together, these results suggest that although IFN-γ still appears to be the main effector cytokine driving the cell-transfer colitis model, IL-23 and T_h17 responses are essential to support the development of chronic inflammation.

6.2 Contributions of IL-17A and IL-17F to IBD

There are multiple lines of evidence to suggest that blocking IL-17A and IL-17F would prevent intestinal inflammation as both cytokines robustly induce neutrophil recruitment and pro-inflammatory cytokines, blocking IL-23 prevents development of pathogenic T_h17 cells and colitis in animal models, and blocking IL-23 signaling is beneficial for treating CD. Along these same lines, IL-17R-deficient mice are significantly protected from TNBS-induced colitis, despite no change in the levels of IL-23 or IL-12 and IFN-γ (Z. Zhang et al., 2006). Thus, it was unexpected that neutralization of IL-17A exacerbated intestinal inflammation in the dextran sodium sulfate (DSS) colitis model (Ogawa et al., 2004). Animals treated with an IL-17A monoclonal antibody had enhanced inflammatory cell infiltrates into the mucosa and submucosa, more severe mucosal injury and drastically increased weight loss. Moreover, addition of IL-17A attenuated the response (Ogawa et al, 2004). These results were confirmed in IL-17A knockout mice, which also developed more severe DSS-induced colitis (X. Yang et al., 2008). Interestingly, this same study showed that IL-17F knockout mice, unlike IL-17A knockouts, were protected from DSS-induced colitis. Colons of IL-17F deficient mice showed little pathology and extremely low levels of pro-inflammatory cytokines (Yang et al, 2008). Using a T cell transfer model, IL-17A secretion by T_h17 cells was also protective against the development of intestinal inflammation, as IL-17A deficient T cells transferred into RAG deficient mice caused more severe disease than transferred wildtype T cells (O'Connor et al, 2009). Additionally, IL-17A has been shown to directly inhibit T_h1 cells and suppress T_h1 mediated intestinal inflammation (Awasthi & Kuchroo, 2009). Taken together, these data suggest that IL-17A has protective roles in acute tissue inflammation and that IL-17F has pathogenic functions. However, there has also been some evidence that IL-17A is not protective. T cells deficient in ROR-γt, and therefore unable to differentiate into T_h17 effector cells, were unable to induce colitis when transferred to RAG-deficient mice, but treatment with IL-17A caused colitis after the transfer of ROR-γt-deficient cells (Leppkes et al., 2009). Therefore, additional work on the mechanisms, function, and regulation of IL-17A/F in the context of intestinal inflammation is required before confident and definitive conclusions can be drawn.

7. Conclusion

Knowledge of T_h17 cells and their characteristic cytokines IL-17A and IL-17F has rapidly progressed. Likewise, significant progress has been made towards understanding their role in regulating the gut environment. However, there are numerous outstanding questions.
The T_h17 subset is unequivocally associated with chronic inflammatory bowel diseases, and the current belief is that they are instigated by a loss of tolerance to the intestinal microflora.

In addition to T_h17 cells, dysregulated T_h1 and Foxp3$^+$ iTreg responses are also involved. Yet, the precise nature of the relationship between T_h17 cells and T_h1 *as well as* T_h17 cells and Foxp3$^+$ iTregs is unclear. Furthermore, in the gut there appears to be multiple cellular sources of IL-17A and IL-17F, in addition to heterogeneous expression of their receptors, IL-17RA and IL-17RC. Our understanding of how IL-17A and IL-17F mediate their cell specific effects and how this plays out during steady states, infectious disease and chronic inflammation in the intestinal tract is currently in progress. Beneficial results have been obtained using antibodies to neutralize IL-12p40 in Crohn's disease and genome wide association studies implicate the IL-23-T_h17 axis in both Crohn's disease and ulcerative colitis. Together these data suggest therapies specifically targeting T_h17 responses might provide better treatments. However, animal models have also shown IL-17A and IL-17F to critically mediate host protection and components of normal barrier function. Thus given these roles, targeted interventions of IL-17A and IL-17F will need careful consideration.

Inflammatory bowel diseases are a complex set of diseases involving pre-disposing genetic factors and environmental triggers. The emerging IL-23-T_h17 axis represents one significant component of these diseases among several. Though progress has been made, a substantial amount of work remains to identify pathways and mechanisms that connect T_h17 cells, IL-17A and IL-17F to the etiology of inflammatory bowel diseases. In particular, genome wide association studies have established a key role for innate immunity in these diseases. Most well known are *NOD2* and autophagy genes *ATG16L* and *IRGM* involved in bacterial detection and processing. In this regard, much less is known about IL-23, IL-17A and IL-17F in aberrant innate immune responses. For now we can ascertain that both innate and adaptive immunity coordinate an imbalanced relationship between host and microflora that leads to chronic intestinal inflammation, and that T_h17 cells and the IL-17A/F cytokine network participate in both arms of the immune system that has gone awry.

8. References

Aggarwal, S., Ghilardi, N., Xie, M., de Sauvage, F. J. & Gurney, A. L. (2003). Interleukin-23 Promotes a Distinct CD4 T Cell Activation State Characterized by the Production of Interleukin-17. *Journal of Biological Chemistry*. Vol:278, No:3, pp. 1910-1914

Alex, P., Zachos, N. C., Nguyen, T., Gonzales, L., Chen, T. E., Conklin, L. S., Centola, M. & Li, X. (2009). Distinct Cytokine Patterns Identified from Multiplex Profiles of Murine DSS and TNBS-Induced Colitis. *Inflammatory Bowel Disease*. Vol:15, No:3, pp. 341-352

Angkasekwinai, P., Park, H., Wang, Y.H., Wang, Y.H., Chang, S. H., Corry, D. B., Lui, Y.J., Zhu, Z. & Dong, C. (2007). Interleukin 25 Promotes the Initiation of Proallergic Type 2 Responses. *Journal of Experimental Medicine*. Vol:204, No:7, pp. 1509-1517

Arisawa, T., Tahara, T., Shibata, T., Nagasaka, M., Nakamura, M., Kamiya, Y., Fujita, H., Nakamura, M., Yoshioka, D., Arima, Y., Okubo, M., Hirata, I. & Nakano, H. (2008). The Influence of Polymorphisms of Interleukin-17A and Interleukin-17F Genes on the Susceptibility to Ulcerative Colitis. *Journal of Clinical Immunology*. Vol:28, No:1, pp. 44-49

Arrieta, M. C., Bistritz, L. & Meddings, J. B. (2006) Alterations in Intestinal Permeability. *Gut*. Vol:55, pp. 1512-1520

Artis, D. (2008). Epithelial-Cell Recognition of Commensal Bacteria and Maintenance of Immune Homeostasis in the Gut. *Nature Reviews Immunology*. Vol:8, No:6, pp. 411-420

Awasthi, A. & Kuchroo, V. K. (2009). IL-17A Directly Inhibits Th1 Cells and Thereby Suppresses Development of Intestinal Inflammation. *Nature Immunology*. Vol:10, No:6, pp. 568-570

Barnes, M. J. & Powrie, F. (2009). Regulatory T Cells Reinforce Intestinal Homeostasis. *Immunity*. Vol:31, pp. 401-411

Belkaid, Y. & Oldenhove, G. (2008). Tuning Microenvironments: Induction of Regulatory T Cells by Dendritic Cells. *Immunity*. Vol:29, No:3, pp. 362-371

Billiau, A., Heremans, H., Vandekerckhove, F., Dijkmans, R., Sobis, H., Meulepas, E. & Carton, H. (1988). Enhancement of Experimental Allergic Encephalomyelitis in Mice by Antibodies Against IFN-γ. *Journal of Immunology*. Vol:140, No:5, pp. 1506-1510

Buonocore, S., Ahern, P. P., Uhlig, H. H., Ivanov, I. I., Littman, D. R., Maloy, K. J. & Powrie, F. (2010). Innate Lymphoid Cells Drive Interleukin-23-Dependent Innate Intestinal Pathology. *Nature*. Vol:464, pp. 1371-1375

Burchill, M. A., Yang, J., Vang, K. B., Moon, J. J., Chu, H. H., Lio, C. J., Vegoe, A. L., Hsieh, C., Jenkins, M. K. & Farrar, M. A. (2008). Linked T Cell Receptor and Cytokine Signaling Govern the Development of the Regulatory T Cell Repertoire. *Immunity*. Vol:28, pp. 112-121

Chang, S. H., Park, H. & Dong, C. (2006). Act1 Adaptor Protein Is an Immediate and Essential Signaling Component of Interleukin-17 Receptor. *Journal of Biological Chemistry*. Vol:281, No:47, pp. 35603-35607

Chen, Y., Chou, K., Fuchs, E., Havran, W. L. & Boismenu, R. (2002). Protection of the Intestinal Mucosa by Intraepithelial γδ T Cells. *PNAS*. Vol:99, No:22, pp. 14338-14343

Chen, Y., Thai, P., Zhao, Y., Ho, Y., DeSouza, M. M. & Wu, R. (2003). Stimulation of Airway Mucin Gene Expression by Interleukin (IL)-17 through IL-6 Paracrine/Autocrine Loop. *Journal of Biological Chemistry*. Vol:278, No:19, pp. 17036-17043

Cher, D. J. & Mosmann, T. R. (1987). Two Types of Murine Helper T Cell Clone. II. Delayed-Type Hypersensitivity is Mediated by Th1 Clones. *Journal of Immunology*. Vol:138, No:11, pp. 3688-3694

Chieppa, M., Rescigno, M., Huang, A. Y. & Germain, R. N. (2006). Dynamic Imaging of Dendritic Cell Extension into the Small Bowel Lumen in Response to Epithelial Cell TLR Engagement. *Journal of Experimental Medicine*. Vol:203, No:13, pp. 2841-2852

Coombes, J. L., Siddigui, K. R., Arancibia-Cárcamo, C. V., Hall, J., Sun, C. M., Belkaid, Y. & Powrie, F. (2007). A Functionally Specialized Population of Mucosal CD103+ DCs Induces Foxp3+ Regulatory T cells via a TGF-beta and Retinoic Acid-Dependent Mechanism. *Journal of Experimental Medicine*. Vol:204, No:8, pp. 1757-1764

Cua, D. J., Sherlock, J., Chen, Y., Murphy, C. A., Joyce, B., Seymour, B., Lucian, L., To, W., Kwan, S., Churakova, T., Zurawski, S., Wiekowski, M., Lira, S. A., Gorman, D., Kastelein, R. A. & Sedgwick, J. D. (2003). Interleukin-23 rather than Interleukin-12 is the Critical Cytokine for Autoimmune Inflammation of the Brain. *Nature*. Vol:421, pp. 744-748

Cua, D. J. & Tato, C. M. (2010). Innate IL-17-Producting Cells: The Sentinels of the Immune System. *Nature Reviews*. Vol:10, pp. 479-489

Doisne, J. M., Soulard, V., Bécourt, C., Amniai, L., Henrot, P., Havenar-Daughton, C., Blanchet, C., Zitvogel, L., Ryffel, B., Cavaillon, J. M., Marie, J. C., Couillin, I. & Benlagha, K. (2011). Cutting Edge: Crucial Role of IL-1 and IL-23 in the Innate IL-17 Response of Peripheral Lymph Node NK1.1- Invariant NKT Calls to Bacteria. *Journal of Immunology*. Vol:186, pp. 662-666

Duerr, R. H., Taylor, K. D., Brant, S. R., Rioux, J. D., Silverberg, M. S., Daly, M. J., Steinhart, A. H., Abraham, C., Regueiro, M., Griffiths, A., Dassopoulos, T., Bitton, A., Yang, H., Targan, S., Datta, L. W., Kistner, E. O., Schumm, L. P., Lee, A. T., Gregersen, P. K., Barmada, M. M., Rotter, J. I., Nicolae, D. L. & Cho, J. H. (2006). A Genome-Wide Association Study Identifies *IL23R* as an Inflammatory Bowel Disease Gene. *Science*. Vol:314, pp. 1461-1463

Elson, C. O., Cong, Y., Weaver, C. T., Schoeb, T. R., McClanahan, T. K., Fick, R. B. & Kastelein, R. A. (2007). Monoclonal Anti-Interleukin 23 Reverses Active Colitis in a T Cell-Mediated Model in Mice. *Gastroenterology*. Vol:132, No:7, pp. 2359-2370

Ely, L. K., Fischer, S. & Garcia, K. C. (2009). Structural Basis of Receptor Sharing by Interleukin 17 Cytokines. *Nature Immunology*. Vol:10, No:12, pp. 1245-1251

Fossiez, F., Djossou, O., Pascale, C., Flores-Romo, L., Ait-Yahia, S., Maat, C., Pin, J., Garrone, P., Garcia, E., Saeland, S., Blanchard, D., Gillard, C., Mahapatra, B. D., Rouvier, E., Golstein, P. & Banchereau, J. (1996). T Cell Interleukin-17 Induces Stromal Cells to Produce Proinflammatory and Hematopoietic Cytokines. *Journal of Experimental Medicine*. Vol:183, pp. 2593-2603

Fujino, S., Andoh, A., Bamba, S., Ogawa, A., Hata, K, Araki, Y., Bamba, T. & Fujiyama, Y. (2003). Increased Expression of Interleukin-17 in Inflammatory Bowel Disease. *Gut*. Vol:52, pp. 65-70

Fuss, I. J., Neurath, M., Boirivant, M., Klein, J. S., de la Motte, C., Strong, S. A., Fiocchi, C. & Strober, W. (1996). Disparate CD4+ Lamina Propria (LP) Lymphokine Secretion Profiles in Inflammatory Bowel Disease. Crohn's Disease LP Cells Manifest Increased Secretion of IFN-gamma whereas Ulcerative Colitis LP Cells Manifest Increased Secretion of IL-5. *Journal of Immunology*. Vol:157, No:3, pp. 1261-1270

Fuss, I. J., Heller, F., Boirivant, M., Leon, F., Yoshida, M., Fichtner-Feigl, S., Yang, Z., Exley, M., Kitani, A., Blumberg, R. S., Mannon, P. & Strober, W. (2004). Nonclassical CD1d-Restricted NK T Cells that Produce IL-13 Characterize an Atypical Th2 Response in Ulcerative Colitis. *Journal of Clinical Investigation*. Vol:113, No:10, pp. 1490-1497

Gaffen, S. L. (2009). Structure and Signaling in the IL-17 Receptor Superfamily. *Nature Reviews Immunology*. Vol:9, No:8, 556-585

Geddes, K., Rubino, S. J., Magalhaes, J. G., Streutker, C., Bourhis, L. L., Cho, J. H., Robertson, S. J., Kim, C. J., Kaul, R., Philpott, D. J. & Girardin, S. E. (2011). Identification of an Innate T Helper Type 17 Response to Intestinal Bacterial Pathogens. *Nature Medicine*. Advanced Online Publication.

Gerhardt, S., Abbott, W. M., Hargreaves, D., Pauptit, R. A., Davies, R. A., Needham, M. R. C., Langham, C., Barker, W., Aziz, A., Snow, M. J., Dawson, S., Welsh, F., Wilkinson, T., Vaugan, T., Beste, G., Bishop, S., Popovic, B., Rees, G., Sleeman, M., Tuske, S. J., Coales, S. J., Hamuro, Y. & Russell, C. (2009). Structure of IL-17A in

Complex with a Potent, Fully Human Neutralizing Antibody. *Journal of Molecular Biology*. Vol:394, pp. 905-921

Godinez, I., Raffatellu, M., Chu, H., Piaxão, T. A., Haneda, T., Santos, R. L., Bevins, C. L., Tsolis, R. M. & Bäumler, A. J. (2009). Interleukin-23 Orchestrates Mucosal Responses to *Salmonella enterica* Serotype Typhimurium in the Intestine. *Infection and Immunity*. Vol:77, No:1, pp. 387-398

He, B., Xu, W., Santini, P. A., Polydorides, A. D., Chiu, A., Estrella, J., Shan, M., Chadburn, A., Vilanacci, V., Plebani, A., Knowles, D. M., Rescigno, M. & Cerutti, A. (2007). Intestinal Bacteria Trigger T Cell-Independent Immunoglobulin A(2) Class Switching by Inducing Epithelial-Cell Secretion of the Cytokine APRIL. *Immunity*. Vol:26, No:6, pp. 812-826

Hemdan, N. Y. A., Birkenmeier, G., Wichmann, G. El-Saad, A. M. A., Krieger, T., Conrad, K. & Sack, U. (2010). Interleukin-17-Producing T Helper Cells in Autoimmunity. *Autoimmunity Reviews*. Vol:9, pp. 785-792

Hinoda, Y., Akashi, H., Suwa, T., Itoh, F., Adachi, M., Endo, T., Satoh, M., Xing, P. X. & Imai, K. (1998). Immunohistochemical Detection of MUC2 Mucin Core Protein in Ulcerative Colitis. *Journal of Clinical Laboratory Analysis*. Vol:12, pp. 150-153

Hoentjen, F. & van Bodegraven, A. A. (2009). Safety of Anti-Tumor Necrosis Factor Therapy in Inflammatory Bowel Disease. *World Journal of Gastroenterology*. Vol:15, No:17, pp. 2067-2073

Hue, S., Ahern, P., Buonocore, S., Kullberg, M. C., Cua, D. J., McKenzie, B. S., Powrie, F. & Maloy, K. J. (2006). Interleukin-23 Drives Innate and T-Cell Mediated Intestinal Inflammation. *Journal of Experimental Medicine*. Vol:203, No:11, pp. 2473-2483

Hugot, J. P. & Cho, J. H. (2002). Update on Genetics of Inflammatory Bowel Disease. *Current Opinion in Gastroenterology*. Vol:18, No:4, pp. 410-415

Hymowitz, S. G., Filvaroff, E. H., Yin, J., Lee, J., Cai, L., Risser, P., Maruoka, M., Mao, W., Foster, J., Kelley, R. F., Pan, G., Gurney, A. L., de Vos, A. M. & Starovansnik, M. A. (2001). IL-17s adopt a cystine knot fold: structure and activity of a novel cytokine, IL-17F, and implications for receptor binding. *The EMBO Journal*. Vol:20, No:19, pp. 5332-5341

Ishigame, H., Kakuta, S., Nagai, T., Kadoki, M., Nambu, A., Komiyama, Y., Fujikado, N., Tanahashi, Y., Akitsu, A., Kotaki, H., Sudo, K., Nakae, S., Sasakawa, C. & Iwakura, Y. (2009). Differential Roles of Interleukin-17A and -17F in Host Defense against Mucoepithelial Bacterial Infection and Allergic Responses. *Immunity*. Vol:30, pp. 108-119

Ismail, A. S., Behrendt, C. L. & Hooper, L. V. (2009). Reciprocal Interactions between Commensal Bacteria and γδ Intraepithelial Lymphocytes during Mucosal Injury. *Journal of Immunology*. Vol:182, pp. 3047-3054

Ito, H. & Fathman, C. G. (1997). CD45RBhigh CD4+ T Cells from IFN-gamma Knockout Mice Do Not Induce Wasting Disease. *Journal of Autoimmunity*. Vol:10, No:5, pp. 455-459

Ivanov, I. I., McKenzie, B. S., Zhou, L., Tadokoro, C. E., Lepelley, A., Lafaille, J. J., Cua, D. J. & Littman, D. R. (2006). The Orphan Nuclear Receptor RORγt Directs the Differentiation Program of Proinflammatory IL-17^{+} T Helper Cells. *Cell*. Vol:126, pp. 1121-1133

Iwakura, Y., Ishigame, H., Saijo, S. & Nakae, S. (2011). Functional Specialization of Interleukin-17 Family Members. *Immunity*. Vol:34, pp. 149-162

Jacob, C. O., Holoshitz, J., van der Meide, P., Strober, S. & McDevitt, H. O. (1989). Heterogeneous Effects of IFN-γ in Adjuvant Arthritis. *Journal of Immunology*. Vol:142, No:5, pp. 1500-1505

Johansson, M. E. V., Phillipson, M., Petersson, J., Velcich, A., Holm, L. & Hansson, G. C. (2008). The Inner of the Two Muc2 Mucin-Dependent Mucus Layers in Colon is Devoid of Bacteria. *PNAS*. Vol:105, No:39, pp. 15064-15069

Kelsall, B. (2008). Recent Progress in Understanding the Phenotype and Function of Intestinal Dendritic Cells and Macrophages. *Mucosal Immunology*. Vol:1, No:6, pp. 460-469

Kinugasa, T., Sakaguchi, T., Gu, X. & Reinecher, H. C. (2000). Claudins Regulate the Intestinal Barrier in Response to Immune Mediators. *Gastroenterology*. Vol:118, No:6, pp. 1001-1011

Kleinschek, M. A., Boniface, K., Sadekova, S., Grein, J., Murphy, E. E, Turner, S. P., Raskin, L., Desai, B., Faubion, W. A., de Waal Malefyt, R., Pierce, R. H., McClanahan, T. & Kastelein, R. A. (2009). Circulating and Gut-Resident Human Th17 Cells Express CD161 and Promote Intestinal Inflammation. *Journal of Experimental Medicine*. Vol:206, No:3, pp. 525-534

Kuestner, R. E., Taft, D. W., Haran, A., Brandt, C. S., Brender, T., Lum, K., Harder, B., Okada, S., Ostrander, C. D., Kreindler, J. L., Aujla, S. J., Reardon, B., Moore, M. Shea, P., Schreckhise, R., Bukowski, T. R., Presnell, S., Guerra-Lewis, P., Parrish-Novak, J., Ellsworth, J. L., Jaspers, S., Lewis, K. E., Appleby, M., Kolls, J. K., Rixon, M., West, J. W., Gao, Z. & Levin, S. D. (2007). Identification of the IL-17 Receptor Related Molecule IL-17RC as the Receptor for IL-17F. *Journal of Immunology*. Vol:179, pp. 5462-5473

Kullberg, M. C., Jankovic, D., Feng, C. G., Hue, S., Gorelick, P. L., McKenzie, B. S., Cua, D. J., Powrie, F., Cheever, A. W., Maloy, K. J. & Sher, A. (2006). IL-23 Plays a Key Role in Helicobacter hepaticus-Induced T Cell-Dependent Colitis. *Journal of Experimental Medicine*. Vol:203, No:11, pp. 2485-2494

Lee, J., Ho, W., Maruoka, M., Corpuz, R. T., Baldwin, D. T., Foster, J. S., Goddard, A. D., Yansurat, D. G., Vandlen, R. L., Wood, W. I. & Gurney, A. L. (2001). IL-17E, a Novel Proinflammatory Ligand for the IL-17 Receptor Homolog IL-17Rh1. *Journal of Biological Chemistry*. Vol:276, No:2, pp. 1660-1662

Leppkes, M., Becker, C., Ivanoc, I. I., Hirth, S., Wirtz, S., Neufert, C., Pouly, S., Murphy, A. J., Valenzuela, D. M., Yancopoulos, G. D., Becher, B., Littman, D. R. & Nurath, M. F. (2009). RORgamma-expressing Th17 Cells Induce Murine Chronic Intestinal Inflammation via Redudant Effects of IL-17A and IL-17F. *Gastroenterology*. Vol:136, No:1, pp. 257-267

Li, H., Chen, J., Huang, A., Stinson, J., Heldens, S., Foster, S., Dowd, P., Gurney, A. L. & Wood, W. I. (2000). Cloning and characterization of IL-17B and IL-17C, two new members of the IL-17 cytokine family. *PNAS*. Vol:97, No:2, pp. 773-778

Li, L., Huang, L., Vergis, A. L., Ye, H., Bajwa, A., Narayan, V., Strieter, R. M., Rosin, D. L. & Okusa, M. D. (2010). IL-17 Produced by Neutrophils Regulates IFN-γ-Mediated Neutrophil Migration in Mouse Kidney Ischemia-Reperfusion Injury. *Journal of Clinical Investigation*. Vol:120, No:1, pp. 331-342

Lim, H. W., Lee, J., Hillsamer, P. & Kim, C. H. (2008). Human Th17 Cells Share Major Trafficking Receptors with Both Polarized Effector T cells and FOXP3+ Regulatory T Cells. *Journal of Immunology*. Vol:180, No:1, pp. 122-129

Linden, S. K., Sutton, P., Karisson, N. G., Korolik, V. & McGuckin, M. A. (2008). Mucins in the Mucosal Barrier to Infection. *Mucosal Immunology*. Vol:1, No:3, pp. 183-197

Liu, Z., Geboes, K., Heremans, H., Overbergh, L., Mathieu, C., Rutgeerts, P. & Ceuppens, J. L. (2001). Role of Interleukin-12 in the Induction of Mucosal Inflammation and Abrogation of Regulatory T Cell Function in Chronic Experimental Colitis. *European Journal of Immunology*. Vol:31, No:5, pp. 1550-1560

Loftus, E. V. Jr. (2004). Clinical Epidemiology of Inflammatory Bowel Disease: Incidence, Prevalence, and Environmental Influences. *Gasterenterology*. Vol:126, pp. 1504-1517

Maele, L. V., Carnoy, C., Cayet, D., Songhet, P., Dumoutier, L., Ferrero, I., Janot, L., Erard, F., Bertout, J., Leger, H., Sebbane, F., Beneche, A., Renauld, J., Hardt, W., Ryffel, B. & Sirad, J. (2010). TLR5 Signaling Stimulates the Innate Production of IL-17 and IL-22 by $CD3^{neg}CD127^{+}$ Immune Cells in Spleen and Mucosa. *Journal of Immunology*. Vol:185, pp. 1177-1185

Maloy, K. J., Salaum, L., Cahill, R., Dougan, G., Saunders, N. J. & Powrie, F. (2003). CD4+CD25+ Tr Cells Suppress Innate Immune Pathology Through Cytokine-dependent Mechanisms. *Journal of Experimental Medicine*. Vol:197, No:1, pp. 111-119

Mannon, P. J., Fuss, I. J., Mayer, L., Elson, C. O., Sandborn, W. J., Present, D., Dolin, B., Goodman, N., Groden, C., Homung, R. L., Quezado, M., Yang, Z., Neurath, M. F., Salfeld, J., Veldman, G. M., Schwertschlag, U. & Strober, W. (2004). Anti-Interleukin-12 Antibody for Active Crohn's Disease. *New England Journal of Medicine*. Vol:351, No:20, pp. 2069-2079

Meresse, B. & Cerf-Bensussan, N. (2009). Innate T Cell Responses in Human Gut. *Seminal Immunology*. Vol:21, No:3, pp. 121-129

Michel, M., Keller, A. C., Paget, C., Fujio, M., Trottein, F., Savage, P. B., Wong, C., Schneider, E., Dy, M. & Leite-de-Moraes, M. C. (2007). Identification of an IL-17-Producing $NK1.1^{neg}$ iNKT Cell Population Involved in Airway Neutrophilia. *Journal of Experimental Medicine*. Vol:205, No:5, pp. 995-1001

Mosmann, T. R., Cherwinski, H., Bond, M. W., Giedlin, M. A. & Coffman, R. L. (1986). Two Types of Murine Helper T Cell Clone. I. Definition According to Profiles of Lymphokine Activities and Secreted Proteins. *Journal of Immunology*. Vol:136, No:7, pp. 2348-2357

Mowat, A. M. (2003). Anatomical Basis of Tolerance and Immunity to Intestinal Antigens. *Nature Reviews Immunology*. Vol:3, No:4, pp. 331-341

Mundy, R., MacDonald, T. T., Dougan, G., Frankel, G. & Wiles, S. (2005). *Citrobacter rodentium* of Mice and Man. *Cellular Microbiology*. Vol:7, No:12, pp. 1697-1706

Murphy, C. A., Langrish, C. L., Chen, Y., Blumenschein, W., McClanahan, T., Kastelein, R. A., Sedgwick, J. D. & Cua, D. J. (2003). Divergent Pro- and Antiinflammatory Roles for IL-23 and IL-12 in Joint Autoimmune Inflammation. *Journal of Experimental Medicine*. Vol:198, No:12, pp. 1951-1957

Nakajima, H., Takamori, H., Hiyama, Y. & Tsukada, W. (1991). The Effects of Treatment with Recombinant Gamma-Interferon on Adjuvant-Induced Arthritis in Rats. *Agents and Actions*. Vol:34, No:1-2, pp. 63-65

Neurath, M. F., Fuss, I., Kelsall, B. L., Stuber, E. & Strober, W. (1995). Antibodies to Interleukin 12 Abrogate Established Experimental Colitis in Mice. *Journal of Experimental Medicine*. Vol:182, No:5, pp. 1281-1290

O'Connor, W. Jr., Kamanaka, M., Booth, C. J., Town, T., Nakae, S., Iwakura, Y., Kolls, J. K. & Flavell, R. A. (2009). A Protective Function for Interleukin 17A in T Cell-Mediated Intestinal Inflammation. *Nature Immunology*. Vol:10, No:6, pp. 603-609

O'Connor, W. Jr., Zenewicz, L. A. & Flavell, R. A. (2010). The Dual Nature of Th17 Cells: Shifting the Focus to Function. *Nature Immunology*. Vol:11, No:6, pp. 471-476

Ogawa, A., Angoh, A., Araki, Y., Bamba, T. & Fujiyama, Y. (2004). Neutralization of Interleukin-17 Aggravates Dextran Sulfate Sodium-Induced Colitis in Mice. *Clinical Immunology*. Vol:110, No:1, pp. 55-62

Oppmann, B., Lesley, R., Blom, B., Timans, J. C., Xu, Y., Hunte, B., Vega, F., Yu, N., Wang, J., Singh, K., Zonin, F., Vaisberg, E., Churakova, T., Liu, M., Gorman, D., Wagner, J., Zurawski, S., Liu, Y., Abrams, J. S., Moore, K. W., Rennick, D., de Waal-Malefyt, R., Hannum, C., Bazan, J. F. & Kastelein, R. A. (2000). Novel p19 Protein Engages IL-12p40 to Form a Cytokine, IL-23, with Biological Activities Similar as well as Distinct from IL-12. *Immunity*. Vol:13, No:5, pp. 715-725

Pan, G., French, D., Mao, W., Maruoka, M., Risser, P., Lee, J., Foster, J., Aggarwal, S., Nicholes, K., Guillet, S., Schow, P. & Gurney, A. L. (2001). Forced Expression of Murine IL-17E Induces Growth Retardation, Jaundice, a Th2-Biased Response, and Multiorgan Inflammation in Mice. *Journal of Immunology*. Vol:167, pp. 6559-6567

Park, H., Li, Z., Yang, X. O., Chang, S. H., Nurieva, R., Wang, Y. H., Wang, Y., Hood, L., Zhu, Z., Tian, Q. & Dong, C. (2005). *Nature Immunology*. Vol:6, No:11, pp. 1133-1141

Porras, M., Martin, M. T., Yang, P., Jury, J., Perdue, M. H. & Vergara, P. (2006). Correlation Between Cyclical Epithelial Barrier Dysfunction and Bacterial Translocation in the Relapses of Intestinal Inflammation. *Inflammatory Bowel Disease*. Vol:12, No:9, pp. 843-852

Powrie, F., Correa-Oliveira, R., Mauze, S. & Coffman, R. L. (1994a). Regulatory Interactions Between CD45RBhigh and CD45RBlow CD4+ T Cells are Important for the Balance Between Protective and Pathogenic Cell-Mediated Immunity. *Journal of Experimental Medicine*. Vol:179, No:2, pp. 589-600

Powrie, F., Leach, M. W., Mauze, S., Menon, S., Caddie, L. B. & Coffman, R. L. (1994b). Inhibition of Th1 Responses Prevents Inflammatory Dowel Disease in SCID Micce Reconstituted with CD45RBhi CD4+ T cells. *Immunity*. Vol:1, No:7, pp. 553-562

Raffatellu, M., Santos, R. L., Verhoeven, D. E., George, M. D., Wilson, R. P., Winter, S. E., Godinez, I., Sankaran, S., Paixao, T. A., Gordon, M. A., Kolls, J. K., Dandekar, S. & Bäumler, A. J. (2008). Simian Immunodeficiency Virus-Induced Mucosal Interleukin-17 Deficiency Promotes *Salmonella* Dissemination from the Gut. *Nature Medicine*. Vol:14, No:4, pp. 421-430

Raffatellu, M. George, M. D., Akiyama, Y., Hornsby, M. J., Nuccio, S., Paixao, T. A., Butler, B. P., Chu, H., Santos, R. L., Berger, T., Mak, T. W., Tsolis, R. M., Bevins, C. L., Solnick, J. V., Dandekar, S. & Bäumler, A. J. (2009). Lipocalin-2 Resistance Confers an Advantage to *Salmonella enterica* Serotype Typhimurium for Growth and Survival in the Inflamed Intestine. *Cell Host & Microbe*. Vol:5, pp. 476-486

Read, S., Malmström, V. & Powrie, F. (2000). Cytotoxic T Lymphocyte-associated Antigen 4 Plays an Essential Role in the Function of CD25+CD4+ Regulatory Cells that

Control Intestinal Inflammation. *Journal of Experimental Medicine*. Vol:192, No:2, pp. 295-302

Rescigno, M., Wrbano, M., Valzasina, B., Francolini, M., Rotta, G., Bonasio, R., Granucci, F., Kraehenbuhl, J. P. & Ricciardi-Castagnoli, P. (2001). Dendritic Cells Express Tight Junction Proteins and Penetrate Gut Epithelial Monolayers to Sample Bacteria. *Nature Immunology*. Vol:2, No:4, pp. 361-367

Rouvier, E., Luciani, M., Mattei, M., Denizot, F. & Golstein, P. (1993). CTLA-8, Cloned from an Activated T Cell, Bearing AU-Rich Messenger RNA Instability Sequences, and Homologous to a Herpesvires Saimiri Gene. *Journal of Immunology*. Vol:150, No:12, pp. 5445-5456

Rutgeerts, P., Van Assche, G. & Vermeire, S. (2006). Review Article: Infliximab Therapy for Inflammatory Bowel Disease—Seven Years On. *Aliment Pharmacology Therapy*. Vol:23, No:4, pp. 451-463

Rovedatti, L., Kudo, T., Biancherri, P., Sarra, M., Knowles, C. H., Rampton, D. S., Corazza, G. R., Monteleone, G., Di Sabatino, A. & MacDonald, T. T. (2009). Differential Regulation of Interleukin 17 and Interferon γ Production in Inflammatory Bowel Disease. *Gut*. Vol:58, pp. 1629-1636

Sakaguchi, S., Sakaguchi, N., Asano, M., Itoh, M. & Toda, M. (1995). Immunologic Self-Tolerance Maintained by Activated T Cells Expressing IL-2 Receptor α-Chains (CD25). *Journal of Immunology*. Vol:155, pp. 1151-1164

Sakaguchi, S. (2000). Regulatory T cells: Key Controllers of Immunologic Self-Tolerance. *Cell*. Vol:101, pp. 455-458

Sandborn, W. J., Feagan, B. G., Fedorak, R. N., Scherl, E., Fleisher M. R., Katz, S., Johanns, J., Blank, M. & Rutgeerts, P. (2008). A Randomized Trial of Ustekinumab, a Human Interleukin-12/23 Monoclonal Antibody, in Patients with Moderate-to-Severe Crohn's Disease. *Gastroenterology*. Vol:135, No:4, pp. 1130-1141

Savage, D. C. (1977). Microbial Ecology of the Gastrointestinal Tract. *Annual Reviews in Microbiology*. Vol:31, pp. 107-133

Schutyser, E., Struyf, S. & van Damme, Jo. (2003). The CC Chemokine CCL20 and it's Receptor CCR6. *Cytokine and Growth Factor Reviews*. Vol:14, pp. 409-426

Schwandner, R., Yamaguchi, K. & Cao, Z. (2000). Requirement of Tumor Necrosis Factor Receptor-associated Factor (TRAF)6 in Interleukin 17 Signal Transduction. *Journal of Experimental Medicine*. Vol:191, No:7, pp. 1233-1239

Shen, F., Ruddy, M. J., Plamondon, P. & Gaffen, S. L. (2005). Cytokines Link Osteoblasts and Inflammation: Microarray Analysis of Interleukin-17 and TNF-alpha-Induced Genes in Bone Cells. *Journal of Leukocyte Biology*. Vol:77, No:3, pp. 388-399

Shen, L. & Turner, J. R. (2006). Role of Epithelial Cells in Initiation and Propagation of Intestinal Inflammation. Eliminating the Static: Tight Junction Dynamics Exposed. *America Journal of Physiology Gastrointestinal Liver Physiology*. Vol:290, No:4, pp. G577-582

Shibata, K., Yamada, H., Hara, H., Kishihara, K. & Yoshikai, Y. (2007). Resident Vδ1+ γδ T Cells Control Early Infiltration of Neutrophils after *Escherichia coli* Infection via IL-17 Production. *Journal of Immunology*. Vol:178, pp. 4466-4472

Starnes, T., Robertson, M. J., Sledge, G., Kelich, S., Nakshatri, H., Broxmeyer, H. E. & Hromas, R. (2001). Cutting Edge: IL-17F, a Novel Cytokine Selectively Expressed in

Activated T Cells and Monocytes, Regulates Angiogenesis and Endothelial Cell Cytokine Production. *Journal of Immunology*. Vol:167, pp. 4137-4140

Starnes, T., Broxmeyer, H. E., Robertson, M. J. & Hromas, R. (2002). Cutting Edge: IL-17D, a Novel Member of the IL-17 Family, Stimulates Cytokine Production and Inhibits Hemopoiesis. *Journal of Immunology*. Vol:169, pp. 642-646

Steinman, L. (2007). A brief history of Th17, the first major revision in the Th1/Th2 hypothesis if T cell-mediated tissue damage. *Nature Medicine*. Vol:13, No:2, pp. 139-145

Symonds, E. L., Riedel, C. U., O'Mahony, D., Lapthorne, S., O'Mahony, L. & Shanahan, F. (2009). Involvement of T Helper Type 17 and Regulatory T Cell Activity in *Citrobacter rodentium* Invasion and Inflammatory Damage. *Clinical & Experimental Immunology*. Vol:157, pp. 148-154

Takahashi, M., Vanlaere, I., de Rycke, R., Cauwels, A., Joosten, L. A. B., Lubberts, E., van den Berg, W. B. & Libert, C. (2006). IL-17 Produced by Paneth Cells Drives TNF-Induced Shock. *Journal of Experimental Medicine*. Vol:205, No:8, pp. 1755-1761

Takatori, H., Kanno, Y., Watford, W. T., Tato, C. M., Weiss, G., Ivanov, I. I., Littman, D. R. & O'Shea, J. J. (2008). Lymphoid tissue inducer-like cells are an innate source of IL-17 and IL-22. *Journal of Experimental Medicine*. Vol:206, No:1, pp. 35-41

Tytgat, K. M. A. J., van der Wal, J. G., Einerhand, A. W. C., Büller, H. A. & Dekker, J. (1996). Quantitative Analysis of MUC2 Synthesis in Ulcerative Colitis. *Biochemical and Biophysical Research Communications*. Vol:224, pp. 397-405

Uhlig, H. H., McKenzie, B. S., Hue, S., Thompson, C., Joyce-Shaikh, B., Stepankova, R., Robinson, N., Buonocore, S., Tiaskalova-Hogenova, H., Cua, D. J. & Powrie, F. (2006). Differential Activity of IL-12 and IL-23 in Mucosal and Systemic Innate Immune Pathology. *Immunity*. Vol:25, pp. 309-318

Umesaki, Y., Setoyama, H., Matsumoto, S., Imaoka, A. & Itoh, K. (1999). Differential Roles of Segmented Filamentous Bacteria and Clostridia in Development of the Intestinal Immune System. *Infection and Immunity*. Vol:67, pp. 3504-3511

Van de Keere, F. & Tonegawa, S. (1998). CD4+ T Cells Prevent Spontaneous Experimental Autoimmune Encephalomyelitis in Anti-Myelin Basic Protein T Cell Receptor Transgenic Mice. *Journal of Experimental Medicine*. Vol:188, No:10, pp. 1875-1882

Veldhoen, M., Hocking, R. J., Atkins, C. J., Locksley, R. M. & Stockinger, B. (2006). TGFbeta in the Context of an Inflammatory Cytokine Milieu Supports de novo Differentiation of IL-17-Producing T Cells. *Immunity*. Vol:24, No:2, pp. 179-189

Voorthuis, J. A. C., Uitdehaag, B. M. J., de Groot, C. J. A., Goede, P. H., van der Meide, P. H. &Dijkstra, C. D. (1990). Suppression of Experimental Allergic Encephalomyelitis by Intraventricular Administration of Interferon-Gamma in Lewis Rats. *Clinical and Experimental Immunology*. Vol:81, pp. 183-188

Wang, X., Lupardus, P., LaPorte, S. L. & Garcia, K. C. (2009). Structural Biology of Shared Cytokine Receptors. *Annual Review of Immunology*. Vol:27, pp. 29-60

Wells, J. M., Loonen, L. M. P. & Karczewski, J. M. (2010). The Role of Innate Signaling in the Homeostasis of Tolerance and Immunity in the Intestine. *International Journal of Medical Microbiology*. Vol:300, pp. 41-48

Wilson, C. B., Rowell, E. & Sekimata, M. (2009). Epigenetic Control of T-Helper-Cell Differentiation. *Nature Reviews Immunology*. Vol:9, No:2, 91-105

Wright, J. F., Guo, Y., Quazi, A., Luxenberg, D. P., Bennett, F., Ross, J. F., Qui, Y., Whitters, M. J., Tomkinson, K. N., Dunussi-Joannopoulos, K., Carreno, B. M., Collins, M. & Wolfman, N. M. (2007). Identification of an Interleukin 17F/17A Heretodimer in Activated Human CD4+ T Cells. *Journal of Biological Chemistry*. Vol:282, No:18, pp. 13447-13455

Wright, J. F., Bennett, F., Li, B., Brooks, J., Luxenberg, D. P., Whitters, M. J., Tomkinson, K. N., Fitz, L. J., Worlfman, N. M., Collins, M., Dunussi-Joannopoulos, K., Chatterjee-Kishore, M. & Carreno, B. M. (2008). The Human IL-17F/IL-17A Heterodimeric Cytokine Signals through the IL-17RA/IL-17RC Receptor Complex. *Journal of Immunology*. Vol:181, pp. 2799-2805

Wyatt, J., Vogelsang, H., Hübl, W., Waldhöer, T. & Lochs, H. (1993). Intestinal Permeability and the Prediction of Relapse in Crohn's Disease. *Lancet*. Vol:341, No:8858, pp. 1437-1439

Yamazaki, T., Yang, X. O., Chung, Y., Fukunaga, A., Nurieva, R., Pappu, B., Martin-Orozco, N., Kang, H. S., Ma, L., Panopoulos, A. D., Craig, S., Watowich, S. S., Jetten, A. M., Tian, Q. & Dong, C. (2008). CCR6 Regulates the Migration of Inflammatory and Regulatory T Cells. *Journal of Immunology*. Vol:181, pp. 8391-8401

Yang, L., Anderson, D. E., Baecher-Allan, C., Hastings, W. D., Bettelli, E., Oukka, M., Kuchroo, V. K. & Hafler, D. A. (2008). IL-12 and TGF-beta and Required for Differentiation of Human T(H)17 Cells. *Nature*. Vol:424, No:7202, pp. 350-352

Yang, X. O., Chang, S. H., Park, H., Nurieva, R., Shah, B., Acero, L., Wang, Y. H., Schluns, K. S., Boarddus, R. R., Zhu, Z. & Dong, C. (2008). Regulation of Inflammatory Responses by IL-17F. *Journal of Experimental Medicine*. Vol:205, No:5, pp. 1063-1075

Yao, Z., Painter, S. L., Fanslow, W. C., Ulrich, D., Macduff, B. M., Spriggs, M. K. & Armitage, R. J. (1995a). Human IL-17: A Novel Cytokine Derived from T Cells. *Journal of Immunology*. Vol.155, pp. 5483-5486

Yao, Z., Fanslow, W. C., Seldin, M. F., Rousseau, A. M., Painter, S. L., Comeau, M. R., Cohen, J. I. & Spriggs, M. K. (1995b). Herpesvirus Saimiri Encodes a New Cytokine, IL-17, which Binds to a Novel Cytokine Receptor. *Immunity*. Vol:3, No:6, pp. 811-821

Zhang, X., Angkasekwinai, P., Dong, C. & Tang, H. (2011). Structure and Function of Interleukin-17 Family Cytokines. *Protein and Cell*. Vol:2, No:1, pp. 26-40

Zhang, Z., Zheng, M., Bindas, J., Schwarzenberger, P. & Kolls, J. K. (2006). Critical Role of IL-17 Receptor Signaling in Acute TNBS-Induced Colitis. *Inflammatory Bowel Disease*. Vol:12, No:5, pp. 382-388

Zheng, Y. & Rudensky, A. Y. (2007). Foxp3 in Control of the Regulatory T Cell Lineage. *Nature Immunology*. Vol:8, No:5, pp. 457-462

Zheng, Y., Valdez, P. A., Danilenko, D. M., Hu, Y., Sa, S. M., Gong, Q., Abbas, A. R., Modrusan, Z., Ghilardi, N., de Sauvage, F. J. & Ouyang, W. (2008). Interleukin-22 Mediates Early Host Defense Against Attaching and Effacing Bacterial Pathogens. *Nature Medicine*. Vol:14, No:3, pp. 282-290

Zhu, J. & Paul, W. E. (2010). Peripheral CD4+ T-Cell Differentiation Regulated by Networks of Cytokines and Transcription Factors. *Immunological Reviews*. Vol:238, pp. 247-262

6

Pathogenesis of Inflammatory Bowel Diseases

Yutao Yan
Emory University
Georgia State University
United States

1. Introduction

Ulcerative colitis (UC) and Crohn's disease (CD), collectively called inflammatory bowel disease (IBD), are idiopathic, chronic, and relapsing intestinal inflammatory disorder, characterized by abdominal pain and diarrhea. UC differs dramatically from CD with the respects of disease distribution, morphology, and histopathology; for example, CD can affect any part of the gastrointestinal (GI) tract, usually discontinuously. UC is confined to the colon, it is characterized by continuous inflammation, invariably involving the rectum, and is classified according to its proximal limit (proctitis, distal, or extensive colitis). Further, unlike CD, inflammation in UC is restricted to the mucosal surface, perhaps giving weight to the emerging concept of a defective mucosal barrier in disease pathogenesis. Histologically active UC typically consists of a neutrophilic mucosal infiltrate, goblet cell depletion, "cryptitis," and prominent crypt abscesses. Acute inflammatory process in UC is associated with mucosal (particularly epithelial) cell destruction. Meantime, UC and CD share a lot of inflammatory similarities, such as epithelial barrier dysfunction, genetic susceptibility etc. IBD may result in significant morbidity and mortality, with compromised quality of life and life expectancy. While there is no cure for IBD, the last two decades have seen tremendous advances in our understanding of the pathophysiology of this intestinal inflammation. Even though the precise etiology of IBD remains elusive, it is accepted (Figure 1) that IBD arises from abnormal host–microbe interactions, including qualitative and quantitative changes in the composition of the microbiota, host genetic susceptibility, barrier function, as well as innate and adaptive immunity. In more detail, some defects occur in luminal bacterial antigen sampling by the epithelium, possibly mediated by toll-like receptors (TLRs) or nucleotide binding oligomerisation domain family (NODs), controlled by genetic factors (including NOD2 for CD etc). An over-response to the antigens then stimulates activated dendritic cells to generate Th1-type /Th17 T cells or Th2-type /NK T cells, which then generate cytokines, initiating a cascade of immunologic events resulting in tissue damage. Thus, the factors participating in what manifests as inflammation in UC and CD are part of a dynamic process in which autoantibodies are generated against mucosal antigens in a susceptible host. The autoantibodies are not primarily responsible for disease pathogenesis; rather, they mark for disease-related autoantigens, which likely cross react with bacterial antigens from the normal intestinal flora. In a genetically susceptible host, the interaction results in an exaggerated inflammatory response in which either a lack of regulatory cells or enhanced numbers of effector cells initiates disease. With time, antigenic spreading to host antigens (the autoantigens) occurs; therefore, removal of these bacteria would no longer affect disease activity (Vanderlugt et al., 1996).

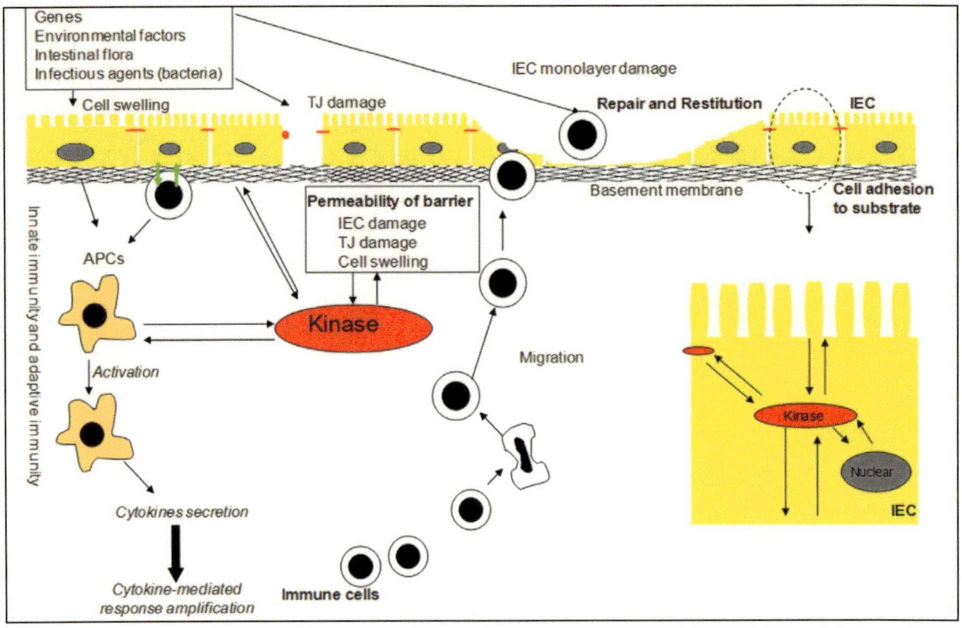

Fig. 1. Pathogenesis of IBD. Many different factors, such as genetic factors, environmental factors, and intestinal non-pathogenic or pathogenic bacteria can damage the mucus, epithelium, or the tight junction, to initiate the inappropriate regulation or deregulation of the immune response, leading to the secretion of pro-inflammatory cytokines, decrease in epithelial barrier function and initiation of the inflamma tion-related signaling pathways. IEC: Intestinal epithelial cell; APC: Antigen presenting cell; TJ: Tight junction. This model adapted from the model presented previously (Yan 2008)

In this chapter, we are going to focus on the involvement of diverse of factors in the pathogenesis of IBD, try to shed some light on the clues of intervention of IBD.

2. Genetic factor

Population-based studies provided compelling evidence that genetic susceptibility plays an essential role in the pathogenesis of IBD, evidence including an 8- to 10-fold greater risk among relatives of UC and CD and greater rates of concordance between twins in UC patients (15.4% in monozygotic vs 3.9% in dizygotic twins) and CD patients (30.3% in monozygotic vs 3.6% in dizygotic twins) (Cho & Brant, 2011). Some of genes encoding protein kinases like ERK1 (Hugot et al., 1996) and p38α (Hampe et al., 1999) are located in major IBD susceptibility regions on chromosome 16 and 6. Recently, substantial advances have been achieved in defining the genetic architecture of IBD since the genome-wide association study (GWAS) analysis heralded a new era of complex disease gene discovery with notable success in CD initially and latterly also in UC. To date, near 99 published IBD susceptibility loci have been discovered and replicated, of which minimum 28 are associated with both UC and CD, although 47 are specific to UC and 24 to CD (Thompson & Lees, 2011). Generally, these genetic loci could be grouped into different categories. Importantly, most of the genes have been linked to defects in innate and adaptive immunity and epithelial barrier function. The first susceptible locus identified in IBD is the major histocompatibility complex (MHC) class II region on chromosome 6 has been clearly demonstrated to be associated with UC (Toyoda et al., 1993).

Gene *NOD2* is the breakthrough discovery whose mutations are associated with CD lying either within or near the C-terminal, leucine-rich repeat domain, which is required for microbial sensing. NOD2 is expressed by many leukocytes, including antigen presenting cells, macrophages, and lymphocytes, as well as ileal Paneth cells, fibroblasts, and epithelial cells. Activation of NOD2 by microbial ligands activates the transcription factor nuclear factor κB (NF-κB) and mitogen activated protein kinase (MAPK) signaling, and functions as a positive regulator of immune defense (Hugot et al., 2001; Ogura et al., 2001). The NOD2 ligand muramyl dipeptide (MDP) is ubiquitous, indicating that broad classes of bacteria are capable of activating NOD2. However, the N-glycolyated form of muramyl dipeptide found in mycobacteria and actinomycetes more potently activates NOD2 compared to the N-acetylated form, found more frequently in gram-positive and gram-negative bacteria (Coulombe et al., 2009). Autophagy 16-like 1 (*ATG16L1*) has been strongly associated with CD and encodes a protein component of the autophagy complex (Levine & Deretic, 2007). ATG16L1 is broadly expressed, including in small intestinal Paneth cells (Cadwell et al., 2008) where it mediates exocytosis of secretory granules that contain antimicrobial peptides.

IL-10 gene SNPs were found to be involved in the UC by GWAS analysis (Franke et al., 2008), and IL-10$^{-/-}$ mouse is one of the oldest and most widely used animal models of UC, in which spontaneous colitis develops in specific pathogen-free conditions (Kuhn et al., 1993). IL10 is expressed by many different cells of the adaptive and innate immune system including Th1, 2, and 17 cells, subsets of regulatory T cells, dendritic cells, macrophages, mast cells, and natural killer cells (Mosser et al., 2008). It has pleiotropic effects on T and B cells, and importantly limits the release of proinflammatory cytokines like TNF-a and IL-12. In the IL-10$^{-/-}$ mouse model, defective counter regulatory anticytokine responses result in inflammation affecting intestinal mucosa which is characterized by enlarged and branched crypts, reduced number of goblet cells, degeneration of superficial epithelial cells, and increased expression of MHC class II molecules in mouse colon. But these IL-10$^{-/-}$ mice require gut microbia to develop inflammation, giving rise to an attractive theory that IL10 could be involved in restricting the mucosal immune response to enteric flora (Louis et al., 2009, Sellon et al., 1998). Interestingly, this IL-10$^{-/-}$ model of UC have, in another hand, elegantly shown a protective role of IL10: transfer of IL10 producing regulatory T cells to immunodeficient mice prevents or cures colitis (Uhlig et al., 2006). Further, IL10 has been shown to exert a protective effect on carcinogenesis in mice (Erdman et al., 2003). The anti-inflammatory response of IL-10 is mediated through IL10 receptor (IL10R) and subsequent activation of signal transducer and activator of transcription 3 (STAT3). IL10R is a heterotetrameric molecule; while IL10R1 is specific to IL10R, IL10R2 is found as a subunit of receptors to other cytokines, notably IL22, IL26, and IFNγ. Extracellular matrix gene 1 (ECM1) (Festen et al., 2010), E-cadherin gene (CDH1), Hepatocyte nuclear factor 4 alpha gene (HNF4a), and laminin B1 (Barrett et al., 2009) are another four genes implicated in mucosal barrier function, conferring risk of UC; ECM1 interacts with the basement membrane, inhibits matrix metalloproteinase 9 (MMP9), and strongly activate NFκB (Chan et al., 2007; Matsuda et al., 2003). The Wnt/beta-catenin signal transduction pathway has been shown to influence ECM1 expression (Kenny et al., 2005). E-cadherin is the first genetic correlation between colorectal cancer and UC, Chimeric mice with impaired E-cadherin function due to expression of dominant-negative N-cadherin developed colitis despite possessing an intact immune system (Hermiston & Gordon 1995a, 1995b). Notably, all of

these 4 genes are regulated or related to protein kinases, for example, HNF4alpha-DNA binding activity is dependent on its phosphorylation by protein kinase A (PKA) (Viollet et al., 1997), while its transcription activity was dependent on AMP-activated protein kinase(AMPK) (Hong et al., 2003).
Similarly, by GWAS analysis, the strongest association in CD was found in interleukin-12 receptor (IL23R) (Duerr et al., 2006)—as well as the previously identified NOD2 gene. Knockout of or antibodies to IL23 prevent the development of intestinal inflammation in such models (McGovern & Powrie, 2007). It is now evident that much of the function previously ascribed to IL12 appears to relate to IL23, both of these cytokines sharing a p40 subunit in their heterodimeric structures. The IL23/IL12 pathway has become the subject of intensive study in the field of immunology as it plays a key role in determining differentiation of naıve T cells into effector Th1 cells (driven by IL12) or Th17 cells (driven by IL23). Some specific bacterial components such as peptidoglycan can differentially induce antigen presenting cells to produce IL23 rather than IL12, leading to distinct patterns of inflammatory response (Begum et al., 2004). Th17 cells are particularly interesting for their role in organ-specific inflammation—raising the hope that therapeutic disruption of the IL23 pathway will control such inflammation without impairing systemic immunity.

3. Microbiota and immune responses

The human GI tract contains as many as 10^{14} individual bacteria, comprising over 500 different species. These commensal bacteria serves as a primary barrier between the intestinal epithelial cells and the external environment, which is critical to the healthy host, as it modulates intestinal development, maintains a healthy intestinal pH, promotes immune homeostasis, and enhances metabolism of drugs, hormones and carcinogens. Evidence from immunologic, microbiologic, and genetic studies implicates abnormal host-microbial interactions in the pathogenesis of UC. But the mechanisms underlying the involvement of microbiota are elusive, and the effects of microbiota are due to their interaction with other factors, such as immunologic factors, genetic factor or epithelial junction proteins. The postulated mechanisms (Packey & Sartor, 2008) are as followed with little modification: (A) Pathogenic bacteria or abnormal microbial composition. A traditional pathogen or functional alterations in commensal bacteria, including enhanced epithelial adherence, invasion, and resistance to killing by phagocytes or acquisition of virulence factors, can result in increased stimulation of innate and adaptive immune responses. Luminal bacterial concentrations are increased in IBD, microbial diversity is diminished, particularly in patients with active disease. The involvement of pathogen mycobacterium avium subspecies paratuberculosis (MAP) in the pathogenesis of IBD is still controversial. Commensal bacteria that undergo functional alterations might contribute to the pathogenesis of IBD. Escherichia coli are commensal aerobic Gram-negative bacteria that play an important role in maintaining normal intestinal homeostasis. Modifications of luminal bacteria concentrations, including E. coli, have been observed in Crohn's disease patients (Frank et al., 2007). Reduced numbers of *Bacteroides fragilis* might also contribute to inflammation because this prominent human symbiont has protective effects: it protects mice from colitis induction by *Helicobacter hepaticus*, a murine commensal bacterium with pathogenic properties (Mazmanian et al., 2005). *Faecalibacterium prausnitzii* has anti-inflammatory properties; its numbers are reduced in patients with CD and associated with risk of postresection recurrence of ileal CD (Sokol et al., 2008). There is a decreased ratio of protective commensal bacterial species compared to aggressive species in patients with IBD.

Decreased concentrations of bacteria that produce butyrate and other short-chain fatty acids (SCFA) may compromise epithelial barrier integrity. (B) Defective host containment of commensal bacteria. Increased mucosal permeability can result in overwhelming exposure of bacterial to TLR ligands and antigens that activate pathogenic innate and T cell immune responses. (C) Defective host immunoregulation. Inflammation might arise from lack of tolerance to antigens present in autologous microflora; cells derived from inflamed intestinal tissues of patients with IBD are activated by exposure to sonicated samples of autologous or heterologous GI microflora, whereas cells from normal individuals respond only to sonicates of heterologous microflora (Duchmann et al., 1997). Antigen-presenting cells and epithelial cells overproduce cytokines due to ineffective down regulation, which results in TH1 and TH17 differentiation and inflammation. Dysfunction of regulatory T cells (Treg) leads to decreased secretion of IL-10 and TGF-β, and loss of immunological tolerance to microbial antigens (an overly aggressive T cell response.).

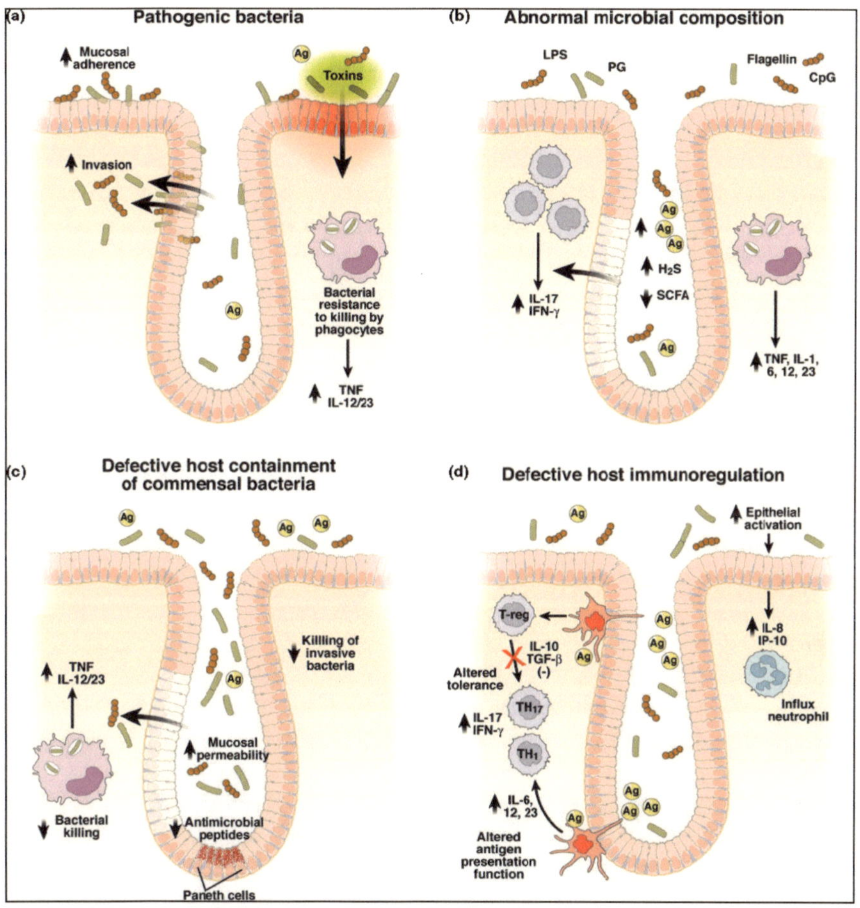

Fig. 2. Proposed mechanisms by which bacteria and fungi induce chronic immune-mediated inflammation and injury of the intestines. This model adapted from the model presented in the work by Dr Sartor (Packey & Sartor 2008) (a) Pathogenic bacteria. (b) Abnormal microbial compostion. (c) Defective host containment of commensal bacteria. (d) Defective host immunoregulation.

The bowel is the largest immunological organ of the body, with continuous interaction between the mucosal immune system and the intestinal flora. IBD is commonly regarded as the consequences of an enhanced inflammatory response or the lack of a down regulatory response to bacteria abnormality (Sartor et al., 2008; Xavier et al., 2007). The dysregulated immune response involving the innate (for example, TLR, DC, etc) and the adaptive immune system (e.g. effector T-cells, regulatory T-cells, eosinophils, neutrophils, etc) may follow or precede the macroscopic lesions. Th-1 and Th17 immune responses play a role in the pathogenesis of Crohn's disease (Sartor, 2008; Strober et al., 2007). The Th1 cytokine profile, which includes IFN-γ and IL-12 p40, is dominant in patients with Crohn's disease. Traditional Th1 responses are mediated by IFN-γ, the production of which is stimulated by IL-12, produced by antigen-presenting cells (APCs). Most experimental colitis models also have a dominant Th1 response, although in several models Th1 responses can change into Th2 (type 2 T-helper lymphocyte) responses as the inflammatory process matures (Spencer et al., 2002; Bamias et al., 2005). How we think about Th1 responses has been influenced by the discovery of an additional Th17 pathway. IL-17 mediates Th17 responses (Kolls & Linden, 2004). The production of this cytokine is stimulated by the production of IL-6, TGFβ and IL-23 by innate immune cells and APCs, especially dendritic cells. Bacterial colonization stimulates IL-23 expression by ileal dendritic cells (Becker et al., 2003). The levels of both IL-23 and IL-17 are increased in Crohn's disease tissues and most forms of experimental colitis (Fujino et al., 2003; Schmidt et al., 2005; Yen et al., 2006). Of pathogenic importance, the IL-12–IFN-γ and IL-23–IL-17 pathways seem to be mutually exclusive, since IFN-γ suppresses IL-17, and vice versa (Kolls et al., 2004). The immunopathogenesis of UC has been a more difficult disease to ascertain, neither IFN-γ (a major Th1 cytokine) nor IL-4 (the major Th2 cytokines) was increased (Fuss et al., 2008). In fact, IL-4 production was found to be decreased in cells extracted from UC tissue and only the fact that an additional Th2 cytokine IL-5 secretion by these cells was somewhat increased hinted that the disease may have a Th2 character. A further, enhanced level of IL-13 was noticed in lamina propria from UC specimens, whereas those from Crohn's disease specimens were producing IFN-γ (Fuss et al., 1996). Fuss (Fuss et al., 2004) found that antigen-presenting cells bearing a CD1d construct (and thus expressing CD1d on its surface, which presents lipid rather than protein antigens to T cells.) could only induce lamina propria mononuclear cells from UC patients but not that of Crohn ' s disease to produce IL-13. Thereby, the cytokine secretion profile seen in UC was produced from a non-classical CD1 dependent NK T cell whereas the cytokines produced in Crohn's disease were from that of an activated classical Th1 CD4 + T cell. In addition, Lamina propria cells enriched for NK T cells from the patients could be shown to be cytotoxic for epithelial cells and such cytotoxicity was further enhanced by IL-13. Antigens in the mucosal microflora activate NK T cells because of barrier dysfunction that, in turn, cause cytolysis of epithelial cells and the characteristic ulcerations associated with the disease. As suggested, enhancement of cytolytic activity was observed *in vitro* in the presence of IL-13. Further, IL-13 was shown to have direct effects on activation of cytokine, transcription. These studies demonstrated that TGF-β transcription was dependent upon IL-13. In short, UC is associated with an atypical Th-2 response mediated by a distinct subset of NK T cells that produce IL- 13 and are cytotoxic for epithelial cells (Fuss et al., 2008). Further, UC is characterized by the presence of various types of autoantibodies which confirm a key role of defect of host/bacterial interface to this disease. Approximately 70% of patients were diagnosed in the traditional manner with ulcerative colitis express pANCA (Saxon et al., 1990). The site of production of pANCA has been localized to the gastrointestinal mucosa (Targan et al., 1995). pANCA-primed B cells have been demonstrated in the mesenteric nodes and were not found in detectable amounts in the periphery (Targan et al., 1995). These findings represent further confirmation that the pANCAreactive antigen(s) also originates in the mucosa. Despite the fact that pANCA can be found in the peripheral circulation, the mucosal origin is the evidence that the antigen(s) to which pANCA reacts is mucosa specific and thus is more closely related to mucosal immune responses and mucosal inflammation. This finding corroborates that disease results from a defect in the hosts reaction to bacteria. The antigens to pANCA have been localized to the nucleus of neutrophils by the use of electron microscopy (Billing et al., 1995).

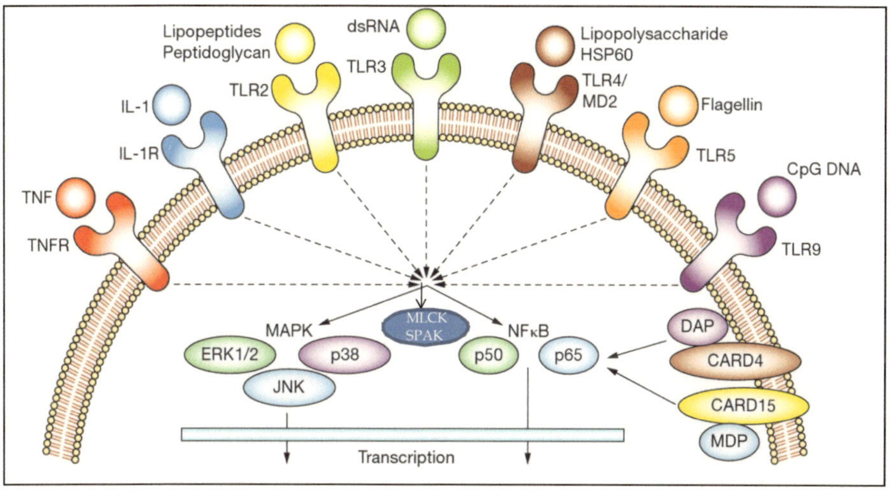

Fig. 3. Binding of microbial adjuvants to extracellular and intracellular patter-recognition receptros and initiate their function by activating preotein kinases. Toll-like receptors on the cell membrane selectively bind to various bacterial, viral or fungal components. This ligation activates conserved signaling pathways that activate NF?B and mitogen-activated protein kinases. These transcription factors stimulate the expression of a number of proinflammatory and antiinflammatory genes. This model adapted and modified from the model presented previously.
http://www.nature.com/nrgastro/v3/n7/full/ncpgasther0528.html

The intestinal mucosa must rapidly recognize detrimental pathogenic threats to the lumen to initiate controlled immune responses but maintain hyporesponsiveness to omnipresent harmless commensals. Pattern recognition receptors (PRRs) may play an essential role in allowing innate immune cells to discriminate between "self" and microbial "non-self" based on the recognition of broadly conserved molecular patterns. Toll-like receptors (TLRs), a class of transmembrane PRRs, play a key role in microbial recognition, induction of antimicrobial genes, and the control of adaptive immune responses. Polymorphisms in TLRs have been linked to Crohn's disease (Franchimont et al., 2004; Torok et al., 2004), and immunofluorescence studies reveal that epithelial TLR expression is markedly upregulated in IBD (Cario et al., 2000). TLR4, for example, is induced by proinflammatory cytokines and is highly expressedin IECs, resident macrophages and dendritic cells in active IBD (Cario, 2000; Hausmann et al., 2002). The functional variant Asp299Gly of TLR4 is associated with IBD and increased susceptibility to Gram-negative infections (Franchimont et al., 2004). Disrupted

TLR4 signalling could engender an inappropriate innate and adaptive immune response necessary to eradicate pathogens, which would result in severe inflammation. Polymorphisms of TLRs 1, 2 and 6 are associated with more extensive disease localization in IBD (Pierik et al., 2006). UC patients have an association between a TLR7 variant and the prevalence of pANCA antibodies, which crossreact with enteric bacterial antigens (Vermeire et al., 2004; Seibold et al., 1998). Blockade of bacterial signalling through NFκB in IECs potentiates chemically induced colitis in TLR4 and TLR9-deficient mice (Fukata et al., 2006; Lee et al., 2006). Individual TLRs differentially activate distinct signaling events via diverse cofactors and adaptors. To date, at least five different adaptor proteins have been identified in humans: MyD88, Mal/TIRAP, TRIF/TICAM-1, TRAM/Tirp/TICAM-2, and SARM (O'Neill et al., 2003). The first identified so-called "classical" pathway (Cario, 2005) involves recruitment of the adaptor molecule MyD88, activation of the serine/threonine kinases of the interleukin 1 receptor associated kinase (IRAK) family, subsequently leading to degradation of inhibitor kB (IkB) and translocation of nuclear factor kB (NFkB) to the nucleus, then result in activation of specific transcription factors, including NFkB, AP-1, Elk-1, CREB, STATs, and the subsequent transcriptional activation of genes encoding pro- and anti-inflammatory cytokines and chemokines as well as induction of costimulatory molecules. All of these various downstream effects are critically involved in the control of pathogen elimination, commensal homeostasis, and linkage to the adaptive immunity. Signaling through different TLRs can result in considerable qualitative differences in TH dependent immune responses by differential modulation of MAPKs and the transcription factor c-FOS (Agrawal et al., 2003). So TLR signalling protects intestinal epithelial barrier and maintains tolerance, but aberrant TLR signalling may stimulate diverse inflammatory responses leading to UC. TLR comprise a family of (so far) 11 type-I transmembrane receptors. Different pathogen associated molecular patterns selectively activate different TLRs: (Lipoptroteins) TLR1, 2 and 6; (dsRNA) TLR3; (LPS) TLR4; (Flagellin) TLR5; (ssRNA) TLR7 and 8; (CpG DNA) TLR9. These signals all converge on a single pathway via myeloid differentiation primary response protein MyD88, which activates NFκB. the NFκB pathway was thought to have predominantly pro inflammatory activities and NFκB is activated in the tissues of UC patients and its inhibition can attenuate experimental colitis (Neurath et al., 1996). In intestine, tolerance is an essential mucosal defence mechanism maintaining hyporesponsiveness to harmless lumenal commensals and their products. Several molecular immune mechanisms that ensure tolerance via TLRs in intestinal epithelial cells (IEC) have recently been described, for example, low expression of TLRs at resting conditions in IEC can maintain hyporesponsiveness to microbiota; high expression levels of the downstream signaling suppressor Tollip which inhibits IRAK activation (Otte et al., 2004), ligand induced activation of peroxisome proliferator activated receptor c (PPARc) which uncouples NFkB dependent target genes in a negative feedback loop (Dubuquoy et al., 2003. Kelly et al., 2004), and external regulators which may suppress TLR mediated signalling pathways. Commensal bacteria may assist the host in maintaining mucosal homeostasis by suppressing inflammatory responses and inhibiting specific intracellular signal transduction pathways (Neish et al., 2000), uncoupling NFkB dependent target genes in a negative feedback loop (Dubuquoy et al., 2003) which may lead to attenuation of colonic inflammation (Kelly et al., 2004).

NODs comprise at present more than 20 different members with C terminal ligand recognition (LRR) domain, central nucleotide binding domain (NBD), and N terminal caspase recruitment domains (CARDs). Recent research has mostly focused on two cytosolic receptors of this family, NOD1 and NOD2, which both play a major role in intestinal regulation of proinflammatory signalling through NFκB in response to distinct bacterial ligands. NOD2 is constitutively or inducibly expressed in all kinds of cells throughout the gasterintestinal tract. MDP has been identified as (so far) the sole ligand of NOD2 (Inohara et al., 2003; Girardin et al., 2003). NOD2 has been found to exert antibacterial activity in intestinal epithelial cells limiting survival of enteric bacteria after invasion. Bacterial clearance of Salmonella typhimurium is strongly accelerated in IEC expressing a functional NOD2 protein, whereas L1007fsinsC mutant expressing IEC are virtually unable to clear the pathogen *in vitro* (Hisamatsu et al., 2003). NOD2 (Chin et al., 2002) knockout mice, exhibit a profoundly decreased ability to clear intracellular Listeria monocytogenes, inducing persistent immune activation by combined loss of antibacterial activity, dysregulation of cytokine production, and imbalance of T cell activation. Emerging studies have started to reveal the molecular mechanisms by which NOD2 influences innate immune responses in the intestinal mucosa. It seems that different NOD2 mutations may span a spectrum of diverse phenotypes, ranging from complete "loss of function" to maximal "gain of function". NOD2 mutations within NBD lead to constitutive ligand independent NFκB activation, causing a chronic systemic inflammatory disorder known as "Blau syndrome"(Inohara et al., 2003a). Conversely, it has been suggested that CD associated NOD2 mutants which are predominantly found in the microbial ligand dependent LRR domain rather reflect "loss of function" phenotypes. Several *in vitro* transfection studies showed that human CD associated NOD2 mutants significantly abolish NFκB activation in response to MDP (Inohara et al., 2003b; Girardin et al., 2003; Chamaillard, 2003). However, paradoxically, macrophages within the intestinal lamina propria of CD patients overproduce NFκB targets, including exaggerated production of proinflammatory cytokines, such as TNF-a and IL-1β (Podolsky, 2002). Accordingly, a recent *in vivo* study now demonstrates that MDP stimulated macrophages isolated from mice generated with a murine NOD22932iC variant, homologous to the human NOD23020insC (=L1007fsinsC) variant, exhibit enhanced NFκB activation, increased apoptosis, and elevated IL-1β secretion (Maeda et al., 2005), possibly implying an important mechanism of how dysfunctional NOD2 may trigger intestinal inflammation in some types of CD. Thus this murine NOD2 frame-shift mutation in the LRR region may imbalance functions of both terminal parts of the whole protein: bacterial dysrecognition through the impaired LRR domain, ligand independent NFκB activation, as well as uncontrolled apoptosis and subsequent induction of IL-1β processing and release through the hyperactive CARD domains. The NOD2 gene product is most abundant in ileal Paneth cells (Lala et al., 2003; Ogura et al., 2003) which express a diverse population of microbicidal defensins restricting colonization or invasion of small intestinal epithelium by bacteria (Ouellette et al., 1994). Stimulation with MDP elicits cryptidin secretion from Paneth cells (Ayabe et al., 2000).

In addition, NF-κB is normally grouped into one of the pro-inflammatory mediators, a protective role for epithelial NF-κB signaling by either bacteria, IL-1, or TNF stimulation of TLRs, or cytokine receptors is demonstrated by conditional ablation of NEMO (IκB kinase) in intestinal epithelial cells causing spontaneous severe colitis (Nenci et al. 2007). Blockade of epithelial NF-κB signaling led to increased bacterial translocation across the injured epithelium, similar to TLR4-deficient mice treated with DSS (Fukata et al., 2006).

4. Barrier dysfunction

Generally, intestinal barrier function consists of different level of defense lines, the mucus layer, commensal microbiota, epithelial cells themselves, the junction between lateral epithelial cells, innate and adaptive immune systems and enteric nerve system. Any stresses which interfere with any level of this defense lines could potentially lead to intestinal barrier dysfunction and result in intestinal inflammation.

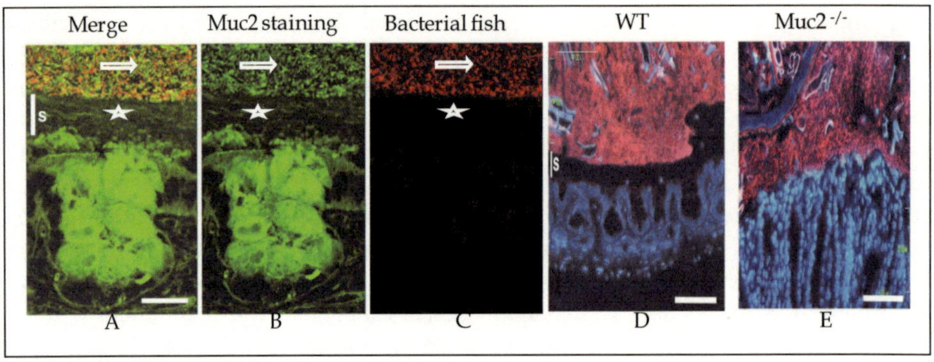

Fig. 4. Merged figure (A) of Muc2immunostaining (green, B) *and FISH analysis using the general bacterial probe EUB338-Alexa Fluor* 555 (red, C) of distal colon, it was shown muc2-postive goblet cells and the outer mucus layer (Arrow) and inner mucus layer (Star) on the epithelium. The inner layer (Star) is devoid of bacteria, which can only be detected in the outer mucus layer. The inner mucus generates a spatial separation between the cells and the microflora. (Scale bar: 20μm.). (D) FISH using the EUB338-Alexa Fluor 555 probe staining bacteria and DAPI DNA staining in colon show a clear separation of the bacterial DNA and epithelial surface in WT mice, but not in Muc2 -/- mice. This separation corresponds to the inner mucus layer (s). (Scale bar: 100μm.). These models adapted from the models presented previously (Johansson 2008).

Epithelial cells form a continuous, polarized monolayer that is linked together by a series of dynamic junctional complexes. Except function as a physical barrier, epithelial cells maintain a mucosal defense system through the expression of a wide range of PRRs, such as TLRs and NODs. These PRRs form the backbone of the innate immune system through the rapid response and recognition of the unique and conserved microbial components, (Medzhitov & Janeway. 2002; Akira et al., 2006). Tight junctions are composed of transmembrane proteins (claudins, occludins, and junctional adhesion molecule [JAM]), peripheral membrane or scaffolding proteins (zonula occludens [ZO]), and intracellular regulatory molecules that include kinases and actin. An anatomically and immunologically compromised intestinal epithelial barrier allows direct contact of the intestinal mucosa with the luminal bacteria and plays a crucial role in the development and maintenance of IBD by initiating chronic inflammatory responses, although it is unclear whether this is a primary pathogenic process or secondary to inflammation. Since the contribution of genetic factors, microbiota and immune responses to the pathogenesis to IBD, we high light the involvement of mucus layer, tight junction itself in the pathogenesis of IBD.

4.1 Mucus layer

As mentioned in previous part of this chapter, the digestive tract is home to 10^{14} bacteria and bacteria genome is as many 10 times as human genome, which has evolved to ensure homeostasis. How to manage this enormous bacterial load without overt immune responses from the adaptive and innate systems is not well understood. When the equilibrium is altered, as in CD and UC, inflammatory responses are initiated against the commensal bacteria. An important component, often neglected due to lack of understanding, is the mucus layer that overlies the entire intestinal epithelium as a protective gel-like layer (Johansson et al., 2008). This thick and hyperviscous mucus layer secreted by goblet cells overlies the entire intestinal epithelium as a protective gel-like layer that can extend up to as much as 150 μm thick in mouse colon (and 800 μm thick in rat colon). There exist two different kinds of mucus layer-out layer and inner layer. The majority of microorganisms in the lumen can be found in the outer mucus layer, there is an inner, protected, and unstirred layer that is directly adjacent to the epithelial surface and is relatively sterile. The sterility of this layer contributes to the retention of a high concentration of antimicrobial proteins (such as cathelicidiens, defensins, and cryptidens) produced by various intestinal epithelial lineages, including enterocytes and Paneth cells. The inner firmly attached mucus layer forms a specialized physical barrier that excludes the resident bacteria from a direct contact with the underlining epithelium. This organization of the colon mucus, as based on the properties of the Muc2 mucin, should be ideal for excluding bacteria from contacting the epithelial cells and thus also the immune system. Alterations or the absence of these protective layers, as in the $Muc2^{-/-}$ mouse colon, allow bacteria to have a direct contact with epithelial cells, to penetrate lower into the crypts and also translocate into epithelial cells. That such a close contact between bacteria and epithelia can trigger an inflammatory response (Johansson et al., 2008; Shen et al., 2009). The surface mucus layer also impacts mucosal permeability, as demonstrated by spontaneous colitis in Muc-2- deficient mice (Bergstrom et al., 2010), and increased dextran sulphate sodium-induced colitis in intestinal trefoil factordeficient mice (Mashimo et al., 1996) and in human UC, particularly in mucus composition and concentration in phospholipids (Braun et al., 2009). Aberrant mucin assembly causes endoplasmic reticulum stress and spontaneous inflammation that resembles UC in mice (Kaser et al., 2008, Heazlewood et al., 2008); defects in the mucus layer could also influence the pattern of microbial colonization and the maintenance of microbial community structure and function. The importance of the Muc2 mucin in organizing the colon mucus protection is further strengthen by the report that two mouse strains with diarrhea and colon inflammation were shown to have two separate spontaneous mutations in the Muc2 mucin (Heazlewood et al. 2008). Importantly, the production of mucin is regulated by protein kinases, for example, resistin and resistin-like molecule (RELM) beta upregulated mucin expression which dependent on the kinase activities of protein kinase C (PKC), tyrosine kinases, and extracellular-regulated protein kinase (Krimi et al., 2008); Cathelicidin stimulates colonic mucus synthesis by up-regulating MUC1 and MUC2 expression through a mitogen-activated protein kinase pathway (Tai et al., 2008).

4.2 Epithelial cell and its tight junction

The intestinal defect was first reported in studies showing that the intestinal mucosa of patients with CD had a decreased ability to exclude large molecules (Hollander et al., 1986). The cellular components of the intestinal barrier consist of the complete array of columnar epithelial cell types (enterocyte, paneth cells, enteroendorine cells, and goblet cells) present within the intestine. These cells are polarized with an apical membrane and a basolateral membrane, and apical membrane composition is distinct from the basolateral membrane, for example, the nutrient transporters are located on the apical membrane; they use Na^+ ions cotransport to provide the energy and directionality of transport. In contrast, the Na^+K^+-ATPase, which establishes the Na^+ electrochemical gradient, is present on basolateral, but not apical membranes. In addition, the lipid composition of the membrane differs; the apical membrane is enriched in sphingolipids and cholesterol relative to the basolateral membrane. One result of this cellular polarization is that the apical membranes of intestinal epithelial cells are generally impermeable to hydrophilic solutes in the absence of specific transporters. Thus, the presence of epithelial cells, particularly the apical membranes, contributes significantly to the mucosal barrier (Shen et al., 2009). Among the most important structures of the intestinal barrier are the epithelial tight junctions (TJs) that connect adjacent enterocytes together to determine paracellular permeability. The tight junction is composed of multiple proteins including transmembrane proteins such as occludin, tricellulin, claudins and junctional adhesion molecule (JAM). The intracellular portions of these transmembrane proteins interact with cytoplasmic peripheral membrane proteins, including zona occludens (ZO)-1,-2,-3 and cingulin (Mitic & Anderson. 1998). These tight junction and cytoplasmic proteins then interact with F-actin and myosin II, thereby anchoring the tight junction complex to the cytoskeleton. Once thought to be static, the association of these proteins with the tight junction is highly dynamic (Shen et al., 2009) and may play a role in epithelial barrier regulation. Occludin was the first tight junction-associated integral membrane protein identified (Furuse et al., 1993). Although occludin knockout mice exhibit intact intestinal epithelial tight junctions and display no observable barrier defect (Schulzke et al., 2005, Saitou et al., 2000). But *in vitro* studies demonstrate crucial roles in tight junction assembly and maintenance (Yu et al., 2005; Suzuki et al., 2009; Elias et al., 2009). This suggests that further analysis of occludin knockout mice under stressed condition may reveal *in vivo* functions of occludin and provide new insight into mechanisms of tight regulation (Turner, 2006). Given the phylogenetic and structural similarities between occludin and tricellulin (Ikenouchi et al., 2005), it may be that the tricellulin accounts for normal intestinal barrier function in occludin knockout mice. This hypothesis could also be applied to inflammatory bowel disease, where intestinal epithelial occludin expression is reduced (Heller et al., 2005). The fact that occludin knockout mice exhibit intact intestinal epithelial barrier function led to the search for additional tight junctional components and ultimately to the discovery of the claudins (Furuse et al., 1998). The claudins are a large family of proteins that also interact with partners on neighboring cells to affect junctional adhesions via extracellular loops. At least 24 different claudin proteins are present in mammals (Van Itallie et al., 2003, 2004, 2006), and these proteins are the primary component of tight junction strands (Furuse et al., 2006). Claudins are expressed in a tissue-specific manner, studies on human intestine confirm the expression of claudins-1, -2, -3, -4, -5, -7, and -8 in the colon, expression of claudins-1, -2, -3, and -4 in the duodenum, and expression of claudins-2 and -4 in the jejunum (Burgel et al., 2002; Escaffit et al., 2005, Szakal et al., 2010; Wang et al., 2010; Zeissing et al., 2007).

The molecular anatomy of transport through tight junction is not yet clear, at least two routes allow transport across the tight junction, and the relative contributions of different paracellular transport are regulated independently (Fihn et al., 2000; Van Itallie, 2008; Watson et al., 2005). One route, the size-dependent pathway, allows paracellular transport of large solutes, including limited flux of proteins and bacterial lipopolysaccharides (Van Itallie 2008; Watson et al., 2005). Although at what size particles are excluded from the leak pathway has not been precisely defined, it is clear that materials as large as whole bacteria cannot pass. Flux across the leak pathway may be increased by cytokines and protein kinases, including IFNγ, TNF (Watson et al., 2005; Wang et al., 2005; Clayburgh et al., 2006), MAPKs, myosin II light chain kinase (MLCK) (Turner 2006) and SPAK (Yan et al., 2011). A second pathway is charge-dependent pathway, characterized by small pores that are defined by tight junction-associated pore-forming claudin proteins (Amasheh et al., 2002; Colegio et al., 2003; Simon et al., 1999). These pores have a radius that excludes molecules larger than 4 A (Van Itallie 2008; Watson et al., 2005). Thus, tight junctions show both size selectivity and charge selectivity, and these properties may be regulated individually or jointly by physiological or pathophysiological stimuli. It need to point out that barrier dysfunction may be caused by increased paracellular permeability, but mainly by epithelial damage, including erosion, and ulceration (Zeissig et al., 2004; Schulzke et al., 2006). In addition, in epithelial cells, the site of claudin protein polymerization to form strands depends on ZO family protein expression (Furuse & Tsukita, 2006), and cells lacking ZO-1 and ZO-2 fail to form tight junctions at all.

Generally, TJ proteins can be subdivided into "tightening" TJ proteins that strengthen epithelial barrier properties (such as occluding and claudin-1 and -4 etc) and "leaky" TJ proteins (like claudin-2) that selectively mediate paracellular permeability. Dysfunctional intestinal barrier is a feature of gut inflammation in humans and has been implicated as a pathogenic factor in IBD for the last 30 years. The factors responsible for barrier dysfunction in UC are similar to those in CD, including an increase in epithelial antigen transcytosis and a change in TJ structure with a reduction in TJ strand count and in the depth of the TJ main meshwork; although, in contrast to CD, strand breaks are not as frequent as in UC (Schmitz et al., 1999; Schurmann et al., 1999). Again, the downregulation of occludin and downregulation of several "tightening" TJ proteins like claudin-1 and -4, together with an upregulation of the pore-forming TJ protein claudin-2 contribute to the barrier defect observed in UC (Heller et al., 2005; Oshima et al., 2008). These disruptions of tight junction proteins could lead to a breakdown in the protective barrier and can be used as a portal of entry by the luminal bacteria. This breach in intestinal barrier can result in inflammatory infiltrate and enhanced production of cytokines and other mediators (such as neutrophil) that can further contribute to the altered barrier function.

Mucosal permeability is influenced by several factors. The surface mucus layer also impacts mucosal permeability, as demonstrated by spontaneous colitis in Muc-2- deficient mice (Van der Sluis et al., 2006), and increased dextran sulphate sodium-induced colitis in intestinal trefoil factordeficient mice (Mashimo et al., 1996). Luminal microbiota can also compromise the intestinal barrier function (Packey & Sartor, 2008). The third is the integrity of the epithelial cell layer and the basement membrane. Molecularly this can be compromised by downregulating tight junction components Claudins 5 and 6, upregulating pore-forming Claudin 2 (Zessig et al., 2007), which can be accomplished by TNF and IL-13, or increasing epithelial apoptosis, which has been achieved in mice by blocking nuclear factor kappa-B (NFκB) signalling. Genetic factors are involved in the loss of intestinal barrier function (Cho & Brant, 2011). Dysregulated innate and adaptive immune system can lead to the enhanced epithelial permeability (Fuss, 2008). Finally, autonomic nerve system function affects epithelial permeability, as demonstrated by mice that develop fulminant jejunoileitis following ablation of enteric glial cells (Bush et al., 1998).

The increased uptake of antigens and macromolecules from the intestinal lumen mediated through this epithelial barrier dysfunction can further exacerbate the inflammatory process, ending up in a vicious circle. In this manner, barrier dysfunction is a perpetuating principle during gastrointestinal inflammation. Since epithelial TJs are important in the maintenance of barrier function, regulatory changes in their function that are commonly found during intestinal inflammation can have severe consequences. For example, the resulting passive loss of solutes into the intestinal lumen and the subsequent osmotically driven water flow results in "leak flux diarrhea", one of the main consequences of UC. The tight junction is, therefore, the rate-limiting step in transepithelial transport and the principal determinant of mucosal permeability. But it has to be pointed out that barrier dysfunction itself is not sufficient to cause intestinal diseases, such as in MLCK (Turner 2006) and SPAK (Yan et al., 2011) transgenic mouse models, these two different transgenic mice revealed increased transepithelial permeability, but neither of them demonstrated any UC characterization, for example, these mice develop normal, no significant weight loss, histologically normal crypts were found, no abscesses was noticed.

Recent molecular advances as well as studies of cellular physiology in model epithelia have instead revealed that both the permeability and selectivity of tight junctions can be modulated dynamically by a variety of signals (Mitic et al., 2000). Much of the progress in this field has rested on a significantly enhanced understanding of the proteins that make up the junction itself, as well as those components of the junction on its cytoplasmic face that link the junctional region both to the cellular cytoskeleton and to signal transduction modules (González-Mariscal et al., 2003).

5. Protein kinase and pathogenesis of IBD

5.1 mitogen activated protein kinases (MAPK)

Interestingly, protein kinases are associated with all different level of aspects, demonstrated promising potential as intervention targets against UC. Intracellular signaling cascades are the main route of communication between the plasma membrane and regulatory targets in various intracellular compartments. The evolutionarily conserved mitogen activated protein kinases (MAPK) signaling pathway plays an important role in transducing signals from diverse extra-cellular stimuli (including growth factors, cytokines and environmental stresses) to the nucleus in order to affect a wide range of cellular processes, such as proliferation, differentiation, development, stress responses and apoptosis. MAPK (Coskun et al., 2011) signaling cascades, which comprise up to seven levels of protein kinases, are sequentially activated by phosphorylation and also involved in intestinal inflammation. These families can be divided into two groups: the classical MAPKs, consisting of ERK1/2, p38, JNK and ERK5, and the atypical MAPKs, consisting of ERK3, ERK4, ERK7 and NLK (Coulombe & Meloche, 2007). The signalling pathways which the members of these families influence can be independent of each other or overlapping. The classical pathway leading to activation of ERK1/2 is through the upstream activation of the Raf MAPKKKs, which activate sequentially the MAPKKs, MEK1/2, which can specifically bind and phosphorylate ERK1/2. At this stage, and depending upon the signal being propagated, the ERK1/2 proteins commonly then phosphorylate the downstream MAPK activated proteins (MAPKAP) 1/2. However, other proinflammatory proteins such as cytosolic phospholipase A_2 can be activated, as well as several transcription factors including Ets-1, Elk and c-myc. These transcription factors aid the inflammatory process by inducing other related cellular processes such as cell migration and proliferation. Interestingly, a role for ERK1/2, using an ERK1/2 inhibitor, was found in cells of the immune system and colonocytes in the development and progression of IBD, through its mediation in the signalling pathways induced by various cytokines, for example IL-21, and IL-1 (Caruso et al., 2007; Kwon et al., 2007). Indeed, several studies, cell line cultures and isolated crypts from human biopsies, have shown that it is not only over-expressed in IBD tissue (both colonocytes and cells in the underlying lamina propria), but that its phosphorylation state and therefore activation state is increased significantly during the active stages of IBD (Waetzig et al., 2002; Dahan et al., 2008). Study also found that Erk activation is involved in claudin-4 protein expression and claudin-4 is involved in the maintenance of the intestinal epithelial cell barrier function (Pinton et al., 2010) as a "tightening" junction protein. Activation of p38/MAPK and Akt signal transduction pathways in the epithelial cells have also been implicated as key mediators of these protective effects (Resta-Lenert & Barrett. 2006). For example, *Lactobacillus GG* (LGG) prevents cytokine-induced apoptosis in both human and mouse intestinal epithelial cells through activating antiapoptotic Akt in a phosphatidylinositol-3κ-kinase (PI3K)-dependent manner and inhibiting proapoptotic p38/MAPK activation (Yan & Polk. 2002). The p38 family is composed of four members: α, β, γ and δ. Expression of the isoforms varies between tissues. Different ligands, via their respective receptors, are able to activate one or several of p38 targets TAK1, ASK1, MLK3, MEKK1-4 and TAO1-3 (Thalhamer et al., 2008). Several studies using the p38 inhibitor, SB203580, have indicated that p38 phosphorylation is increased significantly in IBD tissue (Waetzig et al., 2002; Dahan et al., 2008). This finding is substantiated further by an *in vitro* study, indicating that inhibition of p38 using the natural IL-1 receptor antagonist, in a colonocyte cell line, leads to reduced IL-6 and -8 production, and an *in vivo* study using a murine model of IBD, where inhibition of p38 reduced significantly cytokine mRNA and NFκB activation (Garat et al., 2003; Hollenbach et al., 2004). However, Heat-killed *L. brevis* SBC8803 induced Hsps, phosphorylated p38 MAPK, regulated the expression of tumor necrosis factor alpha (TNF-α), interleukin (IL)-1β and IL-12, and improved the barrier function of intestinal epithelia under oxidant stress (Ueno et al., 2011).

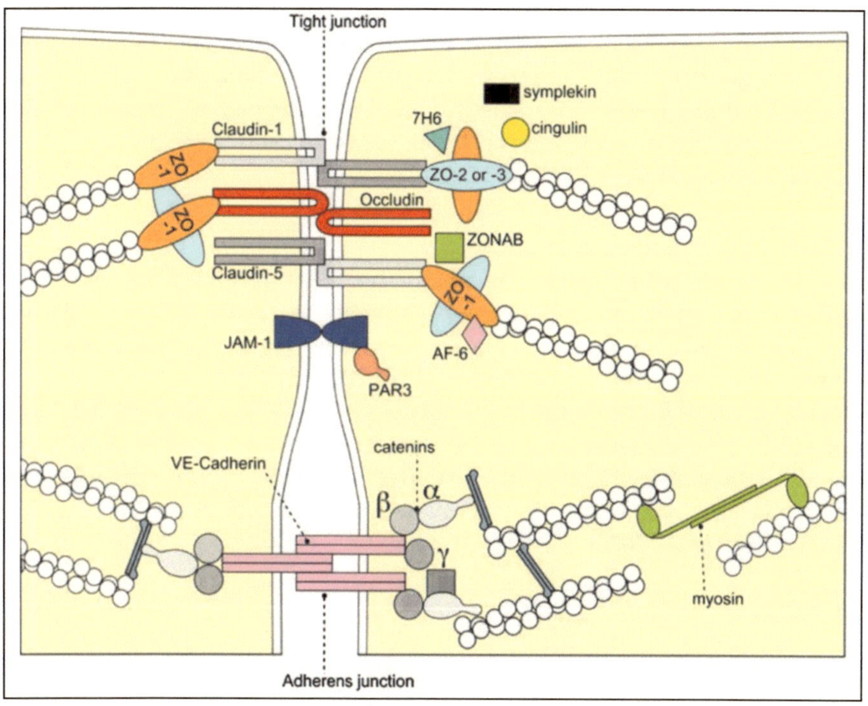

Fig. 5. Molecular compostion of tight junctions. This model adapted from the model presented previously:
http://www.ncbi.nlm.nih.gov/pmc/articles/PMC2413111/?tool=pubmed.

There are three JNK isoforms, JNK1, 2 and 3, of which there are 10 splice forms in total. Studies using a specific inhibitor against JNK1/2 in induced IBD in rodent models or with isolated colonic tissue found that proinflammatory cytokine production was reduced in conjunction with reduced inflammatory cell infiltration. Similarly, increased phosphorylation of JNK1/2 was seen in inflamed tissue from IBD patients (Dahan et al., 2008; Assi K et al., 2006; Mitsuyama et al., 2008). RDP58 (Loftberg et al., 2002) is a peptide consisting of 9 D-amino acids blocking p38 and JNK, further attenuate UC.

5.2 Serine and threonine kinase

5.2.1 Ste20 related proline/alanine rich kinase (SPAK)

SPAK is defined as a ste20-like proline-/alanine rich kinase that contains an N-terminal series of proline and alanine repeats (PAPA box) followed by a kinase domain, a nuclear localization signal, a consensus caspase cleavage motif, and a C-terminal regulatory region (Johnston et al., 2000). Colonic SPAK exists as a unique isoform that lacks the PAPA box and F-α helix loop in the N-terminus (Yan et al., 2007). The diversity of domains present in SPAK protein might be associated with a variety of biological roles. For example, SPAK has been shown to play roles in cell differentiation, cell transformation and proliferation, and regulation of chloride transport (Piechotta et al., 2002; Gagnon et al., 2006). More importantly, a linkage has been established between SPAK and inflammation, SPAK, as an upstream kinase to Na^+-K^+-$2Cl^-$ co-transporter 1 (NKCC1), can phosphorylate Thr203, Thr207, and Thr212 amino acids on NKCC1, which play an important role in inflammation (Topper et al., 1997). Furthermore, we have demonstrated that SPAK can activate p38 pathway (Yan et al., 2007) that is well known involving inflammation. SPAK caused an increase in intestinal permeability, and SPAK transgenic (TG) mice were more susceptible to experimental colitis. Additionally, increased cytokine production and bacterial translocation were associated with the increased colitis susceptibility (Yan Y et al., 2011).

5.2.2 Myosin II light chain kinase (MLCK)

MLCK is a specific Serine and threonine kinase which can phosphorylate MLC. It has been found that MLCK activity is required for TNF-induced acute diarrhea. Further, TNF treatment resulted in increased myosin light chain kinase expression (Wang et al., 2005), as a result of transcriptional activation (Graham et al. 2006) *in vitro* and *in vivo*. Constitutive MLCK activation accelerates onset and increases severity of experimental UC. MLCK inhibition, either pharmacologically or by genetic knockout, prevented both intestinal epithelial MLC phosphorylation and barrier dysfunction. More remarkably, MLCK inhibition also restored net water absorption, and therefore corrected the TNF-dependent diarrhea (Clayburgh et al., 2006).

6. Conclusions

Different aspects of factors are implicated in the pathogenesis of a variety of human intestinal inflammatory disorders including IBD, continuing progress in the understanding of the involvement of these factors in intestinal barrier dysfunction, further in IBD pathogeneses offers hope for a new generation of therapeutic strategies targeted at the modulation of transcription factor activity.

7. References

Agrawal, S., Agrawal, A., & Doughty, B.(2003). Cutting edge: different Toll-like receptor agonists instruct dendritic cells to induce distinct Th responses via differential modulation of extracellular signal-regulated kinase-mitogenactivated protein kinase and c-Fos. *J Immunol.* 171: 4984–9.

Akira, S., Uematsu, S., & Takeuchi O.(2006). Pathogen recognition and innate immunity. *Cell.* 124: 783–801.

Amasheh, S., Meiri, N., & Gitter A.(2002). Claudin-2 expression induces cation-selective channels in tight junctions of epithelial cells. *J Cell Sci.* 115: 4969-76.

Assi, K., Pillai, R., & Gomez-Munoz A. (2006). The specific JNK inhibitor SP600125 targets tumour necrosis factor-alpha production and epithelial cell apoptosis in acute murine colitis. *Immunology.* 118: 112–21.

Ayabe, T., Satchell, D.P., & Wilson, C.L.(2000). Secretion of microbicidal alphadefensins by intestinal Paneth cells in response to bacteria. *Nat Immunol.* 1:113–18.

Bamias, G., Martin, C., & Mishina, M. (2005). Proinflammatory effects of TH2 cytokines in a murine model of chronic small intestinal inflammation. *Gastroenterology.* 128: 654–666

Barrett, J.C., Lee, J.C., & Lees, C.W. (2009). Genome-wide association study of ulcerative colitis identifies three new susceptibility loci, including the HNF4A region. *Nat Genet.* 41:1330–4.

Becker, C., Wirtz, S., & Blessing, M. (2003). Constitutive p40 promoter activation and IL-23 production in the terminal ileum mediated by dendritic cells. *J Clin Invest.* 112: 693–706.

Begum, N.A., Ishii, K., & Kurita-Taniguchi, M.(2004). Mycobacterium bovis BCG cell wallspecific differentially expressed genes identified by differential display and cDNA subtraction in human macrophages. *Infect Immun.* 72, 937–948.

Bergstrom, K.S., Kissoon-Singh, V., & Gibson, L.(2010). Muc2 protects against lethal infectious colitis by disassociating pathogenic and commensal bacteria from the colonic mucosa. *PLoS Pathog.* 6: e1000902.

Billing, P., Tahir, S., & Calfin, B. (1995). Nuclear localization of the antigen detected by ulcerative colitis-associated perinuclear antineutrophil cytoplasmic antibodies. *Am J Pathol.* 147: 979-87.

Braun, A., Treede, I., & Gotthardt, D.(2009). Alterations of phospholipid concentration and species composition of the intestinal mucus barrier in ulcerative colitis: a clue to pathogenesis. *Inflamm Bowel Dis.* 15:1705–1720.

Burgel, N., Bojarski, C., & Mankertz, J.(2002). Mechanisms of diarrhea in collagenous colitis. *Gastroenterology.* 123: 433-43.

Bush, T.G., Savidge, T.C., & Freeman, T.C. (1998). Fulminant jejuno-ileitis following ablation of enteric glia in a adult transgenic mice. *Cell.* 93: 189–201.

Cadwell, K., Liu, J.Y. & Brown, S.L. (2008). A key role for autophagy and the autophagy gene Atg16l1 in mouse and human intestinal Paneth cells. *Nature.* 456:259–63.

Cario, E. (2005). Bacterial interactions with cells of the intestinal mucosa: Toll-like receptors and NOD2. *Gut.* 54:1182-93.

Cario, E., Podolsky, D.K. (2000). Differential alteration in intestinal epithelial cell expression of toll-like receptor 3 (TLR 3) and TLR 4 in inflammatory bowel disease. *Infect Immun.* 68:7010–7.

Caruso, R., Fina, D., & Peluso, I.(2007). A functional role for interleukin-21 in promoting the synthesis of the T-cell chemoattractant, MIP-3alpha, by gut epithelial cells. *Gastroenterology.* 132:166–75.

Chamaillard, M., Philpott, D., & Girardin, S.E.(2003). Gene-environment interaction modulated by allelic heterogeneity in inflammatory diseases. *Proc Natl Acad Sci U S A.* 100:3455–60.

Chan, I., Liu, L., & Hamada, T.(2007). The molecular basis of lipoid proteinosis: mutations in extracellular matrix protein 1. *Exp Dermatol.* 16:881–90.

Chin, A.I., Dempsey, P.W., & Bruhn, K. (2002). Involvement of receptor-interacting protein 2 in innate and adaptive immune responses. *Nature.*416:190–4.

Cho, J.H., & Brant, S.R. (2011). Recent insights into the genetics of inflammatory bowel disease. *Gastroenterology.* 140: 1704–1712.

Clayburgh, D. R., Musch, M.W., & Leitges, M. (2006). Coordinated epithelial NHE3 inhibition and barrier dysfunction are required for TNF-mediated diarrhea *in vivo*. *J Clin Invest.* 116: 2682–2694.

Colegio, O. R., Van Itallie, C., & Rahner, C.(2003). Claudin extracellular domains determine paracellular charge selectivity and resistance but not tight junction fibril architecture. *Am J Physiol Cell Physiol.* 284: C1346–C1354.

Coskun, M., Olsen, J., & Seidelin, J.B.(2011). MAP kinases in inflammatory bowel disease. *Clin Chim Acta.* 412:513-20.

Coulombe, P., & Meloche, S. (2007). Atypical mitogen-activated protein kinases: structure, regulation and functions. *Biochim Biophys Acta.* 1773:1376–87.

Coulombe, F., Divangahi, M., & Veyrier, F. (2009). Increased NOD2-mediated recognition of N-glycolyl muramyl dipeptide. *J Exp Med.* 206:1709–16.

Dahan, S., Roda, G., & Pinn, D.(2008). Epithelial : lamina propria lymphocyte interactions promote epithelial cell differentiation. *Gastroenterology.*134:192–203.

Dubuquoy, L., Jansson, E.A., & Deeb, S.(2003). Impaired expression of peroxisome proliferator-activated receptor gamma in ulcerative colitis. *Gastroenterology,* 124:1265–76.

Duchmann, R., Neurath, M.F., & Meyer, zum. (1997). Responses to self and non-self intestinal microflora in health and inflammatory bowel disease. *Res Immunol.* 148:589–594.

Duerr, R.H., Taylor, K.D., Brant, S.R.(2006). A genome-wide association study identifies IL23R as an inflammatory bowel disease gene. *Science.* 314: 1461-3.

Elias, B.C., Suzuki, T., & Seth, A. (2009). Phosphorylation of Tyr-398 and Tyr-402 in occludin prevents its interaction with ZO-1 and destabilizes its assembly at the tight junctions. *J Biol Chem.* 284:1559-69.

Erdman, S.E., Rao, V.P., & Poutahidis, T. (2003). CD4(þ)CD25(þ) regulatory lymphocytes require interleukin 10 to interrupt colon carcinogenesis in mice. *Cancer Res.* 63:6042–6050.

Escaffit, F., Boudreau, F., & Beaulieu, J.F.(2005). Differential expression of claudin-2 along the human intestine: Implication of GATA-4 in the maintenance of claudin-2 in differentiating cells. *J Cell Physiol.* 203: 15–26.

Festen, E.A., Stokkers, P.C., & Van Diemen, C.C. (2010). Genetic analysis in a Dutch study sample identifies more ulcerative colitis susceptibility loci and shows their additive role in disease risk. *Am J Gastroenterol.*105: 395–402.

Fihn, B.M., Sjoqvist, A., & Jodal, M. (2000). Permeability of the rat small intestinal epithelium along the villus- crypt axis: effects of glucose transport. *Gastroenterology,* 119, 1029–36

Franchimont, D., Vermeire, S., & El Housni, H.(2004) Deficient host-bacteria interactions in inflammatory bowel disease? The toll-like receptor (TLR)-4 Asp299gly polymorphism is associated with Crohn's disease and ulcerative colitis. *Gut.* 53: 987–92.

Frank, D.N., St. Amand, A.L., & Feldman, R.A.(2007). Molecular-phylogenetic characterization of microbial community imbalances in human inflammatory bowel diseases. *Proc Natl Acad Sci U S A.* 104: 13780–5.

Franke, A., Balschun, T., & Karlsen, T.H.(2008). Sequence variants in IL10, ARPC2 and multiple other loci contribute to ulcerative colitis susceptibility. *Nat Genet.*40:1319–1323.

Fujino, S., Andoh, A., & Bamba, S. (2003). Increased expression of interleukin 17 in inflammatory bowel disease. *Gut.* 52: 65–70.

Fukata, M., Chen, A., & Klepper, A. (2006). Cox-2 is regulated by Toll-like receptor-4 (TLR4) signaling: role in proliferation and apoptosis in the intestine. *Gastroenterology.* 131:862–77.

Furuse, M., Hirase, T., & Itoh, M. (1993). Occludin: a novel integral membrane protein localizing at tight junctions. *J Cell Biol.* 123:1777-88.

Furuse, M., Sasaki, H., & Fujimoto, K.(1998). A single gene product, claudin-1 or -2, reconstitutes tight junction strands and recruits occludin in fibroblasts. *J Cell Biol.* 143:391-401.

Furuse, M., & Tsukita, S.(2006). Claudins in occluding junctions of humans and flies. *Trends Cell Biol.* 16:181–8.

Fuss, I.J., Neurath, M., & Boirivant, M.(1996) Disparate CD4+ lamina propria (LP) lymphokine secretion profiles in inflammatory bowel disease. Crohn's disease LP cells manifest increased secretion of IFN-γ, whereas ulcerative colitis LP cells manifest increased secretion of IL-5. *J Immunol.* 157: 1261–70.

Fuss, I.J., Heller, F., & Boirivant, M.(2004). Nonclassical CD1d-restricted NK T cells that produce IL-13 characterize an atypical Th2 response in ulcerative colitis. *J Clin Invest.* 113:1490–7.

Fuss, I.J.(2008). Is the Th1/Th2 paradigm of immune regulation applicable to IBD? *Inflamm Bowel Dis.* Suppl 2:S110-2.

Gagnon, K.B., England, R., & Delpire, E.(2006). Characterization of SPAK and OSR1, regulatory kinases of the Na-K-2Cl cotransporter. *Mol Cell Biol.* 26:689–698.

Garat, C., & Arend, W.P.(2003). Intracellular IL-1Ra type 1 inhibits IL-1-induced IL-6 and IL-8 production in Caco-2 intestinal epithelial cells through inhibition of p38 mitogen-activated protein kinase and NF-kappaB pathways. *Cytokine.* 23: 31–40.

Girardin, S.E., Boneca, I.G., & Viala, J.(2003). Nod2 is a general sensor of peptidoglycan through muramyl dipeptide (MDP) detection. *J Biol Chem.* 278: 8869–72.

González-Mariscal, L., Betanzos, A., & Nava, P.(2003). Tight junction proteins. *Prog Biophys Mol Biol.* 81: 1-44.

Graham, W.V., Wang, F., & Clayburgh, D.R. (2006). Tumor necrosis factor-induced long myosin light chain kinase transcription is regulated by differentiation-dependent signaling events. Characterization of the human long myosin light chain kinase promoter. *J Biol Chem.* 281: 26205–15.

Hampe, J., Shaw, S.H., & Saiz, R. (1999). Linkage of inflammatory bowel disease to human chromosome 6p. *Am J Hum Genet.* 65:1647–55.

Hausmann, M., Kiessling, S., & Mestermann, S.(2002). Toll-like receptors 2 and 4 are up-regulated during intestinal inflammation. *Gastroenterology.* 122: 1987–2000.

Heazlewood, C. K., Cook, M.C., & Eri, R.(2008). Aberrant mucin assembly in mice causes endoplasmic reticulum stress and spontaneous inflammation resembling ulcerative colitis. *PLoS Med.* 5: e54.

Heller, F., Florian, P., & Bojarski, C., (2005). Interleukin-13 is the key effector Th2 cytokine in ulcerative colitis that affects epithelial tight junctions, apoptosis, and cell restitution. *Gastroenterology.* 129:550-64.

Hermiston, M.L., Gordon, J.I. (1995). Inflammatory bowel disease and adenomas in mice expressing a dominant negative N-cadherin. *Science*. 270:1203–1207.

Hermiston, M.L., Gordon, J.I. (1995). *In vivo* analysis of cadherin function in the mouse intestinal epithelium: essential roles in adhesion, maintenance of differentiation, and regulation of programmed cell death. *J Cell Biol*. 129:489–506.

Hisamatsu, T., Suzuki. M., & Reinecker. H.C.(2003). CARD15/NOD2 functions as an antibacterial factor in human intestinal epithelial cells. *Gastroenterology*. 124:993–1000.

Hollander, D., Vadheim, C.M., & Brettholz, E. (1986). Increased intestinal permeability in patients with Crohn's disease and their relatives. A possible etiologic factor. *Ann Intern Med*.105:883–885.

Hong, Y.H., Varanasi, U.S., & Yang, W. (2003). AMP-activated protein kinase regulates HNF4alpha transcriptional activity by inhibiting dimer formation and decreasing protein stability. *J Biol Chem*. 278: 27495-501.

Hugot, J.P., Laurent-Puig, P., & Gower-Rousseau, C. (1996). Mapping of a susceptibility locus for Crohn's disease on chromosome 16. *Nature*. 379:821–23.

Hugot, J.P., Chamaillard, M., & Zouali, H. (2001). Association of NOD2 leucine-rich repeat variants with susceptibility to Crohn's disease. *Nature*. 411:599–603.

Ikenouchi, J., Furuse, M., & Furuse, K.(2005). Tricellulin constitutes a novel barrier at tricellular contacts of epithelial cells. *J Cell Biol*. 171:939-45.

Inohara, N., Ogura, Y., & Fontalba, A. (2003). Host recognition of bacterial muramyl dipeptide mediated through NOD2. Implications for Crohn's disease. *J Biol Chem*. 278:5509–12.

Inohara, N., Nunez, G. (2003). NODs: intracellular proteins involved in inflammation and apoptosis. *Nat Rev Immunol*.3:371–82.

Johansson, M. E., Phillipson, M., & Petersson, J.*(2008)*. The inner of the two Muc2 mucin-dependent mucus layers in colon is devoid of bacteria. *Proc Natl Acad Sci USA* 105: 15064–9.

Johnston, A.M., Naselli, G., & Gonez, L.J. (2000). SPAK, a STE20/SPS1-related kinase that activates the p38 pathway. *Oncogene*. 19:4290–4297.

Kaser, A., Lee, A.H., & Franke, A.(2008). XBP1 links ER stress to intestinal inflammation and confers genetic risk for human inflammatory bowel disease. *Cell*. 134:743–756.

Kelly, D., Campbell, J.I., & King, T.P. (2004). Commensal anaerobic gut bacteria attenuate inflammation by regulating nuclear-cytoplasmic shuttling of PPARgamma and RelA. *Nat Immunol*. 5:104–12.

Kenny, P.A., Enver, T., & Ashworth, A. (2005). Receptor and secreted targets of Wnt-1/beta-catenin signaling in mouse mammary epithelial cells. *BMC Cancer*.5:3.

Kolls, J.K. & Linden, A. (2004). Interleukin-17 family members and inflammation. *Immunity* 21: 467–476

Krimi, R.B., Kotelevets, L., & Dubuquoy, L.(2008). Resistin-like molecule beta regulates intestinal mucous secretion and curtails TNBS-induced colitis in mice. *Inflamm Bowel Dis*. 14:931-41.

Kuhn, R., Lohler, J., & Rennick, D., (1993). Interleukin-10-deficient mice develop chronic enterocolitis. *Cell*. 75:263–274.

Kwon, K.H., Ohigashi, H., & Murakami, A.(2007). Dextran sulfate sodium enhances interleukin-1 beta release via activation of p38 MAPK and ERK1/2 pathways in murine peritoneal macrophages. *Life Sci*. 81:362–71.

Lala, S., Ogura, Y., & Osborne, C.(2003). Crohn's disease and the NOD2 gene: a role for paneth cells. *Gastroenterology*. 125:47–57.

Lee, J., Mo, J.H., & Katakura, K.(2006). Maintenance of colonic homeostasis by distinctive apical TLR9 signaling in intestinal epithelial cells. *Nat Cell Biol.* 8: 1327–36.

Levine, B. & Deretic, V. (2007). Unveiling the roles of autophagy in innate and adaptive immunity. *Nat Rev Immunol.* 7:767–77.

Loftberg, R., Neurath, M., & Ost, A.(2002). Topical NFkB antisense oligonucleotides in patients with active distal colonic IBD. A randomised controlled pilot trial. *Gastroenterology.* 122: A60.

Louis, E., Libioulle, C., & Reenaers, C.(2009). Genetics of ulcerative colitis: the come-back of interleukin 10. *Gut.*58:1173–6.

Maeda, S., Hsu, L.C. &Liu, H. (2005). Nod2 mutation in Crohn's disease potentiates NF-kappaB activity and IL-1beta processing. *Science.* 307:734–8.

Mashimo, H., Wu, D.C., & Podolsky, D.K. (1996). Impaired defense of intestinal mucosa in mice lacking intestinal trefoil factor. *Science.* 274: 262–5

Matsuda, A., Suzuki, Y., & Honda, G.(2003). Large-scale identification and characterization of human genes that activate NF-kappaB and MAPK signaling pathways. *Oncogene.* 22:3307–18.

Mazmanian, S.K., Liu, C.H., & Tzianabos, A.O. (2005). An immunomodulatory molecule of symbiotic bacteria directs maturation of the host immune system. *Cell.* 122:107–118.

McGovern, D., Powrie, F. (2007). The IL23 axis plays a key role in the pathogenesis of IBD. *Gut.* 56: 1333–1336.

Medzhitov, R., & Janeway, C.A. Jr.(2002). Decoding the patterns of self and nonself by the innate immune system. *Science.* 296:298–300.

Mitic, L.L., & Anderson, J.M. (1998). Molecular architecture of tight junctions. *Annu Rev Physiol.* 60:121-42.

Mitsuyama, K., Suzuki, A., & Tomiyasu, N.(2006). Pro-inflammatory signaling by Jun-N-terminal kinase in inflammatory bowel disease. *Int J Mol Med.* 17:449–55.

Mosser, D.M., Zhang, X. (2008). Interleukin-10: new perspectives on an old cytokine. *Immunol Rev.* 226:205–218.

Neurath, M.F., Pettersson, S., & Meyer zum Büschenfelde, K.H.(1996) Local administration of antisense phosphorothioate oligonucleotides to the p65 subunit of NF-κB abrogates established experimental colitis in mice. *Nat Med.* 2: 998–1004.

Nenci, A., Becker, C., & Wullaert, A.(2007). Epithelial NEMO links innate immunity to chronic intestinal inflammation. *Nature.* 446: 557–561.

Neish, A.S., Gewirtz, A.T., & Zeng, H.(2000). Prokaryotic regulation of epithelial responses by inhibition of IkappaB-alpha ubiquitination. *Science.* 289:1560–3.

Ogura, Y., Bonen, D.K., & Inohara, N. (2001). A frameshift mutation in NOD2 associated with susceptibility to Crohn's disease. *Nature.* 411:603–6.

Ogura, Y., Lala, S., & Xin, W. (2003). Expression of NOD2 in Paneth cells: a possible link to Crohn's ileitis. *Gut.* 52:1591–7.

O'Neill, L.A., Fitzgerald, K.A., & Bowie, A.G.(2003). The Toll-IL-1 receptor adaptor family grows to five members. *Trends Immunol.* 24:286–90.

Oshima T, Miwa H, Joh T (2008). Changes in the expression of claudins in active ulcerative colitis. *J Gastroenterol Hepatol.*23(suppl 2): S146–150.

Otte, J-M., Cario, E., & Podolsky, D.K.(2004). Mechanisms of cross hyporesponsiveness to Toll-like receptor bacterial ligands in intestinal epithelial cells. *Gastroenterology.* 126:1054–70.

Ouellette, A.J., Hsieh, M.M., & Nosek, M.T.(1994). Mouse Paneth cell defensins: primary structures and antibacterial activities of numerous cryptdin isoforms. *Infect Immun.* 62:5040–7.

Packey, C.D., & Sartor, R.B. (2008). Interplay of commensal and pathogenic bacteria, genetic mutations, and immunoregulatory defects in the pathogenesis of inflammatory bowel diseases. *J Intern Med.* 263:597-606.

Piechotta, K., Lu. J., & Delpire, E. (2002). Cation chloride cotransporters interact with the stress-related kinases Ste20-related proline-alanine-rich kinase (SPAK) and oxidative stress response 1 (OSR1). *J Biol Chem.* 277:50812–50819.

Pierik, M., Joossens, S., & Van Steen, K. (2006). Toll-like receptor- 1, -2, and -6 polymorphisms influence disease extension in inflammatory bowel diseases. *Inflamm Bowel Dis.* 12: 1–8.

Pinton, P., Braicu, C., & Nougayrede, J.P.(2010). Deoxynivalenol impairs porcine intestinal barrier function and decreases the protein expression of claudin-4 through a mitogen-activated protein kinase-dependent mechanism. *J Nutr.* 140:1956-62

Podolsky, D.K.(2002). Inflammatory bowel disease. *N Engl J Med.*347:417–29.

Resta-Lenert, S., & Barrett, K.E. (2006). Probiotics and commensals reverse TNFalpha-and IFN-gamma-induced dysfunction in human intestinal epithelial cells. *Gastroenterology.* 130:731–746.

Saitou, M., Furuse, M., & Sasaki, H.(2000). Complex phenotype of mice lacking occludin, a component of tight junction strands. *Mol Biol Cell.* 11:4131-4142.

Sartor, R.B.(2008). Microbial influences in inflammatory bowel diseases. *Gastroenterology.* 134: 577–94.

Saxon, A., Shanahan, F., & Landers, C. (1990). A distinct subset of antineutrophil cytoplasmic antibodies is associated with inflammatory bowel disease. *J Allergy Clin Immunol.* 86: 202–210.

Schmidt, C., Giese, T., & Ludwig, B.(2005). Expression of interleukin-12-related cytokine transcripts in inflammatory bowel disease: elevated interleukin-23p19 and interleukin-27p28 in Crohn's disease but not in ulcerative colitis. *Inflamm Bowel Dis.* 11: 16–23.

Schulzke, J.D., Gitter, A.H., & Mankertz, J. (2005). Epithelial transport and barrier function in occludin-deficient mice. *Biochim Biophys Acta.* 1669:34-42.

Schulzke, J.D., Bojarski, C., & Zeissig, S.(2006). Disrupted barrier function through epithelial cell apoptosis. *Ann NY Acad Sci.* 1072:288-299.

Schmitz, H., Barmeyer, C., & Fromm, M.(1999). Altered tight junction structure contributes to the impaired epithelial barrier function in ulcerative colitis. *Gastroenterology.* 116: 301–9.

Schurmann, G., Bruwer, M., & Klotz, A. (1999). Transepithelial transport processes at the intestinal mucosa in inflammatory bowel disease. *Int J Colorectal Dis.* 14: 41–6.

Seibold, F., Brandwein, S., & Simpson, S. (1998). pANCA represents a cross-reactivity to enteric bacterial antigens. *J Clin Immunol.* 18: 153–60.

Sellon, R.K., Tonkonogy, S., & Schultz, M. (1998). Resident enteric bacteria are necessary for development of spontaneous colitis and immune system activation in interleukin-10-deficient mice. *Infect Immun.* 66:5224–5231.

Shen, L., Su, L., & Turner, J.R.(2009). Mechanisms and functional implications of intestinal barrier defects. *Dig Dis.* 27:443-9.

Simon, D.B., Lu, Y., & Choate, K.A.(1999). Paracellin-1, a renal tight junction protein required for paracellular Mg2+ resorption. *Science.* 285: 103–106.

Sokol, H., Pigneur, B., & Watterlot, L. (2008). *Faecalibacterium prausnitzii* is an anti-inflammatory commensal bacterium identified by gut microbiota analysis of Crohn disease patients. *Proc Natl Acad Sci USA.*105:16731–16736.

Spencer, D.M., Veldman, G.M., & Banerjee, S. (2002). Distinct inflammatory mechanisms mediate early versus late colitis in mice. *Gastroenterology.* 122: 94–105.

Strober, W., Fuss, I., & Mannon, P.(2007). The fundamental basis of inflammatory bowel disease. *J Clin Invest.*117: 514–21.

Suzuki, T., Elias, B.C., & Seth, A. (2009). PKC eta regulates occluding phosphorylation and epithelial tight junction integrity. *Proc Natl Acad Sci USA.* 106:61-66.

Szakal, D.N., Gyorffy, H., & Arato, A. (2010). Mucosal expression of claudins 2, 3, and 4 in proximal and distal part of duodenum in children with coeliac disease. *Virchows Arch.* 456: 245–250.

Tai, E.K., Wong, H.P., & Lam, E.K.(2008). Cathelicidin stimulates colonic mucus synthesis by up-regulating MUC1 and MUC2 expression through a mitogen-activated protein kinase pathway. *J Cell Biochem.* 104:251-8.

Targan, S.R., Landers, C.J., & Cobb, L. (1995). Perinuclear anti-neutrophil cytoplasmic antibodies are spontaneously produced by mucosal B cells of ulcerative colitis patients. *J Immunol.* 155:3262–3267.

Thalhamer, T., McGrath, M.A., & Harnett, M.M.(2008). MAPKs and their relevance to arthritis and inflammation. *Rheumatology (Oxf).* 47:409–14.

Thompson, A.I., & Lees, C.W.(2011). Genetics of ulcerative colitis. *Inflamm Bowel Dis.* 17:831–48.

Topper, J.N., Wasserman, S.M., & Anderson, K.R. (1997). Expression of the bumetanide-sensitive Na-K-Cl cotransporter BSC2 is differentially regulated by fluid mechanical and inflammatory cytokine stimuli in vascular endothelium. *J Clin Invest.* 99:2941–49.

Torok, H.P., Glas, J., & Tonenchi, L. (2004). Crohn's disease is associated with a toll-like receptor-9 polymorphism. *Gastroenterology.* 127: 365–6.

Toyoda, H., Wang, S.J., & Yang, H.Y.(1993). Distinct associations of HLA class II genes with inflammatory bowel disease. *Gastroenterology.*104:741-748.

Turner, J.R.(2006). Molecular basis of epithelial barrier regulation: from basic mechanisms to clinical application. *Am J Pathol.* 169:1901-9.

Ueno, N., Fujiya, M., & Segawa, S. (2011). Heat-killed body of lactobacillus brevis SBC8803 ameliorates intestinal injury in a murine model of colitis by enhancing the intestinal barrier function. *Inflamm Bowel Dis.* 17:2235-50.

Uhlig, H.H., Coombes, J., & Mottet, C.(2006). Characterization of Foxp3þCD4þCD25þ and IL-10-secreting CD4þCD25þ T cells during cure of colitis. *J Immunol.*177:5852–5860.

Van der Sluis, M., De Koning, B.A., & De Bruijn, A.C. (2006). Muc 2-deficient mice spontaneously develop colitis, indicating that Muc 2 is critical for colonic protection. *Gastroenterology.* 131: 117–29.

Van Itallie, C.M., Fanning, A.S., & Anderson, J.M.(2003). Reversal of charge selectivity in cation or anion-selective epithelial lines by expression of different claudins. *Am J Physiol Renal Physiol.* 285:F1078-1084.

Van Itallie, C.M., & Anderson, J.M.(2004). The molecular physiology of tight junction pores. *Physiology(Bethesda).*19:331-8.

Van Itallie, C.M., & Anderson, J.M.(2006). Claudins and epithelial paracellular transport. *Annu Rev Physiol.* 68:403-429.

Van Itallie C.M., Holmes, J., & Bridges, A., (2008). The density of small tight junction pores varies among cell types and is increased by expression of claudin-2. *J Cell Sci.* 121:298-305.

Vanderlugt, C.J., Miller, S.D. (1996).Epitope spreading. *Curr Opin Immunol.* 8:831–836.

Vermeire, S., Rutgeerts, P. (2004). Antibody responses in Crohn's disease. *Gastroenterology.* 126: 601–4.

Viollet, B., Kahn, A., & Raymondjean, M.(1997). Protein kinase A-dependent phosphorylation modulates DNA-binding activity of hepatocyte nuclear factor 4. *Mol Cell Biol.* 17: 4208-4219.

Wang, F., Graham, W.V., & Wang, Y.(2005). Interferon-γ and tumor necrosis factor-α synergize to induce intestinal epithelial barrier dysfunction by up-regulating myosin light chain kinase expression. *Am J Pathol.* 166: 409–419.

Wang, N., Yu, H., & Ma, J.(2010). Evidence for tight junction protein disruption in intestinal mucosa of malignant obstructive jaundice patients. *Scand J Gastroenterol.* 45: 191–9.

Watson, C.J., Hoare, C.J., & Garrod, D.R. (2005). Interferon-γ selectively increases epithelial permeability to large molecules by activating different populations of paracellular pores. *J Cell Sci.* 118: 5221–30.

Waetzig, G.H., Seegert, D., & Rosenstiel, P., (2002). p38 Mitogen-activated protein kinase is activated and linked to TNF-alpha signaling in inflammatory bowel disease. *J Immunol.* 168:5342–51.

Xavier, R.J., Podolsky, D.K. (2007). Unraveling the pathogenesis of inflammatory bowel disease. *Nature.* 448: 427–34.

Yan, F., & Polk, D.B. (2002). Probiotic bacterium prevents cytokine-induced apoptosis in intestinal epithelial cells. *J Biol Chem.* 277:50959–65.

Yan, Y., Nguyen, H., & Dalmasso, G.(2007). Cloning and characterization of a new intestinal inflammation-associated colonic epithelial Ste20-related protein kinase isoform. *Biochim Biophys Acta.* 1769:106–116.

Yan, Y., Laroui, H., & Ingersoll, S.A. (2011). Overexpression of Ste20-Related Proline/Alanine-Rich Kinase Exacerbates Experimental Colitis in Mice. *J Immunol.* 187:1496-505.

Yen, D., Cheung, J., & Scheerens, H. (2006). IL-23 is essential for T-cell mediated colitis and promotes inflammation via IL-17 and IL-6. *J Clin Invest.* 116: 1310–1316

Yu, A.S., McCarthy, K.M., & Francis, S.A.(2005). McCormack JM, Lai J, Rogers RA, Lynch RD, Schneeberger EE: Knockdown of occludin expression leads to diverse phenotypic alterations in epithelial cells. *Am J Physiol Cell Physiol.* 288:C1231-1241.

Zeissig, S., Bojarski, C., & Buergel, N. (2004). Downregulation of epithelial apoptosis and barrier repair in active Crohn's disease by tumour necrosis factor alpha antibody treatment. *Gut.* 53:1295-1302.

Zeissig, S., Burgel, N., & Gunzel, D.(2007). Changes in expression and distribution of claudin 2, 5 and 8 lead to discontinuous tight junctions and barrier dysfunction in active Crohn's disease. *Gut.* 56: 61–72.

Part 2

Advances in Diagnosis of Inflammatory Bowel Disease

7

The Role of Imaging in Inflammatory Bowel Disease Evaluation

Rahul A. Sheth and Michael S. Gee
Massachusetts General Hospital, Harvard Medical School, Boston, Massachusetts USA

1. Introduction

The evaluation of the digestive tract through radiologic techniques represents a cornerstone in the management of patients with inflammatory bowel disease (IBD). Historically, a central facet in the diagnostic evaluation for IBD was the double contrast barium enema, which provided a non-invasive method for assessing the mucosal pattern of the large bowel. In the modern era, this approach has been supplanted by endoscopic procedures such as colonoscopy that offer direct mucosal inspection and biopsy capabilities. However, while endoscopy offers unparalleled visualization of the large bowel lumen, the small bowel remains essentially wholly inaccessible by conventional endoscopic techniques (D. D. T. Maglinte, 2006). Thus, one important role that imaging plays in the care of patients with IBD is the evaluation of the small bowel, both to help discriminate between ulcerative colitis (UC) and Crohn's disease (CD), as well as to identify active versus inactive disease.

Moreover, the role of imaging has greatly expanded with the advancement of cross-sectional imaging techniques such as computed tomography (CT) and magnetic resonance imaging (MRI) that can assess the extramural manifestations of IBD. For example, UC almost always affects the colon in a stereotyped way, extending from the rectum proximally in a continuous manner, without skip areas. The superficial erosions in early or mild UC are below the resolution of CT and MRI. However, one severe complication of UC, and a leading cause of death, is toxic megacolon, in which inflammation leads to destruction of ganglion cells and consequent colonic dilation (Elsayes et al., 2010). In these acutely ill patients, non-invasive methods are preferred to endoscopy. Likewise, the urgent and emergent sequelae of CD such as abscesses, fistulae, perforations, and strictures are best identified by radiologic modalities. Additionally, the pre-surgical delineation of disease extent and the post-surgical investigation for operative complications revolve around cross-sectional imaging. Finally, techniques such as MRI that provide superior soft tissue contrast allow for both the improved visualization of the perianal disease manifestations of CD such as fistulae and abscesses, as well as the precise anatomic localization for treatment planning (Schreyer et al., 2004).

Multiple radiologic modalities, including fluoroscopy, CT, MRI, ultrasound, and nuclear medicine techniques, have been applied towards imaging IBD. In this chapter, we will discuss technical considerations, appropriate indications, and key imaging findings for each imaging modality. We will also discuss special considerations in pediatric patients, in particular the risks of recurrent exposure to ionizing radiation.

2. Fluoroscopic imaging

Fluoroscopic imaging traditionally has been considered as the "gold standard" approach to imaging the small bowel. Despite the promotion of newer endoscopic technologies such as video capsule endoscopy and double balloon endoscopy, as well as the development of cross-sectional methods such as CT and MR enterography, fluoroscopy remains a staple tool for the identification of small bowel pathology, particularly pathology involving the terminal ileum.

2.1 Patient preparation and imaging technique

In fluoroscopic imaging, conventional two-dimensional radiographs are obtained with the patient lying on an examination table. The patient is kept nil per os (NPO) for several hours prior to the examination; a bowel cleansing regimen is rarely employed. Bowel visualization is achieved following the administration of radio-opaque contrast agents, a large class of solutions that generally contain varying concentrations of barium. The benefits of fluoroscopic imaging include the ability to visualize peristaltic loops of small bowel in real time, a feature that allows for the discrimination between true abnormalities and transient changes in configuration related to motion. Additionally, with optimal contrast opacification, inspection of the mucosal surface along the entire length of the small bowel in relief is feasible. The patient's position can be adjusted by the fluoroscopist to any desirable obliquity with respect to the X-ray source so that the outline of every loop of small bowel is visualized. The fluoroscopist also employs compressive maneuvers using paddles, balloons, and gloves to spread out the loops of bowel so that they are individually visible.

Fluoroscopic imaging of the small bowel may be performed in two manners, either as a small bowel follow through or as a small bowel enteroclysis. In the former, the patient is asked to drink approximately 500cc of a barium-containing oral contrast solution. Serial spot radiographs are obtained until the bolus has passed the terminal ileum into the cecum; this takes approximately 45-60 minutes, though pro-peristaltic agents such as metoclopramide may be administered to accelerate the process. Fluoroscopy with compression is then performed to identify areas of pathology.

In enteroclysis, a naso-jejunal catheter is placed such that the tip of the catheter terminates in the proximal jejunum, distal to the ligament of Treitz. A barium-containing solution is then infused at a uniform rate through the catheter. One variation is to infuse methylcellulose after a small amount of barium; this "double contrast" technique offers an improved inspection of the mucosal surface pattern (D. D. Maglinte et al., 1987). Advantages of naso-jejunal intubation include bypassing the regulatory mechanisms of the pylorus and a more uniform distention and opacification of the entire small bowel, particularly in patients who are unable to drink an adequate volume of contrast by their own volition. Enteroclysis is particularly effective in provoking radiographic evidence of low-grade partial obstructions in patients with intermittent symptoms, findings that may have been undetectable by small bowel follow through. The process of naso-jejunal intubation and infusion of contrast, however, can be very uncomfortable, and in some cases intolerable, for patients; some institutions provide conscious sedation for that reason.

2.2 Imaging findings in IBD by fluoroscopy

Much of the fluoroscopic imaging of UC, which predominantly involves the large bowel, has been replaced by colonoscopy. However, approximately 20% of patients with severe UC have associated "backwash" ileitis. Fluoroscopy demonstrates a patulous, incompetent ileocecal valve with a granulated mucosal relief pattern of the terminal ileum. This finding is in contrast to CD, which is characterized by a stenotic ileocecal valve with luminal narrowing and ulceration of the terminal ileum. Backwash ileitis usually resolves following total colectomy (Carucci & Levine, 2002).

Crohn's disease can affect the digestive tract anywhere from the mouth to the anus; approximately 80% of these patients have small bowel involvement (Figure 1). Unlike UC, "skip areas" of uninvolved bowel may be interspersed between segments of affected bowel. However, CD has a predilection for affecting the terminal ileum. The earliest radiographic sign of CD is aphthous ulcers, which appear as shallow collections of contrast with surrounding radiolucent haloes due to adjacent mucosal edema. Aphthous ulcers are not specific to CD and may be seen in a number of diseases. However, as CD progresses, the ulcers coalesce to form linear, curvilinear, or spiculated areas of ulceration along the mesenteric border of the small bowel. There is resultant retraction of the bowel wall, leading to pseudodiverticula and pseudosacculation of the anti-mesenteric bowel wall. These active inflammatory changes can lead to intermittent small bowel obstruction, which is best diagnosed by enteroclysis technique. Severe disease produces a classic "cobblestone" appearance, with deep transverse and longitudinal ulcerations bordered by areas of edema creating a checkered mucosal relief pattern. Chronic CD leads to circumferential bowel wall thickening and irreversible stricture formation.

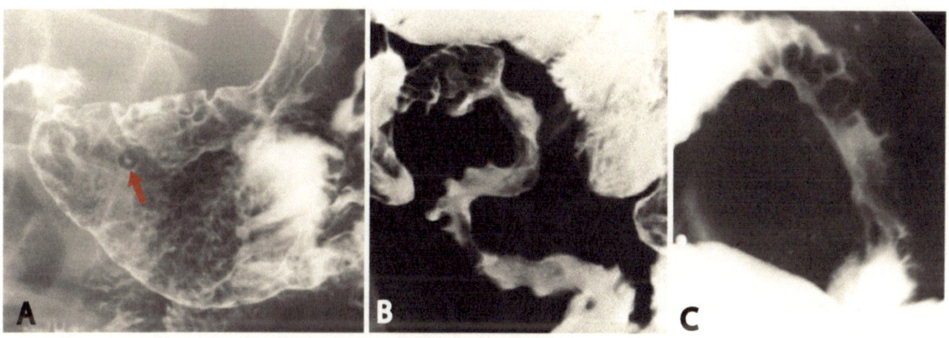

Fig. 1. Fluoroscopic imaging findings in Crohn's disease. A, Aphthous ulcers, which appear as focal collections of contrast with surrounding haloes of mucosal edema, are present in early CD (red arrow). B, Progressive disease results in longitudinal ulcerations on the mesenteric bowel surface with pseudosacculation formation on the anti-mesenteric surface. C, Severe disease can have a "cobblestone" mucosal relief pattern due to intersecting transverse and longitudinal ulcers.

Though fluoroscopic examination of the small bowel is still widely used, trans- and extramural disease are poorly detected with this technique. Moreover, the exposure of patients to ionizing radiation with this modality should be taken into consideration, particularly in patients who are likely to undergo frequent imaging examinations.

3. Computed tomographic imaging

Computed tomography remains the work-horse imaging modality for IBD and its complications in the United States. As a high-resolution cross-sectional technique, CT can visualize not only the bowel lumen, but also the bowel wall, visceral fat, intra-abdominal lymph nodes, and mesenteric vasculature supplying the bowel. Extraintestinal disease manifestations such as nephrolithiasis, sacroiliitis, and primary sclerosing cholangitis can readily be evaluated. Computed tomography can additionally be performed rapidly, and CT scanners are present in most emergency rooms, rendering it an ideal choice in the urgent or emergent setting.

The past two decades have witnessed a revolution in the technology of CT scanners. The introduction of the helical CT scanner has permitted the acquisition of volumetric data sets in a continuous, uninterrupted manner. The source data is obtained isotropically, meaning that the image voxel size is equivalent in all three dimensions. Because of this, the data can be reconstructed from the source axial plane into standard coronal or sagittal planes, or any other plane desired by the radiologist. Also, the advent of multidetector row scanners, initially with 4-slice devices in 1998, followed by 8-, 16-, 64-, and most recently 320-slice devices, has had a dramatic effect on reducing scanning time. This, in turn, has shortened the requisite breath hold for the patient, making the examination more comfortable and less often degraded by respiratory motion artifact (Kalra et al., 2004).

3.1 Patient preparation and imaging technique

There exist a variety of CT protocols for abdominal indications. With regards to IBD, a common reason to pursue imaging is for the assessment of small bowel pathology. As such, CT enterography is usually the imaging protocol of choice. For this imaging examination, patients are kept NPO for several hours prior; similar to fluoroscopy, a bowel cleansing regimen is not routinely required. Intravenous contrast is always used when possible. Enteral contrast is an indispensible component of the technique. Initial CT enterography relied on "positive" enteral contrast agents, usually barium containing solutions whose higher attenuation characteristics opacify the bowel lumen. However, differentiating the thin line of mucosal enhancement due to intravenous contrast from the opaque enteral contrast in the bowel lumen can be challenging. Therefore, a more popular approach is to use "neutral" enteral contrast agents that distend but do not opacify the bowel lumen. In this manner, mucosal enhancement patterns are well seen, as are areas of non-distensibility such as strictures. Water is a commonly used neutral enteral agent, but since this has the disadvantage of being absorbed by the body, commercially available preparations that are isodense to water on CT imaging but are non-absorbable are also prevalent (Horsthuis et al., 2008).

The volume of enteral contrast administered to the patient and the duration over which they are asked to ingest contrast vary by institution. However, the overall goal is to maximize uniform distention of the small bowel. Patients are first instructed to drink the enteral contrast, generally over approximately 45 to 60 minutes. They then lie down on the CT scanner; intravenous contrast is administered; and the CT scan is performed 50-60 seconds later, when mucosal enhancement is at its peak.

The CT analog to fluoroscopic enteroclysis, known at CT enteroclysis, is also used as a method to achieve optimal luminal filling. Contrast is usually administered under fluoroscopic guidance followed by the CT scan. Unlike fluoroscopy, though, a real-time assessment of bowel distensibility cannot be made by CT, as the patients are usually only imaged after the contrast has been fully administered. The disadvantage of patient discomfort caused by naso-jejunal intubation is no different.

An important concern with CT is the use of ionizing radiation. Recent studies suggest that CT exams account for the vast majority of ionizing radiation exposure to IBD patients from imaging, especially among patients diagnosed at an early age. An informed analysis of the associated risks, especially for the pediatric patient, should be performed prior to each examination. This topic is further addressed in section 6.

3.2 Imaging findings in Crohn's disease by CT

A principal clinical question for which CT is utilized in IBD is the determination of active versus inactive disease in the small bowel. This distinction is of high clinical significance: patients with active inflammation are treated medically with immuno-modulatory therapy, while symptomatic patients with inactive, fibrosed strictures often require surgical intervention. Areas of actively inflamed bowel on CT most commonly demonstrate pathologic bowel thickening, which is defined as bowel wall greater than 3mm in thickness. A 3mm cutoff was selected by consensus as the best compromise between sensitivity and specificity and is for the most part used universally for all cross-sectional modalities including MRI and ultrasound. Another differentiating characteristic of active disease is mucosal hyperenhancement, which appears as a pencil-thin line outlining the luminal surface of the bowel wall and reflects the hyperemia of inflammation (Figure 2A). This finding is considered the most sensitive for active disease, and the degree of hyperenhancement may correlate with the degree of underlying inflammation. Active inflammation also results in submucosal edema, which manifests on CT examination as a lower attenuation submucosal layer interposed between mucosal and serosal layers. This mural stratification is also referred to as the "target sign" due to its characteristic appearance (Figure 2C). The most specific feature for active CD is engorgement of the vasa recta adjacent to an inflamed loop of bowel, a finding known as the "comb sign" (Figure 2B). Secondary signs for active inflammation include mesenteric fat stranding and lymphadenopathy. Of note, while mucosal hyperenhancement and abnormal bowel thickening are frequent features of active CD, they are not specific and may be seen in infectious enteritis or mesenteric ischemia. Similarly, mural stratification can be seen in UC as well as bowel ischemia. On the other hand, the "comb sign" is considered fairly specific for CD (Elsayes, et al., 2010; Horsthuis, et al., 2008).

The presence of mucosal hyperenhancement, abnormal bowel wall thickening, mural stratification, and prominent adjacent vasa recta in an area of poorly distensible bowel suggests that the stricture is due to active inflammation and is thus potentially reversible by medical interventions. The strictures of chronic CD, conversely, are fibrotic, irreversible, and do not demonstrate the features of active disease described above. The presence of luminal narrowing with proximal bowel dilation is suggestive of fibrosis. Long-standing inflammation leads to fat deposition within the submucosa of the bowel wall; this apparent mural stratification should not be confused with the "target sign" of active disease and can be differentiated based on the Hounsfield attenuation characteristics of fat, which is less that 0 Hounsfield units (Figure 3A). Secondly, the fibrotic retraction preferentially affects the mesenteric bowel wall, leading to the pseudosacculation appearance on the anti-mesenteric side that can also be seen by fluoroscopy. Finally, chronic transmural CD, possibly due to chronic inflammatory stimulation, produces a fibrofatty proliferation of the mesenteric fat, also known on CT examinations as the "creeping fat sign" (Figure 3B).

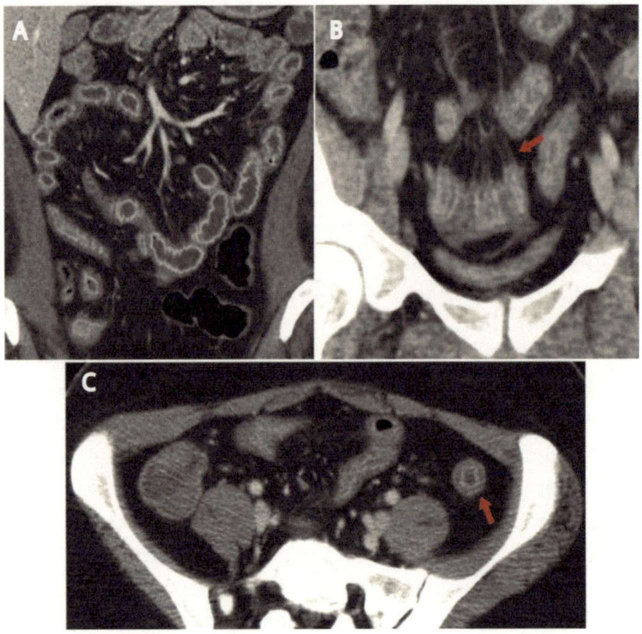

Fig. 2. CT findings in acute Crohn's disease. A, Active inflammation causes mucosal hyperenhancement and bowel wall thickening greater than 3mm. B, Engorgement of the vasa recta adjacent to an inflamed loop of bowel is a specific finding in active CD and has been coined the "comb sign." C, Submucosal edema yields a characteristic "target sign."

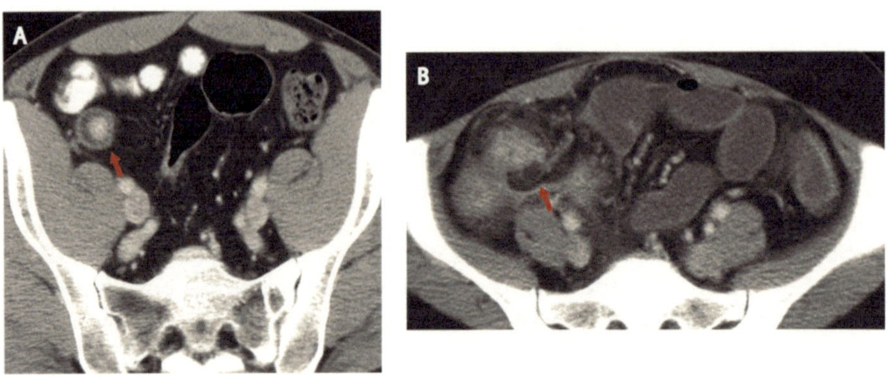

Fig. 3. CT findings in chronic Crohn's disease. A, Fatty depositions in the submucosal layer may mimic the "target sign" of active disease (red arrow). B, Fibrofatty proliferation of the mesenteric fat, or "creeping fat," (red arrow) is seen in chronic, transmural disease.

The extra-mural complications of CD are excellently depicted by CT. Penetrating disease is present in approximately 20% with CD, with fistulas representing the most common pathology in this category (Schreyer, et al., 2004). Fistulous tracts may form between any two epithelially lined viscera in the abdomen, such as other loops of bowel (entero-enteric), the bladder (entero-vesicular), and the skin (entero-cutaneous). A communicating tract that fills with enteral contrast is diagnostic (Figure 4A). Evaluation with CT is highly sensitive for the detection of fistulae, though certain anatomic locations such as the perianal region are better imaged by MRI, as discussed below.

Intra-abdominal abscesses are extra-luminal fluid collections that do not communicate with the bowel (Figure 4B). The discontinuity of the abscess collection with the bowel lumen is important to verify but can occasionally be challenging, as neural enteral contrast within the bowel mimics the attenuation characteristics of the infected fluid within the abscess cavity. For this reason, positive enteral contrast is often preferred to neutral contrast in patients with suspected abscess.

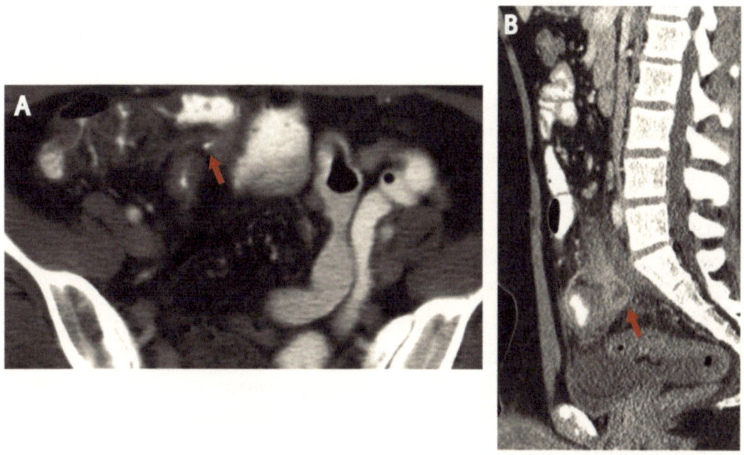

Fig. 4. Complications of Crohn's disease on CT. A, A fistula between two loops of small bowel is well depicted by CT as a thin tract of oral contrast connecting the lumens of the two loops. B, An intra-abdominal abscess posterior to the distal large bowel, likely due to a microperforation, was identified in this patient.

3.3 Imaging findings in ulcerative colitis by CT

As discussed previously, colonoscopy remains the primary approach for diagnosing and determining extent of disease in UC. However, severe complications of UC such as toxic megacolon are an important indication for imaging, with CT representing the mainstay modality in these unstable patients. CT findings include thinning of the colonic wall, luminal distension, and pneumatosis; severe cases can lead to perforation and free intraperitoneal gas.

4. Magnetic resonance imaging

Magnetic resonance imaging enjoys many inherent advantages over other cross-sectional imaging modalities. These include the ability to acquire images in any imaging plane, the lack of ionizing radiation, and excellent soft tissue resolution. Because of the lack of ionizing radiation, imaging may be performed at multiple time points during an examination, for example at different phases of contrast enhancement, providing a multiparametric assessment of any particular pathology. Additionally, "cine" images can be obtained sequentially over time, in an MRI analog to fluoroscopy.

The intrinsic spatial resolution of MRI, however, is inferior to that of CT. An MRI examination also takes longer to complete than a CT exam. However, the widespread adoption of new, faster MRI pulse sequences, described in the subsequent section, has significantly reduced scanning time and opened the door for small bowel imaging. For specific clinical scenarios, such as perianal disease, MRI is the recognized gold standard non-invasive technique.

4.1 Patient preparation and imaging technique

As with CT, multiple different MRI protocols exist for examining the abdomen. In the realm of IBD, one very useful MR examination is magnetic resonance enterography (MRE). Although an in-depth discussion of the various pulse sequences used in abdominal MRI imaging is beyond the scope of this text, a familiarity with the commonly used sequences is valuable in understanding the applicability of MRE. Sequences with T2 weighting are the best for evaluating the bowel wall. Intravenous contrast enhancement appears bright on T1 weighted sequences; however, as feces can occasionally be bright on T1 imaging too, pre-contrast T1 image sets are obtained to help identify true enhancement. Conventional spin echo pulse sequences do not afford the requisite temporal resolution to image the abdomen during a single breath hold; as such, the resulting images are often degraded by respiratory motion artifact. Beyond that, high temporal resolution is made all the more critical when investigating a moving target as the bowel. For these reasons, MRE capitalizes on customized MR pulse sequences that offer improved temporal resolution and are able to image the entire abdomen during a single breath hold. For example, single-shot turbo spin echo (e.g. SSFSE or HASTE) sequences produce high quality, motion-free T2 weighted images of the entire bowel (Fidler, 2007). Balanced steady state free precession sequences (e.g. FIESTA or TrueFISP) are T1 and T2 intermediate-weighted sequences that that are rapid and demonstrate increased conspicuity of the mesentery for detection of inflammatory changes or fistula formation (Chalian et al., 2011). These sequences, due to their rapidity, can be performed as thick slab cinematic acquisitions to evaluate bowel peristalsis, known as MR fluoroscopy. Fat suppression is routinely employed during both T2-weighted and T1-weighted post-contrast sequences, to highlight areas of bowel wall edema and enhancement. The post-contrast T1 fat-suppressed sequences are performed using 3-D techniques to accelerate image acquisition and enable dynamic evaluation of bowel enhancement at multiple timepoints post-contrast. An average imaging time for MRE, exclusive of the time required for enteral contrast administration, is approximately 30-45 minutes.

There is no specific bowel preparation prior to MRE, but patients generally are kept NPO for several hours prior to the exam. Anti-peristaltic agents such as glucagon may help improve image quality and are often administered just prior to imaging. Intravenous contrast with a gadolinium-chelate containing agent is standardly administered. There are several options in enteral contrast, which can be categorized by their MRI signal characteristics. "Negative" agents are intrinsically T1 and T2 dark compounds that usually contain superparamagnetic iron oxide particles. Their principle advantage is that they emphasize mucosal enhancement and bowel wall edema. "Positive" agents are intrinsically T1 and T2 bright compounds; these, similar to positive CT contrast agents, may obscure mucosal enhancement findings and thus are infrequently used. The most commonly used class of MR enteral contrast agents is the "biphasic" type, which are T1 dark and T2 bright. With these agents, one can readily assess the pattern of bowel wall folds on T2 weighted images without losing mucosal enhancement data on T1 weighted images (Tolan et al., 2010). Contrast agents are often hyperosmolar to maximize luminal distention; an important side effect for patients to be aware of is diarrhea.

Enteral contrast is primarily administered orally, though MR enteroclysis is also an option. The attendant patient discomfort and added radiation from the fluoroscopy-guided placement of the naso-jejunal tube are identical to the CT analog. However, one benefit of MR enteroclysis is the ability to perform MR fluoroscopy during the instillation of enteral contrast, a technique that provides dynamic information regarding bowel distensibility.

4.2 Imaging findings in Crohn's disease by MR enterography

The strengths of MRI when applied towards IBD are best suited for investigating the small bowel and the perianal region, anatomic locations towards which CD demonstrates a tropism. Magnetic resonance imaging of the large bowel, an examination that would have increased relevance in UC, is not routinely performed. Therefore, in this section, emphasis will be placed on the findings of CD in the small bowel by MRI.

Many of the imaging characteristics of active CD on MRI, as one may expect, are morphologically identical to those appreciated on CT. For example, bowel wall thickening greater than 3mm is considered abnormal and evidence of active inflammation. Active disease with intramural edema manifests as T2 hyperintensity between the mucosa and muscularis propria (Figure 5A) (Sinha et al., 2009). Mucosal hyperenhancement is also an important marker of active disease. Diffuse, avid, homogeneous mucosal enhancement is suggestive of active disease (Figure 5B). Alternatively, low-level, heterogeneous mural enhancement without a mucosal component favors the diagnosis of chronic fibrosis (Figure 5C). Ulceration may be difficult to identify without proper bowel distention; ulcers appear as thin lines of high signal intensity within thickening loops of bowel. Both MRI and CT are insensitive for early aphthous ulcers, for which fluoroscopy or endoscopy should be considered as more sensitive.

Additional evidence of active disease such as the "comb sign," in which there is engorgement of the mesenteric vessels adjacent to an inflamed loop of bowel, are well identified by MRI. Strictures appear as a focal narrowing in the bowel lumen and are considered significant if there is a pre-stenotic dilation of the proximal bowel. The so-called "creeping fat sign" occurs in chronic, transmural inflammation, in which hypertrophy of the mesenteric fat produces mass effect and surrounds viscera; this sign is specific for CD. Another sign of chronic inflammatory fibrosis is T2 hypointensity within the bowel wall.

Extramural disease is as conspicuous, if not more so, on MRI as it is on CT. Fistulae appear as T2 hyperintense tracts that avidly enhance and extend from bowel to a second epithelial lined organ such as another segment of bowel, the skin, or the bladder. Sinuses are blind-ending tracts that extend from bowel and typically terminate within the mesentery. Both fistulae and sinuses cause translocation of gut flora out of the bowel and can be associated with abscess formation.

4.3 Imaging findings in perianal disease

In addition to evaluating the small bowel with enterography, MRI is a powerful tool in the investigation of perianal fistulae. The lifetime risk of developing fistulous disease in CD is approximately 20-40%. Anorectal fistulae are common and are classified based on their location relative to the anal sphincter complex and pelvic floor musculature, as anatomic location impacts upon treatment options. The most common type of anorectal fistula is the intersphincteric fistula (Figure 6A), followed by the transphincteric fistula (Figure 6B). The accuracy of MRI for diagnosing and classifying anorectal fistulae is comparable to exam under anesthesia (Schreyer et al., 2004).

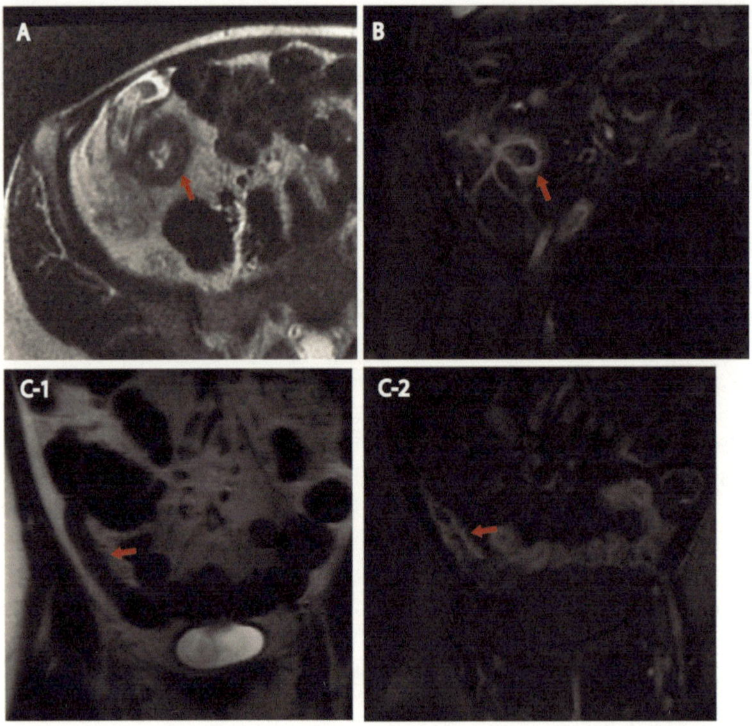

Fig. 5. Findings of Crohn's disease by MR enterography. A) Submucosal edema appears as T2 hyperintensity interposed between the mucosa and muscularis propria (red arrow). B) Homogeneous, avid mucosal enhancement on T1-weighted imaging is suggestive of active disease (red arrow). C) Conversely, fixed lumimal narrowing on a T2 weighted image (red arrow, C-1) that demonstrates delayed mural enhancement on a post contrast T1 weighted image (red arrow, C-2) without a mucosal component is seen in chronic fibrosis.

5. Ultrasound

Ultrasound is a cross-sectional imaging technique that has been used extensively in the imaging of IBD. As with other technologies, ultrasound has its own unique set of advantages, such as low relative cost, lack of ionizing radiation, and real-time imaging capability. Disadvantages include the inability to visualize portions of small bowel, rectum, and sigmoid, as well as operator dependence, with the quality of the examination contingent on the technical skill of the ultrasonographer. Ultrasound has been shown to possibly be as accurate in the diagnosis of IBD as CT and MRI based on detection of wall thickening and hypervascularity by Doppler. However, a high sensitivity is likely achievable only in the hands of an expert ultrasonographer, a resource that is not widely available or easy to standardize. Ultrasound is particularly relevant in pediatric imaging: the smaller body habitus in this patient population allows for a more complete examination, and the lack of ionizing radiation is likely safer compared to CT.

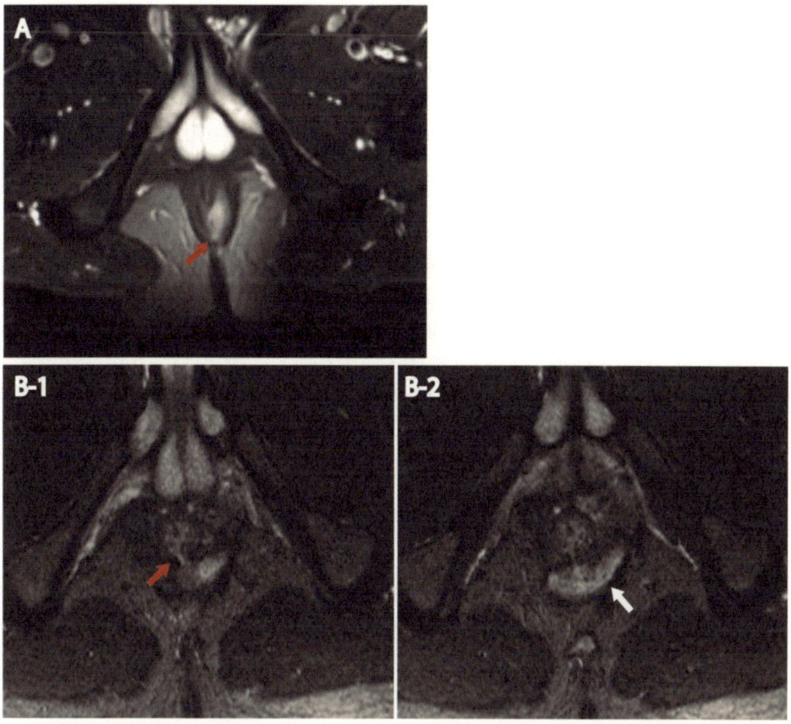

Fig. 6. MRI findings of anorectal fistulae. A, T2 hyperintensity that extends between the external and internal sphincter complexes is diagnostic of a intersphincteric fistula (red arrow). B, Two sequential T2 weighted images demonstrate a linear hyperintense focus traversing through the internal and external sphincter complexes consist with a transsphincteric fistula (red arrow, B-1). The subsequent image demonstrates an associated fluid collection extending into the left ischioanal fossa (white arrow, B-2).

5.1 Patient preparation and imaging technique

Similar to the previously described modalities, minimal patient preparation is required in ultrasound. Since luminal gas can cause artifacts that obscure underlying structures, non-effervescent liquid may be administered to displace bowel gas distally and provide some luminal distension. The choice of ultrasound transducer is predicated by the patient's body size. Higher frequency transducers produce higher resolution images but have poorer tissue penetration compared to lower frequency transducers. Practically, an ultrasonographer will begin the examination with the highest frequency transducer available, which is usually a 15 megahertz transducer; if there are structures that are not well seen, the ultrasonographer can change to a lower frequency one.

The approach to handling the ultrasound transducer and physically tracing it across the abdomen is of paramount importance. A key technique in imaging the bowel is known as "graded compression." Increasing pressure is applied with the transducer head as it is swept across the surface of the abdomen. This has the effect of displacing bowel gas and overlying bowel loops so that the area of interest can be inspected with the greatest possible clarity (Darge et al., 2010).

5.2 Imaging findings in IBD by ultrasound

A normal segment of bowel on ultrasound exhibits five discrete layers. The inner-most layer is a thin hyperechoic line that demarcates the interface between the lumen and the mucosa. The next layer is a hypoechoic line at the interface between the mucosa and submucosa. The third layer is a hyperechoic line between submucosa and the muscularis propria; this is the most commonly involved layer in IBD. The fourth layer is the muscularis propria itself and is hypoechoic. The fifth and final layer is hyperechoic and represents the serosa (Migaleddu et al., 2008).

Inflammatory bowel disease is manifested on ultrasound as abnormal bowel wall thickening, defined as greater than 3mm, and loss of definition of the discrete bowel wall layers. Both UC and CD result in bowel wall thickening. However, in UC the bowel wall layers are preserved, as opposed to CD; this distinction though may not be sufficiently accurate to differentiate the two diseases by US alone. Intra-mural edema appears as generalized hypoechogenicity within the bowel wall. Conversely, fibrostenoic disease exhibits hyperechogenicity of the submucosal layer. Superficial ulcers may be detected as hypoechoic interruptions within the innermost bowel wall layer.

Doppler ultrasound can provide useful adjunct data to the structural information from conventional ultrasound. Normal bowel wall, as well as fibrostenotic bowel wall, does not usually demonstrate detectable Doppler blood flow. Therefore, the presence of intramural blood flow is suggestive of the hyperemia of active disease.

6. Special considerations in the pediatric population

Performing diagnostic imaging examinations on pediatric patients requires consideration of several important factors. For example, pediatric patients may not be able to tolerate prolonged examinations such as MR enterography, necessitating the use of sedation to obtain satisfactory images. Moreover, not only are pediatric patients with IBD committed to a lifetime of imaging studies, but also their increased percentage of actively dividing tissue and relatively smaller body habitus render them inherently more sensitive to radiation injury and mutagenesis compared an adult. When these risks are coupled with their baseline increased risk of malignancy due to IBD, the importance of radiation dose reduction becomes apparent.

The association between diagnostic radiation and cancer risk is controversial. Directly studying the effects of ionizing radiation on malignancy risk is extremely challenging. Frequently cited epidemiologic data are based on atomic bomb survivors and nuclear power plant workers who were exposed to radiation levels that exceed those in diagnostic imaging. Moreover, the deleterious effects of radiation likely have a prolonged incubation time, perhaps on the order of decades, before they are clinically apparent. On the other hand, there is little doubt that every effort should be made to reduce the radiation exposure in pediatric patients to minimize any potential risk.

Estimating the magnitude of absorbed radiation during a CT examination can be made through the use of phantoms. Though no patient, and especially no pediatric patient, is identical to the standard, adult-sized body phantom, this approach remains the most quantitative means of estimating radiation levels within the body during a CT exam. However, extrapolating malignancy risk from these data is difficult, as different organs exhibit unique susceptibilities to radiation exposure. For example, the gonads are far more radio-sensitive than muscle tissue. For this reason, the concept of "effective dose" was introduced. This term, measured in millisieverts (mSv), reflects an attempt to create a standard metric that quantifies the impact of the absorbed radiation (Peloquin et al., 2008). Effective dose is calculated by multiplying the absorbed radiation dose by a conversion factor for the body segment that was imaged; this conversion factor varies based upon the radiosensitivity of the exposed organs.

The choice of imaging modality for IBD over the past two decades has trended towards an increase in the use of CT. Pediatric patients may undergo multiple CT examinations over their lifetime, and the cumulative effective dose they receive may exceed 75 mSv, a level beyond which radiation-induced malignancy is felt to become an increasing concern. Patients with Crohn's disease are imaged far more frequently than those with UC. Also, patients who require immunosuppressive therapy or surgery are also at a higher risk of frequent imaging. Additional risk factors include stricturing or penetrating disease (Desmond et al., 2008).

The most important avenue for reducing radiation dose is the eradication of unnecessary examinations. Minimizing exposure time during fluoroscopy should be standard practice. Multiple techniques for reducing radiation dose in CT examinations have been developed and should be implemented when imaging pediatric patients. Finally, substituting non-ionizing radiation imaging modalities such as MRI and ultrasound should be considered when appropriate.

7. Imaging recommendations in IBD

The modalities described in this chapter each demonstrate their own unique set of advantageous and disadvantageous features. While fluoroscopy may show superficial mucosal disease better than any cross-sectional technique, extra-luminal disease is poorly visualized. The high spatial and temporal resolution of CT has driven its rise in popularity over the past two decades; however, this examination requires the use of ionizing radiation, and an appreciation of the possible associated risks is paramount prior to selecting this modality. While MRI is more costly and time consuming, it may be the best choice in a clinical situation where minimizing radiation dose is important or when soft tissue characterization is required.

For the evaluation of a suspected complication or acute exacerbation of previously diagnosed Crohn's disease in an adult patient, we recommend the use of CT enterography, with MR enterography as the next best option. Urgent and emergent complications such as abscess formation and acute bowel obstruction are best imaged with CT. On the other hand, perianal disease should be investigated with MRI. Early manifestations of IBD may be below the sensitivity of cross-sectional imaging but can be well identified by fluoroscopy. Enteroclysis techniques should generally be reserved for those patients with remitting-relapsing mild symptoms such as partial intermittent small bowel obstructions as a provocative examination to detect short strictures. In pediatric patients, MR enterography is becoming the preferred primary imaging modality due to lack of ionizing radiation. There is likely to be an increasing role for ultrasound in surveillance imaging in the future given its low cost and lack of requirement of sedation or oral contrast preparation.

8. References

Carucci, L. R., & Levine, M. S. (2002). Radiographic imaging of inflammatory bowel disease. *Gastroenterol Clin North Am, 31*(1), 93-117, ix.

Chalian, M., Ozturk, A., Oliva-Hemker, M., Pryde, S., & Huisman, T. A. G. M. (2011). MR Enterography Findings of Inflammatory Bowel Disease in Pediatric Patients. *American Journal of Roentgenology, 196*(6), W810-816.

Darge, K., Anupindi, S., Keener, H., & Rompel, O. (2010). Ultrasound of the bowel in children: how we do it. *Pediatr Radiol, 40*(4), 528-536.

Desmond, A. N., O'Regan, K., Curran, C., McWilliams, S., Fitzgerald, T., Maher, M. M., et al. (2008). Crohn's disease: factors associated with exposure to high levels of diagnostic radiation. *Gut, 57*(11), 1524-1529.

Elsayes, K. M., Al-Hawary, M. M., Jagdish, J., Ganesh, H. S., & Platt, J. F. (2010). CT enterography: principles, trends, and interpretation of findings. *Radiographics, 30*(7), 1955-1970.

Fidler, J. (2007). MR imaging of the small bowel. *Radiol Clin North Am, 45*(2), 317-331.

Horsthuis, K., Stokkers, P. C. F., & Stoker, J. (2008). Detection of inflammatory bowel disease: diagnostic performance of cross-sectional imaging modalities. *Abdom Imaging, 33*(4), 407-416.

Kalra, M. K., Maher, M. M., D'Souza, R., & Saini, S. (2004). Multidetector computed tomography technology: current status and emerging developments. *J Comput Assist Tomogr, 28 Suppl 1*, S2-6.

Maglinte, D. D., Lappas, J. C., Kelvin, F. M., Rex, D., & Chernish, S. M. (1987). Small bowel radiography: how, when, and why? *Radiology, 163*(2), 297-305.

Maglinte, D. D. T. (2006). Small bowel imaging-- a rapidly changing field and a challenge to radiology. *European Radiology, 16*(5), 967-971.

Migaleddu, V., Quaia, E., Scano, D., & Virgilio, G. (2008). Inflammatory activity in Crohn disease: ultrasound findings. *Abdom Imaging, 33*(5), 589-597.

Peloquin, J. M., Pardi, D. S., Sandborn, W. J., Fletcher, J. G., McCollough, C. H., Schueler, B. A., et al. (2008). Diagnostic ionizing radiation exposure in a population-based cohort of patients with inflammatory bowel disease. *Am J Gastroenterol, 103*(8), 2015-2022.

Schreyer, A. G., Seitz, J., Feuerbach, S., Rogler, G., & Herfarth, H. (2004). Modern imaging using computer tomography and magnetic resonance imaging for inflammatory bowel disease (IBD) AU1. *Inflamm Bowel Dis, 10*(1), 45-54.

Sinha, R., Murphy, P., Hawker, P., Sanders, S., Rajesh, A., & Verma, R. (2009). Role of MRI in Crohn's disease. *Clin Radiol, 64*(4), 341-352.

Tolan, D. J. M., Greenhalgh, R., Zealley, I. A., Halligan, S., & Taylor, S. A. (2010). MR enterographic manifestations of small bowel Crohn disease. *Radiographics, 30*(2), 367-384.

8

Health-Related Quality of Life in Inflammatory Bowel Disease

Ramiro Veríssimo
University of Porto Faculty of Medicine
Portugal

1. Introduction

There is a generalized conviction that morbidity and mortality indexes commonly used to assess health outcomes are scarce in information. Furthermore, the accelerated rate at which new means of therapeutic intervention emerge has stressed the interest in other ways to assess the health status; namely the subjective health status while depicting the functional ability. Which, given the exponential growth of studies coming to light, became indexed in MEDLINE since 1977 under the keywords Quality-of-Life. But although much has been written on the use of this sort of questionnaires in several areas of research, and particularly in epidemiological studies and in clinical trials, it is also true that its infiltration in clinical practice is little more than shy.

2. Conceptualization

2.1 Model

In fact, clinicians have always kept some reserve towards adopting in daily practice aspects related with human characteristics that they somehow consider subjective and personal; especially when compared with laboratory data or endoscopic findings. They seem reluctant to adopt variables of this type in order to quantify their interventions' outcomes. That is, insofar as Quality of Life is considered a relatively vague concept and not in the least in accordance with medical requirements. However, in this sense it is meant to be stripped of all generic notions such as satisfaction with lifestyle, involving instead mostly aspects related with health and medical care related experiences.

This is why it is usually considered equivalent to health status in terms of symptoms and functional ability; further specifying **Health-related Quality of Life** (HR-QoL), thus aiming at limiting the concept's scope and cleansing the acknowledged multidimensionality of its content from the refuse of aspects less related with medical intervention objectives, as is the case, for example, of aspects concerned with financial or housing situation.

2.2 Applications

As mentioned above, in recent years there has been a growing interest in evaluating Health-related Quality of Life [1, 2], particularly when it concerns chronic conditions which are not curable, but also have considerably remote prospects of death. This way one can assume that one of the main goals of the therapeutic intervention is somehow to improve patients'

Quality of Life; and this must be in a final analysis the touchstone by which to assess the outcomes of those interventions.

Therefore, the main goal is to achieve an accurate assessment of the health status, either at individual or population level, in order to consider the outcomes of care more positively or negatively. In fact, it has been observed that activity indexes used in chronic Inflammatory Bowel Disease (IBD) are no exception, turning out to be insufficiently sensitive and even differing from the patients' perception of their own status [3, 4]. Moreover, these Quality of Life indexes have been shown to be more heavily related with well-being and fewer requests of health services than the clinical evaluation of the disease's activity [5].

Hence some of the applications that one can infer for this type of assessment. For example, where **clinical trials** are concerned, they usually focus on physiological reactions; however the assessment of Quality of Life is by far a much better way to assess functional ability. Therefore, if functional ability is indeed an important outcome, then it must be evaluated directly. In other words, clinical trials should include more information of this type in order to properly assess the therapeutic effectiveness.

In fact, **patients in particular** and society in general care more about symptomatic complaints and functional ability than laboratorial findings and physiological responses. However, given that these complaints frequently take an emotional aspect, they are often ignored. Faced with increasingly incapacitated patients, the clinicians continually report "improvement" in their notes on patient status. This only stresses the importance of a standardized assessment of functional ability and the need to translate this added interest from the field of research to that of clinical practice. In other words, this will allow triages aimed at identifying patients who stand out in terms of need for special attention or certain differentiated healthcare; namely through the potential involvement of certain problems of psychosocial nature, liable to be identified or determined by these instruments. Furthermore, it may allow monitoring clinical assessment and suggesting alternative therapeutic solutions; thus contributing to a more adequate clinical intervention. As previously stated, Quality of Life may often collide with clinical assessment, but what has been observed is that this type of data, whether on grounds of mistrust, inadequacy, or the unavailability on the opportune moment, is often ignored in decision making at this level [6]. It all comes down, in the specific context of the therapeutic relationship, to meet patient's expectations; which this process somehow makes more explicit.

Systematic research at the **population level** may determine with some precision which areas of healthcare intervention, if untended by conventional epidemiological measures, may be considered especially problematic, as perceived by patients. Furthermore, the quality of services rendered can and should be assessed in terms of results attained in this domain, allowing the elaboration, and result comparison, of alternative strategies.

3. Methods

3.1 Dimensions

The notion of Health-related Quality of Life (HR-QoL) is nonetheless an encompassing notion, as it includes patients' perceptions of their own health condition and their experience of the disease. From this **multidimensionality** stem the main obstacles in conceiving, analyzing and interpreting studies on Quality of Life. As such, although it integrates disease-related factors, it is also shaped by a psycho-affective dimension and influenced by aspects of socio-cultural nature. It is in this sense that disease activity is understood in the context of a somatic dimension, of which Quality of Life is a part, but differs in two fundamental aspects; namely, the fact that the assessment must take into account factors not only disease-related but also psychosocial, and the consequent aspect that the assessment is necessarily subjective as it is based on the patients' account of those factors. However, just as in the disease assessment in the form of histopathological typification and determination of location and extent, the Quality of Life assessment aims at quantifying the multiple factors that contribute to the illness status. In other words, the goal is to assess not only the disease but also the patients' perception of the disease.

3.2 Requirements

The trustworthiness clinicians usually attribute to their data, as opposed to those based on elements given by patients, rests upon three types of factors: their quantifiable nature, their objectivity (observable by third parties), and their susceptibility to material storage (histopathology, radiology) for future consultation or verification. But above everything else, what is at stake is their coherence and repeatability; which to a great extent include all other aspects. However, the possibility of obtaining the same results in different observations, regardless of the observer, is precisely one of the criteria in the elaboration of the psychometric instruments, among which are those aimed at Quality of Life; and this lends them the same reliability as in the abovementioned laboratorial results [7].

In order to assess Quality of Life some aspects must be taken in consideration first [8]. The instrument must have **validity**, as well as coherence and reliability. In other words, it must be specific in the sense that it assesses what it is meant to assess, and thus allowing to separate the cases from the non-cases within the context of the model on which it is based. This issue may be addressed by the concurrency method, which consists in comparing the results with those obtained by other previously validated or commonly used methods, such as clinical and laboratorial results. These external criteria, although they may evaluate partial aspects of the problem, should not yield overlapping results; which would indicate the redundancy of the new method. In fact, the goal is a quantifiable means of approaching in a more significant manner the issue of patient's Quality of Life. Additionally, in the absence of a validation capable of providing standardized data from which to interpret the results, these should always be referred to the population from which they were drawn, in order to allow a careful weighing of all inferences, as population specificities and idiosyncrasies may be an important source of artifacts.

The instrument must have coherence, which may be tested by the split-half method, as well as **reliability**, in the sense that observations are repeatable; which may be tested by the test-retest method, somehow granting the basic postulate of all scientific processes that under the same circumstances the same results will be obtained regardless of the observer. As far as this aspect is concerned, that is, in order to ensure repeatability, stability is paramount. However, to provide for any **utility** regarding the abovementioned applications, an instrument such as this must have enough **sensitivity** to allow for discrimination. In other words, it must be able not only to differentiate among people with more or less Quality of Life, but also to detect Quality of Life variations in a given patient or group of patients. This type of sensitivity to change, crucial in clinical trials and cost/benefit analysis, is also known as reactivity.

Specificity may be seen, to a certain extent, as a characteristic varying reversely to sensitivity. That is to say that a greater sensitivity, which allows an identification of most cases, is useful mostly in studies of epidemiological triage. In clinical practice, however, it is detrimental in the sense that a lower specificity leads to many false positives. High specificity, although it yields more false negatives, which is to say that many cases go undetected on account of insufficient sensitivity, is more useful in clinical practice in the sense that it provides a higher degree of certainty in a particular case. In this aspect as well, Quality of Life is not different from other assessment methods being used in other areas of biomedical intervention. Consider for instance the methods used to detect tuberculosis as compared to the tests used instead to corroborate the therapeutic intervention for the same disease. Additionally, an instrument well suited in a research context may prove impractical as an administrative routine or hard to read in the daily rush of clinical practice. Although patients usually enjoy answering to questionnaires whose contents they believe to be important for their clinician [9]. Still, although it is known that abridged versions are prone to be less valid, aspects such as time-consuming implementation or difficult interpretation of results must be taken into account, given that, added to their unfamiliarity, their significance is less intuitively grasped than clinical or laboratorial data obtained through more conventional means [10]. Therefore the **adequacy** of the instruments to their goal, that is, the rigorous construction and selection in terms of the aims to be achieved, is also a crucial requirement to meet.

Finally, there are issues remaining such as the assessment of illiterate patients, for whom self-assessment is not an option. It is known that interviewing, regardless of its degree of structure, deviates from the standard procedure required for repeatability; forcing the assessment of aspects such as inter-rater reliability.

3.3 Instruments

The scales for assessment of patient functional ability date back to the 1940s. Some noteworthy examples are the *American Rheumatism Association Function Scale* [11], the *Karnofsky Score* [12] created for cancer patients – from which has somehow derived the V axis of the Diagnostic and Statistical Manual of Mental Disorders (DSM) as used in present days –, or the *New York Heart Association Functional Classes*. These early instruments aimed at combining several dimensions into a single scale. In the 1950s appeared the *Daily Activities Scales* to assess the degree of incapacitation of patients interned in tertiary healthcare units. By their own nature they were less useful regarding psychosocial aspects; and the first instruments capable of assessing health status as we understand it today, appeared only in the 1970s. However, despite the studies of validation and reproducibility, they were still hard to implement; mainly due to questionnaire length, which came to be reduced only in the 1980s. A few examples of this trend are the *Nottingham Health Profile* [13], the *Dartmouth COOP Charts* [14], the *Medical Outcome Study Short Form* [15, 16] and the *Mini-Duke Health Profile* [17].

The trend throughout the 1990s was towards specificity, granting them more face value with clinicians and added on sensitivity to changes in patient status in terms of clinical progression. Furthermore, their multidimensionality allows for more detailed information on certain aspects. Ulterior psychometric refinement and improvements in adequacy progressively contributed to spread out the interest about its implementation in daily use.

1. **Global assessment**

The simplest method consists in posing patients a single question; the patients themselves somehow include in the answer the various implicit dimensions. There lies also its main shortcoming: single point assessments do not give us any information whatsoever on the factors leading to this or that answer.

Such is the case, for example, of questions like "On a scale from 0 to 4, how would you describe your general health status and well-being?"; to which patients must reply either "good", "reasonable", "poor", "bad" or "very bad". The obtained answer has proven to be a clinically effective way of globally assessing health status. In patients with Inflammatory Bowel Disease (IBD) it was even shown to be a strong indicator of the number of consultations taken [18].

2. Generic assessment

Generic assessments [8, 19] are characterized by the fact that they do not take into account aspects pertaining to specific diseases. From the start this allows for obtained scores to be compared between different groups of patients and even different pathologies. Furthermore, as they represent the answers of a group of patients, they are especially useful in epidemiological studies or as a mean to analyze factors to be considered in decisions regarding healthcare policy and guidelines.

i. Time Trade-off Technique (TTOT)

Defined as a utilitarian assessment, the *Time Trade-off Technique* [20] is an application issuing from the clinical decision model. It consists in assessing patients' perception of their health status in relation to death. Ranging from 0 (death) to 1 (perfect health), the score is obtained by asking the patient to choose (hypothetically, of course) between living with their present health status, with all it may imply in terms of physical and psychosocial limitations, and living less time with perfect health. For example, let us consider two thirty-year-old patients with Crohn's disease whose life expectancy is 75 years: the healthier one may be willing to give up on 5 years in order to live with perfect health to the age of 70, while the less healthy one may be willing to give up on 30 years to live with perfect health to the age of 45. The utilitarian score would then be 0.93 (70/75) for the former and 0.60 (45/75) for the latter.

Variation in this type of score may be used, for example, to assess how a patient deals with the efficacy of a certain therapy. However, as in the case of global assessment, it does not make explicit in which particular sector was improvement or deterioration felt. For this reason, as a method it is more evaluative than discriminative.

ii. Sickness Impact Profile (SIP)

Health profiles, of which *Sickness Impact Profile* [21] is an example, encompass several aspects of patients' life and behavior, both somatic and psychosocial, in terms of the disease perceived impact. This profile not only has a global score, but also has three sub-scores for physical aspects, four for psychosocial aspects and five for autonomous areas.

As a generic scale with discriminative capability, it can be used in planning healthcare policies, as it allows functional status comparisons between patients with different illnesses [5, 17].

iii. Psychosocial Adjustment to Illness Scale (PAIS)

The *Psychosocial Adjustment to Illness Scale* [22], proposed by the author of the SCL-90, is another well-studied generic health profile [23] which may be used to explore several intervening factors in the psychosocial adjustment to illness. Besides a global score, it covers aspects of health orientation, vocational environment — work, school and home activities,— domestic environment, sexual relationships, extended family relationships, social environment, and psycho-affective disturbance. It can be applied either by patients themselves or some other person; and being a generic profile, it can be applied to patients with different pathologies, allowing comparison studies. However, existing standard groups refer to patients with lung cancer, renal dialysis, severe burns and essential hypertension.

Moreover, the 4 possible answers to each of the 46 questions offer some difficulty of application in clinical practice; either because of its lengthy and time-consuming format – necessary to ensure the data validation required to explore the several areas it is meant to assess –, or because of its elaborate and numerous nuances, which may constitute a serious obstacle for patients with a low cultural background and little academic qualification.

iv. Quality of Life Scale

The *Self-Assessment Quality of Life Scale* [24] is yet another generic instrument that has also been proposed, with the particularity of having a version which uses a computer as means of implementation as well as archive and automatic processing of the resulting data [25].

3. Specific assessment

Specific assessment uses instruments capable of evaluating certain statuses and worries of patients with a specific disease. This ought to be the case of an assessment aimed for instance, at Crohn's disease; which must include issues related to intestinal functioning, abdominal pain and sexual aspects. Whereas another assessment aimed at rheumatoid arthritis may instead evaluate prehensile strength and mobility.

The advantages of such specificity lie on the added sensitivity to variation in clinical status, which may occur with the passing of time [26]. This aspect, combined with the fact that the issues and areas explored overlap those usually performed and evaluated by clinicians, makes it readily applicable in clinical trials.

The disadvantages concern the inability to differentiate between patients with different diseases or even in the context of the same disease, on account that, as was previously noted, the population used to develop the instrument must be taken into account. This aspect is well illustrated by the "ceiling effect" [7]: a Quality of Life scale developed in IBD in-patients may not be sensitive enough to Quality of Life variations in ambulatory patients, as these are expected to belong to a less severe clinical condition. The same goes for the "floor effect", which undermines the sensitivity/reactivity of an instrument used on patients with low Quality of Life, as they can hardly present lower values in further assessments.

Generally speaking, it can be said that all instruments available in the context of Inflammatory Bowel Disease (IBD) have content validation, that is, the questions they explore represent effectively the aspects they propose to assess. The same can be said of concurrent validation, given that the respective scores correlate with those of other previously validated Health-related Quality of Life instruments. Finally, there is also construct validation regarding scales constructed following a hypothetical model and then put to test in groups of patients with certain characteristics, or whose health status was assessed by other means; thus confirming the model.

i. Inflammatory Bowel Disease Questionnaire (IBDQ)

The *Inflammatory Bowel Disease Questionnaire* (IBDQ) [27, 28, 29, 30], conceived for use in therapeutic trials, is a questionnaire covering intestinal and systemic symptoms as well as affective and social behavior aspects, which was initially meant to be applied as a structured interview. Widely used and translated into many different languages [31] – Dutch [32, 33], Portuguese [34, 35, 36], Spanish [37, 38, 39], Korean [40], UK English [41, 42], Greek [43, 44], Swedish [45, 46], Norwegian [47], Japanese [48, 49], German [50, 51, 52], Chinese [53], Lebanese [54], Brazilian [55], Italian [56] –, it has shown its cross-cultural stability, while also being recognized as robust in psychometric terms, with proven reproducibility, stability and sensitivity to variations among Inflammatory Bowel Disease (IBD) affected patients, both in ambulatory regime and as in-patients.

Aiming to improve its adequacy, some modified versions came to light. One of those first modified versions, a self-applied questionnaire with 36 Likert-type questions [57], although using many questions from the IBDQ, from which it was derived – contributing to a certain degree of concurrent validation –, should not be considered properly standardized, given that the control study was performed only on a group of healthy people. Moreover, its application was aimed at a sample of patients only mildly affected by Inflammatory Bowel Disease (IBD). Some other versions and new modes of administration [58] came forward later on; ultimately agreeing upon a light-footed 32-item revised version (IBDQ-R) with proven psychometrics and adequacy [59].

ii. Cleveland Clinic Inflammatory Bowel Disease Questionnaire

The *Cleveland Clinic Questionnaire* [60] is a structured interview with 47 questions evaluated on a Likert-type scale which was shown to be correlated with the *Sickness Impact Profile*. Its focus is less on clinical symptoms and more on functional aspects of patient daily life. This allows to some extent its use in generic terms, going so far as to discriminate, in a slightly altered version, Inflammatory Bowel Disease (IBD) patients from multiple sclerosis and rheumatoid arthritis patients; the latter showing lower values of HR-QoL [61].

Specifically conceived to be used with Inflammatory Bowel Disease (IBD) patients, it can discriminate between patients with Ulcerative Colitis and patients with Crohn's disease, as well as tell apart patients with more severe forms from those with less severe ones; as is the case, respectively, for those with and without a history of prior surgical intervention.

iii. Rating Form of IBD Patients Concerns (RFIPC)

Although it does not assess symptoms or functional statuses, as it was not specifically conceived to assess Health-related Quality of Life, the *Rating Form of IBD Patients Concerns* [62] was shown to correlate with well-being reports, the psycho-affective disturbance degree assessed by the SCL-90, and daily functioning. It is based on a self-applied questionnaire with 25 questions answered by means of an analogical scale and oriented towards patient fears and concerns. It was applied to a large sample of American IBD patients and claims to be an index capable of evaluating results from psychotherapeutic interventions or simple counseling.

In other cultural contexts this questionnaire showed a much more random and less reliable behavior; which gave rise to an explanation, put forward after further probing, that physicians dealing with these patients may be less prone to enlighten them about the implications of their condition [63].

iv. Ulcerative Colitis and Crohn's Disease Health Status Scales (UC/CD HSS)

Based on the assumption that health status and its evolution depend both on disease-related factors and psychosocial factors [3], the *UC/CD Health Status Scales* [64] were conceived integrating aspects related with medical assistance, daily functioning and psycho-affective discomfort to differentiate situations of mild affliction from more severe cases and to predict the outcome.

They would benefit from prospective validation in order to strengthen its warrant for correct predictions in terms of prognosis or therapeutic response. However, the included symptoms have revealed from the start, through a nation-wide American study, that they have a better predictive power than that of *Crohn's Disease Activity Index* (CDAI) [65].

4. Quality of life findings in inflammatory bowel disease

Despite the vast number of published studies claiming to have assessed the Quality of Life, for the most part they were based on clinical evaluations or questionnaires of which there is insufficient data concerning their standardization. This lends their possible conclusions a great degree of relativity and leads to restricted information available in this area. However, the general rule is that ambulatory Inflammatory Bowel Disease (IBD) patients have a reasonably good Health-related Quality of Life [5, 18, 60, 66].

In a wide-range study [18], Drossman's workgroup has studied a great deal of aspects related to Inflammatory Bowel Disease (IBD) in 997 members of the Crohn's & Colitis Foundation of America. This study concluded that, as compared to the general population, only a slight increase in psychological distress can be observed. Nevertheless, while the daily functional status was overall quite good, disturbances, if any, stemmed less from physical aspects and more from psychological or social functioning factors. Additionally, when compared to Ulcerative Colitis, Crohn's disease patients showed more psychosocial difficulties and resorted to healthcare services more often; although the differences are not significant when adjusted to the greater severity of their symptoms.

As for coping mechanisms, considering that strategies focused on the problem have been considered more adaptive in the sense that they dampen the psychosocial disturbances, it is exactly to this type of strategies that these patients resort more often: facing problems and making their positive reassessment, while resisting interference from emotional distress and also seeking social support.

Assuming that the common ground for a better or worse Health-related Quality of Life is the underlying personality, a study [67] was conducted among IBD patients aiming at disclosing any particular characteristics relevant to this population in terms of relationships with QoL dimensions as assessed by the IBDQ-R [60]. The framework considered to do so was the psychobiological model of temperament and character [68, 69], of which variables even have the proven ability to predict independent DSM diagnoses of personality disorders [70]. Just to conclude that QoL – both IBDQ Global score and all its dimensions –, is significantly modulated and may be predicted to some extent through a recognizable distressed type of personality. But also further suggest an adjustment typology relying on different aspects of personality. Namely, that harm avoidance by temperament is the main predictor of bowel symptoms, systemic symptoms and emotional status; while the relative strength of dimensionally assessed character disorder – after controlling for harm avoidance – mainly accounted for social malfunctioning [67].

Quality of Life and psychosocial factors – well-being, psychological disturbances and functional status – were shown to be much better predictive factors, in terms of the number of consultations taken, than the commonly used disease activity indexes; which are not even significant. But these latter indexes – severity of symptoms, steroid dosage and weight loss – are otherwise quite good predictors of hospital admission and surgery.

Moreover, the *Rating Form of IBD Patients Concerns* (RFIPC) has allowed to conclude that these patients' main worries and fears are: incertitude regarding the disease evolution, medication effects, energy level, surgery and having an ostomy bag, being a burden on others, loss of bowel control and the possibility of cancer. Furthermore, within this concern spectrum some differences have been established between patients with Crohn's disease and Ulcerative Colitis. The former are more concerned with their energy level, being a burden to others, full development, pain and suffering, expenses and the risk of contagion to others. While the latter fear mostly the possibility of cancer. Finally, there is a relation between these concerns and the psychological well-being and daily functioning; suggesting that a psycho-educational intervention aimed at these concerns can play an important role in improving these patients' health status and Quality of Life.

In yet another study [5] conducted by the same workgroup using the *Sickness Impact Profile* (SIP) among both in-patients and ambulatory as well , the results came to confirm that the psychological and social factors have a greater effect on the daily functioning status than do physical aspects. This is more so in Crohn's disease than in Ulcerative Colitis, but above all among in-patients as compared to those in ambulatory care. This also came out as a result from a study using *Cleveland Clinic Questionnaire* in ambulatory patients [60], which has shown a poorer Quality of Life among patients with Crohn's disease when compared to those with Ulcerative Colitis; and the same goes for patients with a surgery history when compared to those without surgery. This is hard to interpret in the case of Ulcerative Colitis patients, where colectomy is presumed to heal. However, the high rank of the health care facilities where the study has been conducted allows to conjecture that the sample may have been selected focusing on patients with postoperative complications.

While being aware that different questionnaires lead to different interpretations about Quality of Life after restorative proctocolectomy [71], the question raised here is knowing to what extent the colectomy may improve the Health-related Quality of Life; or whether there are significant differences according to the chosen procedure. In fact a study with such a focus, using utilitarian methods such as the *Time Trade-off Technique* (TTOT) [72], confirmed such improvement. In yet another study conducted one year after surgery, the authors found no differences among the several used procedures: conventional ileostomy, Kock pouch and ileal pouch anal anastomosis. Although the difference in methodologies prevents any direct comparisons, going as far back as 1981 another study which engaged 1000 patients operated for Ulcerative Colitis came to slightly different conclusions [73]. This study concluded, using a suitable questionnaire to assess Health-related Quality of Life, that, when compared to patients with Kock pouch, patients with ileal pouch anal anastomosis felt fewer difficulties both sexually and in sport activities. The same was true when compared to ileostomy patients; although these mentioned fewer problems with travelling. Drossman's workgroup also approached this issue with their *Rating Form of IBD Patients Concerns* (RFIPV) [74], reinforcing these studies' conclusions on the positive response in terms of Quality of Life among colectomized Ulcerative Colitis patients. Furthermore concluding that ostomies reduce the level of concern regarding cancer, surgery and ostomy itself; without significantly raising those related with bodily image – sexuality, intimacy, attraction –. The same cannot be said about Crohn's disease; possibly due to the post-operatory severity of these patients condition [60].

5. Conclusions

The level of interest seen recently in assessing the Health-related Quality of Life led to the creation of a number of assessment instruments with applications in several areas of intervention, such as clinical practice, research and healthcare policy guidelines. However, in order to make an adequate choice and/or a correct use of these instruments, it is necessary to have some knowledge of the characteristics and limitations of both generic instruments and IBD-specific instruments. As for the countless studies published which refer to this concept, the main conclusion to be drawn still is the scarcity of standardized conditions. However, overall they all point to a relatively good Health-related Quality of Life among these patients.

An increase in the interest for this type of instruments is foreseeable in the near future, towards a better assessment of Inflammatory Bowel Disease (IBD) impact both on an individual – clinical orientation in medical or surgical contexts – and a population levels – therapeutic efficacy, budget planning –.

6. References

[1] Ware J, Brook R, Rogers W, *et al.* Comparison of health outcomes at a health maintenance organization with those of fee for service care. *Lancet.* 1986; 848: 1017-22

[2] Jenkinson C. Quality of life measurement: does it have a place in routine clinical assessment? *Journal of Psychosomatic Research.* 1994; 38(5): 377-81.

[3] Garrett JW, Drossman DA. Health status in inflammatory bowel disease: biological and behavioral considerations. *Gastroenterology.* 1990; 99: 90-6

[4] Buxton MJ, Lacey LA, Feagan BG, *et al.* Mapping from disease-specific measures to utility: an analysis of the relationship between the Inflammatory Bowel Disease Questionnaire and Crohn's Disease Activity Index in Crohn's disease and measures of utility. *Value Health.* 2007; 10(3): 214-20 [United States]

[5] Drossman DA, Patrick DL, Mitchell CM, et al. Health related quality of life in inflammatory bowel disease: Functional status and patient worries and concerns. *Dig Dis Sci.* 1989; 34: 1379-86

[6] Rubenstein L, Calkins D, Young R, *et al.* Improving patient functions: a randomized trial of functional disability screening. *Ann Intern Med.* 1989; 111: 836-42

[7] Feinstein AR. An additional basic science for clinical medicine: IV. The development of clinimetrics. *Ann Intern Med.* 1983; 99: 843-8

[8] Guyatt GH, Feeny DH, Patrick DL. Measuring health-related quality of life. *Ann Intern Med.* 1993; 118: 622-9

[9] Nelson E, Berwick D. The measurement of health status in clinical practice. *Med Care.* 1989; 27: 77-90

[10] Tugwell P, Bombardier C, Buchanan W, et al. Methotrexate in rheumatoid arthritis: impact of quality of life assessed by traditional standard item and individualized patient preference health status questionnaires. *Arch Intern Med.* 1990; 150: 59-62

[11] Steinbrocker O, Traeger C, Battman R. Therapeutic criteria in rheumatoid arthritis. *JAMA* 1949; 140: 659-62

[12] Karnofsky D, Burchenal J. The clinical evaluation of chemotherapeutic agents in cancer. *In*: MacLeod C (ed). *Evaluation of chemotherapeutic agents.* New York: Columbia University Press. 1949; pp 191-205

[13] Hunt S, McEwen J, McKenna S. *Measuring health status.* London: Croom Helm, 1986

[14] Nelson EV, Landgraf JM, Wasson JH, *et al.* The functional status of patients: how can it be measured in physicians offices? *Med Care* 1990; 28: 1111-26

[15] Stewart AL, Hays RD, Ware JE Jr. The MOS short-form general health survey: reliability and validity in a patient population. *Med Care* 1988; 26: 724-35

[16] Ware JE Jr, Sherbourne CD. The MOS 36-item short-form health surveu (SF-36). I. Conceptual framework and item selection. *Med Care* 1992; 30: 473-83

[17] Parkerson GR, Broadhead WE, Tse CK. Development of the 17-item Duke Health Profile. *Family practice* 1991; 8(4): 396-401

[18] Drossman DA, Leserman J, Mitchell CM, *et al.* Health status and health care use in persons with inflammatory bowel disease: A national sample. *Dig Dis Sci* 1991; 36: 1746-55

[19] Patrick DL, Deyo RA. Generic and disease specific measures in assessing health status and quality of life. *Med Care* 1989; 27: 217-32
[20] Torrance GW, Thomas WH, Sackett DL. A utility maximization model for evaluation of health care program. *Health Serv Res* 1972; 7: 118-33
[21] Bergner M, Bobbitt RA, Carter WB, *et al.* The Sickness Impact Profile: development and final revision of a health status measure. *Med Care* 1981; 19: 787-805
[22] Derogatis LR. The Psychosocial Adjustment to Illness Scale (PAIS). *J Psychosom Res* 1986; 30(1): 77-91
[23] Derogatis LR, Lopez M. *Psychosocial Adjustment to Illness Scale (PAIS & PAIS - SR): Scoring, Procedures & Administration Manual - I.* Baltimore: Clinical Psychometric Research, 1983
[24] Stocker MJ, Dunbar GC and Beaumont G. The SmithKline Beecham 'quality of life' scale: a validation and reliability study in patients with affective disorder. *Quality of Life Research* 1992; 1: 385-95
[25] Novo Nordisk A/S. Novo Nordisk Park, 2760. Måløv. Denmark
[26] Guyatt GH, Walter S, Norman G. Measuring change over time: assessing the usefulness of evaluative instruments. *J Chron Dis* 1987; 40: 171-8
[27] Guyatt GH, Mitchell A, Irvine EJ *et al.* A new measure of health status for clinical trials in inflammatory bowel disease. *Gastroenterology* 1989; 96: 804-10
[28] Irvine E. Quality of Life - Rationale and Methods for Developing a Disease Specific Instrument for Inflammatory Bowel Disease *Scand J of Gastroenterology* 1993; 28(sup 199): 22-7
[29] Irvine E. Quality of Life - Measurement in Inflammatory Bowel Disease *Scand J of Gastroenterology* 1993; 28(sup 199): 36-9
[30] Irvine E, Feagan B, Rochon J, *et al.* Quality of Life: A valid and reliable measure of therapeutic efficacy in the treatment of Inflammatory Bowel Disease. *Gastroenterology* 1994; 106(2): 287-96
[31] Pallis AG, Mouzas IA, *et al.* The Inflammatory Bowel Disease Questionnaire: a review of its national validation studies. *Inflamm Bowel Dis* 2004; 10(3): 261-9
[32] deBoer AJ, Wijker W, *et al.* Inflammatory Bowel Disease Questionnaire: cross-cultural adaptation and further validation. *Eur J Gastroenterol Hepatol* 1995; 7(11): 1043-50
[33] Russel MG, Pastoor CJ, *et al.* Validation of the Dutch translation of the Inflammatory Bowel Disease Questionnaire (IBDQ): a health-related quality of life questionnaire in inflammatory bowel disease. *Digestion* 1997; 58(3): 282-8
[34] Verissimo R. *Chronic Inflammatory Bowel Disease: Psychological Factors* (Doctoral thesis). Porto, University of Porto, 1997 [Portuguese]
[35] Verissimo R, Mota-Cardoso R, Taylor G. Relationships between Alexithymia, Emotional Control and Quality of Life in Patients with Inflammatory Bowel Disease. *Psychother Psychosom* 1998; 67(2): 75-80
[36] Pontes RM, Miszputen SJ, *et al.* Quality of life in patients with inflammatory bowel diseases: translation to Portuguese language and validation of the Inflammatory Bowel Disease Questionnaire (IBDQ). *Arq Gastroenterol* 2004; 41(2): 137-43 [Portuguese]
[37] López-Vivancos J, Casellas F, Badia X, *et al.* Validation of the Spanish Version of the Inflammatory Bowel Disease Questionnaire on Ulcerative Colitis and Crohn's Disease. *Digestion* 1999; 60(3): 274-80

[38] Masachs M, Casellas F, *et al.* Spanish translation, adaptation and validation of the 32-item questionnaire on quality of life for inflammatory bowel disease (IBDQ-32). *Rev Esp Enferm Dig* 2007; 99(9): 511-9 [Spanish]

[39] Vidal A, Gomez-Gil E, *et al.* Psychometric properties of the original Inflammatory Bowel Disease Questionnaire, a Spanish version. *Gastroenterol Hepatol* 2007; 30(4): 212-8

[40] Kim WH, Cho YS, *et al.* Quality of life in Korean patients with inflammatory bowel diseases : ulcerative colitis, Crohn's disease and intestinal Behcet's disease. *Int J Colorectal Dis* 1999; 14(1): 52-7

[41] Han SW, McColl E, *et al.* The inflammatory bowel disease questionnaire: a valid and reliable measure in ulcerative colitis patients in the North East of England. *Scand J Gastroenterol* 1998; 33(9): 961-6

[42] Cheung WY, Garratt AM, Russell IT and Williams JG. The UK IBDQ — A British version of the inflammatory bowel disease questionnaire: development and validation. *J Clin Epidemiol* 2000; 53(3): 297-306

[43] Pallis AG, Vlachonikolis IG, *et al.* Quality of life of Greek patients with inflammatory bowel disease. Validation of the Greek translation of the inflammatory bowel disease questionnaire. *Digestion* 2001; 63(4): 240-6

[44] Vlachonikolis IG, Pallis AG, *et al.* Improved validation of the Inflammatory Bowel Disease Questionnaire and development of a short form in Greek patients. *Am J Gastroenterol* 2003; 98(8): 1802-12

[45] Hjortswang H, Jarnerot G, *et al.* Validation of the inflammatory bowel disease questionnaire in Swedish patients with ulcerative colitis. *Scand J Gastroenterol* 2001; 36(1): 77-85

[46] Stjernman H, Granno C, *et al.* Evaluation of the Inflammatory Bowel Disease Questionnaire in Swedish patients with Crohn's disease. *Scand J Gastroenterol* 2006; 41(8): 934-43

[47] Bernklev T, Moum B, *et al.* Quality of life in patients with inflammatory bowel disease: translation, data quality, scalling assumptions, validity, reliability and sensitivity to change of the Norwwegian version of IBDQ. *Scand J Gastroenterol* 2002; 37(10): 1164-74

[48] Hashimoto H, Green J, *et al.* Reliability, validity and responsiveness of the Japanese version of the Inflammatory Bowel Disease Questionnaire. *J Gastroenterol* 2003; 38(12): 1138-43

[49] Watanabe K, Funayama Y, *et al.* Assessment of the Japanese Inflammatory Bowel Disease Questionnaire in patients after ileal pouch anal anastomosis for ulcerative colitis. *J Gastroenterol* 2006; 41(7): 662-7

[50] Hauser W, Dietz N, Grandt D *et al.* Validation of the inflammatory bowel disease questionnaire IBDQ-D, German version, for patients with ileal pouch anal anastomosis for ulcerative colitis. *Z Gastroenterol* 2004; 42(2): 131-9

[51] Janke KH, Klump B, *et al.* Validation of the German version of the Inflammatory Bowel Disease Questionnaire (Competence Network IBD, IBDQ-D) *Psychother Psychosom Med Psychol* 2005; 56(7): 291-8 [German]

[52] Janke KH, Steder-Neukamm U, *et al.* Quality of life assessment in Inflammatory Bowel Disease (IBD): German version of the Inflammatory Bowel Disease Questionnaire (IBDQ-D; disease-specific instrument for quality of life assessment) — first application and comparison with international investigations. *Gesundheitswesen* 2006; 67(8-9): 656-64 [German]

[53] Ren WH, Lai M, Chen Y, Irvine EJ, Zhou YX. Validation of the Mainland Chinese Version of the Inflammatory Bowel Disease Questionnaire (IBDQ) for Ulcerative Colitis and Crohn's Disease. *Inflamm Bowel Dis* 2007; 13(7): 903-10

[54] Abdul-Baki H, ElHajj I, *et al.* Clinical epidemiology of inflammatory bowel disease in Lebanon. *Inflamm Bowel Dis* 2007; 13(4): 475-80

[55] Oliveira S, Zaltman C, *et al.* Quality-of-life measurement in patients with inflammatory bowel disease receiving social support. *Inflamm Bowel Dis* 2007; 13(4): 470-4

[56] Ciccocioppo R, Klersy C, Russo ML, et al. Validation of the Italian translation of the Inflammatory Bowel Disease Questionnaire. *Digestive and Liver Disease* 2011; 43(7): 535-41

[57] Love JR, Irvine EJ, Fedorak RN. Quality of life in inflammatory bowel disease. *J Clin Gastroenterol.* 1992; 14: 15-19.

[58] Lam MY, Lee H, Bright R, et al. Validation of interactive voice response system administration of the Short Inflammatory Bowel Disease Questionnaire. *Inflamm Bowel Dis* 2009; 15(4): 599-607

[59] Verissimo R. Quality of Life in Inflammatory Bowel Disease: Psychometric evaluation of an IBDQ cross-culturally adapted version. *J Gastrointestin Liver Dis* 2008; 17(4): 439-44

[60] Farmer RG, Easley KA, Farmer JM. Quality of life assessment by patients with inflammatory bowel disease. *Cleve Clin J Med* 1992; 59: 35-42

[61] Rudick RA, Miller D, Clough JD, *et al.* Quality of life in multiple sclerosis: comparison with inflammatory bowel disease and rheumatoid arthritis. *Arch Neurol* 1992; 49: 1237-42

[62] Drossman DA, Leserman J, Li Z, *et al.* The rating form of IBD patient concerns: a new measure of health status. *Psychosom Med* 1991; 53: 701-12

[63] Verissimo R. Quality of Life in Inflammatory Bowel Disease: specific concerns and functional status (abstract 34). *J Port Gastroenterol* 1996; 3(2) supl: 18 [Portuguese]

[64] Drossman DA, Li Z, Leserman J, Patrick DL. Ulcerative colitis and Crohn's disease health status scales for research and clinical practice. *J Clin Gastroenterol* 1992; 15: 104-12

[65] Best WR, Becktel JM, Singleton JW, *et al.* Development of a Crohn's disease activity index. National Cooperative Crohn's disease study. *Gastroenterology* 1976; 70: 439-44

[66] Mitchell A, Guyatt G, Singer J, *et al.* Quality of life in patients with inflammatory bowel disease. *J Clin Gastroenterol* 1988; 10: 306-10

[67] Verissimo R. Personality and Quality of Life among Inflammatory Bowel Disease patients (abstract). *Psychosom Med* 2002; 64: 143

[68] Cloninger C. A systematic method for clinical description and classification of personality variants. A proposal. *Arch Gen Psychiat* 1987 June; 44: 573-588.

[69] Verissimo R. Psychobiological model of personality: temperament and character dimensions. Arq Psiquiatria 2008; 5(1/2): 61-73 [Portuguese]

[70] Svrakic D, Whitehead C, Przybeck T, Cloninger C. Differential diagnosis of personality disorders by the seven factor Model of Temperament and Character. *Arch Gen Psychiatry* 1993 Dec; 50(12): 991-999.

[71] Scarpa M, Ruffolo C, Polese L, *et al.* Quality of life after restorative proctocolectomy for ulcerative colitis : different questionnaires lead to different interpretations. *Arch Surg* 2007; 142(2): 158-65

[72] McLeod RS, Churchill DN, Lock AM, *et al.* Quality of life of patients with ulcerative colitis preoperatively and postoperatively. *Gastroenterology* 1991; 101: 307-13

[73] Kohler LW, Pemberton JH, Zinsmeister AR, *et al.* Quality of life after proctocolectomy. A comparison of Brook ileostomy, Kock pouch, and ileal pouch-anal anastomosis. *Gastroenterolgy* 1991; 101: 679-84

[74] Drossman DA, Mitchell CM, Appelbaum MI, *et al.* Do IBD ostomates do better? A study of symptoms and health-related quality of life (abstract). *Gastroenterology* 1989; 96: 130

9

Validation of a Quantitative Determination Method of Paramino-Salicylic Acid by High-Performance Liquid Chromatography and Its Application in Rat Plasma

Ibrahima Youm, Malika Lahiani-Skiba and Mohamed Skiba
Laboratoire de Pharmacie Galénique, UMR CNRS 5007
UFR Médecine et Pharmacie, Université de ROUEN, Rouen
France

1. Introduction

The non steroid anti-inflammatory drugs (NSAID) are among the most prescribed because of their analgesic and anti-inflammatory properties [1].The derivatives of the acid aminosalicylic (4ASA and 5-ASA) are used since many years in the treatment of the intestinal chronic inflammatory diseases: Crohn disease and colitis. Aminosalicylic acids exert a direct anti- inflammatory action on the intestinal mucous membranes. They do not have any link with the drugs of cortisone family, or with traditional NSAID used for pain and rheumatism. They are also different from the acetylsalicylic acid (Aspirine®).
4ASA also known under the name of paramino benzoïc acid (PABA) or paramino salicylic acid (PASA) (figure 1) is employed for the treatment of the ulcerative colitis and Crohn disease. These diseases are characterized by an ignition of the colorectal mucous membrane [2].

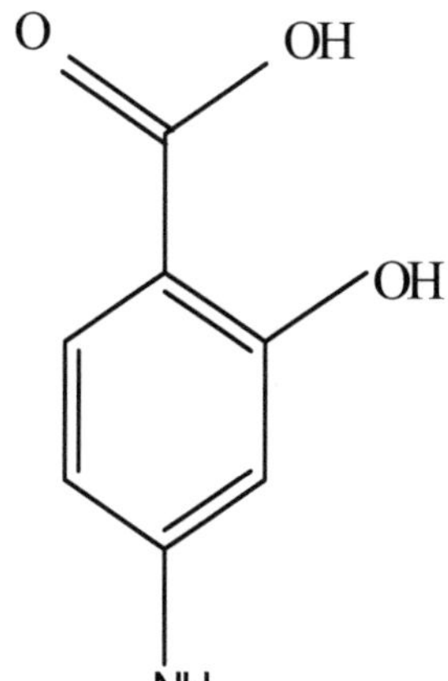

Fig. 1. Molecular structure of 4ASA

In the literature, several analytical methods primarily based on separation were described. Therefore, quantitative methods to assay, for instance a drug substance or its impurities, have needed to be fully validated after development. Depending on the type of analytical method and its intended use, a check for linearity, precision, accuracy, specificity, range, limits of detection and quantification, and/or robustness, is required [3-7], gas chromatography coupled with the mass spectrometry were the most usually used methods for analytes separation [8]. A capillary method of electrophoresis was developed for 4ASA determination and its metabolites: acid N-acetyl-p-aminosalicylic (N-acetyl-PASA) in urine. Good separation of analytes was carried out with a 12 min retention time for15min [9]. 4ASA is also quantified by HPLC in the biological fluids [10, 11]. In this present article, we describe the development of a new RP-HPLC method for the determination of 4ASA at the same time in both aqueous medium and plasma.

2. Material and methods

4ASA was supplied by Merck (Hohenbrunn, Germany). Formic acid (99-100%) was provided by Prolabo. Potassium dihydrogene phosphate (KH2PO4), acetonitrile (MeCN) and potassium hydroxide (KOH) were provided by SDS (Peypin, France). Alpha cyclodextrine was purchased from Waker and Gelucire® from Gattefossé (France). Sodium citrate was obtained from Sigma chemical Co (USA). Water purified on Milli-Q system (Millipore, USA) was used. All other chemicals were of analytical grade.

2.1 Instrumentation

The liquid chromatographic system used in the present study, consisted of a pump (880-Jasco, Japan), an automatic injector (autosampler HPLC -360Kontron, Brehme, Germany) and a detector (Jasco 875-UV). All the parameters of HPLC were controlled by the Azur software: version 3.0 coupled to an acquisition box (Azur PAD).

2.2 Chromatographic conditions

The mobile phase was prepared by mixing water, formic acid and acetonitrile in varied proportions. The optimum mobile phase used in the validation studies consisted of water-formic acid-acetonitrile 67:3:30, (v/v/v). Before analysis the mobile phase was filtered through a 0.45µm membrane and degassed by ultra sonication (Transsonic 950, Prolabo). Solvent delivery was employed at a flow rate of 1.0 ml min $^{-1}$. A Kromasil column: C-18µm, 250mm ×4.6mm (Chromato, France HAS) was used and maintained at room temperature. Detection of the analytes was carried out at 300nm.The appropriate wavelength for the detection of the drug was determined by wavelength scanning over the range of 200-400nm. Injection volume of the analytes was set to a constant volume of 50µl.

2.3 Validation of the method

The described method has been validated in terms of specificity, precision, linearity, accuracy, limit of detection (LOD) and limit of quantification (LOQ).

2.3.1 Precision

Precision was expressed with respect to the intra and inter-day variations in the expected drug concentrations.

2.3.2 Linearity

Data were obtained using a stock solution of 4ASAS at 0.5 $mg.ml^{-1}$ as concentration. This solution was then diluted using highly purified water to obtain the standard solutions from 1 to 125µg/ml concentrations. Five injections were made for each concentration. The linearity of the calibration curves was determined on three different days for intra or inter-day variation.

2.3.3 Accuracy

Accuracy of the proposed method was established by recovery experiments using standard addition method. This study was employed by addition of a standard reference (pure marketed product whose purity was tested beforehand by Differential Scanning Calorimetry (DSC) and Fourier transformed Infrared Spectrometry (FT-IR).

2.3.4 Robustness

An experimental design was used to evaluate the influence of selected factors. Two-level factorial design was used (Table **1**).

	1	2	3	123
	MeCN (%)	Wavelength (nm)	Flow rate (ml/min)	pH
1	-	-	-	-
2	+	-	-	+
3	-	+	-	+
4	+	+	-	-
5	-	-	+	+
6	+	-	+	-
7	-	+	+	-
8	+	+	+	+

Low level	-	27	297	0,8	2
High level	+	33	303	1,2	2,4

n=5

Table 1. Influence of selected factors: MeCN (%), Wavelength (nm), Flow rate (ml/min) and pH on the robustness of the method:

For this method only factors were examinated: acetonitrile ratio, wavelength, flow rate and pH.

2.3.5 Limit of detection and limit of quantification

Several approaches were used to determine the detection and quantitation limits. These include visual evaluation, signal-to-noise ratio, the use of standard deviation of the response and the slope of the calibration curve.
In the present study, the LOD was related to signal / noise of the system and was defined as a peak whose report/ration signal background noise was at least equal to 3/1. The LOQ was defined as a peak whose report/ ratio signal background noise was at least equal to 10/1.

The determination of these values was made starting from the line of the range standard. These two values were calculated from the Response Factor (Rf) according to formulas (1) and (2): the initial concentration corresponds to the intersection of the right-hand side to the y-axis [12].

$$\mathrm{Fr} = \frac{\text{Standard area}}{\text{Initial Concentration}} \tag{1}$$

$$\text{Sample concentration} = \frac{Sample\ area}{Fr} \tag{2}$$

2.3.6 Stability

Experiments were carried out under the same conditions as the samples analysis.

2.3.7 Recovery test

Recovery test was carried out by weighing three batches of pellets (containing 50% of 4ASA) compared with a powder sample of pure active ingredient. Amounts representing 120,100 and 80% of 4ASA were used as equivalent concentrations. Each batch is crushed using a mortar then filtered before being solubilized in 250ml water with respect of sink conditions. The release properties of the active ingredient from the extruded formulations matrix were studied by using a process of the delayed release. The medium of dissolution was maintained at 37°C with 100 rpm stirring. After 6 hours, three samples of 1 ml were taken in each sample of buffer solution of phosphate potassium (0.2 M) whose pH was adjusted to 7.5 using a potassium hydroxide buffer (KOH 1M).

3. Application to biological samples

The proposed method was applied to the determination of 4ASA in plasma samples from the bioequivalence study. *In vivo* studies of 4ASA blood concentration were carried out by using established methods of the literature [10]. Male Sprague-Dawley rats weighing 200–250g (n = 4) were purchased from Charles Rivers Enterprise (France) and kept in laboratory conditions before experiments.

3.1 Linearity and precision

Linearity was assessed by analyzing seven standards with concentrations over the range of 10-100µg/ml in plasma (n=5). Precision and accuracy were tested comparing to the values obtained previously in aqueous solution. Aliquot of 1000µl plasma were mixed with 500µl of standard solution of 4ASA. The mixture was vortexed for 2 min and transferred into the vial for HPLC analysis (n=8).

3.2 Recovery test in plasma

For recovery test, three samples of 1000µl plasma were mixed with 250µl of standard solution (25, 50 and 100µg/ml) of 4ASA. The mixture was vortexed for 2 min and transferred into the vial for HPLC analysis (n=5).

3.3 Stability test in plasma

Drug stability during sample collection and processing is an important factor for clinical bioanalysis. Three samples of 1000µl plasma were mixed with 500µl of standard solution of 4ASA and analyzed at 0 and 24hours at room temperature and at 4°C (n=5).

3.4 Blood-plasma partition ratio

Blood-plasma partition ratio would predict plasma concentration-time courses following 4ASA oral doses to rats.

Partition test was carried out using three fresh samples of blood (1ml) mixed with 500µl of 100µg/ml standard solution of 4ASA. The mixture was maintained in constant stirring at room temperature for ten minutes and analyzed by HPLC.

3.5 Bioavailability

Each rat received an oral dose of minigranules containing 25mg of 4ASA. Three hours after administration of minigranules, the rats were anesthetized with an intra peritoneal pentobarbital 10% (ABBOT, Ringis, France) at the dose of 100µl/100g (re-injected with 10µl/100g as necessary). The internal carotid artery was cannulated via 4cm paratracheal incision, and blood samples were taken at 0.5, 1, 2, 3 and 4 hours after anesthesia.

Rats were killed at the end of experiments by exsanguinations. These samples were collected into eppendorf tubes containing 500µl of citrate buffer (0.129M) and kept on ice for at least 30 min.

Plasma was obtained by centrifugation (Eppendorf centrifuge, Germany) at 3500 rpm for 10 min and transferred to clean test tubes. After vortexing for 1 min using a Heidolph Top-mix 94323 (Bioblock scientific, Germany), plasma samples were analyzed by HPLC method. Analyte concentrations were calculated by using an account of the factor of dilution.

4. Results and discussion

4.1 Chromatographic conditions

Experiments were carried out with 10 up to 90% of acetonitrile and water as a mobile phase. The best peak shape and the maximum of separation were obtained with a binary mixture: water - acetonitrile (70% and 30% respectively). A minimum of retention time (Rt=4.3-4.8) with good peak resolution was obtained under a flow of $1ml.min^{1}$.

The optimum wavelength for analyte detection with adequate sensitivity was found to be 300nm.

Retention time was very sensitive to the freshness or ageing of mobile phase.

4.2. Validation of the method

4.2.1 Specificity/selectivity

A chromatogram was obtained from blank samples. No peak corresponding to the endogenous compounds was detected at the analyte retention time (4.3-4.8min) at 300nm. It means that the developed method is selective in relation of the used carrier for pellet formulation.

4.2.2 Linearity

Seven-point linearity curve was constructed for three consecutive days. Samples were quantified using

concentrations – peak area relationships and were calculated by the simple regression analysis. The plots of peak area ratios versus concentrations of all analytes were found to be linear within the concentration range (Figure **2**).

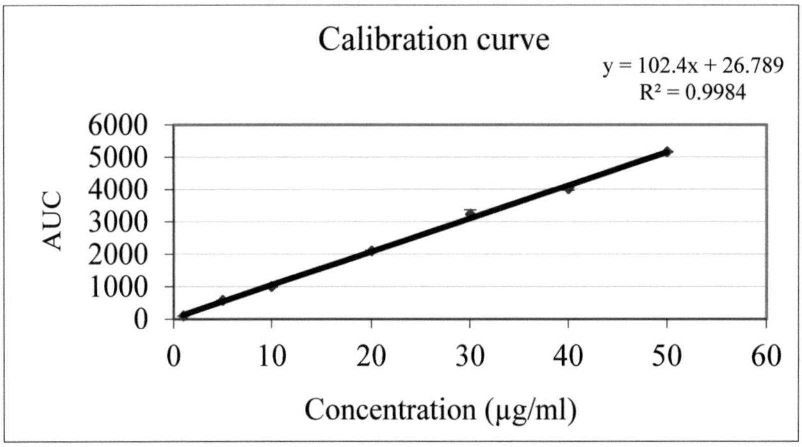

Fig. 2. Linearity of quantitative method by HPLC. Bars represent standard deviations of the mean (n = 5)

4.2.3 Accuracy and precisions

The results were expressed as percent recoveries of the particular components in the samples. The average percent recoveries (±RSD) were respectively in the range of 97.3±0.9 - 99±1.7 (Table **2**).

Concentration (mg/ml)	0,005	0,0075	0,01
Mean of AUC	329,747	489,049	725,458
RSD (%)	0,740	1,874	0,51

Table 2. Accuracy of the proposed method (n =10). AUC: Area Under Curve

The results of intra-day and inter-day precision experiments are indicated according to the averages and relative standard deviations (RSD). Inter-day and intra-day precision given by relative standard deviation (%R.S.D.) of quality control samples were ≤ 3.3%. The calculated values are presented onto (Table **3**).

Concentration (µg/ml)	Intra-day		Inter-day	
	Area (UA)	RSD (%)	Area (UA)	RSD (%)
1	98,47	0,98	94,57	2,20
5	551,00	0,60	563,31	3,35
10	998,01	0,61	990,82	0,76
20	2058,66	0,18	2090,11	0,51
30	3189,39	2,29	3246,26	1,19
40	4059,34	3,19	4046,40	1,26
50	4843,45	1,01	4939,88	3,24

Table 3. Intra and inter-day precision of 4ASA quantification with area (UA) andRelative Standard Deviation (RSD) (n=3).

4.2.4 Limit of Detection (LOD) and Limit of Quantification (LOQ)
The results showed a less significant limit of detection (105ng/ml) compared to the limit of quantification (305ng/ml).

4.2.5 Recovery test
The overall mean recoveries calculated were 80, 100 and 120 for low, medium and high quality control samples respectively. A linear curve was obtained meaning proportional analyte amount (Figure 3).

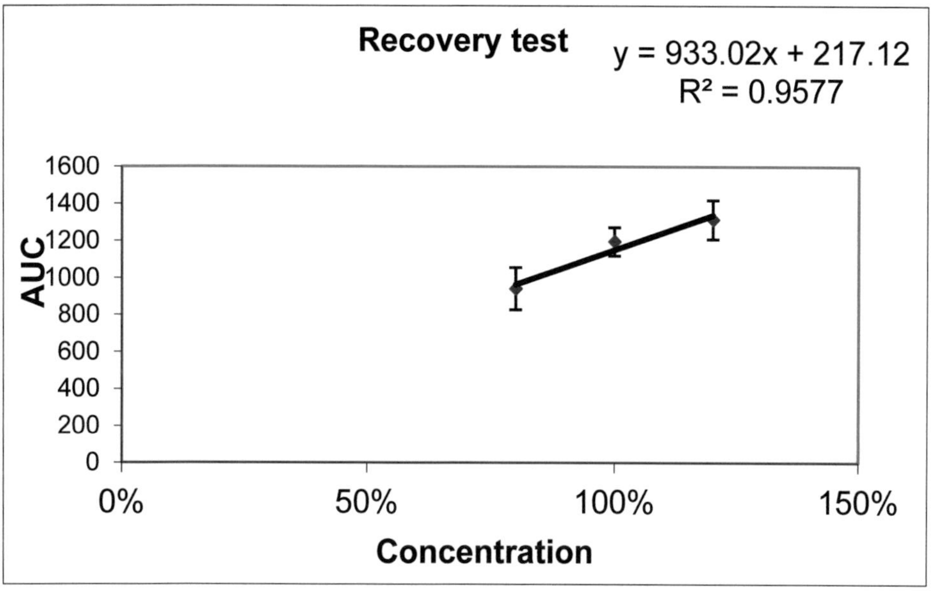

Fig. 3. Chart of the test of recovering: Bars represent standard deviations of the mean (n=9).

4.2.6 Robustness
Two-level fractional factorial design were applied in this method. The operational parameters do not lead to essential changes of the performance of the chromatographic system except the wavelength. Only the wavelength seemed to influence the robustness of the method. The interaction between the acetonitrile ratio and the flow rate didn't seem to have any effect on the robustness (Figure 4).
The obtained values were accurate and RSD values didn't exceed 3.3%. On the other hand the retention time varied quickly from 2.98 to 5.28 min for each modified parameter. Acetonitrile change ratio would change the polarity of the mobile phase while pH could modify the analyte protonation.

4.2.7 Study of 4ASA stability
Three aliquots were used during this experiment which lasted 6 hours. The medium of dissolution was maintained with 37°C, in constant stirring with 100 rpm to simulate gastrointestinal conditions. The results showed a relative stability of 93.5% (Figure 5).

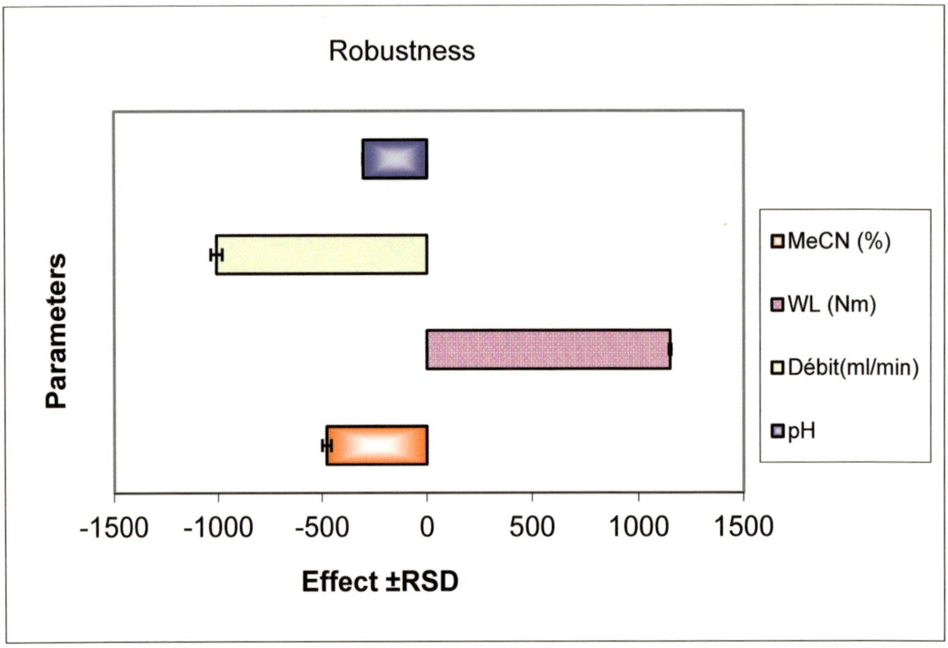

Fig. 4. Histogram representing robustness test of the method. Bars represent standard deviations of the mean (n=5).

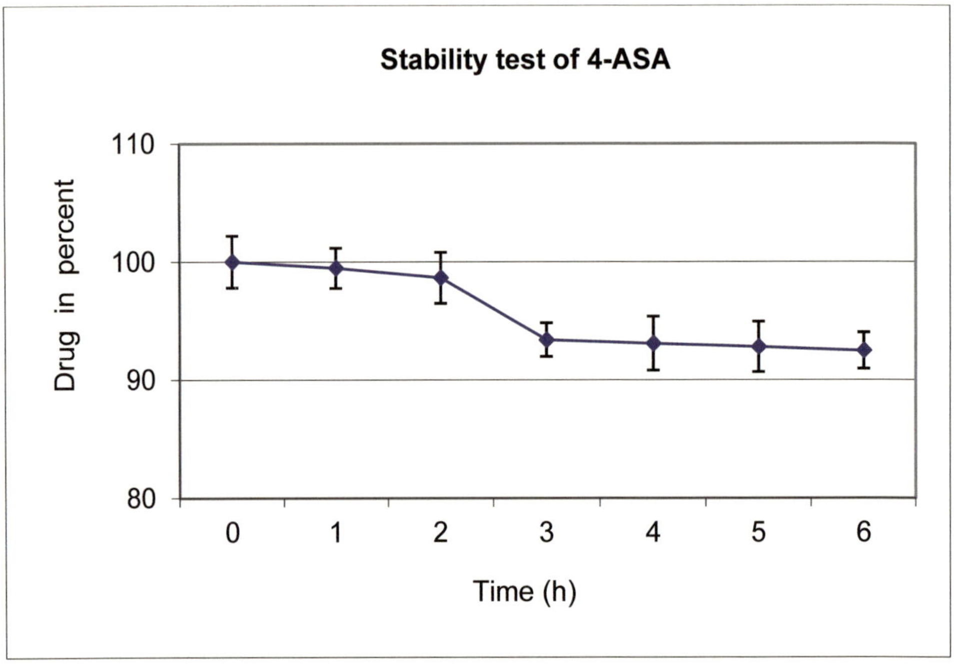

Fig. 5. Study of 4ASA stability during 6h. Bars represent standard deviations of the mean (n=3)

The determination of 4ASAconcentration following the degradation, was a positive point on the specificity of the drug.
It would mean that the first breackdowned products did not absorb at 300nm. However new peaks at lower retention time (<3min) were detected on seven day-old samples at 300nm.The later consideration deals with the specificity of the method and its ability to separate degradation products for pure drug.

4.3 Application to biological samples

The validated analytical method was applied to male Sprague-Dawley rats.
Compared to the results given by working standard solutions, good peak shape and acceptable sensitivity were obtained with the same mobile phase (acetonitrile /water 30:70) from diluted plasma samples containing 4ASA. Good precision (CV=3.39%) and reproducibility were also observed during 4ASA quantification in plasma samples (Table **4**).

	Area	%
Mean	8849,978	100,7479
RSD	152,8166	2,718627

Table 4. Evaluation of the Intra assay precision (n=8)

The accuracy of these values was confirmed by back calculating the concentration of the calibrations standards.
The retention time was from 4.3 to 5.2 min and did not interfer with other compounds from plasma. This period was closed to that obtained with those obtained with aqueous solution (4.3-4.8min). The concentration range (10-100µg/ml) in plasma is shorter than the aqueous medium concentration (1 to 125µg/ml). The regression equation was Y=88.72 x-88.38 and coefficient of correlation (r^2) was 0,999.With regard to the partition test, plasma level of 4ASA reached a maximum of 101.95% (Figure 6).

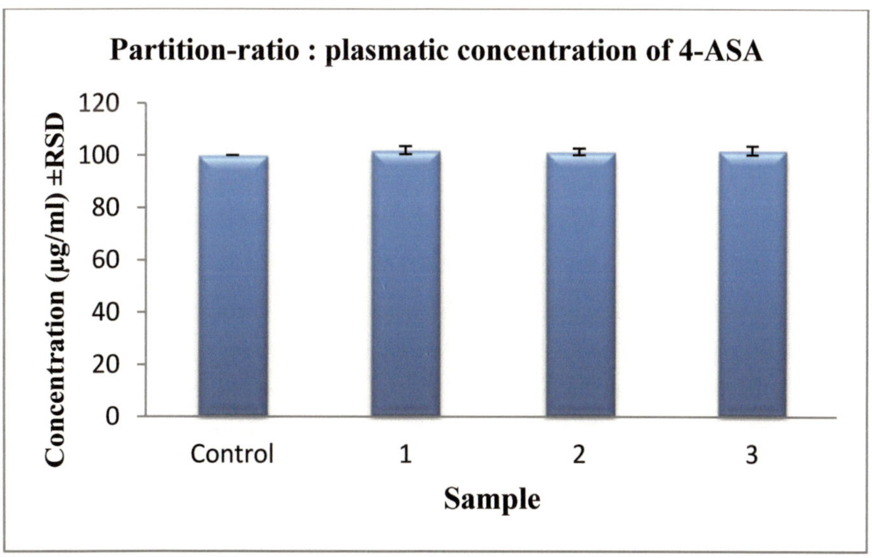

Fig. 6. Plasmatic concentration of 4ASA after partition-ratio.
Bars represent standard deviations (n=5)

The average recovery of assay was 93.54%, 100.89% and 100.23% for low, medium and high concentrations of 4ASA in plasma respectively (Table **5**).

Concentration (µg/ml)	RSD (%)	
Expected	Measured	
25	23,39	1,74
50	51,45	3,28
100	100,3	1,65

Table 5. Responses in recovery tests at low, mean and high value. Mean ±RSD

Stability tests were investigated using the procedure described above. The results indicated that 4ASA was stable in plasma at -4°C for 24h (Figure **7**).

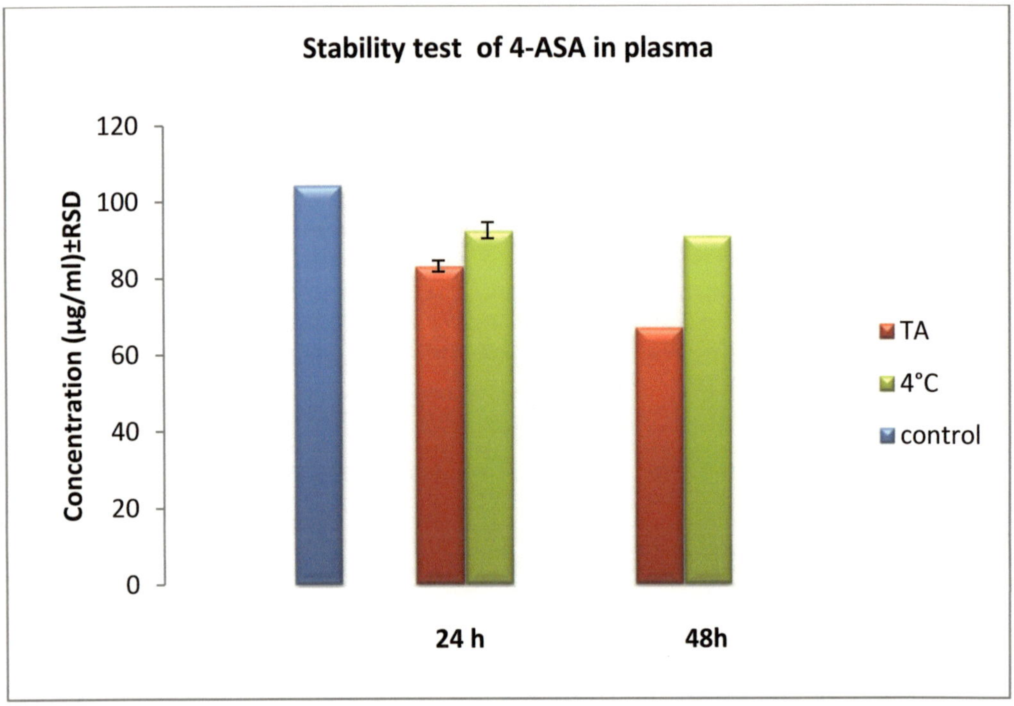

Fig. 7. Stability test of 4ASA in plasma after 48h at room temperature (RT) and at 4°C. Bars represent standard deviations of the mean (n=5).

Since 4ASA was degraded in human plasma in 24 hours at room temperature and would be useful for immediate-release solid oral dosage forms. The profile of bioavailability test curve was characteristic of a dosage form with extended release. Because the plasma content of 4ASA was almost constant, it could mean that equilibrium of the balance absorption/ degradation was maintained (Figure **8**).

We notice that stability of the analyte during sample collection was investigated using the procedure described above. In connection with bioavailability, these results were unexpected because the concentration remains relatively constant.

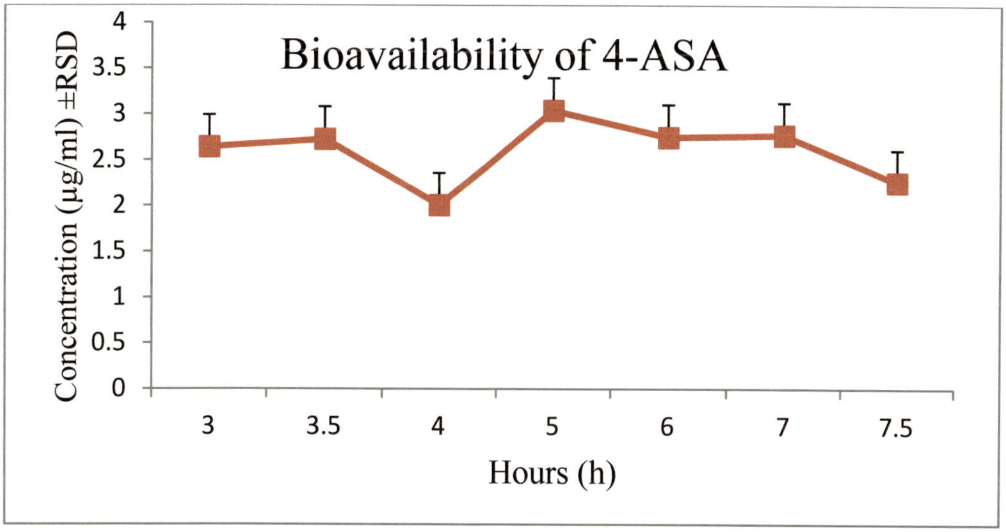

Fig. 8. Plasma concentration-time profile after i.v. administration of 25 mg/kg 4- ASA after 7.5h. Bars represent standard deviations of the mean (n=4).

5. Conclusion

In pharmaceutical analysis, often a method validation is required in order to meet the strict regulations, set by the regulatory authorities. This method was then developed and validated for the determination of 4ASA. Thus specificity, precision, accuracy, linearity, recovery and the limits were acceptable with the execution run time for control studies. It would be very useful for release profile study in simulated intestinal medium of the analyte in question. These results indicated that the RP-HPLC method was specific for the determination of 4ASA in plasma, under the chromatographic conditions employed.
Through this method the retention time was reduced considerably compared to previous results obtained by Gennaro *et al* [13]. With these present results it is possible to save time and solvents used to constitute the mobile phase. In addition, studies in plasma indicated that this method is suitable for pharmacokinetic studies.

6. Acknowledgements

The authors thank also In-Cyclo Society for his financial support.

7. References

[1] Wolfe, M.M.; Lichtenstein, D.R, Singh, G. *N Engl J Med.*, 1999, 340, 1888-99.
[2] GETAID. Intest info "les derives amino-salicylés"., 2005
[3] Defilippi, A.; Piancone, G.; Costa Laia, R. Tibaldi, G.P. Chromatographia., 1995, 40-170.
[4] Defilippi, A.; Piancone, G.; Costa Laia, R. ; Balla, S.; Tibaldi, G.P. J. Chromatogr., 1994, 656-466.
[5] Sadeg, N.; Pertat, N.; Dutertre, H.; Dumontet, M. J. Chromatogr., 1996, 675,113.

[6] Seifart, H.I.; Kruger, P.B.; Parkin, D.P; Van Jaarsveld, P.P.; Donald, P.R., J. Chromatogr., 1993, 619,285.
[7] Hansen Jr. E.B.; Dooley, K.L.; Thompson Jr. H.C. J. Chromatogr., 1995, 670, 259.
[8] Karlaganis, G.; Peretti, E.; Lauterburg, B.H.; J. Chromatogr., 1987, 420,171.
[9] Cummins, C. L.; O' Neil, W.; Soo, E. C.; Lloyd, D. K.; Wainer I.W. Newspaper chromatography B., 1997, 697, 283-288.
[10] Song, M.; Xia, B.; Li J. Postgrad Med J., 2006, 82, 130–135.
[11] Vernia, P.; Cittadini, M. ; Caprilli, R. Dig Dis Sci., 1995, 40,305–307.
[12] Mocak, J.; Bond, A. M.; Mitchell, S.; Scollary, G. *Pure* & *Appl. Chern.,* 1997, 69, 297-328.
[13] Gennaro, M.C.; Calvino, R.; Abrigo, C. Journal of Chromatography B., 2001, 754, 477–486.

10

Approach to the Management of the Pregnant Inflammatory Bowel Disease Patient: Successful Outcome

Flavio M. Habal
University Health Network
University Of Toronto
Canada

1. Introduction

Inflammatory bowel disease (IBD) encompasses Crohn's disease (CD) and ulcerative colitis (UC) and it affect young adults in their reproductive years (Andres & Friedman, 1999).

Approximately 25% of these patients will conceive after the diagnosis is made. Many women with IBD raise concerns related to the effects of both the disease and medical therapy on fertility, pregnancy and foetal outcomes. On the basis of prospective and registry data, it is known that women with IBD have a higher risk of low-birth-weight deliveries and pre-term deliveries (Cornish J, 2007). With the exception of patients who have had previous pelvic surgery, the majority of these patients are able to conceive, have a normal pregnancy and a good foetal outcome. Maintaining remission, with drug therapy, prior to conception and during pregnancy is of prime importance. Control of disease activity before conception and during pregnancy is critical to optimize both maternal and fetal health (Mountfield, 2010). Normal maternal weight gain during pregnancy appears to protect against adverse outcome. The majority of drugs used in IBD appear to be safe and their benefit appears to outweigh the risk of disease exacerbation and poor foetal outcome. The newer biologic anti TNF alpha drugs appear to be safe during pregnancy.

Although there are reports of some traces of drugs in breast milk in women taking medications no major undue complication has been reported.

Treatment of IBD patients who are contemplating conception should be tailored to each patient, taking into accounts the patient wishes and concerns. The patient should be followed by a multidisciplinary team including the family physician, the gastroenterologist and the obstetrician.

Preconception advice and counselling

Preconception care aims to ensure the optimal physical and mental well-being of women and their partners at the onset of and during early pregnancy, to increase the likelihood of normal pregnancy and the delivery of a healthy infant. Pre pregnancy counselling should be an integral part of IBD consultation. Patient understanding of the disease and its changes during pregnancy and breastfeeding is vital for a successful outcome. In a recent abstract from England the authors showed that there was a lack of knowledge and understanding in the women of reproductive age about their disease, medication and effects of these on pregnancy. It is important to discuss the issues related to pregnancy and conception either at diagnosis or when medication is initially prescribed. In our experience some pregnant women tend to stop their medication in fear of the side effect of the drugs on the developing foetus, with an inherent risk of disease flare up. A questionnaire study by Mountfield et al found that a large proportion of subjects (84%) reported concerns that IBD medications would harm their pregnancy, whereas only 19% women reported concerns about the effect of active IBD on pregnancy. The author reported that patients with active disease had higher risks of adverse outcome with a better outcome if they are in remission (Mountfield, 2010).

It is estimated that more than 50% of pregnancies are not planned hence as soon as the diagnosis is made this issue should be brought up. See table 1, for general pre-pregnancy recommendations.

Folic acid is an important vitamin that should be taken prior to conception since neural tube defect occurs as soon as conception is discovered. It is interesting in the British abstract only 43 women (65.15%) knew the beneficial effect of folic acid pre-conception and during the first trimester of pregnancy (Chakrabarty & Poullis, 2011).

The patient, her partner and her physician should discuss the possibility of disease exacerbation during pregnancy while off treatment and the necessary courses of action in such an event. Treatment choices depend on individual preference, disease severity and potential for drug toxicity. Risks and benefits of maintenance therapies during pregnancy with the best available evidence should be addressed. In addition, breastfeeding should be presented as a favourable option since it confers numerous benefits to both mother and child. The likelihood of medication secretion in breast milk and impact on foetal wellbeing should be approached and encouraged.

General advice pre pregnancy
1. Discuss potential pregnancy outcome, breast feeding, and drug therapy
2. Diet and nutrition
3. Folic acid supplementation 5 mg daily
3. Stop smoking
4. Decrease alcohol intake
5. Establish a record of vaccination and update

Table 1.

Dietary supplementation and nutritional therapy

Nutritional therapy: The average weight gain during pregnancy is 11-16 kg. Early nutritional intervention is indicated in pregnant women with active IBD who may not be gaining weight. Enteral feeding has been anecdotally shown to be associated with normal pregnancy outcome (Teahon, 1991) and total parenteral nutrition (TPN) may be required in very sick IBD patients.

TPN proved to be helpful and lifesaving in malnourished pregnant women and promoted foetal growth, as shown by the longitudinal ultrasonographic evaluations (Caruso, 1998).

2. Folic acid, calcium and vitamin D

Folic acid supplementation is recommended for all pregnant women. Women with IBD may have folic acid deficiency or be taking medications that interfere with folic acid metabolism such as Sulfasalazine (Alstead, 2002). Certain patients with Cohn's disease are on low residue diet and may be folate deficient. Thus, pregnant women with IBD should be encouraged to take 5 mg of folic acid per day instead of 1 mg/d as recommended for the general population. Also, patients with IBD on steroid therapy should be encouraged to take calcium and vitamin D supplementation to prevent bone loss.

3. Alcohol

Heavy drinking throughout pregnancy can result in what is known as foetal alcohol syndrome. Patients contemplating pregnancy should be educated about the adverse effects of alcohol. Foetal Alcohol Syndrome (FAS) is a pattern of mental and physical defects clinically defined by growth deficiency, central nervous system damage and dysfunction, and a unique cluster of facial abnormalities. on foetal development. Prenatal alcohol exposure can also cause less pronounced mental, learning and behavioural disabilities in the child, commonly termed as Foetal Alcohol Spectrum Disorders (FASDs) (Davies & Bledsoe, 2005).

4. Smoking

Smoking increases the risk of developing CD and worsens its course, increasing the need for steroids, immunosuppressants and re-operations. It appears that smoking cessation improves CD and aggravates ulcerative colitis (Lakatos P Let al, 2007).

Tobacco smoking during pregnancy has been associated with placenta previa, placental abruption, premature rupture of membranes (Shah & Bracken, 2000; Mercer, 2008). It can result in small foetal size at 10-19 weeks and may result in early premature birth, low birth weight, and poor foetal outcome. Smoking cessation should be encouraged in the patient prior to, during and after pregnancy.

5. Heredity

Genetic factors appear to play a role in the pathogenesis of Crohn's disease (CD) and ulcerative colitis (UC) (Thompson N et al. 1996).

In association with environmental triggers, heredity increases the risk of developing IBD; however, studies of twins also indicate the involvement of multiple factors (Orholm M, 2000; Tysk C et al 1988). Offspring of patients with IBD are two to 13 times more likely to develop IBD than the general population. The risk of an infant developing IBD is 8% to 11% if one parent has IBD and 20% to 35% if both parents have the disease. Data suggest, however, that the risk is decreased in breastfed infants (Yang H et al 1983).

In the general population, approximately 4% of babies born every year have congenital abnormalities, an outcome similar to what is seen in retrospective studies of women whose IBD is treated during their pregnancy. Studies that report prematurity and small-for-gestational-age infants did not document maternal smoking, alcohol consumption, disease status and medication use.

6. Effect of IBD on fertility, pregnancy and foetal outcomes

6.1 IBD and fertility

Infertility rates in women with inactive CD appear to be similar to those of the general population (8% to 10%) (Khosla et al 1984).

Active disease decreases fertility, possibly as a result of decrease libido, fatigue and concerns regarding the disease. Other factors may be caused by inflammation or adhesions in the fallopian tubes or ovaries, and may cause painful intercourse (Steinlauf & Present DH **2004)**.

Some women choose not to bear children secondary to fear of pregnancy (Marri, 2007) and the risk of inheritance of the disease and the possible harmful effect of drug therapy. Patient education preconception may alleviate this fear and may lead to successful pregnancy.

Women who have undergone ileal pouch-anal anastomosis are less fertile. In a recent meta-analysis of ileal pouch-anal anastomosis (IPPPA) resulted in a threefold increased risk of infertility as opposed to those treated medically (Waljee J et al 2006).

Some of the evidence suggests that extensive pelvic surgery and rectal resection with the creation of J pouch lead to scarring, adhesions and tubal infertility (Arkuran & McComb, 2000; Oresland et al, 1994).

Despite these suggestions it appears that the majority of these patients can still conceive with IVF (Kwan & Mahadevan, 2010). In patients with active Crohn's disease there appear to be decreased fertility, which can be restored upon induction of remission (Baiocco & Korelitz, 1984).

It is recommended that female patients who are planning to conceive and require colectomy for acute ulcerative not undergo IPPPA and instead undergo ileostomy and rectal sparing. IPPPA should then be performed after conception. Despite this recommendation, there is no data as yet to support such an approach (Janneke, 2010). Patients, who undergo IPPPA, are more likely to have a Caesarean section following RPC (Cornish, 2011).

6.2 IBD and pregnancy outcomes

Due to the lack of prospective studies clinical outcomes in IBD and pregnancy has been controversial with data showing poor outcome and others showing no effect. Some of these reviews or meta-analysis did not take into account some factors such as drug use by the patients, population age, smoking and alcohol and duration of disease (Dominitz et al, 2002; Fonager et al 1992). Similarly the reviews are variable between ulcerative colitis and Crohn's disease.

In 2007 Cornish et al published a meta-analysis on the influence of IBD on pregnancy. The analysis reviewed 12 studies that met specific inclusion criteria and reported the outcomes of interest. The studies included 1952 women with CD, 1113 with UC and 320,531 controls. For women with IBD, the analysis found a 1.87-fold increase in premature births (less than 37 weeks; P<0.001); more than double the incidence of low birth weight (LBW) (less than 2500 g; P<0.001); a 1.5-fold increase in caesarean section (P<0.001); and a 2.37-fold increase in congenital abnormalities (P<0.001). The analysis was unable to determine which women had a higher risk of adverse outcomes, but the authors concluded that pregnant women with IBD should be treated as a high-risk group. There were significant limits to this study. These studies were of an observational nature which make them vulnerable to bias; the low incidence of adverse outcomes makes statistical precision difficult; and disease activity was not reported in relation to outcomes. In addition, increased risks of congenital abnormalities associated with 5-ASA, azathioprine and anti-TNF-alpha medications seen in a pooled analysis may be associated with the disease and not the medications. The authors also pointed out the need for a definitive study to determine optimal management and to support the development of new guidelines to assist patients and clinicians in decision-making (Cornish et al 2007).

In a recent publication **by** Raatikainen there was a lower birth weight of newborns from mothers with UC as compared to the general population (3317 _ s.d. 658 g vs. 3506 _ s.d. 613 g, P = 0.003;3340 _ s.d. 631 g vs. 3507 _ s.d. 613 g, P = 0.002) respectively. Newborns in the CD group were also smaller than those in the reference group but the difference was not statistically significant (Raatikainen et al 2011).

A Taiwanese, Asian population database from 2001-2003 study found an increase of preterm births (11.73 vs. 6.25%; $p = 0.004$) and LBW (12.76 vs. 5.55%; $p < 0.001$), controlling for maternal characteristics including age, parity and education level (Lin, 2010). In a cohort study from Northern California Kaiser population, pregnant women with IBD were more likely to have a spontaneous abortion (OR: 1.65; 95% CI: 1.09–2.48); an adverse pregnancy outcome (stillbirth, preterm birth or SGA infant; OR: 1.54; 95% CI: 1.00–2.38); or a complication of labour (OR: 1.78; 95% CI: 1.13–2.81). The study did not find a difference in the rate of congenital malformations in control versus IBD patients, either as a group or for UC and CD separately (Mahadevan et al 2007).

In a review in 1998 Subahani et al found that CD, especially active disease, is associated with decreased birth weights, preterm delivery and caesarean section (Subahani & Hamilton, 1998).

In a case-control study published by Bush comparing 116 pregnancies in patients with IBD with 56,398 controls, there were no differences in ante partum complications, including chronic hypertension, hyperemesis gravidarum, preterm labour or pre-eclampsia. Among patients with IBD, however, induction of labour (32% versus 24%; P=0.002), chorioamnionitis (7% versus 3%; P=0.04), and caesarean section (32% versus 22%; P=0.007) were all more frequent. Neonatal complications, including low birth weight (LBW), very low birth weight, intrauterine growth restriction, Apgar scores and congenital anomalies, were similar in both groups. Subgroup analysis found a decreased risk of LBW associated with previous IBD surgery, quiescent disease, and CD compared with UC (Bush et al, 2004).

The most recent and only prospective study has just been published by the ECCO-Epicom study (Bertoli et al, 2011). This study from Europe was prospective case-controlled with 332 patients with IBD both Crohn's disease and Ulcerative colitis who were pregnant and were compared to non-IBD pregnant women in the general population. In this study there was no difference in live births, spontaneous or therapeutic abortions, infant death in utero, preterm deliveries and caesarean sections. There was no difference in congenital anomalies or birth weight as compared to outcome in pregnancy in the general population. The only risk that was demonstrated to be associated with congenital anomaly and preterm delivery was older age ≥ 35 years. Smoking was found to be a factor which increased the risk of preterm delivery.

Dejaco performed a prospective study assessing risk factors for poor pregnancy outcome in 58 patients with IBD (Dejaco, et al 2006). The authors found that active disease during pregnancy represents a significant risk factor for unfavourable birth outcome. These results support the current treatment guidelines, which state that the maintenance of remission during pregnancy is essential (Carter, et al 2004). Pregnant women should be treated as aggressively as women who are not pregnant.

7. Mode of delivery

The decision to have a caesarean section should be made on purely obstetric grounds with a discussion with the gastroenterologist. In a meta-analysis in 2007, a pregnant woman with IBD was 1.5 times more likely to undergo c section (95% CI 1.26-1.79; $p<0.001$) (Cornish et al, 2007). Some surgeons advise elective caesarean section to avoid risk of anal sphincter damage. Vaginal delivery and episiotomy may lead to development or worsening of perianal CD (Brandt LJ, 1995). Current indications for caesarean section are active perianal disease and presence of an ileoanal pouch. There is no absolute contraindication to vaginal delivery in pregnant patients with inactive IBD (Alexandra Ilnyckyet al, 1999).

8. Endoscopy during pregnancy

It is best to avoid any major investigation during pregnancy such as radiation, endoscopy or major surgery. Indications for endoscopy during pregnancy include significant or continued gastrointestinal bleeding, dysphagia, severe or (Qureshi et al, 2005) refractory nausea and vomiting or abdominal pain, and a strong suspicion of a colonic mass. It is best to postpone endoscopy to the second trimester. If endoscopy is indicated it is important to place the patient in lateral decubitus position avoid vena caval or aortic compression by the gravid uterus. This otherwise may lead to decreased uterine blood flow and foetal hypoxemia (Kemmerer, 1979).

No evidence exists that would suggest endoscopy could affect the pregnancy. Obstetrical support should be available in the event of a pregnancy-related complication, and the presence of foetal heart sounds should be confirmed before administering sedation before and after the procedure (Qureshi et al, 2005).

Endoscopy should be done with minimal sedation. Meperidine, FDA class B followed by small doses of midazolam FDA class C. (Qureshi, 2005) Benzodiazepines (D) should be avoided in the first trimester since they have been associated with congenital cleft palate and when used late in pregnancy with neurobehavioral disorders (Ornoy, 1998; Dolovich, et al 1998; Laegreid et al,1989). Propofol, FDA class B, should be administered by an anaesthetist; its safety as yet in first trimester has not been studied (Gin, 1994).

9. Radiology

An excellent guideline regarding pregnancy and radiation has been published by the CDC Radiation and Pregnancy: A Fact Sheet for Clinicians Prenatal Radiation Exposure: A Fact Sheet for Physicians (CDC) 2003 http://www.bt.cdc.gov/radiation/prenatalphysician.asp , and documentations could be found in: Valentin J, 2000.

In certain circumstances radiographic imaging may be needed to rule out obstruction, perforation or toxic mega colon. Investigations that expose the patient to less radiation are preferable specifically plain abdominal films rather than CT or barium studies. Ultrasound is the safest form of radiologic imaging. It can be used to assess abscess formation and can provide information on bowel wall thickness. MRI studies are also safe and have been used to diagnose terminal ileal CD during pregnancy since active disease in the mother has an adverse effect on the foetus; investigation for diagnostic and therapeutic purposes is warranted and should not be delayed. The foetal radiation dose should be estimated by qualified medical personnel to provide a more detailed approximation of risks to the foetus (Osei et al, 1999).

10. Medication and therapy during pregnancy

Aside from Methotrexate and Thalidomide most of the drugs used in IBD appear to be safe during gestation. The US FDA classification of drugs offers a guide to the use of medications during pregnancy. The FDA categories are listed in **table 2**.

Definition	Class
Controlled studies in women fail to demonstrate a risk to the foetus in the first trimester (and there is no evidence of risk in later trimesters) and the possibility of foetal harm appears remote	A
Either animal reproduction studies have not demonstrated a foetal risk, but there are no controlled studies in pregnant women OR animal reproduction studies have shown an adverse effect (other than decrease in fertility) that was not confirmed in controlled studies in women in the first trimester (and there is no evidence of risk in later trimesters)	B
Either studies in animals have repeated adverse effects on the foetus (teratogenic, embryonic or other) and there are no controlled studies in women or studies in women and animals are not available. Drugs should be given only if the potential benefit justifies the potential risk to the foetus	C
There is positive evidence of human foetal risk but the benefits from use in pregnant women may be acceptable despite the risk (e.g. if the drug is needed in a life threatening situation or for a serious disease for which safer drugs cannot be used or are ineffective)	D
Studies in animals or human beings have demonstrated foetal abnormalities OR there is evidence of foetal risk based on human experience OR both, and the risk of the use of the drug in pregnant women clearly outweighs any possible benefit. The drug is contraindicated in women who are or may become pregnant.	X

Table 2. Food and drug administration (FDA) classes in pregnancy

Crohn's disease and ulcerative colitis appear to be mediated by different aspects of immune system. CD is thought to be related to the over expression of T cell helper (Th) 1 cytokines, such as TNF-alpha, which stimulate cell-mediated immunity and result in transmural inflammation of the gut (Neissner & Volk, 1995). In contrast, UC is believed to result from a dysregulation of intestinal immunity involving the Th2 cytokine response. Increased expression of TNF-alpha, however, has been observed in patients with UC. The newer treatment modalities, with biologics, over the past decade, are to target specific inflammatory mediators such as TNFα.

There are several medications used to treat IBD. These include aminosalicylates, such as Mesalamine, and immune modulators, such as Azathioprine and Methotrexate. Other drugs include Corticosteroids which are effective in inducing remission in both CD and UC but ineffective in maintenance therapy. Steroids result in side effects in the majority of patients taking the drug on a long term basis.

Medications	FDA Class
5-Aminosalicylic acid* preparations (sulfasalazine, mesalamine, balsalazide); metronidazole, amoxicillin/clavulanic acid; infliximab; adalimumab; Certolizumab	B
5-Aminosalicylic acid preparations (Olsalazine); fluoroquinolones; corticosteroids; bisphosphonates;cyclosporin; tacrolimus Biphosphonates	C
Azathioprine; 6-MP	D
Methotrexate; thalidomide	X

Table 3. Inflammatory bowel disease medications FDA classes: Summary of safety data during pregnancy* *Asacol (Mesalamine)* Dibutyl phthalate (DBP)
P=PRECAUTIONS

A recent study by Moskovitz et al (2004) assessed the effect of 5-ASA drugs, metronidazole, ciprofloxacin, prednisone, 6-mercaptopurine, azathioprine and cyclosporine on pregnancy outcomes in 113 IBD patients with 207 documented conceptions. The authors reviewed information obtained on smoking history, birth weight, and type of delivery. They also followed the pregnancy outcomes: spontaneous abortion, therapeutic abortion, maternal or foetal illness resulting in abortion, premature birth, healthy full-term birth, multiple births, ectopic pregnancy and congenital defects. The study also analyzed the effect of medications on pregnancy outcomes during the first trimester and at any time during the pregnancy. No significant differences were seen among groups in pregnancy outcomes. A multivariate analysis controlling for maternal age showed no negative influence of any medication on pregnancy outcomes.

11. 5-ASA compounds sulfasalazine/mesalamine/olsalazine

Sulfasalazine has been assigned to pregnancy category B by the FDA. It was one of the earliest therapeutics used in IBD. Sulfasalazine is metabolized by intestinal bacterial flora to sulfapyridine (SP) and 5-ASA. Sulfapyridine crosses the placenta to the fetus with the foetal concentrations being approximately the same as the maternal serum concentrations. Caution should be exercised when Sulfasalazine is administered to a nursing woman. Sulphonamides are excreted in the milk. In the newborn, they compete with bilirubin for binding sites on the plasma proteins and may thus cause kernicterus.
There was no significant increase in prevalence of selected congenital abnormalities in the children of women treated with Sulfasalazine during pregnancy. A review of the medical literature covering 1,155 pregnancies in women with ulcerative colitis suggested that the

outcome was similar to that expected in the general population (Jarnerot, 1982). Sulfapyridine acts as a competitive inhibitor of the enzyme dihydropteroate synthase in the folate metabolism; and this may lead to a deficiency of dihydrofolate and tetrahydrofolate. Patients receiving Sulfasalazine should receive folic acid supplementations.

Oligospermia and infertility have been observed in men treated with Sulfasalazine; this effect is reversed upon discontinuing the drug.

At the 2006 Digestive Disease Week in Los Angeles, USA, Mahadevan reported that the use of 5-ASA and Sulfasalazine during pregnancy was not associated with an increase in adverse outcomes. A trend toward an increased risk of congenital malformations was seen during conception and the first trimester with Sulfasalazine, but not with 5-ASA. On the contrary, an increased risk of adverse outcomes was seen in women not taking 5-ASA during the second and third trimesters, suggesting a protective effect of the medication (Mahadevan &Corley, 2006).

In a recent meta-analysis of seven studies prior to 2007, with a total of 2200 pregnant women with IBD there was an 1.16-fold increase in congenital malformations, an 2.38-fold increase in stillbirth, an 1.14-fold increase in spontaneous abortion, an 1.35-fold increase in preterm delivery, and an 0.93-fold increase in low birth weight (Rahimi R et al 2008; Norgard et al, 2003).

Asacol is covered with an inactive enteric coating of dibutyl phthalate (DBP) that prevents the medication from degrading before it reaches the small intestine. DBP was associated with external and skeletal malformations and adverse effects on the male reproductive of rodents system. Patients who are using Asacol have 50 times higher mean urinary concentration of monobutyl phthalate, the main DBP metabolite, than the mean for nonusers (2,257 microg/L vs. 46 microg/L; $p < 0.0001$) (Hernández-Díaz et al 2009). These results raise concern about potential human health risks, particularly pregnant women and children. Although this has not been shown in any human study, Asacol should be used during pregnancy only if the potential benefit justifies the potential risk to the fetus.FDA 2010 *Safety Labelling Changes Approved By FDA Center for Drug Evaluation and Research (CDER) – May 2010.These patients may need to be switched to non DBP containing Mesalamine* .

Contraindicated	Limited data, potential toxicity	Safe
Thalidomide	Metronidazole	5-ASA preparations
Methotrexate	Fluoroquinolones	(sulfasalazine/mesalamine)
Cyclosporine	Bisphosphonates	Amoxacillin/clavulanic
Tacolimus (FK506)	Azathioprine	Acid
	6-Mercaptopurine (6-MP)	Corticosteroids
	Adalimumab	
	Infliximab	

Table 4. Breastfeeding safety of medications used to treat IBD

12. Immune modulators

12.1 Azathioprine/6 mercaptopurine

6-mercaptopurine (6MP) and its prodrug azathioprine (AZA) are pregnancy category D drugs. These have been proven to be effective in the treatment of steroid-dependent or resistant IBD Crohn's disease (CD) and ulcerative colitis (Gisbert et al, 2009). These drugs are used as immunosuppressive therapies in autoimmune diseases, transplant patients and in leukemia. Azathioprine and 6-mercaptopurine are purine analogues that interfere with the synthesis of adenine and guanine ribonucleosides. These ribonucleosides are important precursors of DNA and RNA and hence act on rapidly producing cells. Following oral intake of AZA 47% of the drug is available to the systemic circulation whereas only 16% of 6-mercaptopurine is available (Zimm, et al, 1983). In animal studies, in mice after intraperitoneal administration of azathioprine, there was evidence of increased frequencies of cleft palate, open-eye, and skeletal anomalies. There was a significant decrease in thymic size. The dose given is equivalent of 4–13 times the maximum human therapeutic dose of AZA.There was no discussion regarding its effect on the immune system development, which is important for future immunity.

The safety of azathioprine in pregnancy comes from studies in transplantation and rheumatology patients (Rosenkrantz et al, 1967.; Gaudier, et al 1988).

The foetus is protected from potential teratogenic effects of azathioprine and 6-MP due to the lack in foetal liver of the enzyme inosinate phosphorylase which is necessary to convert azathioprine and 6-MP to active metabolites. Both these medications when used in small doses in clinical practice do not affect human interstitial cell function or gametogenesis (Golby, 1970; Penn, et al 1971).

13. Should azathioprine/6 mercaptopurine be used in pregnancy?

In a retrospective chart review and telephone recalls of some of the patients who had received 6-Mercaptopurine for IBD before or during conception, there was no statistical difference in abortion secondary to a birth defect, major congenital malformations, neoplasia, or increased infections among male or female patients taking 6-MP compared with controls (RR = 0.85 [0.47-1.55], P = 0.59) (Francella, et al, 2003).

In a retrospective Swedish registry study reviewing patients receiving azathioprine (AZA) during pregnancy by women, the majority of whom were with inflammatory bowel disease, and the rest being with other autoimmune disorders, malignancy, and organ transplantation, the rate of congenital malformations was 6.2% in the AZA group and 4.7% among all infants born (adjusted OR: 1.42, 95% CI: 0.98–2.04) (Cleary& Kallen, 2009).

There was an association between early pregnancy AZA exposure and ventricular/atrial septal defects (adjusted OR: 3.18, 95% CI: 1.45–6.04). Exposed infants were also more likely to be preterm, to weigh <2500 gm, and to be small for gestational age compared to all infants born. The authors pointed in their article regarding the severity of the disease and its association with drug use (Cleary& Kallen, 2009).

In a Danish registry study in women with Crohn's diseases receiving drug therapy during pregnancy the risk of preterm birth and congenital abnormalities was greater when azathioprine/mercaptopurine was prescribed as compared to women who did not used drugs. Preterm births were more prevalent among Thiopurine-exposed women (25%) compared to the reference group (6.5%). Congenital abnormalities were also more prevalent among azathioprine/mercaptopurine-exposed women (15.4 versus 5.7%, adjusted relative risk, 2.9; 95% CI, 0.9–8.9). Among Thiopurine-exposed women, the risk of preterm birth was also increased to 4.2 (95% CI, 1.4–12.5) compared to the control group (Norgard, et al 2007). The conclusion of this study was subsequently challenged, based on bias, the disease activity of the patients and the use of confidential interval (Simpson, et al 2008).

In a prospective, controlled, multicentre study conducted by the Tel Aviv University (Israel), 189 pregnant women on azathioprine were compared to a cohort of 230 pregnant women who did not take Azathioprine. The aim of that study was to determine risk of congenital malformation in pregnant women exposed to azathioprine and to assess the pregnancy outcome (Goldstein, et al, 2007). The rate of congenital malformations did not differ between the two groups; there were more cases noted of prematurity (21% vs. 5%, $P < 0.001$) and low birth weight (23% vs. 6%, $P < 0.001$) in the azathioprine group.

The most recent ECCO consensus guidelines recommend the use of AZA/6-MP in high risk patients where the benefit outweighs the risk of relapse of the disease. The European consensus guidelines consider azathioprine to be safe and well tolerated in pregnant women with no consistent reports of abnormalities of fertility, prematurity, or congenital defects (Van Assche, et al 2010).

Based on the data published in the transplant literature, the American Gastroenterology Association, and The ECCO consensus guidelines, the recommendation is that Azathioprine /6-Mercaptopurine treatment to be continued during pregnancy (Van Assche, et al 2010). The discontinuation of therapy in pregnant women, in remission, may be more harmful (Zlatanic et al, 2003) than precipitating a flare up with more deleterious effect on the neonate (Mahadevan U, Kane S. 2006). Although some negative outcomes in some cases of pregnancy in IBD women have been reported, the majority of case series or cohort studies have not shown an increase in congenital anomalies. Despite this recommendation, the risks and benefits of treatment must be carefully balanced by the patient in consultation with her Doctor and partner.

14. Breast feeding: Azathioprine/6 mercaptopurine

The majority of physicians have not recommended breast feeding of neonates while mothers are receiving thiopurines. The reason for this has been the theoretical potential risks of bone marrow suppression, susceptibility to infection, and pancreatitis in the neonate. In a prospective study in 10 women receiving AZA while breast feeding in 31 samples, there was only one woman who had a low measurable level on AZA in two samples of the breast milk. The concentrations of 6-MP was 1.2 and 7.6 nanograms/mL, as compared with therapeutic immunosuppressant level of 50 nanograms/mL in serum. The conclusion of the authors was that there were no clinical or haematological signs of immunosuppression in any of the ten neonates and that breast feeding should not be withheld (Sau et al, 2007).

Based on the case reports and the presence of low to absent levels of Thiopurine in the breast milk of women receiving thiopurines, breast feeding can be continued. The benefits of breastfeeding outweigh the theoretical risk. A discussion with the mother explaining the risk benefit should be undertaken (*Gardiner al, 2006; Christensen, et al 2008*).

15. Birth outcome in IBD fathers on immunosuppressive drugs

Pregnant women with IBD who are on thiopurines drugs, and who are in remission should continue their medication during their pregnancy (Caprilli, et al 2006; Gisbert et al 2009; Van Assche et al, 2010). The safety of Thiopurine derivatives has been controversial in male patients exposed to thiopurines at the time of conception. In a retrospective study by Rajapakse published in 2000, there was an increase in adverse side effects. In 13 males exposed to Thiopurine at the time of conception, there were two congenital anomalies and two spontaneous abortions. Based on that study there was some concern about continuing the drug in male patients wishing to have children. Further publications did not confirm these findings (Francella, et al, 2003; Truel, et al 2010).

16. Cyclosporine and inflammatory bowel disease

Cyclosporine (CsA) is classified as FDA pregnancy category C. CsA is a selective immunosuppressive drug that has been used mainly in solid organ transplant such as liver, kidney and heart. CsA inhibits the activation of T cells, preventing formation of IL-2.In inflammatory bowel disease, it is mostly used to induce remission in acute ulcerative colitis non responsive to conventional therapy intravenous corticosteroids (Lichtiger et al, 1994; Cohen et al, 1999). Its use has been mostly used to delay surgery in acute ulcerative colitis. The majority of literature in cyclosporine and pregnancy has been reported in transplant publications (Nagy et al, 2003).

Most of the data regarding the use of cyclosporine in pregnancy comes from transplant patients. In a meta-analysis of 15 studies of pregnancy outcomes in 410 transplant patients receiving cyclosporine, showed no significant increase in major malformations. Congenital malformation was 4.1% which was similar to the general population receiving no drugs. (Nagy et al, 2003). 2003). Pregnant transplant patients who are stable while receiving Cyclosporine appear to have a good pregnancy and foetal outcome Nagy et al, 2003). Cyclosporine is secreted in breast milk at high concentrations. Due to its possible toxic effect on the newborn and possible immunosuppression, the American Paediatric association does not recommended breast feeding while taking the drug (Kwan et al, 2010).

17. Corticosteroids (FDA class C)

Corticosteroids are classified as pregnancy category C drugs. They are given to patients via a variety of forms which include oral and topical formulations and those of parental preparations. These include prednisone, prednisolone, dexamethasone and budesonide. Corticosteroids are frequently used to induce remission in both Crohn's disease and ulcerative colitis. These drugs have not been shown to be effective in maintenance therapy although they are associated with side effects in almost 100% of patients taking these medications for a long term (Alstead & Nelson, 2003). The foetal placenta contains the enzyme 11β-hydroxysteroid dehydrogenase type 2 (11β-HSD2), which catalyzes the metabolism of cortisol and corticosterone to inert 11-keto forms (cortisone, 11-dehydrocorticosterone). This placental enzymic barrier allows the maternal cortisol to be inactivated so that the majority of cortisol in the human fetal circulation at term is derived from the fetal adrenals (Murphy et al ,1974; Lopez-Bernal et al,1980; Beitens, et al 1973; Stewart et al, 1995). Dexamethasone is not inactivated by 11β-hydroxysteroid dehydrogenase hence it passes the placenta freely and thus should be avoided during conception.

Corticosteroids have been implicated in oral cleft palate when they are used in the first trimester (Bush et al, 2004; Carmichael, et al 1999; Pradat et al, 2003).

A recent nationwide health registry data study from Denmark between 1996 and 2008, looking at pregnant women receiving corticosteroids, with 832,637 live births was recently published in the Canadian Medical Association journal (CMAJ). This study did not demonstrate that pregnant women receiving corticosteroids during the first trimester were any more likely to have offspring with a cleft lip with or without cleft palate than mothers who did not take the drug (Anders et al, 2011). A prospective study was published by Mogadam reporting on the use of corticosteroids during pregnancy which was used with or without Sulfasalazine. In that study they followed the outcome in two hundred eighty-seven pregnancies on treatment and compared to 244 pregnant IBD on no treatment. There was no increased incidence of prematurity, spontaneous abortion, stillbirth, or developmental defects (Mogadam et al,1981).

Pregnant women with active disease during conception can be safely treated with corticosteroids to induce remission. Although gestational diabetes and hypertension may be precipitated, the benefit outweighs the risk.

18. Budesonide

Budesonide is an enteric coated locally acting glucocorticoid preparation which has a pH- and time-dependent coating that enables its release into the ileum and ascending colon. It is used for the treatment of mild to moderate Crohn's disease with limited systemic bioavailability due to extensive first-pass hepatic metabolism. Budesonide has been shown to be effective for induction of remission in Crohn's disease.

In a limited study using 8 patients with Crohn’s disease at a dose of 6-9 mg daily there was no evidence of foetal abnormality (Beaulieu, et al 2009).

Breast feeding: Corticosteroids

Corticosteroids are secreted in small amounts into breast milk. The maternal: foetal ratio of steroid serum concentrations depends on which steroid the patient is taking. The foetal levels are 10%-12% of that in maternal serum. It has been suggested that infants should be monitored for adrenal suppression if the mothers are taking a more than a daily dose of 40 mg. While breastfeeding is safe with steroid use, mothers are encouraged to defer breastfeeding until 4 h after taking oral dosing of steroids to reduce neonatal exposure. However, systemic effects in the infant are unlikely with doses of up to 40mg of prednisolone or equivalent (Ferguson et al, 2008; Blanford et al, 1977).

Budesonides and Breast feeding

Limited studies are available on budesonide in breast feeding. In a study in asthmatic nursing women on maintenance treatment with inhaled budesonide (200 or 400 microg twice daily) showed negligible systemic exposure to budesonide in breast-fed infants (Fält et al, 2007).

19. Immunobiologic therapy, pregnancy and lactation

Anti-TNF agents fall within the US FDA category B concerning foetal risk, because animal reproduction studies have failed to demonstrate a risk to the foetus but adequate and well-controlled studies of pregnant women have not been conducted.

Biological therapies targeting TNF-α have significantly improved the management of IBD refractory to conventional therapies, in steroids sparing, improvement in perianal disease and maintaining remission. It has been shown to result in mucosal healing. Data regarding their safety are scarce for the other compounds. No increased risks associated with pregnancy have been observed for Infliximab or Adalumimab, but caution in pregnancy and during breast-feeding is currently advocated.

The role of TNF-alpha for embryonic implantation, foetal development and labour has been well studied. TNF-alpha controls arachadonic acid metabolism production through the cyclooxygenase pathway. Subsequently, TNF-alpha plays an important role in implantation and vascular permeability. TNF-alpha production is low in the first gestational trimester, but increases thereafter, reaching a peak at the onset of labour (Daher et al, 1999). These high levels have been shown to play an important role in the induction of the labour process and in delivery via augmenting uterine contractions. It has been reported that blastocyst implantation during early pregnancy may be promoted by TNF-alpha but at the same time it may mediate recurrent spontaneous abortion at a later stage of gestation. The serum levels of TNF-α and those of soluble TNFR-1 were found to be higher in women who had spontaneous early abortions (Yu et al,2005).

Anti-TNF agents include infliximab, a chimeric monoclonal IgG1 anti-TNF antibody, adalimumab, a human monoclonal IgG1 anti-TNF antibody, and etanercept, a soluble TNF receptor fusion protein linked to the Fc portion of a human IgG1. IgG1 antibody do not cross the placenta in the first trimester but cross the placenta by the late second trimester and the third trimester. Certolizumab another anti TNFα antibody, is a PEGylated Fab' fragment of humanized anti TNF alpha monoclonal antibody rather than a whole human immunoglobulin G1 (IgG1) antibody (Stephens 2006). A recent abstract on Certolizumab, reported on placental transfer. The report included 10 IBD women, with one twin delivery. There was a low level on antibodies of Certolizumab confirming the animal reports (Wolf et al, 2010; Stephens et al, 2006).

To date, there have been few comprehensive studies in IBD patients who had conceived while receiving immunobiologic therapy. Most of the publications and reports have been retrospective reviews. Roux et al (2007) reported their experience with three rheumatoid arthritis patients who became pregnant while undergoing anti-TNF-alpha therapy. Although one patient terminated her pregnancy despite no known pregnancy or foetal complications, the other two patients delivered healthy infants. Another study from the infliximab study database showed that 96 patients exposed to infliximab during pregnancy had outcomes no different than in the general population (Katz et al, 2004). In the first reported study of intentional infliximab administration for CD during pregnancy, Mahadevan et al (2005) showed, in acutely ill patients with Crohn's disease, excellent outcomes. All 10 pregnancies ended in live births and there were no congenital malformations, intrauterine growth retardation or small-for-gestational-age infants. In those ten patients, three of the infants were born prematurely and one had low birth weight (LBW).

There has not been adequate and well-controlled studies conducted in pregnant or lactating women. It has been increasingly used in autoimmune diseases such as rheumatoid arthritis, psoriatic arthritis (PsA), juvenile idiopathic arthritis (JIA) ankylosing spondylitis (AS) and in inflammatory bowel disease.

Most of the literature regarding anti-TNF-alpha therapy in pregnancy comes from studies in rheumatoid arthritis. The data have been obtained from retrospective studies, registry studies and case reports. Based on all publications no firm conclusions can be made regarding the long term safety of biologics during pregnancy. Mahadevan et al in the London position statement at the World Congress of Gastroenterogy consensus guideline (2010) considers infliximab to have a low risk and compatible with the use during conception in at least first and second trimester.

Recently, the mother risk program in Canada published a review of 300 pregnancies in women who received anti TNF alpha during conception. The review suggested that infliximab carries low foetal risk and is compatible with use during conception and the first two trimesters of pregnancy (Djokanovic et al, 2011).

A recent observational study by the Leuven, group in Belgium, was published. They assessed pregnancy outcomes in 212 women with IBD. Pregnancy outcome was assessed in 42 pregnancies in women who received anti-TNF treatment (35 IFX, 7 ADA) and were compared with that in 23 pregnancies prior to IBD diagnosis, 78 pregnancies before start of IFX, 53 pregnancies with indirect exposure to IFX, and 56 matched pregnancies in healthy women. Their conclusion was that direct exposure to anti-TNF treatment during pregnancy was not related to a higher incidence of adverse outcomes than IBD overall (Schnitzler et al, 2011).

Vasiliauskas monitored a pregnant patient who continued on standard-dose infliximab therapy during her pregnancy and lactation. The measurement of serum infliximab in the breastfed infant was 39.5 µg/mL or less and the drug was not detected in the breast milk. Importantly, despite continued breast-feeding and adherence to therapy, the levels declined in the infant over the subsequent six months. They concluded that infliximab levels were likely due to placental transfer and less likely the result of breastfeeding (Vasiliauskas et al, 2006). The blood levels in the newborn were within the therapeutic range. The authors recommended that such therapy be avoided after 30 weeks gestation when possible. As of the date of this publication, no increased risk of embryotoxicity, teratogenicity or adverse pregnancy outcome has been reported in patients treated with anti-TNF therapy (Skomsvoll et al, 2007).

The majority of studies regarding breast feeding while receiving anti-TNF therapy has not demonstrated any adverse outcomes. The data, however, appear limited. In a case report publication in which serial sampling of breast milk over a one-month time period failed to detect any concentrations of infliximab. Furthermore, at a follow-up of just over two years, no developmental abnormalities were noted in the child. Ostensen et al (2004) showed that etanercept, a soluble TNF-alpha receptor fusion protein, was detected in breast milk with maximal doses noted the day following the injection. The effect on the developing immune system in the infant - if indeed the levels in breast milk are significant - remains to be seen. The European Panel on the Appropriateness of Crohn's Disease Therapy (EPACT), an international multidisciplinary panel, met recently to develop safety criteria for clinical decision-making related to the use of drugs in pregnant and nursing women with IBD. The panel was cautious about the safety of infliximab, based primarily on label (Mottet et al, 2007) recommendations, and emphasized the need for further large, randomized controlled trials.

At the present time the risk benefit should be always assessed. Pregnant women who are receiving biologics and are in remission should continue the treatment. In the case of Infliximab and Adalumimab it should be held at 32 weeks and restarted after delivery. Breast feeding is compatible with Infliximab treatment. No data so far on breast feeding with Adalumimab although the author does not discourage breast feeding in these women.

20. Bisphosphonates (FDA Class C)

Careful consideration should be undertaken in women of child bearing age who require biphosphonates. As with most drugs used during conception, the risk and benefits of biphosphonates should be carefully weighed in these women.

There are several biphosphonates currently approved for use in osteoporosis including: alendronate (Fosamax ®), etidronate (Didrocal ®), risedronate (Actonel ®) and zoledronic acid (Aclasta®).

Biphosphonates are used to treat and to prevent corticosteroids induced osteoporosis. Approximately 50% of the Biphosphonates binds to the skeleton and the rest is excreted non-metabolized by the kidneys (Papapoulos, 2008). The long-term effects of alendronate, one of the Biphosphonates, on human bone development are unknown and the half-life of alendronate is greater than 10 years. The concern with long-term biphosphonates treatment is that the drug is slowly released from maternal bone and may result in continuous low-level exposure to the foetus during gestation. The released bisphosphonate can cross the placenta and incorporate into foetal bone. In animal studies where biphosphonates were given to pregnant rats, the drug appears to cross the placenta, accumulate in the foetal skeleton, decrease foetal weight, decrease bone growth, and lead to protracted deliveries and neonatal deaths (Patlas et al, 1999).

21. Summary and conclusion

Managing a pregnant woman with inflammatory bowel disease is challenging but often rewarding. This management should include the patient and her partner, in association with the family physician, the gastroenterologist and the obstetrician. Most women with IBD, who are in remission, are as likely as women without IBD to conceive and have a normal pregnancy. These patients should be encouraged to continue the medications throughout the pregnancy and while breast feeding.

Women with ulcerative colitis who have undergone ileal pouch-anal anastomosis operation are less likely to conceive. Women with active ulcerative colitis who require colectomy, and are planning to have a family, should reconsider having a pouch surgery. They should have an ileostomy and postpone a pouch until after conceiving. With the exception of Methotrexate, most drugs used in IBD are relatively safe to administer in pregnancy and can be used while breast feeding.

The newer biologic drugs appear to be quite effective and safe during pregnancy and with breastfeeding. Since these drugs cross the placenta mostly in the third trimester they should not be administered after 32 week of gestation.

Despite all our knowledge and availability of literature the risk benefit should be always weighed. The decision of the mother should always be respected, should she decide on not taking the medications.

Take home messages:

1. Patient education is of primary importance in a successful outcome in IBD women during pregnancy.
2. IBD patients in remission have the same chance in getting pregnant as non IBD patients.
3. Pregnant IBD patients outcomes are better if patients are maintained in remission.
4. Ileoanal pouch patients have a lower rate of conception.
5. Biologics drugs appear to be safe during pregnancy and in lactation.
6. Biologic drugs, if possible, should be withheld at 32 weeks gestation
7. Breast feeding should be encouraged in women receiving most of IBD drugs.

22. References

Alstead EM. Inflammatory bowel disease in pregnancy. Postgrad Med J. 2002; 78:23–26.

Alstead EM, Nelson-Piercy C. Inflammatory bowel disease in pregnancy. Gut. 2161.

Anders Hviid, Ditte Mølgaard-Nielsen. Corticosteroid use during pregnancy and risk of oro facial clefts. CMAJ, 2011,April11.

Andres PG, Friedman LS. Epidemiology and the natural course of inflammatory bowel disease. Gastroenterol. Clin. North Am. 1999;28(2):255–281, vii.

Arkuran C, McComb P. Crohn's disease and tubal infertility: the effect of adhesion formation. Clin. Exp. Obstet. Gynecol. 2000;27(1):12–13 .

Baiocco PJ, Korelitz BI. The influence of inflammatory bowel disease and its treatment on pregnancy and fetal outcome. J. Clin Gastroenterol 1984; 6: 211–16.

Beaulieu DB, Ananthakrishnan AN, Issa M, Rosenbaum L, Skaros S, Newcomer JR, Kuhlmann RS, Otterson MF, Emmons J, Knox J, Binion DG. / Budesonide induction and maintenance therapy for Crohn's disease during pregnancy. Inflamm Bowel Dis. 2009 Jan; 15(1):25-8.

Beitens, IZ, Bayard, F, Ances, IG, Kowarski, A, Migeon, CJ: The metabolic clearance rate, blood production, interconversion and transplacental passage of cortisol and cortisone in pregnancy near term. Pediatr Res 1973 7:509–519.

Bertoli A ,Pedersen N, Duricova D , et al: Pregnancy outcome in inflammatory bowel disease:prospective European case control ECCO-EpiCom study,2003-2006. Aliment Pharmacol Ther.2011:1365 (on-line publication August 2011).

Blanford AT, Murphy BE. In vitro metabolism of prednisolone, dexamethasone, betamethasone, and cortisol by the human placenta. Am J Obstet Gynecol. 1977; 127:264–267.

Brandt LJ, Estabrook SG, Reinus JF. Results of a survey to evaluate whether vaginal delivery and episiotomy lead to perineal involvement in women with Crohn's disease. Am J Gastroenterol. 1995;90:1918–1922.

Bush MC, Patel S, Lapinski RH, Stone JL. Perinatal outcomes in inflammatory bowel disease. J Matern Fetal Neonatal Med. 2004; 15:237–41.

Cantu JM, Garcia-Cruz D. Midline facial defect as a teratogenic effect of metronidazole. Birth Defects 1982; 18:85.

Caprilli R, Gassul MA, Escher JC, Moser G, et al. European evidence based consensus on the diagnosis and management of Crohn's disease: special situation. Gut 2006; 55 (suppl 1):i36-i58.

Carmichael SL, Shaw GM. Maternal corticosteroid use and risk of selected congenital anomalies. Am. J. Med. Genet. 1999; 86(3): 242–244

Carter MJ, Lobo AJ, Travis SPL., IBD Section, British Society of Gastroenterology Guidelines for the management of inflammatory bowel disease in adults. Gut. 2004; 53:V1–16.

Caruso A, De Carolis S, Sergio Ferrazzani, Carmen Trivellini, Carmen Mastromarino, Mauro Pittiruti·· Pregnancy Outcome and Total Parenteral Nutrition in Malnourished Pregnant Women Fetal Diagn Ther 1998; 13:136-140

Chakrabarty, G *, A Poullis Gut 2011; 60:A135 doi:10.1136/gut.2011.239301.287

Chatzinoff M, Guario JM, Corson SL, et al.Sulfasalazine-induced abnormal sperm penetration assay reversed on changing to 5-aminosalicylic acid enemas .Digestive Diseases and Science.1983;33:108-110.

Christensen LA, Dahlerup JF, Nielsen MJ, et al. Azathioprine treatment during lactation. Aliment Pharmacol Ther. 2008; 28: 1209–1213

Cleary BJ, Kallen B. Early pregnancy azathioprine use and pregnancy outcomes. Birth Defects Res A Clin Mol Teratol. 2009; 85: 647–654.

Cohen RD, Stein R, Hanauer SB. Intravenous cyclosporin in ulcerative colitis: a five-year experience. Am J Gastroenterol 1999; 94:1587-1592.

Cornish J, Tan E, Singh B, Bundock H, Mortensen N, Nicholls R, Clark S, Tekkis P. Female infertility following restorative proctocolectomy. Colorectal Dis 2011;1463-1318.

Cornish J, Tan E, Teare J, et al. A meta-analysis on the influence of inflammatory bowel disease on pregnancy. Gut 2007; 56:830-837.

Davies J BJ. Prenatal alcohol and drug exposures in adoption. Pediatr Clin 2005; 52:1369-1393.

Czeizel AE, Dudas I, Paput L, Banhidy F. Prevention of Neural-Tube Defects with Periconceptional Folic Acid, Methylfolate, or Multivitamins? Ann Nutr Metab 2011; 58:263-271.

Daher S, Fonseca F, Ribeiro OG, Musatti CC, Gerbase-DeLima M. Tumor necrosis factor during pregnancy and at the onset of labor and spontaneous abortion. Eur J Obstet Gynecol Reprod Biol 1999; 83:77-79.

Dejaco C, Angelberger S, Waldhoer T, et al. Risk factors for pregnancy outcome in patients with inflammatory bowel disease (IBD) Gastroenterology. 2006; 130(Suppl 2): A-39. (Abst)

Djokanovic N, Klieger-Grossmann C, Pupco A, Koren G. Safety of infliximab use during pregnancy. Reprod Toxicol 2011; 32:93-97.

Dolovich LR, Addis A, Vaillancourt JMR, Power JD, Koren G, EinarsonTR. Benzodiazepine use in pregnancy and major malformations or oral cleft: meta-analysis of cohort and case-controlled studies. BMJ 1998; 317:839-43.

Dominitz JA, Young JC, Boyko EJ. Outcomes of infants born to mothers with inflammatory bowel disease: a population-based cohort study. Am J Gastroenterol. 2002; 97:641–648

Falt A, Bengtsson T, Kennedy BM, Gyllenberg A, et al.Exposure of infants to budesonide through breast milk of asthmatic mothers.J Allergy Clinical Immunol 2007;120(4):798-802.

FDA 2010 Safety Labelling Changes Approved By FDA Center for Drug Evaluation and Research (CDER) - May 2010.

Ferguson BC, Mahsud-Dornan S,and Patterson RN Inflammatory bowel disease in pregnancy. BMJ. 2008; 337(7662): 170–173.

Fonager K, Sorensen HT, Olsen J, Dahlerup JF, Rasmussen SN. Pregnancy outcome for women with Crohn's disease: a follow-up study based on linkage between national registries. Am. J. Gastroenterol.1998; 93(12),:2426–2430 .

Francella A, Dyan A , Bodian C et al. Th e safety of 6-mercaptopurine for childbearing patients with inflammatory bowel disease: a retrospective cohort study . Gastroenterology 2003; 124 : 9 – 17 .

Gardiner SJ, Gearry RB, Roberts RL, et al. Exposure to thiopurine drugs through breast milk is low based on metabolite concentrations in mother-infant pairs. Br J Clin Pharmacol. 2006; 62: 453–456.

Gaudier FL, Santiago-Delpin E, Riveral J, et al.Pregnancy after renal transplantation.Surg Gynecol Obstet.1988;167(6):533-43.

Gin T. Propofol during pregnancy. Acta Anaesthesiol Sin 1994; 32:127-132.

Gisbert JP, Linares PM, McNicholl AG, et al. Meta-analysis: the efficacy of azathioprine and mercaptopurine in ulcerative colitis. AlimentPharmacol Ther. 2009; 30:126–137.

Golby M. Fertility after renal transplantation. Transplantation. 1970;10:201–207

Goldstein LH, Dolinsky G, Greenberg R, et al. Pregnancy outcome of women exposed to azathioprine during pregnancy. Birth Defects Res A Clin Mol Teratol 2007; 79: 696–701.

Hernández-Díaz S, Mitchell AA, Kelley KE, Calafat AM, Hauser R. Medications as a potential source of exposure to phthalates in the U.S. population. Environ Health Perspect 2009; 117:185-189.

Ilnyckyji A, Blanchard JF, Rawsthorne P, Bernstein CN. Perianal Crohn's disease and pregnancy: role of the mode of delivery. Am J Gastroenterol 1999; 94:3274-3278.

Janneke van der Woude C , Sanja Kolacek Iris Dotan et al. European evidenced-based consensus on reproductionin inflammatory bowel disease.Journal of Crohn's and Colitis 2010;4:493–510

Jarnerot G, Fertility, sterility and pregnancy in chronic inflammatory bowel disease. Scand J Gastroenterol 1982; 17:1-4.

Kammerer WS.Non-obstetric surgery during pregnancy. Med Clin North am. 1979; 63:1157-64

Katz JA, Antoni C, Keenan GF, Smith DE, Jacobs SJ, Lichtenstein GR. Outcome of pregnancy in women receiving infliximab for the treatment of Crohn's disease and rheumatoid arthritis. Am J Gastroenterol. 2004; 99:2385–92

Khosla R, Willoughby CP, Jewell DP.Crohn's disease and pregnancy. Gut 1984; 25:52-56

Kornfeld D, Cnattingius S, Ekbom A. Pregnancy outcomes in women with inflammatory bowel disease--a population-based cohort study. Am J Obstet Gynecol 1997; 177:942-946.

Kwan L Y ,Mahadevan U. Inflammatory Bowel Disease and Pregnancy: An Update. Expert Rev Clin Immunol. 2010; 6(4):643-657

Laegreid L, Olegard R, Wahlstrom J, Conradi N. Teratogenic effects ofbenzodiazepine use during pregnancy. J Pediatr 1989; 114:126-31.

Lakatos PL, Szamosi T and Lakatos L. Smoking in inflammatory bowel diseases: good, bad or ugly? World J JGastroenterol. 2007; 13(46):6134-9.

Langagergaard V, Pedersen L, Gislum M, Norgard B, Sorensen HT. Birth outcome in women treated with azathioprine or mercaptopurine during pregnancy: Danish nationwide cohort study. Aliment Pharmacol Ther 2007; 25: 73–81.

Lichtiger S, Present DH, Kornbluth A, et al. Cyclosporine in Severe Ulcerative Colitis Refractory to Steroid Therapy. N Engl J Med 1994; 330:1841-1845

Ligumsky M, Badaan S , Lewis H et al. Eff ects of 6-mercaptopurinetreatment on sperm production and reproductive performance: a study inmale mice . Scand J Gastroenterol 2005; 40: 444 - 9.

Lin HC, Chiu CC, Chen SF et al. Ulcerative colitis and pregnancy outcomes in an Asian population. Am. J. Gastroenterol. 2010;105(2): 387–394

Lopez-Bernal, A, Flint, APF, Anderson, ABM, Turnbull, AC: 11β-Hydroxysteroid dehydrogenase activity (E.C.1.1.1.146) in human placenta and decidua. J Steroid Biochem 1980 13:1081–1087,

Mahadevan U. Fertility and pregnancy in the patient with inflammatory bowel disease. Gut 2006;55:1198–1206.

Mahadevan U, Corley D. Aminosalicylates (ASA) use during pregnancy is not associated with increased adverse events or congenital malformations (CM) in women with inflammatory bowel disease (IBD). Gastroenterology 2006; 130(Suppl 2): A-40. (Abst)

Mahadevan U, Kane S. American gastroenterological association institute technical review on the use of gastrointestinal medications in pregnancy. Gastroenterology 2006; 131: 283–311.

Mahadevan U, Kane S, Sandborn WJ, et al. Intentional infliximab use during pregnancy for induction or maintenance of remission in Crohn's disease. Aliment Pharmacol Ther. 2005;21:733–38.

Mahadevan U, Sandborn WJ, Li DK et al. Pregnancy outcomes in women with inflammatory bowel disease: a large community-based study from Northern California. Gastroenterology2007 133(4), 1106–1112

Marri SR, Ahn C, Buchman AL. Voluntary childlessness is increased in women with inflammatory bowel disease. Inflamm.Bowel Dis 2007;13(5): 591–599

Mercer BM, Merlino AA, Milluzzi CJ, Moore JJ. Small fetal size before 20 weeks' gestation: associations with maternal tobacco use, early preterm birth, and low birthweight. Am J Obstet Gynecol 2008; 198:673.

Mogadam M, Dobbins WO, Korelitz BI, et al. Pregnancy in inflammatory bowel disease: effect of sulfasalazine and corticosteroids on fetal outcome. Gastroenterology 1981; 80: 72–6.

Moretti ME, Verjee Z, Ito S, Koren G. Breast-feeding during maternal use of azathioprine. Ann Pharmacother 2006; 40:2269-2272.Moskovitz DN, Bodian C, Chapman ML, et al. The effect on the fetus of medications used to treat pregnant inflammatory bowel-disease patients. Am J Gastroenterol 2004; 99:656-6

Mottet C, Vader JP, Felley C, et al. Appropriate management of special situations in Crohn's disease (upper gastro-intestinal; extra-intestinal manifestations; drug safety during pregnancy and breastfeeding): Results of a multidisciplinary international expert panel-EPACT II. J Crohn's Colitis 2009; 3:257-263.

Mountifield R, Bampton P, Prosser R, Muller K, Andrews JM. Fear and fertility in inflammatory bowel disease: a mismatch of perception and reality affects family planning decisions. Inflamm Bowel Dis 2009; 15:720-725.

Mountifield RE, Prosser R, Bampton P, Muller K, Andrews JM. Pregnancy and IBD treatment: this challenging interplay from a patients' perspective. J Crohn's Colitis 2010; 4:176-182.

Murphy, BEP, Clark, SJ, Donald, IR, Pinsky, M, Vedady, DL: Conversion of maternal cortisol to cortisone during placental transfer to the human fetus. Am J Obstet Gynecol 1974 118:538–541.

Nagy S, Bush MC, Berkowitz R, Fishbein TM, Gomez-Lobo V. Pregnancy outcome in liver transplant recipients. Obstet Gynecol 2003;102:121-128.

Neissner M, Volk BA. Altered Th1/Th2 cytokine profiles in the intestinal mucosa of patients with inflammatory bowel disease as assessed by quantitative reversed transcribed polymerase chain reaction (RT-PCR) Clin Exp Immunol. 1995;101:428–35.

Norgard B, Fonager K, Pedersen L, Jacobsen BA, Sorensen HT. Birth outcome in women exposed to 5-aminosalicylic acid during pregnancy: a Danish cohort study. Gut 2003;52(2): 243–247.

Norgard B, Pedersen L, Christensen LA, Sorensen HT. Therapeutic drug use in women with Crohn's disease and birth outcomes: a Danish nationwide cohort study. Am J Gastroenterol 2007; 102: 1406–13.

Oresland T, Palmblad S, Ellstrom M et al. Gynaecological and sexual function related to anatomical changes in the female pelvis after restorative proctocolectomy. Int. J. Colorectal Dis. 1994;9(2), 77–81.

Orholm M, Binder V, Sørensen TI, Rasmussen LP, Kyvik KO. Concordance of inflammatory bowel disease among Danish twins. Results of a nationwide study. Scand J Gastroenterol. 2000;35:1075–81.

Ornoy A, Arnon J, Shechtman S, Moerman L, Lukashova I. Is benzodiazepine use during pregnancy really teratogenic? ReprodToxicol 1998;12:511-5.

Osei EK, Faulkner K.Fetal doses from radiological examinations. Br J Radiol. 1999 Aug;72(860):773-80.

Ostensen M, Eigenmann GO. Etanercept in breast milk. J Rheumatol 2004;31:1017-1018.

Paediatric Formulary Committee. BNF for Children 2010. London: BMJ Publishing Group, RPS Publishing, and RCPCH Publications; 2010

Penn I, Makowski E, Droegemueller W, Halgrimson CG, Starzl TE. Parenthood in renal homograft recipients. JAMA. 1971; 216:1755–1761.

Pradat P, Robert-Gnansia E, Di Tanna GL, et al. First trimester exposure to corticosteroids and oral clefts. Birth Defects Res A Clin Mol Teratol 2003; 67:968-970.

Present DH. Pregnancy and inflammatory bowel disease. In: BaylessTM, HanauerSB, eds. Advanced Therapy of Inflammatory Bowel Disease. Hamilton: B.C. Decker Inc., 2001: 613–18.

Qureshi WA, Rajan E, Adler DG et al. ASGE guideline: guidelines for endoscopy in pregnant and lactating women. Gastrointest. Endosc. 2005; 61(3): 357–362.

Raatikainen K, Mustonen J, Pajala_M, Heikkinen M & Heinonen S. The effects of pre- and post-pregnancy inflammatory bowel disease diagnosis on birth outcomes. Aliment Pharmacol Ther 2011; 33: 333–339

Kornfeld D, Cnattingius S, Ekbom A. Pregnancy outcomes in women with inflammatory bowel disease--a population-based cohort study. Am J Obstet Gynecol 1997; 177:942-946.

Rahimi R, Nikfar S, Rezaie A, Abdollahi M. Pregnancy outcome in women with inflammatory bowel disease following exposure to 5-aminosalicylic acid drugs: a meta-analysis. Reprod Toxicol 2008; 25:271-5.

Rajapakse RO, Korelitz BI , Zlatanic J et al. Outcome of pregnancies whenfathers are treated with 6-mercaptopurine for infl ammatory bowel disease .Am J Gastroenterol 2000 ; 95 : 684–8

Rosenkrantz JG, Githens JH, Cox SM, Kellum DL. Azathioprine (Imuran) and pregnancy. Am J Obstet Gynecol 1967; 97:387–394.

Roux CH, Brocq O, Breuil V, Albert C, Euller-Ziegler L. Pregnancy in rheumatology patients exposed to anti-tumour necrosis factor (TNF)-alpha therapy. Rheumatology (Oxford) 2007; 46:695-698.

Sau A, Clarke S, Bass J, Kaiser A, Marinaki A, Nelson-Piercy C. Azathioprine and breastfeeding: is it safe? BJOG 2007; 114:498-501.

Shah NR ,Bracken MB.A systemic review and meta-analysis of prospective studies on the association betwe en cigarette smoking and preterm delivery.Am J Obtstet Gynecol 2000 ;182:465-72.

Schnitzler F, Fidder H, Ferrante M, et al. Outcome of pregnancy in women with inflammatory bowel disease treated with antitumor necrosis factor therapy. Inflamm Bowel Dis 2011; 17:1846-1854.

Simpson PW, Melmed GY, Dubinksy M. The impact of medical therapy for inflammatory bowel disease on pregnancy outcome. Am J Gastroenterol. 2008; 103: 805–806

Skomsvoll JF, Wallenius M, Koksvik HS, et al. Drug insight: Anti-tumor necrosis factor therapy for inflammatory arthropathies during reproduction, pregnancy and lactation. Nat Clin Pract Rheumatol 2007; 3:156-164.

Steinlauf AF, Present DH. Medical management of the pregnant patient with inflammatory bowel disease. Gastroenterol Clin North Am. 2004; 33:361–85.

Stephens P, Nesbitt A, Foulkes R. Placental transfer of the anti-TNF antibody TN3 in rats: comparison of Immunoglobulin G1 and pegylated Fab versions. Gut 2006; 55:A8.Stewart, PM, Rogerson, FM, Mason, JI: Type 2, 11β-hydroxysteroid dehydrogenase messenger RNA and activity in human placenta and fetal membranes: its relationship to birth weight and putative role in fetal steroidogenesis. J Clin Endocrinol Metab 1995; 80:885–890,

Subhani JM, Hamiliton MI. Review article: The management of inflammatory bowel disease during pregnancy. Aliment Pharmacol Ther. 1998; 12:1039–1053.

Teahon K,Pearson M,Levi AJ,Bjarnson I.Elemental diet in the management of Crohn's disease during pregnancy.Gut.1991;32(9):1079-1081

Truel C, Lopez-San Roman A,Bermejo F, Taxonera C et al. Outcomes of pregnancies fathered by inflammatory bowel disease patients exposed to thiopurine. Am J Gastroenterol.2010; 105(9):2003-8.

Thompson N, Driscoll R, Pounder RE, et al. Genetics versus environment in inflammatory bowel disease. Br Med J 1996; 312: 95–6.

Tysk C, Lindberg E, Järnerot G, Flodérus-Myrhed B. Ulcerative colitis and Crohn's disease in an unselected population of monozygotic and dizygotic twins. A study of heritability and the influence of smoking. Gut. 1988; 29:990–6.

Valentin J, Editor, Annals of the ICRP, Publication 84: Pregnancy and Medical Radiation, International Commission on Radiological Protection, Volume 30, No. 1. Tarrytown, New York: Pergamon, Elsevier Science, Inc., 2000.

Van Assche G, Dignass A, Reinisch W, et al. The second European evidence based Consensus on the diagnosis and management of Crohn's disease: special situations. J Crohns Colitis 2010; 4: 63–101.

van der Woude CJ, Kolacek S, Dotan I, Oresland T, Vermeire S, Munkholm P, Mahadevan U, Mackillop L, Dignass A; European Crohn's Colitis Organisation (ECCO). European evidenced-based consensus on reproduction in inflammatory bowel disease. J Crohns Colitis. 2010 Nov;4(5):493-510

Van Domselaar M, Algaba A, Estellés J, López-Serrano P, Linares PM, Muriel A. Outcomes of pregnancies fathered by inflammatory bowel disease patients exposed to thiopurines. Am J Gastroenterol. 2010 Sep; 105(9):2003-8

Vasiliauskas EA, Church JA, Silverman N, Barry M, Targan SR, Dubinsky MC. Case report: evidence for transplacental transfer of maternally administered infliximab to the newborn. Clin Gastroenterol Hepatol 2006; 4:1255-1258.

Waljee J, Morris AM, Higgins PD. Threefold increased risk of infertility: a meta-analysis of infertility after ileal pouch anal anastomosis in ulcerative colitis. Gut 55(11), 1575–1580 (2006).

Wolf D MU. Certolizumab Pegol Use in Pregnancy: Low Levels Detected in Cord Blood. Arthritis Rheum 2010; 62:718.

Yang H, McElree C, Roth MP, Shanahan F, Targan SR, Rotter JI. Familial empirical risks for inflammatory bowel disease: Differences between Jews and non-Jews. Gut. 1993;34:517–24.

Yu XW, Li X, Ren YH, Li XC. Tumour necrosis factor-alpha receptor 1 polymorphisms and serum soluble TNFR1 in early spontaneous miscarriage. Cell Biol Int 2007;31:1396-1399.

Zimm S, Collins JM, Riccardi R, O'Neill D, Narang PK, Chabner B, Poplack DG. Variable bioavailability of oral mercaptopurine.Is maintenance chemotherapy in acute lymphoblastic leukemia being optimally delivered? N Engl J Med. 1983; 308:1005–1009.

Zlatanic J, Korelitz BI, Rajapakse R, et al. Complications of pregnancy and child development after cessation of treatment with 6-mercaptopurine for inflammatory bowel disease. J Clin Gastroenterol. 2003; 36: 303–309.

11

Bone Morphogenetic Proteins and Signaling Pathway in Inflammatory Bowel Disease

Ivana Maric[1], Tamara Turk Wensveen[2], Ivana Smoljan[3], Zeljka Crncevic Orlic[2] and Dragica Bobinac[1]
[1]*Department of Anatomy, Faculty of Medicine, University of Rijeka*
[2]*Department of Internal Medicine, Clinical Hospital Rijeka*
[3]*Psychiatric Hospital Rab*
Croatia

1. Introduction

Inflammatory bowel disease (IBD) is a chronic, relapsing disease of the gastrointestinal (GI) tract of uncertain origin. Its two main phenotypes are Crohn's disease (CD) and ulcerative colitis (UC). CD affects any part of the GI tract and is characterized by transmural inflammation, whereas UC is confined to the colon and affects only the mucosal layer. IBD is thought to occur in genetically predisposed individuals that develop an abnormal immune response to enteric bacteria in the intestinal mucosa (Podolsky, 2002; Xavier RJ & Podolsky, 2007). Disease occurs as a result of complex and dynamic interactions between immune and non-immune cells as well as the cross-talk between intestinal epithelium and mesenchyme (Danese, 2011; MacDonald et al., 2011; Strober & Fuss, 2011). Therefore, factors that are able to influence both interactions may be very important for the pathogenesis and treatment of IBD.

Bone morphogenetic proteins (BMPs) are a large group of structurally related proteins that belong to the transforming growth factor-β (TGF-β) superfamily. Along with their primarily osteogenic function their importance in development, proliferation and morphogenesis of a variety of cells and tissues has been shown (Hogan, 1996; Vukicevic et al., 1989; 1995; Wozney et al., 1988). In addition, association of BMPs with healing processes of different non-skeletal tissues and organs was also described (Lories et al., 2005; Martinovic et al., 2002; Nguyen et al., 2008; Simic & Vukicevic, 2004; Turk et al., 2009; Vukicevic et al., 1996; Vukicevic & Grgurevic, 2009). Due to their wide-range of effects, they are commonly named "body morphogenetic proteins" (Reddi, 2005). Perturbations in BMP expression and BMP signaling pathway have been associated with the pathological conditions linked to several human diseases such as inflammatory bowel disease (IBD) (Allaire et al., 2011; Burke et al., 2007; Krishnan et al., 2011).

In this chapter we will discuss the importance of BMPs in gut development and hereditary diseases as well as their influence on cellular and molecular events that occur in IBD and fibrogenesis, the most common complication of IBD. Furthermore, we will address the therapeutical potential of BMPs, especially BMP7 in treatment of IBD. Finally, we will explore the possibility of BMP pathway components as putative biomarkers of gut tumor development and progression.

2. Bone morphogenetic proteins

BMPs comprise a group of very important signaling molecules, which is demonstrated by the the fact that several of these proteins, as well as their intracellular signaling components have been conserved in *Drosophila* and *Caenorhabditis elegans*. They are originally isolated from bone and major contribution to their isolation and characterization was made by Sampath and Reddi (Sampath & Reddi, 1981; Sampath et al., 1987). BMPs are a large family within the transforming growth factor β (TGFβ) superfamily. Twenty BMP family members have been isolated and characterized so far. BMPs are divided into 4 groups based on their structure and function: the BMP2/4 group consists of BMP2, BMP4 and Decapentaplegic (dpp) in Drosophila, the OP-1 group is made up of BMP5, BMP6, BMP7 or osteogenic protein (OP1), BMP8 (OP2) and 60A in Drosophila, the GDF5 group includes the growth-differentiation factor-5 (GDF5) or cartilage-derived morphogenetic protein-1 (CDMP1), GDF6 (CDMP2 or BMP13) and GDF7 (BMP12), and finally the forth group includes BMP9 and BMP10 (Miyazono, 2000; Miyazono et al., 2010). Grouping of BMPs is continually subject to changes due to studies which reveal their structure.

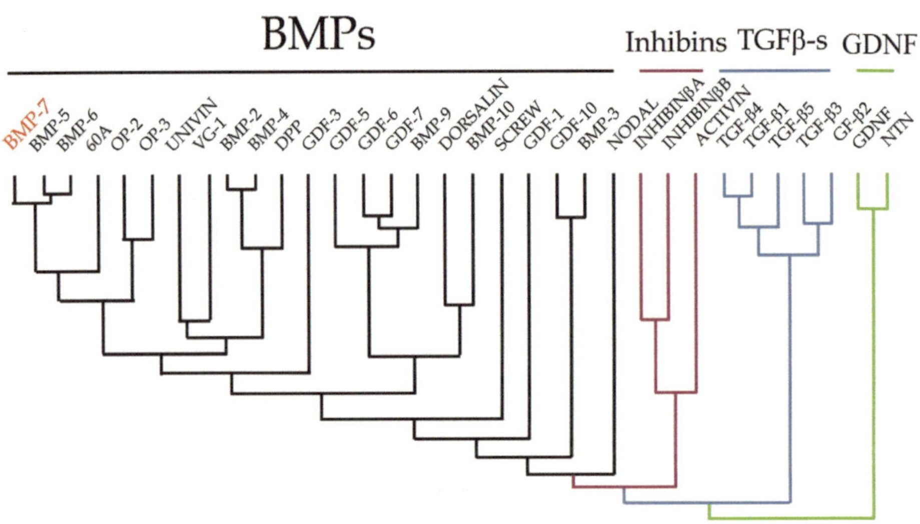

Fig. 1. TGFβ superfamily (according to Celeste et al., 1990).

BMPs are 30-38 kDa dimeric molecules. Their structure is very important for biological activity in vivo. They are synthesized as large precursor proteins in the cytoplasm that are proteolytically processed to yield mature proteins (Kingsley, 1994). Mature BMP molecules are characterized by the formation of a cysteine knot with the seven conserved cysteine domains. Active form of the molecule is dimeric as a homodimer or heterodimer (Rueger, 2002).

BMPs transduce their signals by binding to two different transmembrane serine/threonine kinase receptors, type I (BMPRI) and type II (BMPRII). Three type I and three type II receptors are identified for BMP ligand binding (Fig. 2). Type I receptors include activin receptor type IA (ActRIA or ALK2) and BMP receptors type IA and IB (BRIA or ALK3; BRIB or ALK6), while type II receptors are BMP receptor type II (BRII), activin receptor type IIA and IIB (ActRIIA and ActRIIB) (Miyazono et al., 2005, Sieber et al., 2009). Receptors form heteromeric complexes and activate downstream signaling molecules through Smad and non-Smad signaling pathway (Fig. 3) (Korchynskyi & ten Dijke, 2002; Massague et al., 2005; Miyazono et al., 2005). Both receptors are required to activate the signaling pathway. By BMP ligand binding, type II receptor phosphorylates the type I receptor which propagates the signal (Massague et al., 2005, Wrana et al., 1994).

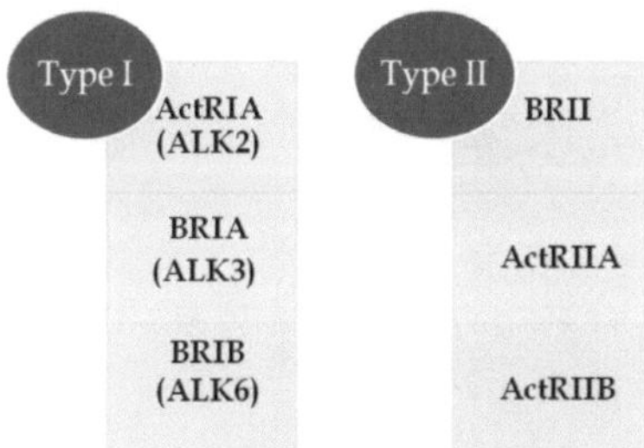

(a) BMP-receptors

Smads		
R-Smads	Co-Smad	I-Smads
Smad 1/5/8 Smad2/3	Smad4	Smad6 Smad7

(b) BR-Smad and AR-Smad proteins

Fig. 2. Components of TGFβ/BMP signaling pathway

The intracellular mediators of BMP signaling transduction are Smad transcription factors. Smad is named after human Sma1 assessment and its identification with similar genes found in *Drosophila* (Drosophile mothers against dpp - Mad) and *Caenorhabditis elegans* (Sma) (Liu et al., 1996). Three subclasses of Smad proteins have been described based on their structure and function: receptor regulated Smads (R-Smads), common mediator Smad (co-Smad), and inhibitory Smads (I-Smads) (Fig. 2). R-Smads are further subdivided into BR-Smads referred to as BMP signaling (Smad1/5/8) and AR-Smads referred to as activin/TGFβ signaling (Smad2/3). They are phyosphorylated by the type I receptors, interact with co-Smad (Smad4) and translocate into the nucleus initiating transcription of BMP response genes (Kawabata et al., 1998; Miyazono et al., 2010). Inhibitory Smads (I-Smad6/7) compete with R-Smads for the activated type I receptor binding site. Smad7 inhibits both activin/TGFβ and BMP signaling pathway while Smad6 preferentially inhibits BMP signaling (Hanyu et al., 2001).

BMP signaling is controlled also by soluble BMP antagonists. They exert their function by direct binding of BMPs and prevent functional receptor/ligand interaction (Lein et al., 2002; Piccolo et al., 1996; Yanagita, 2005; Zimmerman et al., 1995). Several structurally distinct classes of inhibitory BMP binding proteins have been described in vertebrates: twisted gastrulation (TSG), chordin and noggin and the DAN-family of inhibitors. The DAN family includes a large number of members such as DAN, cerebrus, protein related to DAN and cerebrus (PRDC), gremlin, Cer1, USAG-1 and sclerostin (Bouwmeester et al., 1996; Hsu et al., 1998; Stanley et al., 1998). They bind different BMPs with various degrees of affinity and specifity. For instance, noggin and chordin bind BMP2 and -4 with higher affinity than BMP7 whereas sclerostin binds with greater affinity BMP6 and -7 (Lein et al., 2002; Yanagita, 2005).

3. BMPs and their signaling pathway in gastrointestinal tract

3.1 BMPs and their signaling pathway in gastrointestinal tract development

BMPs and their signaling pathways are important for the normal development of the gastrointestinal tract. They are active from the earliest stage of development and revealed to be essential for the intestinal growth and morphogenesis. It has also been shown that BMP

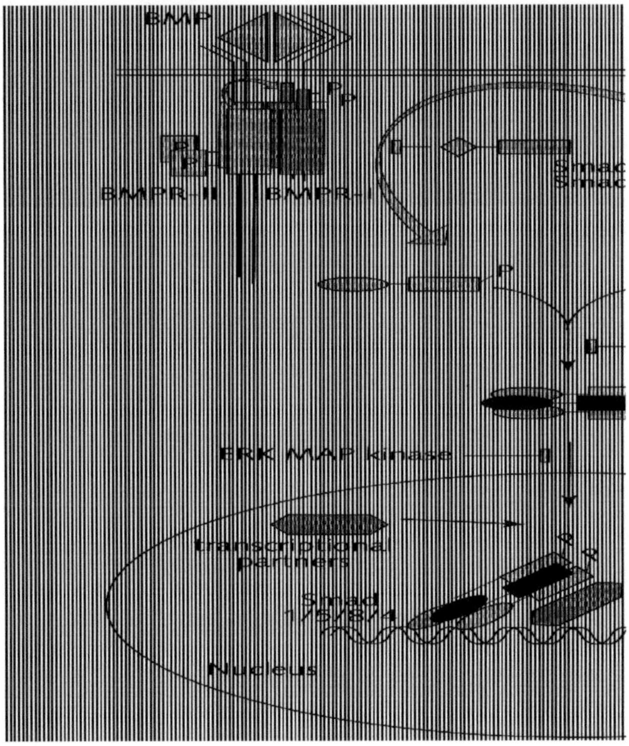

Fig. 3. BMP signaling pathway (with kind permission from Springer Science+Business Media: Bone morphogenetic proteins: from laboratory, to clinical practice, Bone morphogentic protein receptors and their nuclear effectors in bone formation, 2002, pp. 31–60, Korchynskyi, O. & ten Dijke, P. Fig. 3)

signaling is a mediator in epithelial and mesenchymal stroma interaction which is required for the intestinal growth, morphogenesis, differentiation and homeostasis (Batts et al., 2006; de Santa Barbara et al., 2005). Initial investigation of the BMP expression in the GI tract showed limited expression of individual BMP and its receptors during development. BMP6 and BMP7 were found in the developing human and mouse intestine limiting its expression to the smooth muscle cells and intestinal epithelium, respectively (Helder et al., 1995; Perr et al., 1999). Expression of BMP type I receptor (ALK6) was found in the stomach and its pyloric region (Dewulf et al.,1995). It has also been noticed that villus formation depends on high BMP2 and -4 expressions in the condensed mesenchyme underlying sites of future villus formation and may inhibit crypt formation in the overlying epithelium (Karlsson et al., 2000). In addition, BMP2 and its receptors (IB and II) were expressed in the smooth muscle progenitors of mouse embryonic GI tract with evident BMP2-induced smooth muscle differentiation and phenotype (Goldman et al., 2009).
De Santa Barbara et al. (2005) noticed that the BMP signaling pathway showed wider expression than BMP ligands in the chick developing gut. This pathway is activated in all three tissue layers of the GI tract, allowing interaction and reciprocal communication. The BMP signaling activity was found in the mesoderm during the differentiation into visceral smooth muscle and was downregulated by the completion of this process. A similar observation was made for the enteric nervous system (ENS) during its derivation of the ectoderm. BMP

signaling activity is detected also in the endoderm, future epithelium with prominent delay of BMP signaling activation in the colon. Inhibition of BMP activation by Bapx1 misexpression in the chick gut mesoderm results in diminished influence of mesoderm to endoderm-ectoderm signaling. This leads to an altered gut phenotype with marked muscular hypertrophy followed by abnormality in the ENS and epithelium. Decreased BMP signaling in mice overexpressing the BMP-antagonist noggin leads to abnormal villus morphogenesis of mouse proximal intestine. This was associated with stromal and epithelial hyperplasia, and ectopic crypt formation due to low levels of BmprIA and pSmad1/5/8 (Batts et al., 2006). A similar abnormal phenotype was found in the large intestine. These results suggest that BMP signaling restricts the site of crypt formation to the intervillus region and normally suppresses crypt formation in the villus. Human GI diseases which are accompanied by abnormal intestinal morphology, like JP or ENS disorder and even more chronic intestinal diseases associated with muscular hypertrophy such as Hirschprung's disease, could be associated with defects in the BMP signaling pathway (Amiel & Lyonnet, 2001; He et al., 2004).

3.2 BMPs and their signaling pathway in the normal gastrointestinal tract

BMPs and their signaling pathway are expressed in normal intestine and colon. It was shown that BMP2, the BMP receptors (Ia, Ib, II), phosphorylated Smad1 and Smad4 are present in mature colonocytes at the epithelial surface of normal human and mouse colon (Hardwick et al., 2004). The expression of BMP receptors was also found in colonic epithelial cell lines and BMP2 treatment in vitro resulted in inhibition of proliferation and induction of apoptosis. BMPRIA and BMP2 are highly expressed in the villus epithelium and distal/surface epithelium of the adult mouse small and large intestine with increase expression in stroma and crypt epithelium (Batts et al., 2006; Haramis et al., 2004). BMP4 is expressed in stromal cells and mesenchimal cells surrounding the crypt and glands of the small and large intestine (Haramis et al., 2004; He et al., 2004).

The expression profile of genes in the mouse intestine showed a difference between the expression of BMP signaling components in the epithelium and mesenchyme (Li et al., 2007). BMP signaling is observed in both epithelial and mesenchymal compartments, though studies to date have primarily addressed epithelial signal transduction (He et al., 2004). BMP2, BMP4, BMP5, BMP6 and BMPRII are expressed in mesenchymal compartments while only BMP7 showed epithelial enrichment. BMP7 was present in surface epithelial cells and crypts of the normal colon mucosa (Grijelmo et al., 2007). BMP receptors type I (BMPRIA or ALK3 and Acvr1 or ALK2) are present in mesenchymal compartments while the expression of BMPRIB (ALK6) was found in both compartments. Smads are expressed in both epithelial and mesenchymal compartments with slight enrichments in the mesenchyme while Smad4 expression was approximately equal in both compartments. Along the colon crypt, a different pattern of Smad4 expression was observed with high expression in the zone of terminal differentiation (Korchynskyi et al., 1999).

Apart from noggin, the BMP pathway inhibitors are located exclusively in the mesenchyme. The gene expression analysis of normal human colon tops and basal crypts revealed difference in nine hundred and sixty-nine cDNA clones from these two compartments (Kosinski et al., 2007). BMP1, BMP2, BMP5, BMP7, SMAD7 and BMPRII were highly expressed in colon tops while expression of the BMP antagonists gremlin 1, gremlin 2 and chordin-like 1 was found in basal colon crypts originating from myofibroblasts and smooth muscle cells (Fig. 4). It was also shown that activation of extracellular calcium-sensing receptor (CaSR), expressed on the epithelia of the GI tract and myofibroblasts, downregulated BMP4 and noggin expression and raises the effective concentration of BMP2 leading to increased intestine repair and barrier development (Peiris et al., 2007).

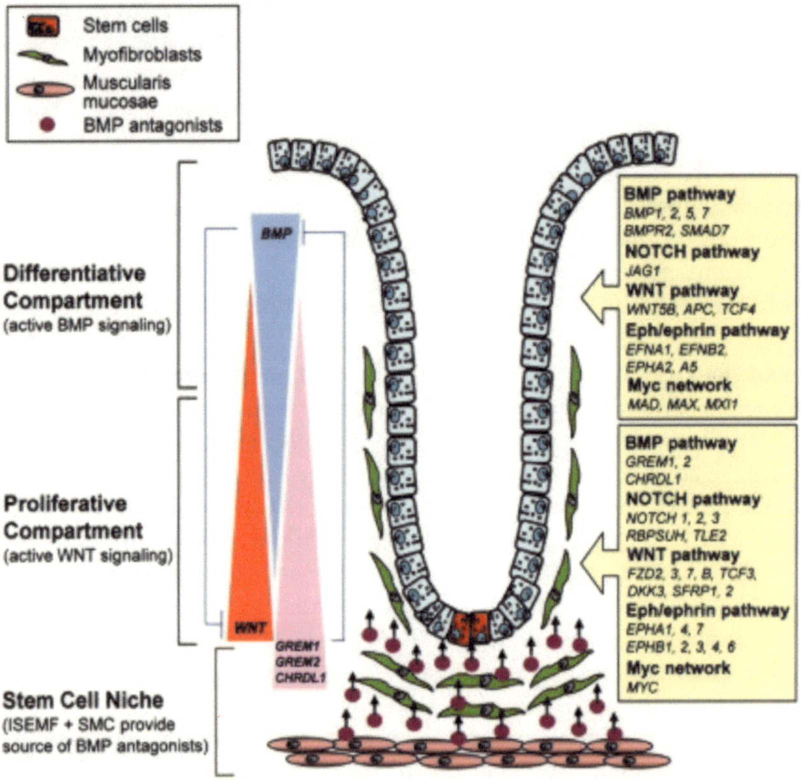

Fig. 4. BMP signaling components in compartments of the normal colon crypt (from Kosinski et al. (2007). Gene expression patterns of human colon tops and basal crypts and BMP antagonists as intestinal stem cell niche factors. *Proc Natl Acad Sci USA* 104:15418-15423. Copyright (2007) National Academy of Science, U.S.A. Used with kind permission).

3.3 BMPs and TGFβ/BMP signaling pathway in inflammatory bowel disease

Animal models of colitis are often used to aid in IBD research. They allow a detailed examination of the pathological process from acute to chronic phase, providing an insight into the immunological disturbances behind the pathogenesis of IBD (Hibi et al., 2008; Mizoguchi & Mizoguchi, 2010; Shi et al., 2011). In these animal models colitis can be induced by chemical, immunological, microbiological and physical factors (Boirivant et al., 1998; Morris et al., 1989; Okayasu et al., 1990). There are also transgenic and knock-out mouse strains that develop colitis, as well as spontaneous colitis models (Matsumoto et al., 1998; Mombaerts et al., 1993; Sadlack et al., 1993; Sundberg et al., 1994). Chemically induced colitis is one of the most utilized animal models. Dextran sulfate sodium (DSS), a heparin-like polysaccharide is often used to induce a UC-like colitis because of its simplicity and reproducibility of the inflammatory intestinal lesions. In the intestine of DSS treated mice epithelial barrier disruption with neutrophil and macrophage infiltration is observed as well as abnormal cytokine production (Dieleman et al., 1994; Kitajima et al., 1999). Trinitrobenzene sulfonic acid (TNBS) dissolved in ethanol induces a CD-like colitis, with transmural inflammation (Elson et al., 1995). Ethanol is thought to cause a transient increase in intestinal permeability, allowing TNBS to invade the musocal layers and act as a hapten to form complete antigens with tissue proteins. This provokes an intense and sustained inflammatory response and breaks T-cell tolerance to mucosal antigens (Boismenu & Chen, 2000). Genetic colitis models such as gene knockout and transgene models offer another approach in experimental IBD research. They imply genetic modifications that favor the development of colitis. IL-2 deficient mice spontaneously develop a UC-like colitis in 100% of cases, while mice lacking the IL-10 gene develop chronic colitis only in the presence of enteric bacteria (Kuhn et al., 1993; Sadlack et al., 1993). Other genetic models include T cell receptor, STAT3 and IL-17 gene manipulation (Alonzi et al., 2004; Hibi et al., 2002; Mombaerts et al., 1993).

Monteleone et al. (2001) were among the first groups to show the disturbance of the TGF-β1 signaling pathway in human IBD. They found that Smad7, an inhibitor of BMP-signaling, was overexpressed, whereas Smad3, an R-Smad of this signaling pathway, was downregulated. Due to Smad7 inhibition, lamina propria mononuclear cells (LPMC) isolated from mucosa of CD patients were not able to respond to TGF-β1 and to downregulate proinflammatory cytokine expression, especially of TNFα and IFNγ. Moreover, Smad7 inhibition by specific antisense oligonucleotides allowed LPMC to respond to TGF-β1 restoring TGF-β1 signaling by increasing pSmad3 and decreasing Smad7, and provide TGF-β1-mediated inhibition of proinflammatory cytokine production in experimentally induced colitis (Boirivant et al., 2006). Previously, it was shown that mice with targeted disruption of the TGF-β1 gene or one of its intracellular signaling components develop multifocal inflammation (Shull et al., 1992). High expression of Smad7, as seen in IBD mucosa, was a consequence of deregulated post-translational modification. Various proteins were shown to be involved, including Smurfs, the transcriptional coactivator p300, Arkadia and Jun activation domain-binding protein 1, which regulate Smad7 nuclear export and/or make the protein resistant to proteasome-mediated degradation (Monteleone et al., 2004a; 2004b; 2005). Targeted blocking of Smad7 gene expression was shown to be an effective way to attenuate the ongoing intestinal inflammation (Monteleone et al., 2008).

The R-Smad, Smad3 plays an important role in TGFβ signaling. Smad3 heterozygous mice, characterized by reduced levels of Smad3, showed accelerated healing of colonic mucosa after experimental induction of colitis with TNBS. The most prominent effects were on re-epithelization and proliferation of the intestinal epithelium, which was associated with reduced production of TGF-β1 (Tokumasa et al., 2004). Another molecule of this pathway, CTGF, which acts as a downstream effector of the TGFβ signaling pathway, was markedly increased in almost 90% of CD tissue samples. CTGF expression is mostly localized in fibroblasts of the submucosal layer while completely lacking in inflammatory cells (di Mola et al., 2004). More recently, it has been reported that deficiency of Smad5 in intestinal epithelial cells leads to an increase of cell migration and villus lengthening followed by disassembly of the apical junctional complex (Allaire et al., 2011). This intestinal epithelial impairment makes $Smad5^{\Delta IEC}$ mice more susceptible to DSS colitis development and reduced healing. Decreased expression of the BR-Smad, Smad5 was also found in intestinal samples from IBD patients, which emphasizes the importance of BMP signaling in IBD.

Several growth factors like TGFβ superfamily, growth hormone, epidermal growth factor, keratinocyte growth factor, teduglutide and granulocyte macrophage/granulocite colony stimulating factors have been involved in clinical studies so far (Krishnan et al., 2010). BMPs as osteoinductive agents are mostly implemented in healing bone damage but the presence of their expression during development and in adulthood indicates their importance during different disease and healing processes. We have previously shown the accumulation of radioactively labeled BMP7 in the GI tract primarily in stomach and intestine with the highest uptake in terminal ileum (Fig. 5)(Maric et al., 2003).

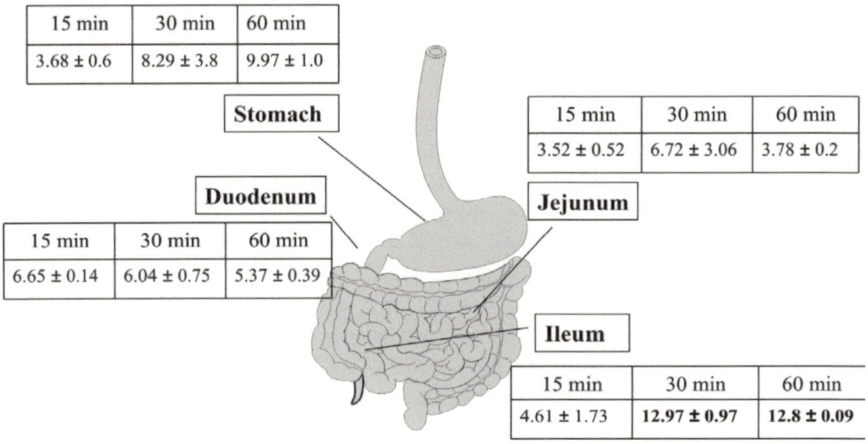

Fig. 5. Biodistrubution of ^{125}I-labeled BMP7 in rat gastrointestinal tract. Rats were analyzed at different time points following i.v. injection of ^{125}I-BMP7 (injected dose was 25 μCi/0.791 μg/kg). Relative uptake of ^{125}I-BMP7 was expressed as ng of radiolabeled BMP7/g wet tissue weight (Maric et al., 2003).

In addition, systemically applied BMP7 reduced the macroscopic and microscopic changes observed in TNBS-induced colitis followed by downregulation of proinflammatory cytokines (i.e. IL-6, TNFα, ICAM-1) and pro-fibrogenic cytokines (i.e. TGFβ). BMP7 accelerated healing of wounded tissue and reduced neutrophil infiltration (Fig. 6, Fig. 7 & Fig. 8).

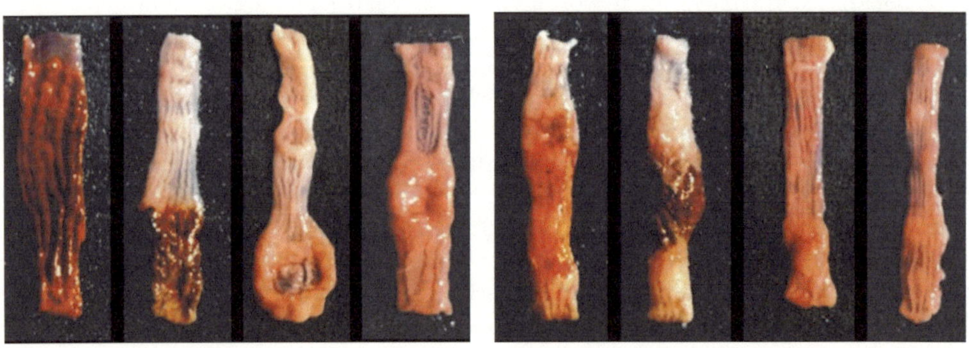

(a) TNBS-colitis (b) TNBS-colitis upon BMP7 treatment

Fig. 6. Macroscopic appearance of colonic mucosa during different days of experimentally induced colitis. The cobblestone-like ulceration in acute (days 2 and 5) and linar ulceration in chronic (days 14 and 30) stage was evident in colon. BMP7, applied systemically reduced macroscopic colon damage.

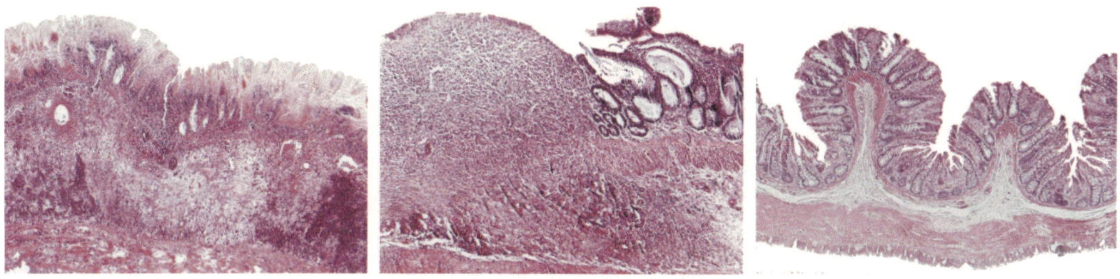

(a) Acute stage of colitis (b) Chronic stage of colitis (c) BMP7 treatment

Fig. 7. Representative histological sections of colon from colitic rats treated with vehicle (a, b) and BMP7 (c). Histologic findings in early stage of TNBS-colitis showed intensive inflammatory cell infiltration associated with colonic mucosa swelling and bleeding. In chronic stage of TNBS-colitis (b), diffuse infiltration with lymphocytes and fibroblasts was observed in ulcus region presenting healing process of colon tissue. The microstructure of colon was restored upon therapeutically application of BMP7 (c) Magnification x100.

BMP2 and BMP7 expression has been found in colon samples during acute and chronic stages of experimental colitis. BMP7 treatment slightly reduced the expression level of BMP2 (Maric et al., 2003; 2008). Beneficial effects of BMP7 were also observed in intestinal ischemia/reperfusion injury and fibrosis associated with chronic intestinal inflammation (Flier et al., 2010; Radhakrishnan et al., 2008).

3.4 BMP and their pathway in intestinal fibrosis

Intestinal fibrosis is a major complication of CD disease which is an outcome of multiple factors. It occurs as a result of different types of chronic inflammation, initiated in various cellular sources, but all result in deregulation of extracellular matrix turnover (Burke 2007, Fiocchi & Lund, 2011). TGFβ is described as the most potent profibrotic factor of several

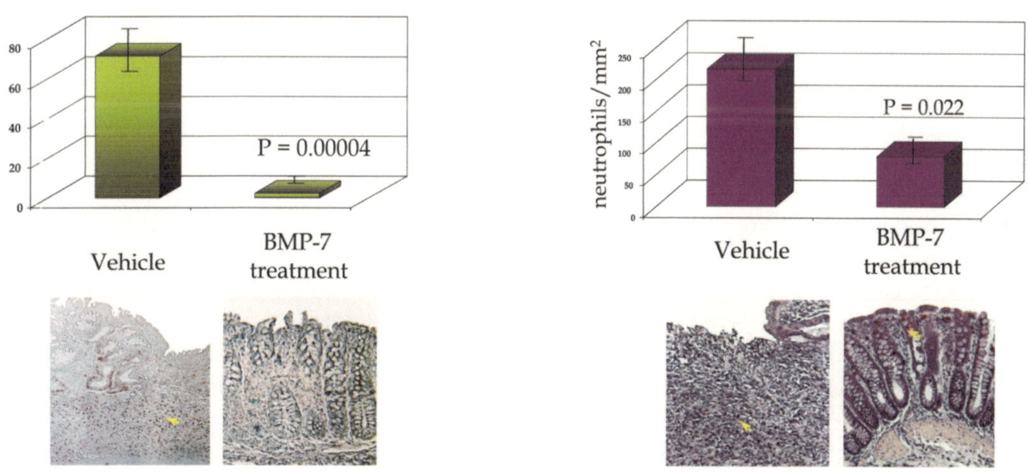

(a) PCNA staining (b) Naphtol AS-D chloroacetate esterase staining

Fig. 8. Effect of BMP7 treatment on cell proliferation and neutrophil accumulation in TNBS-induced colitis. BMP7 significantly reduced cell proliferation and neutrophil accumulation upon 14-day long therapy.

organs including organs of the GI tract. Experimental studies revealed that disruption of the TGFβ/Smad signaling pathway contributed to both chronic tissue inflammation and fibrosis (Flanders 2004; Nguyen & Goldschmeding, 2008; Pucilowska et al., 2000; Rieder et al., 2007). Key molecules of this pathway are Smad3 and Smad7. Smad3 null mice exhibit a significant reduction of intestinal fibrosis, associated with increased intestinal expression of Smad7 and decreased expression of Smad3, CTGF, collagen I-III and TGFβ following TNBS induced colitis (Latella et al., 2009; Zanninelli et al., 2006,). Wild-type mice, on the other hand, showed decreased expression of Smad7 and increased expression of Smad3, similar to the findings of di Sabatino (2009) in biopsies of intestinal strictures from patients suffering from Crohn's disease. Myofibroblasts from mucosa underlying CD strictures produced significantly higher amounts of collagen induced by an increased expression of TGFβ and Smad2/3 but not Smad7 (di Sabatino et al., 2009). It was pointed out that a disturbance of TGFβ/BMP downstream signaling components could contribute to intestinal fibrosis and therefore they were presented as more specific antifibrotic targets than TGFβ. Increased expression of TGFβ, CTGF, collagen-1α, and BMP7 was found in strictured segments of CD intestinal biopsies (Burke et al., 2008), although previous studies showed anti-inflammatory and antifibrotic properties of BMP7 (Maric et al., 2003; Flier et al., 2010). The correlation between steroid treatment and stricture development in CD was also observed followed by increased expression of CTGF in both, *in vivo* and *in vitro* by stimulating intestinal fibroblasts (Burke et al., 2008). The capacity of BMP7 to antagonize the pro-fibrotic effects of TGFβ in various organs including the gut has recently been shown (Fiocchi, 1997; Flier et al., 2010; Zeisberg et al., 2005). Treatment with BMP7 inhibits intestinal fibrosis by downregulation of TNF and by inhibition of TGFβ-induced epithelial to mesenchymal transition of the intestinal epithelial cells, which generates activated fibroblasts and contributes to intestinal fibrosis (Flier et al., 2010).

3.5 BMP and their pathway in other gastrointestinal diseases

Germline mutations in two members of the BMP pathway have been found to cause juvenile polyposis (JP). JP is an autosomal dominant hamartomatous polyposis syndrome. Affected individuals are predisposed to upper gastrointestinal and colorectal cancer. In almost half of the cases, patients have mutations or deletions in *SMAD4* and *BMPR1A* genes (Howe et al., 1998; Houlston et al., 1998; Langeveld et al., 2010; van Hattem et al., 2008; Woodford-Richens et al., 2001; Zhou et al., 2001). Genetic linkage studies of JP patients revealed that Smad4 germline mutation was mapped to chromosome 18q21 while BMPR1A germline mutations were localized on chromosome 10q22-23 (Howe et al., 1998; 2001). In a genotype-phenotype correlation study of JP patients, a significant prevalence of gastric polyposis was found in patients with Smad4 mutations when compared to other subsets of patients (Friedel et al., 2002). Histologically, JP polyps are characterized by dilated glands, abundant stroma and inflammatory infiltrates in a thickened lamina propria with normal epithelial covering (Howe et al., 2004). SMAD4 is a known tumor suppressor gene in pancreatic and colon cancer, but in JP it was hypothesized that SMAD4 gene acts as a susceptibility gene, a „gatekeeper", its loss of function resulting in polyp formation through indirect mechanisms, suggesting an important role of the stromal inflammatory response in the regulation of epithelial tumorigenesis (Moskaluk et al., 1997; Takagi et al., 1996). This theory was supported by a study on homozygous Smad4 knockout mice. The most important histological findings included thickened intestinal musoca with polyp formation, loss of villus architecture and expansion of the stroma with plasma cell infiltrates, while mice with conditional Smad4 deletion in the intestinal epithelial layer did not develop intestinal tumors (Kim et al., 2006). In contrast, polyps from JP patients with a germline SMAD4 mutation showed biallelic inactivation of SMAD4 in both the epithelium and stroma, suggesting a common clonal origin (Woodford-Richens et al., 2000).

Familial adenomatous polyposis (FAP) is an autosomal dominant syndrome characterized by hundreds to thousands of adenomatous colorectal polyps that are caused by a deletion in the adenomatous polyposis coli (APC) gene, localized on chromosome 5q21. Polyps develop in adolescence, and if not treated, malignant alteration inevitably occurs (Morton et al., 1993). Extraintestinal manifestations may also be present in form of osteomas, desmoid tumors, dental abnormalities and extracolonic cancer (Galiatsatos & Foulkes, 2006). APC gene plays an important role in Wnt signaling and is involved in ubiquitine-mediated degradation of β-catenin. Functional defects of APC therefore lead to aberrant Wnt pathway activity, resulting in uncontrolled cell proliferation (Rustgi et al., 2007). In intestinal homeostasis, BMP molecules have a suppresive effect on Wnt-β-catenin pathway and preserved BMP signaling is required for inhibition of intestinal stem cell proliferation and repression of polyp formation (He et al., 2004; Haramis et al., 2004). Conversely, higher expression of Wnt signaling molecules in FAP results in BMP signaling downregulation. In a study on Wnt target genes, in APC mutant mice heterozygous for an allele equivalent to a human APC mutation, more severe polyposis and faster rate of tumor growth was associated with higher expression of the BMP antagonist Gremlin 1 and lower BMP2 and BMP4 expression (Lewis et al., 2010). Analogous results were found in human FAP tissue specimens, with BMP2 expression lost in dysplatic epithelium of mycroadenomas (Hardwick et al., 2004).

Association of JP and FAP with the BMP signaling pathway was confirmed by experiments on BMP-transgenic mice. Transgenic mice which overexpressed the BMP anatagonist noggin or mice with conditional inacativation of BMPRIA which led to disruption of both epithelial and mesenchymal BMP signaling, showed highly increased formation of intestinal polyps morphologically similar to those in JP (Haramis et al., 2004; He et al., 2004). Loss of mesenchymal BMP signaling by conditional inactivation of BMPRII in stroma led to intestinal bleeding, thickness of mucosa due to epithelial hyperplasia and myofibroblast increment and multiple hemartomatous polyp appearance (Beppu et al., 2008; Hardwick et al., 2008). These expression patterns found in human polyposis syndromes indicate that altered BMP expression plays an important role in uncontrolled cell proliferation and tumorigenesis in the intestine.

Finally, alteration of the BMP signaling pathway may be involved in the appearance of intestinal mucosal atrophy due to total parenteral nutrition (Zhang et al., 2009). Expression of BMP2, BMP4, BMPRII and pSmad1/5/8 has been found to be increased in intestinal mucosa without differences in BMP antagonist expression following parenteral nutrition. These alterations were suggested to affect epithelial cell proliferation.

3.6 BMPs and their pathway in gastrointestinal cancers

Extensive research was conducted to explore the genes and factors that may trigger the initiation and progression of colorectal cancers (Ulman & Itzkowitz, 2011). Among a small number of genes known to affect cancer development, BMPs and their signaling pathway have been under intensive research during the last decade (van den Brink & Offerhaus, 2007). So far, studies have revealed contradictory findings. Some of them have shown reduced or complete loss of BMP signaling, while others have shown increased expression of this pathway.

Deregulation of mechanisms controlling expression of Smads was found in human colorectal cancers characterized by selective up-regulation of R-Smads in tumor cells and absence of Smad expression in tumor stroma (Korchynskyi et al., 1999). Co-Smad and I-Smad were expressed in both tumor and normal tissues. BMP2, BMP3 and BMP7 have been found to be growth suppressive for colorectal cancer cells (Beck et al., 2006; Hardwick et al., 2004; Loh et al., 2008). BMP2 exerts growth suppression by increasing $p21^{WAF1}$ protein levels, inducing $p21^{WAF1}$ stabilization and not its transcription (Back et al., 2007). BMP/Smad independent pathways, like the RAS/ERK-mediated signaling cascade, interferes with BMP2-induced $p21^{WAF1}$ stabilization, thus acting as a negative regulator of BMP signaling and arresting growth suppression. The expression of BMPRIA and pSmad1 was found in human colon cancer specimens as well as in several cell lines (Beck et al., 2006). The consequence of the loss of normal feedback inhibition could be seen in the intestinal epithelial cells in JP, where the absence of BMP signaling may lead to enhanced production of BMPs in the lamina propria or in epithelial cells (van den Brink, 2004). In addition, the loss of BMP signaling could also be connected with tumor progression. BMP4 and BMP7 expression has been found to increase with progression of the adenoma-carcinoma sequence and to correlate with a worse prognosis (Deng et al., 2007, Motoyama et al., 2008). The comparison of human adenoma and colorectal cancer specimens revealed the loss of active BMP signaling pathway in 9.1% and 77.7%, respectively, (Kodach et al., 2007; 2008a) which correlated with tumor progression from late adenoma to early carcinoma. The most prominent finding was the loss of BMPRII and Smad4 expression in colorectal carcinoma (Hardwick et al., 2008; Kodach et al., 2007; 2008a) which was confirmed by similar findings in sporadic colorectal carcinoma. The loss of BMPRII expression was strictly correlated with microsatellite instability (Kodach et al., 2008b). On the other hand, it was noticed that BMP signaling was regained in more advanced tumor stages (Kodach et al., 2008a).

Significantly higher BMP7 expression was found in human colorectal cancer than in normal tissues. This expression correlated with parameters of pathological aggressiveness and poorest prognosis (Motoyama et al., 2008). BMP7 showed a divergent role in different pathological changes of colon mucosa (Grijelmo et al., 2007). Whether proinvasive or protective activity will prevail depends on the activity of inflammation, tumor type and grade and the status of the BMP-Smad dependent and independent pathways. BMP7 and its receptors are expressed in normal human colon crypts, aberrant crypt foci in sigmoiditis and in half of colorectal tumors. It is involved in cellular scattering and invasion of premalignant and carcinoma colon epithelial cells probably by BMP-Smad independent pathways. Recent studies have re-emphasized the influence of intact BMP signaling on tumor growth as well as on survival and proliferation of colon carcinoma cells *in vivo* and *in vitro* (Lorente-Trigos et al., 2010). The different levels of BMPs (BMP2, BMP4), Smad proteins (Smad1, Smad4, Smad5, and Smad8) and absence of BMP inhibitor (chordin and gremlin) expression was found in advanced sporadic colon carcinomas. Proliferation and tumor growth of primary colon carcinoma cells *in vivo* can be influenced by altering the activity of BMPRIB. An increase in this activity leads to enhanced tumor growth while its inhibition yields the opposite effect. In this respect BMPs, as members of TGFβ superfamily, resemble the TGFβ signaling pathway in sporadic colorectal cancer (Akiyama et al., 1996; Markowitz et al., 1995).

4. Conclusion

BMPs play a vital role in embryogenesis and in tissue homeostasis of numerous organs including the GI tract and their malfunction may cause different human disorders.

Ubiquitous presence of BMPs and their importance in regeneration of many tissues aroused their name from bone morphogenetic protein to body morphogenetic protein (Reddi AH 2005). The BMP pathway showed complexity by numerous ligands and their antagonists, downstream effectors and/or other signaling mediators. In addition, the interaction of the BMP pathway with other signaling cascades adds another level of regulation.

Animal models of IBD provide a valuable tool in IBD research, and are detrimental for the understanding of the role of BMP signaling in this family of diseases. Since they are readily available and reproducible, they contribute greatly to our knowledge of the complex mechanisms of this chronic and debilitating disease and also facilitate the development of new therapeutic modalities.

The BMPs play an important role in a multitude of physiological processes and alterations in their signaling properties have been associated with various diseases. These include the majority of pathologies of the gastrointestinal tract, among which Crohn's disease, ulcerative colitis and various GI cancers. Not surprisingly, BMP signaling has been under extensive investigation as a therapeutic target. We, for example, have previously shown the beneficial effects of BMP7 therapy in an experimental model for colitis, with both anti-inflammatory and antifibrotic effects on colon damage. In addition, possible targets of the BMP signaling pathway for the prevention or treatment of IBD are Smad proteins, including Smad3, Smad5 or Smad7. However, many of the molecular mechanisms behind their functions are yet to be revealed and are currently under our and other people's investigation.

In summary, the BMP signaling pathway plays a major role in GI diseases and we therefore present it as a group of molecules of high clinical potential for the future.

5. References

Akiyama, Y.; Iwanaga, R.; Ishikawa, T.; Sakamoto, K.; Nishi, N.; Nihei, Z.; Iwama, T.; Saitoh, K. & Yuasa Y. (1996). Mutations of the transforming growth factor-beta type II receptor gene are strongly related to sporadic proximal colon carcinomas with microsatellite instability. *Cancer*, Vol.78, No.12, pp. 2478-2484.

Allaire, J.M.; Darsigny, M.; Marcoux, S.S.; Roy, S.A.; Schmouth, J.F.; Umans, L.; Zwijsen, A.; Boudreau, F. & Perreault, N. (2011). Loss of Smad5 leads to the disassembly of the apical junctional complex and increased susceptibility to experimental colitis. *Am J Physiol Gastrointest Liver Physiol.*, Vol.300, No.4, pp. G586-G597.

Alonzi, T.; Newton, I.P.; Bryce, P.J.; Di Carlo, E.; Lattanzio, G.; Tripodi, M.; Musiani, P. & Poli, V. (2004). Induced somatic inactivation of STAT3 in mice triggers the development of a fulminant form of enterocolitis. *Cytokine*, Vol.26, No.2, pp.45- 56.

Amiel, J. & Lyonnet, S. (2001). Hirschsprung disease, associated syndromes, and genetics: a review. *J Med Genet.*, Vol.38, No.11, pp.729-739.

Batts, L.E.; Polk, D.B.; Dubois, R.N. & Kulessa, H. (2006). Bmp signaling is required for intestinal growth and morphogenesis. *Dev Dyn.*, Vol.235, No.6, pp. 1563-1570.

Beck, S.E.; Jung, B.H.; Fiorino, A.; Gomez, J.; Rosario, E.D.; Cabrera, B.L.; Huang, S.C.; Chow, J.Y. & Carethers, J.M. (2006). Bone morphogenetic protein signaling and growth suppression in colon cancer. *Am J Physiol Gastrointest Liver Physiol.*, Vol.291, No.1, pp. G135-G145.

Beck, S.E.; Jung, B.H.; Del Rosario, E.; Gomez, J. & Carethers, J.M. (2007). BMP-induced growth suppression in colon cancer cells is mediated by p21WAF1 stabilization and modulated by RAS/ERK. *Cell Signal.*, Vol.19, No.7, pp. 1465-1472.

Beppu, H.; Mwizerwa, O.N.; Beppu, Y.; Dattwyler, M.P.; Lauwers, G.Y.; Bloch, K.D. & Goldstein AM. (2008). Stromal inactivation of BMPRII leads to colorectal epithelial overgrowth and polyp formation. *Oncogene*, Vol.27, No.8, pp. 1063-1070.

Bevan, S.; Woodford-Richens, K.; Rozen, P.; Eng, C.; Young, J.; Dunlop, M. & al. (1999). Screening SMAD1, SMAD2, SMAD3, and SMAD5 for germline mutations in juvenile polyposis syndrome. *Gut*, Vol.45, No.3, pp. 406-408.

Boirivant, M.; Fuss, I.J.; Chu, A. & Strober, W. (1998). Oxazolone colitis: A murine model of T helper cell type 2 colitis treatable with antibodies to interleukin 4. *J Exp Med.*, Vol.188, No.10, pp.1929-1939.

Boirivant, M.; Pallone, F.; Di Giacinto, C.; Fina, D.; Monteleone, I.; Marinaro, M.; Caruso, R.; Colantoni, A.; Palmieri, G.; Sanchez, M.; Strober, W.; MacDonald, T.T. & Monteleone, G. (2006). Inhibition of Smad7 with a specific antisense oligonucleotide facilitates TGF-beta1-mediated suppression of colitis. *Gastroenterology*, Vol.131, No.6, pp. 1786-1798.

Boismenu R & Chen Y. (2000). Insights from mouse models of colitis. *J Leukoc Biol.*, Vol.67, No.3, pp. 267–278.

Bouwmeester, T.; Kim, S.; Sasai, Y.; Lu, B. & De Robertis, E.M. (1996). Cerberus is a head-inducing secreted factor expressed in the anterior endoderm of Spemann's organizer. *Nature*, Vol.382, No.6592, pp. 595-601.

Burke, J.P.; Ferrante, M.; Dejaegher, K.; Watson, R.W.; Docherty, N.G.; De Hertogh, G.; Vermeire, S.; Rutgeerts, P.; D'Hoore, A.; Penninckx, F.; Geboes, K.; Van Assche, G. & O'Connell, P.R. (2008). Transcriptomic analysis of intestinal fibrosis- associated gene expression in response to medical therapy in Crohn's disease. *Inflamm Bowel Dis.*, Vol.14, No.9, pp. 1197-1204.

Burke, J.P.; Mulsow, J.J.; O'Keane, C.; Docherty, N.G.; Watson, R.W. & O'Connell, P.R. (2007). Fibrogenesis in Crohn's disease. *Am J Gastroenterol.*, Vol.102, No.2, pp. 439-448.

Centrella, M.; Horowitz, M.C. ; Wozney, J.M. & McCarthy, T.L. (1994). Transforming growth factor-β gene family members and bone. Endocr Rev., Vol. 15, No.1, pp. 27-39. Danese, S. (2011). Immune and nonimmune components orchestrate the pathogenesis of inflammatory bowel disease. *Am J Physiol Gastrointest Liver Physiol.*, Vol.300, No.5, pp. G716-G722.

Deng, H.; Ravikumar, T.S. & Yang, W.L. (2007). Bone morphogenetic protein-4 inhibits heat-induced apoptosis by modulating MAPK pathways in human colon cancer HCT116 cells.*Cancer Lett.*, Vol.256, No.2, pp.207-217.

De Santa Barbara, P.; Williams, J.; Goldstein, A.M.; Doyle, A.M.; Nielsen, C.; Winfield, S.; Faure, S. & Roberts, D.J. (2005). Bone morphogenetic protein signaling pathway plays multiple roles during gastrointestinal tract development. *Dev Dyn.*, Vol.234, No.2, pp. 312-322.

Dewulf, N.; Verschueren, K.; Lonnoy, O.; Morén, A.; Grimsby, S.; Vande Spiegle, K.; Miyazono, K.; Huylebroeck, D. & Ten Dijke, P. (1995). Distinct spatial and temporal expression patterns of two type I receptors for bone morphogenetic proteins during mouse embryogenesis. *Endocrinology.*, Vol.136, No.6, pp. 2652-2663.

Dieleman, L.A.; Ridwan, B.U.; Tennyson, G.S.; Beagley, K.W.; Bucy, R.P. & Elson, C.O. (1994). Dextran sulfate sodium-induced colitis occurs in severe combined immunodeficient mice. *Gastroenterology*, Vol.107, No.6, pp.1643–1652.

di Mola, F.F.; Di Sebastiano, P.; Gardini, A.; Innocenti, P.; Zimmermann, A.; Büchler, M.W. & Friess, H. (2004). Differential expression of connective tissue growth factor in inflammatory bowel disease. *Digestion*, Vol.69, No.4, pp. 245-253.

Di Sabatino, A.; Jackson, C.L.; Pickard, K.M.; Buckley, M.; Rovedatti, L.; Leakey, N.A.; Picariello, L.; Cazzola, P.; Monteleone, G.; Tonelli, F.; Corazza, G.R.; MacDonald, T.T. & Pender, S.L. (2009). Transforming growth factor beta signalling and matrix metalloproteinases in the mucosa overlying Crohn's disease strictures. *Gut*, Vol.58, No.6, pp. 777-789.

Elson, C.O.; Sartor, R.B.; Tennyson, G.S. & Riddell, R.H. (1995). Experimental models of inflammatory bowel disease. *Gastroenterology*, Vol.109, No.4, pp. 1344–1367.

Fiocchi, C. (1997). Intestinal inflammation: a complex interplay of immune and nonimmune cell interactions. *Am J Physiol.*, Vol.273, No.4 Pt 1, pp. G769-G775.

Fiocchi, C. & Lund, P.K. (2011). Themes in fibrosis and gastrointestinal inflammation. *Am J Physiol Gastrointest Liver Physiol.*, Vol.300, No.5, pp. G677-G683.

Flanders, K.C. (2004). Smad3 as a mediator of the fibrotic response. *Int J Exp Pathol.*, Vol.85, No.2, pp.47-64.

Flier, S.N.; Tanjore, H.; Kokkotou, E.G.; Sugimoto, H.; Zeisberg, M. & Kalluri, R. (2010). Identification of epithelial to mesenchymal transition as a novel source of fibroblasts in intestinal fibrosis. *J Biol Chem.*, Vol.28, No.26, pp.20202-20212.

Friedl, W.; Uhlhaas, S.; Schulmann, K.; Stolte, M.; Loff, S.; Back, W.; Mangold, E.; Stern, M.; Knaebel, H.P.; Sutter, C.; Weber, R.G.; Pistorius, S.; Burger, B. & Propping, P. (2002). Juvenile polyposis: massive gastric polyposis is more common in MADH4 mutation carriers than in BMPR1A mutation carriers. *Hum Genet.*, Vol.111, No.1, pp. 108-111.

Galiatsatos, P. & Foulkes, W.D. (2006). Familial adenomatous polyposis. *Am J Gastroenterol.*, Vol.101, No.2, pp. 385-398.

Goldman, D.C.; Donley, N. & Christian, J.L. (2009). Genetic interaction between Bmp2 and Bmp4 reveals shared functions during multiple aspects of mouse organogenesis. *Mech Dev.*,, Vol.126, No.3-4, pp. 117-127.

Grijelmo, C.; Rodrigue, C.; Svrcek, M.; Bruyneel, E.; Hendrix, A.; de Wever, O. & Gespach, C. (2007). Proinvasive activity of BMP-7 through SMAD4/src-independent and ERK/Rac/JNK-dependent signaling pathways in colon cancer cells. *Cell Signal.*, Vol.19, No.8, pp. 1722-1732.

Hanyu, A.; Ishidou, Y.; Ebisawa, T.; Shimanuki, T.; Imamura, T. & Miyazono, K. (2001). The N domain of Smad7 is essential for specific inhibition of transforming growth factor-beta signaling. *J Cell Biol.*, Vol.155, No.6, pp. 1017-1027.

Haramis, A.P.; Begthel, H.; van den Born, M.; van Es, J.; Jonkheer, S.; Offerhaus, G.J. & Clevers, H. (2004). De novo crypt formation and juvenile polyposis on BMP inhibition in mouse intestine. *Science*, Vol.303, No.5664, pp. 1684-1686.

Hardwick, J.C.; van Den Brink, G.R.; Bleuming, S.A.; Ballester, I.; Van Den Brande, J.M.; Keller, J.J.; Offerhaus, G.J.; Van Deventer, S.J. & Peppelenbosch, M.P. (2004). Bone morphogenetic protein 2 is expressed by, and acts upon, mature epithelial cells in the colon. *Gastroenterology*, Vol.126, No.1, pp. 111-121.

Hardwick, J.C.; Kodach, L.L.; Offerhaus, G.J. & van den Brink, G.R. (2008). Bone morphogenetic protein signaling in colorectal cancer. *Nat Rev Cancer.*, Vol.8, No.10, pp. 806-812.

He, X.C.; Zhang, J.; Tong, W.G.; Tawfik, O.; Ross, J.; Scoville, D.H.; Tian, Q.; Zeng, X.; He, X.; Wiedemann, L.M.; Mishina, Y. & Li, L. (2004). BMP signaling inhibits intestinal stem cell self-renewal through suppression of Wnt-beta-catenin signaling. *Nat Genet.*, Vol.36, No.10, pp. 1117-1121.

Helder, M.N.; Ozkaynak, E.; Sampath, K.T.; Luyten, F.P.; Latin, V.; Oppermann, H. & Vukicevic, S. (1995). Expression pattern of osteogenic protein-1 (bone morphogenetic protein-7) in human and mouse development. *J Histochem Cytochem.*, Vol.43, No.10, pp. 1035-1044.

Hibi, T.; Ogata, H. & Sakuraba, A. Animal models of inflammatory boel disease. (2002). *J Gastroenterol.*, Vol.37, No.6, pp. 409-417.

Hogan, BL. (1996). Bone morphogenetic proteins: multifunctional regulators of vertebrate development. *Genes & Dev.*, Vol.10, No.13, pp. 1580-1594.

Houlston, R.; Bevan, S.; Williams, A.; Young, J.; Dunlop, M.; Rozen, P.; Eng, C.; Markie, D.; Woodford-Richens, K.; Rodriguez-Bigas, M.A.; Leggett, B.; Neale, K.; Phillips, R.; Sheridan, E.; Hodgson, S.; Iwama, T.; Eccles, D.; Bodmer, W. & Tomlinson, I. (1998). Mutations in DPC4 (SMAD4) cause juvenile polyposis syndrome, but only account for a minority of cases. *Hum Mol Genet.*, Vol.7, No.12, pp. 1907–1912.

Howe, J.R.; Roth, S.; Ringold, J.C.; Summers, R.W.; Järvinen, H.J.; Sistonen, P.; Tomlinson, I.P.; Houlston, R.S.; Bevan, S.; Mitros, F.A.; Stone, E.M. & Aaltonen, L.A. (1998). Mutations in the SMAD4/DPC4 gene in juvenile polyposis. *Science,* Vol.280, No.5366, pp. 1086-1088.

Howe, J.R.; Bair, J.L.; Sayed, M.G.; Anderson, M.E.; Mitros, F.A.; Petersen, G.M.; Velculescu, V.E.; Traverso, G. & Vogelstein, B. (2001). Germline mutations of the gene encoding bone morphogenetic protein receptor 1A in juvenile polyposis. *Nat Genet.*, Vol.28, No.2, pp. 184–187.

Howe, J.R.; Sayed, M.G.; Ahmed, A.F.; Ringold, J.; Larsen-Haidle, J.; Merg, A.; Mitros, F.A.; Vaccaro, C.A.; Petersen, G.M.; Giardiello, F.M.; Tinley, S.T.; Aaltonen, L.A. & Lynch, H.T. (2004). The prevalence of MADH4 and BMPR1A mutations in juvenile polyposis and absence of BMPR2, BMPR1B, and ACVR1 mutations. *Med Genet.*, Vol.41, No.7, pp. 484-491.

Hsu, D.R.; Economides, A.N.; Wang, X.; Eimon, P.M. & Harland, R.M. (1998). The Xenopus dorsalizing factor Gremlin identifies a novel family of secreted proteins that antagonize BMP activities. *Mol Cell.*, Vol.1, No.5, pp. 673-683.

Karlsson, L.; Lindahl, P.; Heath, J.K. & Betsholtz, C. (2000). Abnormal gastrointestinal development in PDGF-A and PDGFR-α deficient mice implicates a novel mesenchymal structure with putative instructive properties in villus morphogenesis. *Development*, Vol.127, No.16, pp. 3457-3466.

Kawabata, M.; Imamura. T. & Miyazono, K. (1998). Signal transduction by bone morphogenetic proteins. *Cytokine Growth Factor Rev.*, Vol.9, No.1, pp. 49-61.

Kim, B.G.; Li, C.; Qiao, W.; Mamura, M.; Kasprzak, B.; Anver, M.; Wolfraim, L.; Hong, S.; Mushinski, E.; Potter, M.; Kim, S.J.; Fu, X.Y.; Deng, C. & Letterio, J.J. (2006). Smad4 signalling in T cells is required for suppression of gastrointestinal cancer. *Nature,* Vol.441, No.7096, pp. 1015–1019.

Kingsley, DM. (1994). The TGF-beta superfamily: new members, new receptors, and new genetic tests of function in different organisms. *Genes Dev.* Vol.8, No.2, pp. 133-146.

Kitajima, S.; Takuma, S. & Morimoto, M. (1999). Tissue distribution of dextran sulfate sodium (DSS) in the acute phase of murine DSS-induced colitis. *J Vet Med Sci.*, Vol.61, No.1, pp. 67–70.

Kodach, L.L.; Bleuming, S.A.; Musler, A.R.; Peppelenbosch, M.P.; Hommes, D.W.; van den Brink, G.R.; van Noesel, C.J.; Offerhaus, G.J. & Hardwick, J.C. (2008a). The bone morphogenetic protein pathway is active in human colon adenomas and inactivated in colorectal cancer. *Cancer*, Vol.112, No.2, pp. 300-306.

Kodach, L.L.; Wiercinska, E.; de Miranda, N.F.; Bleuming, S.A.; Musler, A.R.; Peppelenbosch, M.P.; Dekker, E.; van den Brink, G.R.; van Noesel, C.J.; Morreau, H.; Hommes, D.W.; Ten Dijke, P.; Offerhaus, G.J. & Hardwick, J.C. (2008b). The bone morphogenetic protein pathway is inactivated in the majority of sporadic colorectal cancers. *Gastroenterology*, Vol.134, No.5, pp. 1332-1341.

Korchynskyi, O.; Landström, M.; Stoika, R.; Funa, K.; Heldin, C.H.; ten Dijke, P. & Souchelnytskyi, S. (1999). Expression of Smad proteins in human colorectal cancer. *Int J Cancer.*, Vol.82, No.2, pp.197-202.

Korchynskyi, O. & ten Dijke, P. (2002). Bone morphogentic protein receptors and their nuclear effectors in bone formation. In: *Bone morphogenetic proteins: from laboratory to clinical practice,* S. Vukicevic, T.K. Sampath, (Ed.), 31–60, Birkhäuser Verlag AG, ISBN 3-7643-6509-9, Basel, Switzerland.

Kosinski, C.; Li, V.S.; Chan, A.S.; Zhang, J.; Ho, C.; Tsui, W.Y.; Chan, T.L.; Mifflin, R.C.; Powell, D.W.; Yuen, S.T.; Leung, S.Y. & Chen, X. (2007). Gene expression patterns of human colon tops and basal crypts and BMP antagonists as intestinal stem cell niche factors. *Proc Natl Acad Sci USA*, Vol.104, No.39, pp. 15418-15423.

Krishnan, K.; Arnone, B. & Buchman, A. (2011). Intestinal growth factor: potential use in the treatment of inflammatory bowel disease and their role in mucosal healing. *Inflamm Bowel Dis.*, Vol.17, No.1, pp. 410- 422.

Kuhn, R.; Lohler, J.; Rennick, D.; Rajewsky, K. & Muller, W. (1993). Interleukin-10-deficient mice develop chronic enterocolitis. *Cell*, Vol.75, No.2, pp. 263–274.

Langeveld, D.; van Hattem, W.A.; de Leng, W.W.; Morsink, F.H.; Ten Kate, F.J.; Giardiello, F.M.; Offerhaus, G.J. & Brosens, L.A. (2010). SMAD4 immunohistochemistry reflects genetic status in juvenile polyposis syndrome. *Clin Cancer Res.*, Vol.16, No.16, pp. 4126-4134.

Latella, G.; Vetuschi, A.; Sferra, R.; Zanninelli, G.; D'Angelo, A.; Catitti, V.; Caprilli, R.; Flanders, K.C. & Gaudio, E. (2009). Smad3 loss confers resistance to the development of trinitrobenzene sulfonic acid-induced colorectal fibrosis. *Eur J Clin Invest.* Vol.39, No.2, pp. 145-156.

Lein, P.; Drahushuk, K.M. & Higgins, D. (2002). Effects of bone morphogenetic proteins on neural tissues. In: *Bone morphogenetic proteins: from laboratory to clinical practice,* S. Vukicevic, T.K. Sampath (Ed.), 289-319, Birkäuser Verlag AG, ISBN 3-7643-6509-9, Basel, Switzerland.

Lewis, A.; Segditsas, S.; Deheragoda, M.; Pollard, P.; Jeffery, R.; Nye, E.; Lockstone, H.; Davis, H.; Clark, S.; Stamp, G.; Poulsom, R.; Wright, N. & Tomlinson, I. (2010). Severe polyposis in Apc (1322T) mice is associated with submaximal Wnt signalling and increased expression of the stem cell marker Lgr5. *Gut*, Vol.59, No.12, pp. 1680-1686.

Li, X.; Madison, B.B.; Zacharias, W.; Kolterud, A.; States, D. & Gumucio, D.L. (2007). Deconvoluting the intestine: molecular evidence for a major role of the mesenchyme in the modulation of signaling cross talk. *Physiol Genomics.*, Vol.29, No.3, pp. 290-301.

Liu, F.; Hata, A.; Baker, J.C.; Doody, J.; Cárcamo, J.; Harland, R.M. & Massagué, J. (1996). A human Mad protein acting as a BMP-regulated transcriptional activator. *Nature*, Vol. 381, No.6583, pp. 620-623.

Lorente-Trigos, A.; Varnat, F.; Melotti, A. & Ruiz i Altaba A. (2010). BMP signaling promotes the growth of primary human colon carcinomas in vivo. *J Mol Cell Biol.*, Vol.2, No.6, pp. 318-332.

Loh, K.; Chia, J.A.; Greco, S.; Cozzi, S.J.; Buttenshaw, R.L.; Bond, C.E.; Simms, L.A.; Pike, T.; Young, J.P.; Jass, J.R.; Spring, K.J.; Leggett, B.A. & Whitehall, V.L. (2008). Bone morphogenic protein 3 inactivation is an early and frequent event in colorectal cancer development. *Genes Chromosomes Cancer*, Vol.47, No.6, pp. 449-460.

Lories, R.J.; Derese, I. & Luyten, F.P. (2005). Modulation of bone morphogenetic protein signaling inhibits the onset and progression of ankylosing enthesitis. *J Clin Invest.*, Vol.115, No.6, pp. 1571-1579.

MacDonald, T.T.; Monteleone, I.; Fantini, M.C. & Monteleone, G. (2011). Regulation of homeostasis and inflammation in the intestine. *Gastroenterology*, Vol.140, No.6, pp. 1768-1775.

Markowitz, S.; Wang, J.; Myeroff, L.; Parsons, R.; Sun, L.; Lutterbaugh, J.; Fan, R.S.; Zborowska, E.; Kinzler, K.W. Vogelstein B, et al. (1995). Inactivation of the type II TGF-beta receptor in colon cancer cells with microsatellite instability. *Science*, Vol.268, No.5215, pp. 1336-1338.

Maric, I.; Poljak, Lj.; Zoricic, S.; Bobinac, D.; Bosukonda, D.; Sampath, K.T. & Vukicevic, S. (2003). Bone morphogenetic protein-7 reduces the severity of colon tissue damage and accelerates the healing of inflammatory bowel disease in rats. *J Cell Physiol.*, Vol.196, No.2, pp. 258-264.

Maric, I.; Kucic, N.; Grahovac, B.; Bobinac, D. & Vukicevic, S. (2008). Expression of bone morphogenetic protein -2 and -7 during experimental inflammatory bowel disease. *Medicina Fluminensis*, Vol.44, No.1, pp. 60-66.

Martinovic, S.; Borovecki, F.; Sampath, T.K. & Vukicevic, S. (2002). Biology of bone morphogenetic proteins. In: *Bone morphogenetic proteins: from laboratory to clinical practice*, S. Vukicevic, T.K. Sampath (Ed.), 87-119, Birkäuser Verlag AG, ISBN 3-7643-6509-9, Basel, Switzerland.

Massague, J.; Seoane, J. & Wotton, D. (2005). Smad transcription factors. *Genes Dev.*, Vol.19, No.23, pp. 2783-2810.

Matsumoto, S.; Okabe, Y.; Setoyama, H.; Takayama, K.; Ohtsuka, J.; Funahashi, H.; Imaoka, A.; Okada, Y. & Umesaki, Y. (1998). Inflammatory bowel disease-like enteritis and caecitis in a senescence accelerated mouse P1/Yit strain. *Gut*, Vol.43, No.1, pp. 71–78.

Miyazono, K. (2000). TGF-beta signaling by Smad proteins. *Cytokine Growth Factor Rev.*, Vol.11, No.1-2, pp. 15-22.

Miyazono, K.; Maeda, S. & Imamura, T. (2005). BMP receptor signaling: transcriptional targets, regulation of signals, and signaling cross-talk. *Cytokine Growth Factor Rev.*, Vol. 16, No.3, pp. 2512-63.

Miyazono, K.; Kamiya, Y. & Morikawa, M. (2010). Bone morphogenetic protein receptors and signal transduction. *J Biochem.*, Vol.147, No.1, pp. 35-51.

Mizoguchi, A. & Mizoguchi, E. (2010). Animal models of IBD: linkage to human disease. *Curr Opin Pharmacol.*, Vol.10, No.5, pp. 578-587.

Mombaerts, P.; Mizoguchi, E.; Grusby, M.J.; Glimcher, L.H.; Bhan, A.K. & Tonegawa, S. (1993). Spontaneous development of inflammatory bowel disease in T cell receptor mutant mice. *Cell*, Vol.75, No.2, pp. 275–282.

Monteleone, G.; Kumberova, A.; Croft, N.M.; McKenzie, C.; Steer, H.W. & MacDonald, T.T. (2001). Blocking Smad7 restores TGF-β1 signaling in chronic inflammatory bowel disease. *J Clin Invest.*, Vol.108, No.4, pp. 523-526.

Monteleone, G.; Pallone, F. & MacDonald, T.T. (2004). Smad7 in TGF-β-mediated negative regulation of gut inflammation. *Trends Immunol.*, Vol.25, No.10, pp. 513-517.

Monteleone, G.; Mann, J.; Monteleone, I.; Vavassori, P.; Bremner, R.; Fantini, M.; Del Vecchio Blanco, G.; Tersigni, R.; Alessandroni, L.; Mann, D.; Pallone, F. & MacDonald, T.T.(2004). A failure of transforming growth factor-beta1 negative regulation maintains sustained NF-kappaB activation in gut inflammation. *J Biol Chem.*, Vol.279, No.6, pp. 3925-3932.

Monteleone, G.; Del Vecchio Blanco, G.; Monteleone, I.; Fina, D.; Caruso, R.; Gioia, V.; Ballerini, S.; Federici, G.; Bernardini, S.; Pallone, F. & MacDonald, T.T. (2005). Post-transcriptional regulation of Smad7 in the gut of patients with inflammatory bowel disease. *Gastroenterology*, Vol.129, No.5, pp. 1420-1429.

Monteleone, G.; Boirivant, M.; Pallone, F. & MacDonald, T.T. (2008). TGF-beta1 and Smad7 in the regulation of IBD. *Mucosal Immunol.*, Vol.1, Suppl.1, pp. S50-S53.

Morris, G.P.; Beck, P.L.; Herridge, M.S.; Depew, W.T.; Szewczuk, M.R. & Wallace, J.L. (1989). Hapten-induced model of colonic inflammation and ulceration in the rat colon. *Gastroenterology*, Vol.96, No.3, pp. 795-803.

Morton, D.G.; Macdonald, F.; Haydon, J.; Cullen, R.; Barker, G.; Hulten. M.; Neoptolemos, J.P.; Keighley, M.R. & McKeown, C. (1993). Screening practice for familial adenomatous polyposis: the potential for regional registers. *Br J Surg .*, Vol.80, No.2, pp. 255-258.

Moskaluk, C.A.; Hruban, R.H.; Schutte, M.; Lietman, A.S.; Smyrk, T.; Fusaro, L.; Lynch, J.; Yeo, C.J.; Jackson, C.E.; Lynch, H.T. & Kern, S.E. (1997). Genomic sequencing of DPC4 in the analysis of familial pancreatic carcinoma. *Diagn Mol Pathol.*, Vol.6, No.2, pp. 85-90.

Motoyama, K.; Tanaka, F.; Kosaka, Y.; Mimori, K.; Uetake, H.; Inoue, H.; Sugihara, K. & Mori, M. (2008). Clinical significance of BMP7 in human colorectal cancer. *Ann Surg Oncol.*, Vol.15, No.5, pp. 1530-1537.

Nguyen, T.Q.; Roestenberg, P.; van Nieuwenhoven, F.A.; Bovenschen, N.; Li, Z.; Xu, L.; Oliver, N.; Aten, J.; Joles, J.A.; Vial, C.; Brandan, E.; Lyons, K.M. & Goldschmeding, R. (2008). CTGF inhibits BMP-7 signaling in diabetic nephropathy. *J Am Soc Nephrol.*, Vol.19, No.11, pp. 2098-2107.

Nguyen, T.Q. & Goldschmeding, R. (2008). Bone morphogenetic protein-7 and connective tissue growth factor: novel targets for treatment of renal fibrosis? *Pharm Res.*, Vol.25, No.10, pp. 2416-2426.

Okayasu, I.; Hatakeyama, S.; Yamada, M.; Ohkusa, T.; Inagaki, Y. & Nakaya, R. (1990). A novel method in the induction of reliable experimental acute and chronic ulcerative colitis in mice. *Gastroenterology*, Vol.98, No.3, pp. 694–702.

Peiris, D.; Pacheco, I.; Spencer, C. & MacLeod, R.J. (2007). The extracellular calcium-sensing receptor reciprocally regulates the secretion of BMP-2 and the BMP antagonist Noggin in colonic myofibroblasts. *Am J Physiol Gastrointest Liver Physiol.*, Vol.292, No.3, pp. G753-G766.

Perr, H.A.; Ye, J. & Gitelman, S.E. (1999). Smooth muscle expresses bone morphogenetic protein (Vgr-1/BMP-6) in human fetal intestine. *Biol Neonate.*, Vol.75, No.3, pp. 210-214.

Piccolo, S.; Sasai, Y.; Lu, B. & De Robertis, E.M. (1996). Dorsoventral patterning in Xenopus: inhibition of ventral signals by direct binding of chordin to BMP-4. *Cell*, Vol.86, No.4, pp. 589-598.

Podolsky, DK. (2002). Inflammatory bowel disease. *N Engl J Med.*, Vol.347, No.6, pp. 417-429.

Pucilowska, J.B.; Williams, K.L. & Lund, P.K. (2000). Fibrogenesis. IV. Fibrosis and inflammatory bowel disease: cellular mediators and animal models. *Am J Physiol Gastrointest Liver Physiol.*, Vol.279, No.4, pp. G653-G659.

Radhakrishnan, R.S.; Radhakrishnan, G.L.; Radhakrishnan, H.R.; Xue, H.; Adams, S.D.; Moore-Olufemi, S.D.; Harting, M.T.; Cox, C.S. Jr. & Kone, B.C. (2008). Pretreatment with bone morphogenetic protein-7 (BMP-7) mimics ischemia preconditioning following intestinal ischemia/reperfusion injury in the intestine and liver. *Shock*, Vol.30, No.5, pp. 532-536.

Reddi, A.H. (2005). BMPs: from bone morphogenetic proteins to body morphogenetic proteins. *Cytokine Growth Factor Rev.*, Vol.16, No.3, pp. 249-250.

Rieder, F.; Brenmoehl, J.; Leeb, S.; Schölmerich, J. & Rogler, G. (2007). Wound healing and fibrosis in intestinal disease. *Gut*, Vol.56, No.1, pp. 130-139.

Rueger, D.C. (2002). Biochemistry of bone morphogenetic proteins, In: *Bone morphogenetic proteins. From laboratory to clinical practice*, S. Vukicevic & T.K. Sampath, (Ed.), 1-18, Birkhäuser Verlag, ISBN 3-7643-6509-9, Basel, Switzerland.

Rustgi, A.K. (2007). The genesis of hereditary colon cancer. *Genes Dev.*, Vol.21, No.20, pp. 2525-2538.

Sadlack, B.; Merz, H.; Schorle, H.; Schimpl, A.; Feller, A.C. & Horak, I. (1993). Ulcerative colitis-like disease in mice with a disrupted interleukin-2 gene. *Cell*, Vol.75, No.2, pp. 253-261.

Sampath, T.K. & Reddi, A.H. (1981). Dissociative extraction and reconstitution of extracellular matrix components involved in local bone differentiation. *Proc Natl Acad Sci USA*, Vol.78, No.12, pp. 7599-7603.

Sampath, T.K.; Muthukumaran, N. & Reddi, A.H. (1987). Isolation of osteogenin, an extracellular matrix-associated, bone-inductive protein, by heparin affinity chromatography. *Proc Natl Acad Sci USA*, Vol.84, No.20, pp. 7109-7113.

Shi, X.Z.; Winston, J.H. & Sarna, S.K. (2011). Differential immune and genetic responses in rat models of Crohn's colitis and ulcerative colitis. *Am J Physiol Gastrointest Liver Physiol.*, Vol.300, No.1, pp. G41-G51.

Shull, M.M.; Ormsby, I.; Kier, A.B.; Pawlowski, S.; Diebold, R.J.; Yin, M.; Allen, R.; Sidman, C.; Proetzel, G.; Calvin, D.; Annunziata, N. & Doetschman, T. (1992).Targeted disruption of the mouse transforming growth factor-beta 1 gene results in multifocal inflammatory disease. *Nature*, Vol.359, No.6397, pp. 693-699.

Sieber, C.; Kopf, J.; Hiepen, C. & Knaus, P. (2009). Recent advances in BMP receptor signaling. *Cytokine Growth Factor Rev.*, Vol.20, No.5-6, pp. 343-355.

Simic, P. & Vukicevic, S. (2004). Bone morphogenetic proteins in development. In: Bone morphogenetic proteins: regeneration of bone and beyond, S. Vukicevic, T.K. Sampath, (Ed.), 73-108, Birkäuser Verlag AG, ISBN 3-7643-7139-0, Basel, Switzerland.

Stanley, E.; Biben, C.; Kotecha, S.; Fabri, L.; Tajbakhsh, S.; Wang, C.C.; Hatzistavrou, T.; Roberts, B.; Drinkwater, C.; Lah, M.; Buckingham, M.; Hilton, D.; Nash, A.; Mohun, T. & Harvey, R.P. (1998). DAN is a secreted glycoprotein related to Xenopus cerberus. *Mech Dev.*, Vol.77, No.2, pp. 173-184.

Strober, W. & Fuss, I.J. (2011). Proinflammatory cytokines in the pathogenesis of inflammatory bowel diseases. *Gastroenterology*, Vol.140, No.6, pp. 1756-1767.

Sundberg, J.P.; Elson, C.O.; Bedigian, H. & Birkenmeier, E.H. (1994). Spontaneous, heritable colitis in a new substrain of C3H/HeJ mice. *Gastroenterology*, Vol.107, No.6, pp. 1726–1735.

Takagi, Y.; Kohmura, H.; Futamura, M.; Kida, H.; Tanemura, H.; Shimokawa, K. & Saji, S. (1996). Somatic alterations of the DPC4 gene in human colorectal cancers in vivo. *Gastroenterology*, Vol.111, No.5, pp. 1369-1372.

Tokumasa, A.; Katsuno, T.; Tanaga, T.S.; Yokote, K.; Saito, Y. & Suzuki, Y. (2004). Reduction of Smad3 accelerates re-epithelialization in a murine model of colitis. *Biochem Biophys Res Commun.*, Vol.317, No.2, pp. 377-383.

Turk, T.; Leeuwis, J.W.; Gray, J.; Torti, S.V.; Lyons, K.M.; Nguyen, T.Q. & Goldschmeding, R. (2009). BMP signaling and podocyte markers are decreased in human diabetic nephropathy in association with CTGF overexpression. *J Histochem Cytochem.*, Vol.57, No.7, pp. 623-631.

Ullman, T.A. & Itzkowitz, S.H. (2011). Intestinal inflammation and cancer. *Gastroenterology*, Vol.140, No.6, pp. 1807-1816.

van den Brink, G.R. (2004). Linking pathways in colorectal cancer. *Nat Genet.*, Vol.36, No.10, pp. 1038-1039.

van den Brink, G.R & Offerhaus, G.J. (2007). The morphogenetic code and colon cancer development. *Cancer Cell*, Vol.11, No.2, pp. 109-117.

van Hatten, W.A.; Brosens, L.A.; de Leng, W.W.; Morsink, F.H.; Lens, S.; Carvalho, R.; Giardiello, F.M. & Offerhaus, G.J. (2008). Large genomic deletions of SMAD4, BMPR1A and PTEN in juvenile polyposis. *Gut*, Vol.57, No.5, pp. 623-627.

Vukicevic, S.; Luyten, F.P. & Reddi, A.H. (1989). Stimulation of the expression of osteogenic and chondrogenic phenotype in vitro by osteogenin. *Proc Natl Acad Sci USA*, Vol.86, No.22, pp. 8793-8797.

Vukicevic, S.; Stavljenic, A. & Pecina, M. (1995). Discovery and clinical applications of bone morphogenetic proteins. *Eur J Clin Chem Clin Biochem.*, Vol.33, No.10, pp. 661-671.

Vukicevic, S.; Kopp, J.B.; Luyten, F.P. & Sampath, T.K. (1996). Induction of kidney mesenchyme by osteogenic protein-1, (bone morphogenetic protein-7). *Proc Natl Acad Sci USA*, Vol.93, No.17, pp. 9021-9026.

Vukicevic, S. & Grgurevic, L. (2009). BMP-6 and mesenchymal stem cell differentiation. *Cytokine Growth Factor Rev.*, Vol.20, No.5-6, pp.:441-448.

Woodford-Richens, K.; Williamson, J.; Bevan, S.; Young, J.; Leggett, B.; Frayling, I.; Thway, Y.; Hodgson, S.; Kim, J.C.; Iwama, T.; Novelli, M.; Sheer, D.; Poulsom, R.; Wright, N.; Houlston, R. & Tomlinson, I. (2000). Allelic loss at SMAD4 in polyps from juvenile polyposis patients and use of fluorescence in situ hybridization to demonstrate clonal origin of the epithelium. *Cancer Res.*, Vol.60, No.9, pp. 2477-2482.

Woodford-Richens, K.L.; Rowan, A.J.; Poulsom, R.; Bevan, S.; Salovaara, R.; Aaltonen, L.A.; Houlston, R.S.; Wright, N.A. & Tomlinson, I.P. (2001). Comprehensive analysis of SMAD4 mutations and protein expression in juvenile polyposis: evidence for a distinct genetic pathway and polyp morphology in SMAD4 mutation carriers. *Am J Pathol.*, Vol.159, No.4, pp. 1293-1300.

Wozney, J.M.; Rosen, V.; Celeste, A.J.; Mitsock, L.M.; Whitters, M.J.; Kriz, R.W.; Hewick, R.M. & Wang, E.A. (1988). Novel regulators of bone formation: molecular clones and activities. *Science*, Vol.242, No.4885, pp. 1528-1534.

Wrana, J.L.; Attisano, L.; Wieser, R.; Ventura, F. & Massagué, J. (1994). Mechanism of activation of the TGF-beta receptor. *Nature*, Vol.370, No.6488, pp. 341-347.

Xavier, R.J. & Podolsky, D.K. (2007). Unravelling the pathogenesis of inflammatory bowel disease. *Nature*, Vol.448, No.7152, pp. 427-434.

Yanagita, M. (2005). BMP antagonists: their roles in development and involvement in pathophysiology. *Cytokine Growth Factor Rev.*, Vol.16, No.3, pp. 309-317.

Zanninelli, G.; Vetuschi, A.; Sferra, R.; D'Angelo, A.; Fratticci, A.; Continenza, M.A.; Chiaramonte, M.; Gaudio, E.; Caprilli, R. & Latella, G. (2006). Smad3 knock-out mice as a useful model to study intestinal fibrogenesis. *World J Gastroenterol.*, Vol.12, No.8, pp. 1211-1218.

Zeisberg, M.; Shah, A.A. & Kalluri, R. (2005). Bone morphogenic protein-7 induces mesenchymal to epithelial transition in adult renal fibroblasts and facilitates regeneration of injured kidney. *J Biol Chem.*, Vol.280, No.9, pp. 8094-8100.

Zhang, C.; Feng, Y.; Yang, H.; Koga, H. & Teitelbaum, D.H. (2009). The bone morphogenetic protein signaling pathway is upregulated in a mouse model of total parenteral nutrition. *J Nutr.*, Vol.139, No.7, pp. 1315-1321.

Zhou, X.P.; Woodford-Richens, K.; Lehtonen, R.; Kurose, K.; Aldred, M.; Hampel, H.; Launonen, V.; Virta, S.; Pilarski, R.; Salovaara, R.; Bodmer, W.F.; Conrad, B.A.; Dunlop, M.; Hodgson, S.V.; Iwama, T., Jarvinen, H.; Kellokumpu, I.; Kim, J.C.; Leggett, B.; Markie, D.; Mecklin, J.P.; Neale, K.; Phillips, R.; Piris, J.; Rozen, P.; Houlston, R.S.; Aaltonen, L.A.; Tomlinson, I.P. & Eng, C. (2001). Germline mutations in BMPR1A/ALK3 cause a subset of cases of juvenile polyposis syndrome and of Cowden and Bannayan-Riley-Ruvalcaba syndromes. *Am J Hum Genet.*, Vol.69, No.4, pp. 704–711.

Zimmerman, L.B.; De Jesús-Escobar, J.M. & Harland, R.M. (1996). The Spemann organizer signal noggin binds and inactivates bone morphogenetic protein 4. *Cell*, Vol.86, No.4, pp. 599-606.

12

Genetic Differentiation of Fungi of the Genus *Candida* Isolated from Patients with Inflammatory Bowel Diseases

Danuta Trojanowska[1], Marianna Tokarczyk[1], Małgorzata Zwolińska-Wcisło[2], Paweł Nowak[1], Sebastian Różycki[1] and Alicja Budak[1]
[1]*Department of Pharmaceutical Microbiology of Jagiellonian University Collegium Medicum*
[2]*Department of Gastroenterology, Hepatology and Infectious Diseases of Jagiellonian University Collegium Medicum*
Poland

1. Introduction

Inflammatory bowel diseases (IBD) constitute a group of incurable, inflammatory GI diseases of unknown etiology and the chronic course, with periods of spontaneous disease remissions and aggravations (Muszyński, 2001). This group of diseases includes Crohn`s disease and ulcerative colitis. They are characterized by inflammatory reactions and changes in the structure of intestinal mucosa (Rzeszutko, 2006). IBD etiopathogenesis is not clearly defined. The most essential etiological issues include environmental factors, genetic conditioning, abnormalities of intestinal immunological mechanisms and the bacterial flora (Konturek, 2001). The inflammation which develops in the intestine is mostly due to improper, low-fiber diet which is based on highly processed products and on the poor physical activity. Familial diseases confirmed in 10% of cases speak for the genetic source. Immunological mechanisms which develop in response to food and bacterial antigens are extremely significant (Muszyński, 2001; Polińska et al., 2009). A markedly increased interest has been observed in the intestinal microflora which is believed to be essential in inducing IBD development and in relapses of its clinical symptoms. Bacteria which are normally resident in the GI tract determine the proper work of intestines and protect from excessive proliferation of undesired microorganisms. The contribution of the intestinal flora to the development of the biofilm, which prevents the colonization of pathogens including fungi of the genus *Candida* in the GI tract, is extremely significant. The area of interest in fungi which are a part of microflora and constitute a potential source of systemic dissemination by colonizing the GI tract has greatly increased lately (Berhardt & Knoke, 1997). In the normal environment fungi are in balance with the bacterial flora and as commensals do not induce the inflammation. The main cause of its development, however, is the immune system impairment and a decrease of immunity. It affects patients with neoplasms and transplant recipients (Pfaller & Diekema, 2007; Warnock & Campbell, 1996). Other diseases causing inflammations are: diabetes and other endocrinopathies, infections due to HIV virus and also surgical procedures, damaged tissues and inflammations of the mucous membrane of the alimentary tract. Aggressive therapies with antibiotics, steroids and immunosuppressants disturb the endogenic bacterial flora and as a result contribute to the development of mycoses (Budak et al., 2003; Schelenz, 2008). The most essential factors affecting the increase of the frequency of fungal infections, especially those with *Candida* etiology, are commonly used invasive medical devices introduced into the human body, such as various catheters, tracheotomy tubes, stents, prostheses, implants and pacemakers which develop the biofilm on their surfaces due to fungi. The formation of the biofilm due to fungi which cause the inflammation has an essential clinical effect because it increases their resistance to drugs as well as the ability of cells which are inside the biofilm to defend themselves againt the immunological reaction of the host. The biofilm formed on the surface of medical devices which have been introduced into the body decreases their effectiveness and is the source of future inflammations (Jain et al., 2007; Ramag et al., 2006).

In the considerable number of healthy individuals fungi of the genus *Candida* colonize the oral cavity and pass through the esophagus, the stomach and the small intestine to reside in the large intestine. A number of healthy carriers of *Candida* in the oral cavity amounts to 30-50%, where *C.albicans* is a predominant species, constituting 70-80%. The most frequent site of candidiasis is the large intestine. Erosions, extensive ulcerations covered by false membranes and thrush-like changes develop within the mucous membrane. The fungal penetration into the submucosal membrane, muscularis and blood vessels is also possible. It includes vascular inoculation and the formation of microabscesses in various organs and tissues. Vascular invasion can lead to the obstruction of the artery and eventually to myocardial infarction.

Fungi of the genus *Candida* which are present in the large intestine were considered as sources of chronic and recurrent infections which can lead to the development of inflammations. Intestinal inflammations are likely to produce favorable conditions for the fungal invasion (Zwolińska-Wcisło et al., 2006). It is difficult to show the border between the colonization and the infection caused by fungi of the genus *Candida* within the oral cavity because asymptomatic carriers frequently develop the abundant increase of fungi in the cultured oral cavity and throat smears. It means that the presence of fungi on the mucous membrane of the oral cavity cannot be treated only as the saprophytic flora. In the healthy individual the stomach and the small intestine have the function of the passage of the fungal flora. In patients from the risk group the initial segment of the small intestine can be the site of the pathological colonization of fungi and the fungal infection develops in the ileocecal segment. Affected patients experience stomach cramps, flatulence, diarrhea and GI bleeding i.e., symptoms frequently reported by patients with acute IBD in the medical history (Mokrowiecka & Małecka-Panas, 2007).

It is difficult to explain the relation between the occurrence of fungi and the development of inflammations because candidiasis of the oral cavity and further segments of the GI tract is not the frequent subject of investigations. Recent studies on the role of fungi of the genus *Candida* in inflammatory bowel diseases were performed in the group of patients with IBD whose clinical samples for mycological investigations were collected by means of colonoscopy (biopsy taken from the large intestine, aspirate from the intestinal contents and brush-smears), as well as the throat smear and the examination of feces. Samples were taken from patients in various periods of symptom aggravation. It was revealed that despite the abundant increase of fungi in throat and feces cultures no essential settlement of fungi on the mucous membrane of the large intestine was noted. However, while performing regular mycological studies of the group of patients with the history of the 5-year- course of the disease fungi were isolated from all clinical samples in each acute stage of the disease. It was shown that the presence of fungi in the oral cavity of this group of patients could affect the significantly frequent fungal colonization of the mucous membrane of the large intestine in the active phase of the disease. The possibility of the transmission of the fungal flora of the oral cavity to other segments of the GI tract was confirmed on the basis of 100% affinity of *C.albicans* strains isolated from the same patient, examined by means of the PCR-RAPD method (Trojanowska et al., 2010).

In the most recent studies the diagnostics of invasive fungal inflammations includes molecular methods based on DNA and RNA analyses. The polymerase chain reaction (PCR) with its various modifications is routinely used. One of them is RAPD (*Random Amplified Polymorphism DNA*), commonly used in epidemiological investigations because of its rapid and simple procedure and the possibility of the simultaneous comparison of a large number of strains.

Strain typing based on PCR-RAPD enables the determination of genetic affinity of investigated strains or their distinctiveness in the particular time. The RAPD method is based on the reaction of amplification using short starters with the randomized base sequence, which bind to the analysed DNA in various sites, depending on the investigated strain. The presence or the lack of differences in the electrophoretic partition signifies the differentiation or compatibility of strains. It is used to perform epidemiological investigations which aim at determining the source of infection and the clonal characterization of distinguished isolates. In addition, it is possible to watch the transmission of strains which cause the inflammation, or monitor the therapy. In case of the infection relapse the analysis of isolated strains enables to detect if it is caused by the same strain which can suggest the ineffective therapy or if it is due to other strains suggesting the recurred infection (Dzierżanowska, 2006).

C.albicans is the most commonly isolated species from the GI tract and as the opportunistic flora can easily adapt itself to many sites of the body. However, as the non-pathogenic intestinal flora it can be replaced by rarely isolated but more virulent non-albicans strains, such as: *C.glabrata, C.tropicalis* and *C.krusei*. It is significant to explain if non-albicans species isolated from various clinical samples of the same patient can constitute one clone transferred from the oral cavity to the lower segments of the GI tract or if various factors affect the genetic diversity of isolated strains?

2. The aim of the study

The aim of the study was the determination of the genetic diversity of *Candida spp.* strains isolated from clinical samples of various segments of the GI tract of the same patient using PCR-RAPD method and the assessment of the transmission of non-albicans strains in the alimentary tract based on the analysis of obtained results of genetic investigations.

3. Materials and methods

The material for the study consisted of 39 *Candida spp.* strains isolated from clinical samples taken by means of colonoscopy and from the oral cavity and feces of patients diagnosed in the Department of Gastroenterology, Hepatology and Infective Diseases of Jagiellonian University Collegium Medicum in Cracow. The strains came from 7 patients. In four of them ulcerative colitis was diagnosed and three of them developed Crohn`s disease. In six patients non-albicans strains were cultured on all clinical samples and in one patient *C.albicans* strains were cultured on samples taken from the GI tract twice, at one-year-interval. Clinical samples for mycological examinations were taken in various periods of symptom aggravation. The smear and feces were examined before preparing the patient for colonoscopy during which the biopsy was taken from the affected mucous membrane of the large intestine as well as the aspirate of intestinal contents and the brush-smear.The identification of fungi was carried out using the CAN2 chromogenic base (bioMerieux) and API Candida tests (bioMerieux). Genetic examinations were performed using the PCR-RAPD technique for 10 *C.albicans* strains isolated from 1 patient, 20 *C.glabrata* strains from 4 patients, 5 *C.tropicalis* strains from 1 patient and 4 *C.krusei* strains from 1 patient.

3.1 DNA isolation

From the 48-hour-culture of strains on the Sabouraud agar (bioMerieux) the suspension in 0.85% NaCl was compounded. Genomic DNA was isolated using Genomic Mini AX YEAST (A&A Biotechnology). DNA concentration was marked spectrophotometrically at the wave length equal to 260nm.

3.2 PCR-RAPD reaction

In the PCR-RAPD reaction 3 primers were used: CD16AS(5`-CTC TTG AAA CTG GGG AGA CTT GA-3`), ERIC2 (5`-AAG TAA GTG ACT GGG GTG AGC G-3`) and HP1247 (5`-AAG AGC CCG T-3`). The reaction was conducted using Promega reagents. The reaction mixture in its final volume of 25 ul contained: 5 ul 5x colourless Go Taq Flexi Buffer (ph 8.5), 1.5 ul 25mM MgCl2, 100 uM of each nucleotide, 100pmol primer and 0.625 U Go Taq DNA polymerase. The following RAPD reaction conditions were stated for the examined strains: initial denaturation at 94°C for 5 min, 45 cycles comprising the true denaturation at 94°C for 1 min, primer attachment at 36°C for 1 min, elongation at 72°C for 1 min and final prolongation at 72°C for 7 min.

3.3 Electrophoresis in the agarose gel

Reaction products were detected during electrophoresis in the 2% agarose gel (Sigma), in the TBE buffer (Tris-Borate Buffer) and the differentiation of the electrophoresis image of PCR-RAPD reaction products in the BIO-PROFIL Bio-ID++ program was analysed (Vilber-Lormat, France).

4. Results

The assessment of the *Candida spp.* strain transmission in the GI tract was performed on the basis of the PCR-RAPD reaction product analysis comprising the determination of a degree of affinity between strains isolated from particular segments of the GI tract of the same patient. The examinations included strains isolated from the following clinical samples: throat smear (1), biopsy of the affected wall of the large intestine (2), aspirate of intestinal contents (3), brush-smear from the intestine (4), feces (5). *C.glabrata* was isolated from clinical samples of 4 patients, *C.tropicalis* and *C.krusei* were isolated from other examined patients and *C.albicans* was isolated from the same patient twice, at one-year-interval. The selective amplification of the genetic material obtained from examined strains with CD16SA, ERIC2 and HP1247 primers confirmed 100% homology among *C.albicans* strains isolated for the first time from the patient No.I (Fig.1) and *C.glabrata* strains from the patient No.II (Fig.2).

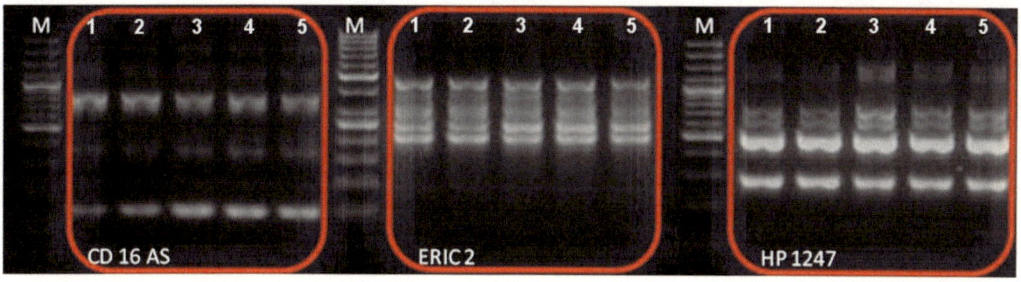

1- throat smear, 2- colonic biopsy, 3- aspirate of intestinal contents, 4- brush-smear from the intestine, 5- feces, M- marker (100bp)

Fig. 1. Distribution of the products of PCR-RAPD reaction with three primers (CD 16 AS, ERIC-2, HP 1247) on agarose gel, showing similarities between *C.albicans* strains isolated from patient No.I (the first isolation).

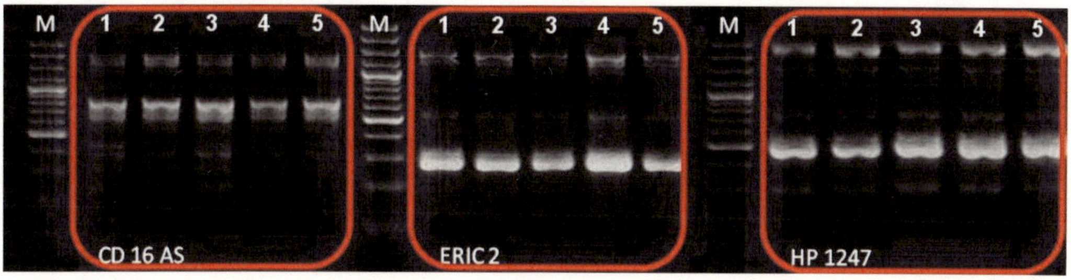

1- throat smear, 2- colonic biopsy, 3- aspirate of intestinal contents, 4- brush-smear from the intestine, 5- feces, M- marker (100bp)

Fig. 2. Distribution of the products of PCR-RAPD reaction with three primers (CD 16 AS, ERIC-2, HP 1247) on agarose gel, showing similarities between *C.glabrata* strains isolated from patient No.II.

100% compatibility was also revealed with two primers (CD16AS and ERIC2) in case of *C.glabrata* from the patient No.III and the HP1247 primer showed 100% compatibility between strains taken from the throat, biopsy, aspirate and feces as well as 80% strain homology from the brush-smear (Fig.3). Similarly, 100% homology with CD16AS and ERIC2 primers was obtained in case of *C.tropicalis* from the patient No.VI and over 80% homology with the HP1247 primer was achieved (Fig.7).

The homology lower than 90% with three primers was found among *C.albicans* cultured a year after the first isolation from the patient No.I (Fig.5), *C.glabrata* derived from the patient No.IV (Fig.6) and the patient No.V (Fig.7) as well as *C.krusei* isolated from the patient No.VII (Fig.8).

A degree of homology equal to or exceeding 90% was assumed as a criterium of the lack of genetic strain diversity (Speijer et al., 1999) (Tab.1).

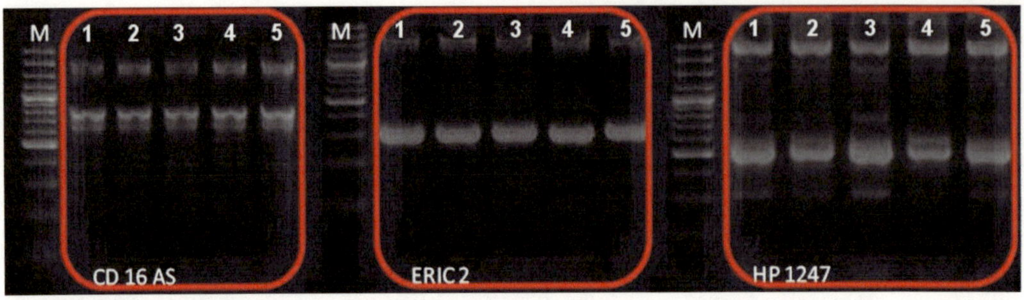

1- throat smear, 2- colonic biopsy, 3- aspirate of intestinal contents, 4- brush-smear from the intestine, 5- feces, M- marker (100bp)

Fig. 3. Distribution of the products of PCR-RAPD reaction with three primers (CD 16 AS, ERIC-2, HP 1247) on agarose gel, showing similarities between *C.glabrata* strains isolated from patient No.III.

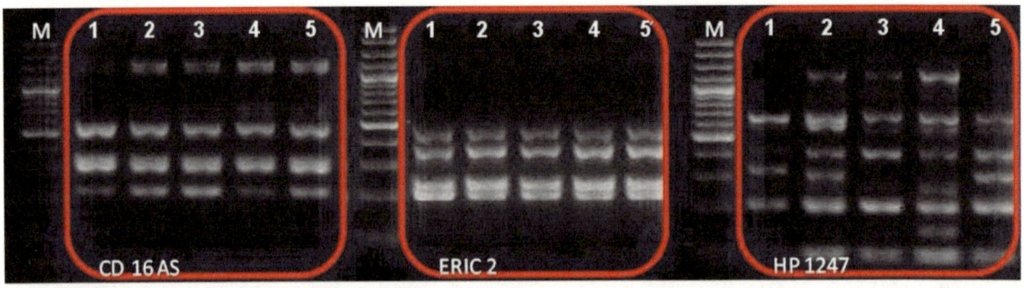

1- throat smear, 2- colonic biopsy, 3- aspirate of intestinal contents, 4- brush-smear from the intestine, 5- feces, M- marker (100bp)

Fig. 4. Distribution of the products of PCR-RAPD reaction with three primers (CD 16 AS, ERIC-2, HP 1247) on agarose gel, showing similarities between *C.tropicalis* strains isolated from patient No.VI.

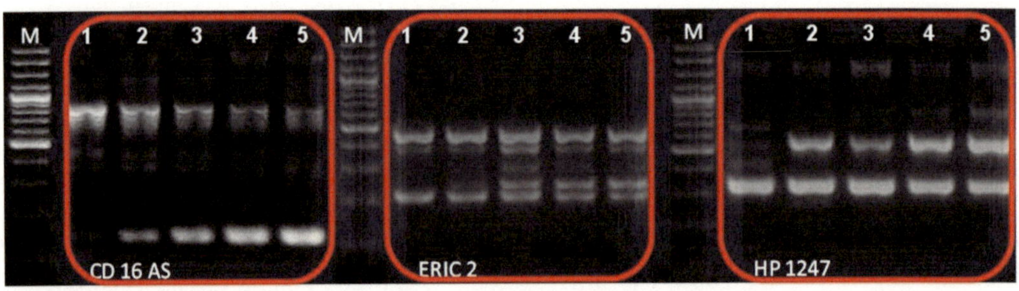

1- throat smear, 2- colonic biopsy, 3- aspirate of intestinal contents, 4- brush-smear from the intestine, 5- feces, M- marker (100bp)

Fig. 5. Distribution of the products of PCR-RAPD reaction with three primers (CD 16 AS, ERIC-2, HP 1247) on agarose gel, showing similarities between *C.albicans* strains isolated from patient No.I (second isolation).

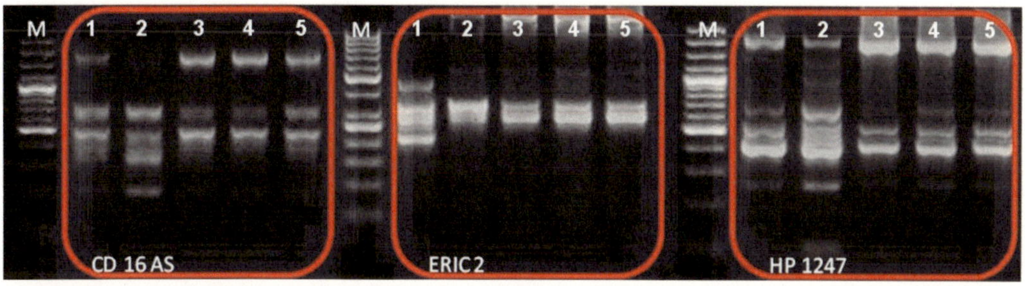

1- throat smear, 2- colonic biopsy, 3- aspirate of intestinal contents, 4- brush-smear from the intestine, 5- feces, M- marker (100bp)

Fig. 6. Distribution of the products of PCR-RAPD reaction with three primers (CD 16 AS, ERIC-2, HP 1247) on agarose gel, showing similarities between *C.glabrata* strains isolated from patient No.IV.

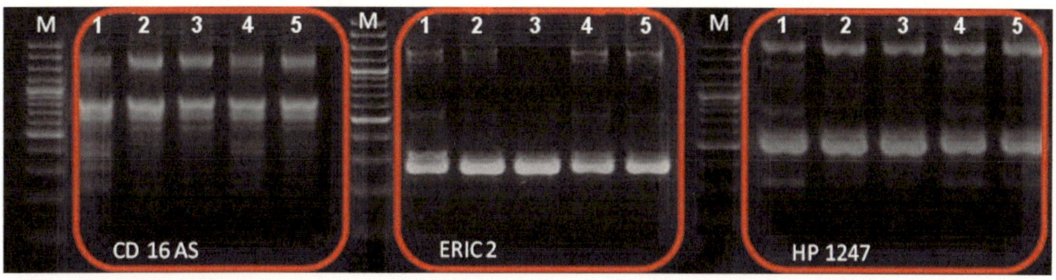

1- throat smear, 2- colonic biopsy, 3- aspirate of intestinal contents, 4- brush-smear from the intestine, 5- feces, M- marker (100bp)

Fig. 7. Distribution of the products of PCR-RAPD reaction with three primers (CD 16 AS, ERIC-2, HP 1247) on agarose gel, showing similarities between *C.glabrata* strains isolated from patient No.V.

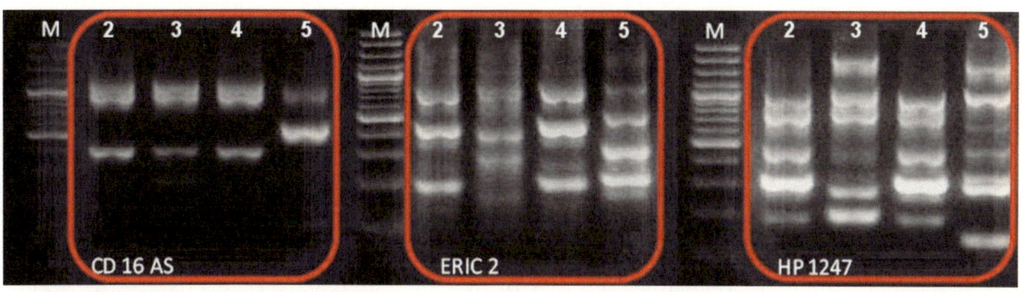

2- colonic biopsy, 3- aspirate of intestinal contents, 4- brush-smear from the intestine, 5- feces, M- marker (100bp)

Fig. 8. Distribution of the products of PCR-RAPD reaction with three primers (CD 16 AS, ERIC-2, HP 1247) on agarose gel, showing similarities between *C.krusei* strains isolated from patient No.VII.

Patient	Strain	Degree of homology
I	*Candida albicans*	>90%
I	*Candida albicans*	<90%
II	*Candida glabrata*	>90%
III	*Candida glabrata*	>90%
IV	*Candida glabrata*	<90%
V	*Candida glabrata*	<90%
VI	*Candida tropicalis*	>90%
VII	*Candida krusei*	<90%

Table 1. A degree of homology among *Candida spp.* strains isolated from clinical samples from patients with IBD.

5. Discussion

Results of earlier investigations performed in a group of patients with IBD confirmed the possibility of the oral cavity fungal flora transmission to further segments of the GI tract on the basis of 100% genetic affinity among isolated *C.albicans* strains in the PCR-RAPD method (Trojanowska et al., 2010). It was an impulse for performing current investigations which include the analysis if non-albicans strains isolated from various clinical samples, taken from the same patient turn out to be one clone or not and if not, which factors cause the genetic diversity among these strains?

The analysis of *C.albicans* genotypes isolated from the patient No.I in the first examination of the acute stage of the disease revealed 100% homology of all strains. The passage of *C.albicans* is highly probable due to the properties of this fungal species. It is the most common opportunistic species having a great ability to adapt itself to various environments of the body, which is determined by the high expression of virulent factors responsible for the pathogen invasion (enzymes, phenotypic variability, adhesion) (Dzierżanowska, 2006). It is extremely interesting that the analysis of *C.albicans* strains isolated from the same patient after one-year-observation showed the larger variability of strains, especially the strain isolated from the oral cavity whose similarity to other strains amounted to 61-90%, depending on the used primer. The change could have been affected by the used therapy and in the result by the selection of the more resistant clone. This finding is confirmed by investigations performed by Tanaka, which enabled to divide strains isolated during the course of candidiasis into three groups. One of them included strains which were replaced by other strains during the course of the disease (Tanaka , 1997). In our investigations, which analysed non-albicans strains, 100% similarity was confirmed in *C.glabrata* strains isolated from patients No.II and III as well as the patient No.IV (*C.tropicalis*), using CD16AS and ERIC2 primers while the HP1247 primer turned out to be more differentiating for investigated strains. Other patients (No.IV, V, VII) developed the larger differentiation between strains. The attention should be focused on the fact that some differences in the *Candida spp.* strain homology can be determined by the limited repeatability of the PCR-RAPD method as well as its considerable susceptibility to changes of reaction conditions, such as: the concentration of the primer and other reaction constituents (Wolinowska, 2002). Moreover, slight genome mutations affecting the RAPD profile change may emerge during the frequent strain passage and a long-term culture (Lehmann et al., 1992). The patient`s condition, susceptibility to infection and the used therapy are also significant in the selection and differentiation of strains.

Inflammatory processes which accompany the main disease are essential factors predisposing to the invasive growth of *Candida* in patients with IBD. These patients develop pathological factors in the structure of the GI wall, disturbed immunological mechanisms and a disproportion in the proper intestinal flora composition, which promote the excessive fungal development (Zwolińska-Wcisło et al., 2009). Patients from this group undergo the complex therapy including glucocorticoids and immunosuppressants which inhibit inflammatory reactions in intestines but suppress the immunity of the body leading to the spread of the fungal flora in areas which are specially favorable for its multiplication.

Inflammatory bowel diseases are still the subject of many publications. It is interesting because of theoretical and cognitive issues in the aspect of discovering new etiopathogenetic mechanisms as well as practical ones concerning the use of new diagnostic and therapeutic methods. The knowledge of IBD mechanisms enables the more precise intervention into particular stages of the inflammatory process and the elaboration of methods to control the inflammation. It also allows to minimize adverse effects and eventually to improve the quality of life of patients affected by these diseases. The chronic character of IBD, periodic aggravations of the disease, the high activity of the inflammatory process as well as not always adequate response to the introduced treatment make these diseases serious clinical problems (Montgomery & Ekbom, 2002; Colombel et al., 2008). Variety of clinical symptoms, complications and systemic effects make that the differential diagnostics comprises numerous diseases (Grzymisławski & Kanikowska, 2010).Apart from some bacterial infections, other inflammatory diseases with the clinical picture resembling IBD, such as: tuberculosis as well as parasitic and fungal inflammations should be taken into consideration (Radwan et al., 2009).

Investigations confirm (Trojanowska et al., 2010) that acute stages of these diseases reveal the presence of fungi in all clinical samples taken from the GI tract. As the endogenic flora fungi can be the cause of abnormal immunological mechanisms in IBD and in consequence can cause the development of systemic candidiasis (Radwan et al., 2009). The diagnostics of GI fungal diseases is based on imaging techniques (endoscopy), microscopic methods (histological preparations), and mycological, serological and genetic investigations (Biliński et al., 2008).The molecular analysis enables to detect the presence of genes determining factors of fungal virulence and genes resistant to antifungal drugs (Wolinowska, 2002). Nowadays, there is an increase of the number of inflammations due to *C.krusei* and *C.glabrata* strains resistant to fluconazole, the drug which is mostly used in the prevention of candidiasis in patients with IBD.

Fungi of the genus *Candida* constitute the essential etiological factors of opportunistic inflammations. The development of medicine and the introduction of new therapeutic strategies paradoxically contribute to the increase of fungal inflammations. It is mostly connected with an increasing number of patients with immunosuppression and disturbed homeostasis (Schelenz, 2008).

6. Conclusions

The transmission of *Candida spp.* strains in the GI tract, especially the most frequently isolated *C.albicans* and *C.glabrata* strains, is possible. Therefore, the fungi in the oral cavity of patients with IBD cannot be regarded exclusively as saprophytic flora, which in the active phase of IBD, can multiply and disseminate to further parts of the GI tract. This fact suggests justifiability of using antifungal therapy, wich can provide the relief of symptoms of candidiasis or decrease in their intensity.

This knowledge can be used in prophylaxis, diagnostics and in monitoring the treatment of GI tract candidiasis. The confirmation of candidiasis with the *C.glabrata* or *C.krusei* etiology requires the elimination of fluconazole which is commonly used in the prevention and the treatment of candidiasis. The introduced therapy which causes the selection of the more resistant clone can affect the genetic diversity of strains.

7. References

Berhardt, H. & Knoke, M. (1997). Mycological aspects of gastrointestinal microflora. *Scandinavian Journal of Gastroenterology*, Vol.32, Suppl. 222, pp. 102-106, 0036-5521.

Biliński, P.; Seferyńska, I. & Warzocha, K. (2008). Diagnostyka i leczenie układowych zakażeń grzybiczych w onkohematologii. *Onkologia w Praktyce Klinicznej*, Vol.4, No.1, pp. 15-24, 1734–3542.

Budak, A.; Bogdał, J. & Zwolińska-Wcisło, M. (2003). Kolonizacja grzybicza przewodu pokarmowego w badaniach klinicznych i doświadczalnych. *Przewodnik Lekarza*, Vol.6, No.9, pp. 81-89, 1505-8409.

Colombel, I.F.; Watson, A.I.M. & Neurath, M. (2008). The 10 remaining mysteries of inflammatory bowel disease. *Gut*, Vol.57, No.4, pp. 429-433, 0017-5749.

Dzierżanowska, D. (Ed.). (2006). *Zakażenia grzybicze: wybrane zagadnienia*, Alfa-Medica Press, 83-88778-99-42006, Bielsko Biała, Poland.

Grzymisławski, M. & Kanikowska, A. (2010). Pozajelitowe manifestacje nieswoistych zapaleń jelit. *Gastroenterologia Praktyczna*, Vol.4, No.5, pp. 40-48, 2080-9956.

Jain, N.; Kohli, R.; Cook, E.; Gialanella, P.; Chang, T. & Fries, B.C. (2007). Biofilm formation and antifungal susceptibility of *Candida* isolates from urine. *Applied and Environmental Microbiology*, Vol.73, No.6, pp. 1697-1703, 0099-2240.

Konturek, S.J. (Ed.). (2001). *Gastroenterologia i hepatologia kliniczna*. Wydawnictwo Lekarskie PZWL, 83-200-2439-0, Warszawa, Poland.

Lehmann, P.F.; Lin, D. & Lasker, B.A. (1992). Genotypic identification and characterization of species and strains within the genus *Candida* by using random amplified polymorphic DNA. *Journal of Clinical Microbiology*, Vol.30, No.12, pp. 3249-3254, 0095-1137.

Mokrowiecka, A. & Małecka-Panas, E. (2007). Różnicowanie i leczenie nieswoistych chorób zapalnych jelit. *Przewodnik Lekarza*, Vol.10, No.1, pp. 56-65, 1505-8409.

Montgomery, S.M. & Ekbom, A. (2002). Epidemiology of inflammatory bowel disease. *Current Opinion in Gastroenterology*, Vol.18, No.4 , pp. 416-420, 0267-1379.

Muszyński, J. (2001). Nieswoiste zapalenia jelit. *Przewodnik Lekarza*, Vol.4, No.6, pp. 22-30, 1505-8409.

Pfaller, M.A. & Diekema, D.J. (2007). Epidemiology of invasive candidiasis: a persistent public health problem. *Clinical Microbiology Reviews*, Vol.20, No.1, pp. 133-163, 0893-8512.

Polińska, B.; Matowicka-Karna, J. & Kemona, H. (2009). The cytokines in inflammatory bowel disease. *Postępy Higieny i Medycyny Doświadczalnej*, Vol. 63, pp. 389-394, 1732-2693.

Radwan, P.; Radwan-Kwiatek, K. & Skrzydło-Radomańska, B. (2009). Rola mikroflory jelitowej w nieswoistych zapaleniach jelit. *Przegląd Gastroenterologiczny*, Vol.4, No.1, pp. 1-6, 1895-5770.

Ramag, G.; Martinez, J.P. & Lopez-Ribot, J.L. (2006). *Candida* biofilms on implantem materials: a clinically significant problem. *FEMS Yeast Research*, Vol.6, No.7, pp. 979-986, 1567-1356.

Rzeszutko, M. (2006). Inflammatory bowel disease - histopathological approach. *Gastroenterologia Polska*, Vol.13, No.6, pp. 485-491, 1232-9886.

Schelenz, S. (2008). Management of candidiasis in the intensive care unit. *Journal of Antimicrobial Chemotherapy*, Vol.61, Suppl.1, pp. 31-34, 0305-7453.

Speijer, H.; Savelkoul, P.H.M.; Bonten, M.J. Stobberingh, E.E. & Tjhie, J.H. (1999). Application of different genotyping methods for *Pseudomonas aeruginosa* in a setting of endemicity in an intensive care unit. *Journal of Clinical Microbiology*, Vol.37, No.11, 3654-3661, 0095-1137.

Tanaka, K. (1997). Strain-relatedness among different populations of pathogenic yeast *Candida albicans* analyzed by DNA typing methods. *Nagoya Journal of Medical Science*, Vol.60, No.(1-2), pp. 1-14, 0027-7622.

Trojanowska, D.; Zwolińska-Wcisło, M.; Tokarczyk, M.; Kosowski, K.; Mach, T. & Budak, A. (2010). The role of *Candida* in inflammatory bowel disease. Estimation of transmission of *C.albicans* fungi in gastrointestinal tract based on genetic affinity between strains. *Medical Science Monitor*, Vol.16, No.6, pp. 451-457, 1234-1010.

Warnock, D.W. & Campbell, C.K. (1996). Medical mycology. *Mycological Research*, Vol.100, No.10, pp. 1153-1162, 0953-7562.

Wolinowska, R. (Ed.). (2002) *Metody molekularne w diagnostyce mikrobiologicznej*. Wydawnictwo Akademii Medycznej w Warszawie, 83-88559-48-6, Warszawa, Poland.

Zwolińska-Wcisło, M.; Budak, A.; Trojanowska D.; Mach, T.; Rudnicka-Sosin, L.; Galicka-Latała, D.; Nowak, P. & Cibor D. (2006). Wpływ kolonizacji grzybów *Candida* na przebieg wrzodziejącego zapalenia jelita grubego. *Przegląd Lekarski*, Vol.63, No.7, pp. 533-538, 0033-2240.

Zwolińska-Wcisło, M.; Brzozowski, T.; Budak, A.; Kwiecień, S.; Sliwowski, Z.; Drozdowicz, D.; Trojanowska, D.; Rudnicka-Sosin, L.; Mach, T.; Konturek, S.J. & Pawlik, W.W. (2009). Effect of *Candida* colonization on human ulcerative colitis and the healing of inflammatory changes of the colon in the experimental model of *colitis ulcerosa* . *Journal of Physiology And Pharmacology*, Vol.60, No.1, pp. 107-118, 0867-5910.

13

A 9-Year Retrospective Study of Hospitalized IBD Patients in Shanghai Rui Jin Hospital

Tianle Ma, Lulu Sheng, Xiaodi Yang, Shuijin Zhu,
Jie Zhong, Yaozong Yuan and Shihu Jiang
Ruijin Hospital affiliated to Medical School of Shanghai Jiao Tong University
China

1. Introduction

Inflammatory bowel disease (IBD), comprising of Crohn's disease (CD) and ulcerative colitis (UC), is a kind of chronic relapsing disorder of unknown etiology, which is characterized clinically of abdominal pain, diarrhea, weight loss, fever, as well as endoscopic, radiologic, histopathologic findings and biochemical changes (e.g. perinuclear anti-neutrophil cytoplasm antibody (p-ANCA), anti-Saccharomyces cerevisiae antibody (ASCA) and IBD-specific p-ANCA markers) (Veluswamy et al., 2010).

IBDs have been shown to be involved with potential factors such as genetic, immunologic, bacterial, and environmental elements; the relative strength of these factors and the importance of their interplay remain largely unknown (Edwards et al., 2008). Differences in incidence rates across age, time, and geographic areas suggest that environmental factors are involved in IBD, while only cigarette smoking and appendectomy have consistently been identified as risk factors (Colombel et al., 2007). Familial aggregation of IBD showed by an epidemiological study first suggested that genetic factors might play an important role in the pathogenesis of IBD. In 2001, the first CD susceptibility gene, NOD2/CARD15 on chromosome 16, was characterized. The gene identification should help us to understand the complex interaction between the environment and the intestinal immune system.

The previous studies of IBD led to a complex overall impression of the disease, with some described patterns in disease prevalence. IBD was considered to be more frequent in the developed countries especially Northern Europe and the United States, usually of colder climates with increased incidence as distance from the equator increases. But now, IBD is increasingly reported in non-classical populations and in developing regions such as Asia, the Mid-East and Africa. More recent data showed significantly higher prevalence in Asians and time trend studies described an increasing trend in the incidence of UC and a similar but lower rise in CD (Goh & Xiao, 2009).

The epidemiological changes that are taking place mirror the experience of Western countries 50 years ago. And the changes seem to occur in parallel with the rapid socioeconomic developments in Asia. It appears that certain racial groups among Asians who are more susceptible to IBD and who will demonstrate a higher frequency of IBD when exposed to putative environment.

In recent years, with the improvement of living standard, the global incidence and prevalence are increasing year by year, which has seriously affected quality of life all over the world.

Because IBDs are chronic, life-long immunologic disorders that frequently require hospitalization or surgery. Such hospitalizations account for a significant portion of the estimated USD 6 billion in healthcare costs annually for IBD in the USA (Cappelman et al., 2008). With regards to the treatments of IBD, it mainly focuses on two aims, one is to induct the ease of acute outbreak; and another is to maintain the alleviation (Domènech, 2006). The traditional drugs used for IBD mainly include 5-aminosalicylic acid, glucocorticoid, and immune inhibitors. In recent years, with the deeper understandings of IBD immunity mechanism, more biological agents have been introduced in the treatment and they have brought new dawn for IBD patients. The advantages of new biological agents in the treatment of IBD spark the clinical debate between the traditional Set-Up way and the new Set-Down strategy (Baert et al., 2007).

Clinically apparent malnutrition is more frequent among IBD admissions than those of non-IBD admissions. Its association with greater mortality and resource utilization may reflect more severe underlying disease that may lead to both malnutrition and worse outcomes. Nevertheless, diagnosable malnutrition may serve as a clinical marker of poor IBD prognosis in hospitalized patients (Nguyen et al., 2008). Therefore, nutrition support for IBD patients plays an important role in the treatment of IBD (Cao et al., 2005). Many previous studies have focused on different aspects of nutrition support, such as nutritional immunology, nutrition pharmacology and so on. The results of the current meta-analysis and multicenter randomized controlled clinical studies have lead to the conclusions that nutrition support especially the enteral nutrition support may induce illness ease, promote mucosal healings, and help maintaining the long-term stability of the disease.

Numerous studies from Europe and North America have provided a wealth of information regarding the epidemiological and clinical characteristics of IBDs in Caucasians. While large clinical material of IBD in China is still limited. The aim of this study is to systematically provide a relatively intact image of IBD patients in our hospital during the past 9 years, which may also be a valuable reference of the situation in China. The reason why we choosing this period of time is because April 2003 was the start of clinical application of double balloon enteroscopy (DBE) in our hospital, and then was also the start when the diagnostic yield of Crohn's Disease in our hospital significantly increased.

2. Patients and methods

2.1 Study population and data collection

The data source of this study was from Shanghai Rui Jin Hospital another from May 2002 to December 2010. It covered all hospitalized IBD patients during a period of 9 years from department of gastroenterology, department of surgery and department of pediatrics. The diagnosis of IBD adhered to the criteria of Lennard-Jones (Lennard-Jones, 1989). Rui Jin Hospital is a tertiary level and first-class public hospital, it serves a well-defined catchment population in Shanghai. Over 96% of the medical care is provided by the public hospital system in this district. About 30% of the hospitalized patients were from the nearby provinces and all over China.

The total hospitalization number enrolled in this retrospective study was 769.The following data were collected and analyzed among the patients: the demographic characteristics (mainly included age and gender), the duration of the disease at diagnosis, the inspection methods used for diagnosis, the location of the lesions involved, the lab data of the patients, and the treatments followed by the convinced diagnosis (medical treatments and/or surgical treatments).

The DBE devices used in the study were manufactured by Fujinon (EN 450P5/20, EN 450T5/20; Fujinon Inc, Saitama, Japan).

2.2 Statistical analysis

We adopt the hierarchical analysis method. All the IBD in-patients during the last 9 years were divided into 3 groups according to the time when they were hospitalized: May 2002 to December 2004 as Group 1, January 2005 to December 2007 as Group 2, January 2008 to December 2010 as Group 3. The study made a longitudinal comparison among the 3 groups, and also made a horizontal comparison between the CD group and the UC group according to the statistical results.

Data analysis was performed using SPSS 17.0 statistical software package (SPSS Inc., Chicago, USA). Continuous variables were summarized using means and standard deviations, while categorical variables were expressed as proportions. Variables were compared with the chi-square test. P value <0.05 was judged of statistical difference, while <0.01 was judged of significantly statistical difference.

3. Results

3.1 Demographic characteristics

Overall, a total number of 769 hospitalized IBD patients were included in this study. Among them, 536 patients suffered CD (69.7%) and 233 patients suffered UC (30.3%), the percentage of CD was significantly higher than that of UC. Mean ages at diagnosis were 36.8±15.4 years old (range 2-88 years) in CD and 44.9±17.3 years old (range 3-83 years) in UC patients. The gender ratio (male/female) was 1.60 in CD and 1.28 in UC, there existed no statistical difference between these two groups (p>0.05). The mean duration of CD at first hospitalization was 5.6±4.7 years (1-70 years), of UC was 5.8±3.8 years (1-25 years).

Group	**CD** (n=536)		**UC** (n=233)		Sum.
	Num. (male: female)	Mean age	Num. (male: female)	Mean age	
Group 1 (2002-2004)	76 (46:30)	42.6±15.2	69 (35:34)	50.0±16.4	145
Group 2 (2005-2007)	186 (119:67)	39.5±15.1	71 (42:29)	46.9±14.7	257
Group 3 (2008-2010)	274 (166:108)	33.4±14.9	93 (54:39)	39.5±18.5	367
Total	536 (331:205)	36.8±15.4	233 (131:102)	44.9±17.3	769

Table 1. Comparison of demographic characteristics among 3 groups

For each stratified period, the results were showed in Table 1. As we could see, the diagnosed numbers of both CD and UC increased with the year, while the ages at diagnosis were decreased. Number of male patients was more than that of female patients in both diseases in each group.

3.2 Diagnostic modalities

With the development and clinical applications of novel techniques for small bowel inspection, such as double balloon enteroscopy (DBE), multisliced CT enterography (MSCTE) and capsule endoscopy (CE), the diagnostic yield of IBD significantly increased in our hospital during the past decade.

Group	MSCTE		Enteroscopy		CE	
	CD (%)	UC (%)	CD (%)	UC (%)	CD (%)	UC (%)
1	4/76 (5.3)	7/69 (10.1)	74/76 (97.4)	66/69 (95.7)	7/76 (9.2)	0/69
2	67/186 (36.1)	6/71 (8.5)	168/186 (90.3)	65/71 (91.5)	22/186 (11.8)	1/71 (1.4)
3	210/274 (76.6)	23/93 (24.7)	266/274 (97.1)	88/93 (94.6)	35/274 (12.8)	2/93 (2.2)

Table 2. Panorama of diagnostic modalities applied in IBD during 2002-2010

The panorama of diagnostic modalities applications was summarized in Table 2. Enteroscopy (in the current study, both colonoscopy and DBE were included) was still the major diagnostic modality in IBD identification. Application of MSCTE became quite common both in CD and UC during year of 2008-2010 (Group 3), the total percentages of patients accepted MSCTE examines raised up to 63.5% (233/367) in all IBDs. Meanwhile, it was revealed that the use of CE was still limited in our hospital.
And we also analyzed the number of patient undertaken more than one single inspection: double inspections and all 3 inspections in different time groups (Tab. 3). In our hospital, the costs of each inspection method were: RMB 300 for colonoscopy, RMB 2,600 for antegrade/retrograde DBE, RMB 1,100 for MSCTE and RMB 2,800 for CE. Though a combination of different inspections may help increasing diagnostic yield, the high expense restricted its clinical application.

Inspection	Group 1		Group 2		Group 3	
	CD (%) (n=76)	UC (%) (n=69)	CD (%) (n=186)	UC (%) (n=71)	CD (%) (n=274)	UC (%) (n=93)
Double	12(15.8)	3(4.3)	31(16.7)	2(2.8)	103(37.6)	17(18.3)
Triple	4(5.3)	0	0	0	0	0

Table 3. Trends of modality combination during the year of 2002-2010

Figure 1 showed the trends of application of enteroscopy, MSCTE, and CE in CD patients during 2002 to 2010. Figure 2 showed the situation in UC. In the histograms, intuitive situation could be observed. During the year of 2008 to 2010, MSCTE became a screening method for CD patients, the application ratio was up to 76.6%.

3.3 Anatomic extent

In this study, we adopted a special scoring method to evaluate the anatomic extent. We scored 1 when the lesion only involved rectosigmoid colon, ileocecal or one segment of small intestine; scored 2 when the lesion extended up to left-sided colon, and scored 3 when

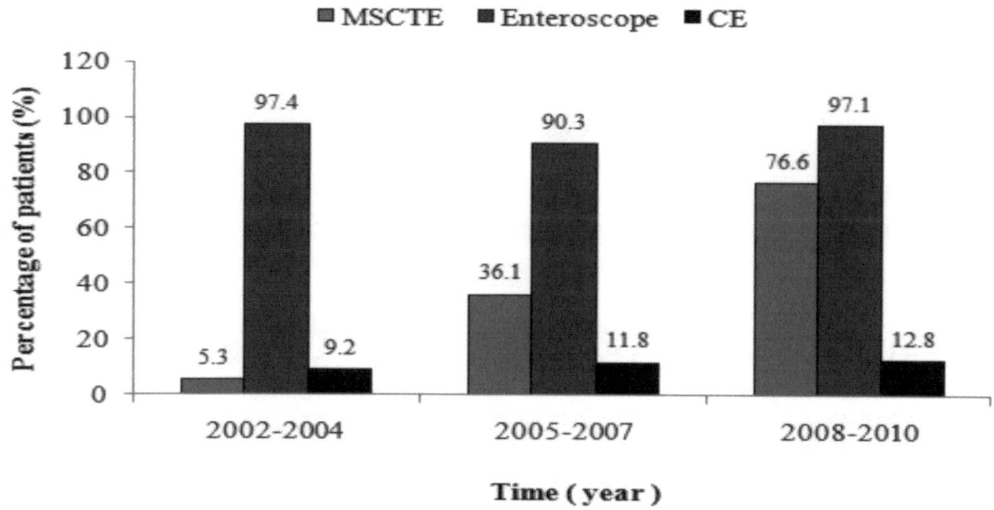

Fig. 1. Application of MSCTE, enteroscope, and CE in CD patients during the retrospective 9 years

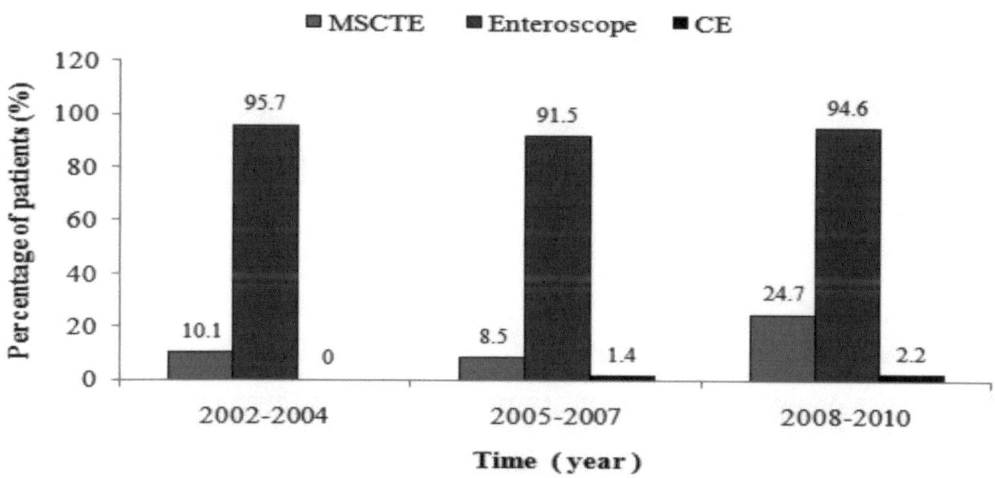

Fig. 2. Application of MSCTE, enteroscope, and CE in UC patients during the retrospective 9 years

the lesion extensively involved the whole length of the colon and/or multiple segments of the small intestine. Then the number of patients of each scoring group was summarized, respectively (Tab. 4).

As we can see, in Group of Score 1, CD was significantly more than UC ($p=0.000<0.001$), which indicated that the anatomic extent of CD is relatively limited comparing with that of UC. While in Group of Score 3, the situation was just the opposite ($p=0.000<0.001$), UC was more likely to involve extensively.

Score	CD (%)	UC (%)	X^2	P value
1	393 (73.3)	137 (58.8)	15.991	0.000
2	85 (15.9)	44 (18.9)	1.065	0.302
3	58 (10.8)	52 (22.3)	17.511	0.000
Total number	536	233		

Table 4. Comparison of anatomic extent in CD and UC

3.4 Laboratory index

Although there are a lot of laboratory parameters believed to have certain relations with the severity of IBDs, the accurate role of each item remains controversial. In the present study, we observed 3 laboratory indexes with more confirming evidence of the clinical value. They are PLT, ESR (erythrocyte sedimentation rate) and CRP (C reactive protein). The criteria of each index were judged according to that of our hospital. PLT concentration higher than $300*10^9/L$, ESR level exceeded 30mm/s, CRP over 0.8mg/L were judged of abnormal.

Primarily research and clinical experience have presented that patients with IBD suffer higher risk of colonic cancer comparing with normal population, thus IBD patients should under the surveillance of tumor marker in order to provide information of the possibility of advancing cancer. Therefore, we also evaluated 3 tumor markers (CEA, CA-125 and CA-199) in all the patients.

According to the results (Tab. 5), we had a rough impression that both ESR level and CRP level were higher in CD than in UC in Group 2 and Group 3. While other lab index showed no obvious difference between CD and UC in all 3 groups.

Lab Index	**Group 1**		**Group 2**		**Group 3**	
	CD (%) (n=76)	**UC** (%) (n=69)	**CD** (%) (n=186)	**UC** (%) (n=71)	**CD** (%) (n=274)	**UC** (%) (n=93)
PLT (>300*10⁹/L)	26 (34.2)	24 (34.8)	96 (51.6)	36 (50.7)	164(59.9)	29 (31.2)
ESR (>30 mm/s)	28 (36.8)	19 (27.5)	142(76.3)	38 (53.5)	143(52.2)	34 (36.6)
CRP (>0.8 mg/L)	12 (15.8)	12 (17.4)	161(86.6)	33 (46.5)	163(59.5)	21 (22.6)
CEA (>5 ng/ml)	8 (10.5)	0	12 (6.5)	2 (2.8)	6 (2.2)	0
CA-125 (>35 U/ml)	9 (11.8)	0	71 (38.1)	31 (43.7)	33 (12.0)	7 (7.5)
CA-199 (>35 U/ml)	0	6 (8.7)	11 (5.9)	8 (11.3)	7 (2.6)	6 (6.5)

Table 5. Comparison of lab index abnormalities between CD and UC in 3 groups

3.5 Clinical manifestation

Patients with IBD usually manifest similar clinical features, but each individual may have his own characteristic. And for CD and UC, the patterns of clinical manifestation are different in some aspect. The major clinical manifestations observed in the study included abdominal mass, abdominal pain, mucous stool, hematochezia, fever (higher than 39°C), small bowel obstruction (SBO), anal fistula, weight loss, surgical intervention and parental manifestations (PM). Parental manifestations mainly included uveitis, episcleritis, stomatitis, erythema nodosum, pyoderma gangrenosum, peripheral arthritis and etc.

The result turned out that the ratios of SBO ($p=0.000<0.01$), anal fistula ($p=0.000<0.01$) and weight loss ($p=0.008<0.01$) in CD were significantly higher than in UC, abdominal pain ($p=0.036<0.05$), surgical intervention ($p=0.025<0.05$) and parental manifestations ($p=0.043<0.05$) also occurred more in CD patients. On the other hand, UC patients were much more common with mucous stool ($p=0.000<0.01$) and hematochezia ($p=0.000<0.01$) (Tab. 6).

Clinical manifestation	**CD** (n=536) (%)	**UC** (n=233) (%)	X^2	P value
Abdominal pain	436 (81.34)	177 (75.9)	4.399	0.036
Abdominal mass	17 (3.17)	3 (1.29)	2.276	0.131
Mucous stool	103 (19.22)	133 (57.08)	109.468	0.000
Hematochezia	175 (32.65)	191 (80.93)	158.415	0.000
Fever	143 (26.68)	59 (25.32)	0.154	0.694
SBO	56 (10.45)	5 (2.15)	15.326	0.000
Anal fistula	45 (8.39)	1 (0.43)	18.326	0.000
Weight loss	210 (39.18)	68 (29.18)	7.028	0.008
Surgery	51 (9.51)	11 (4.72)	5.035	0.025
PM	29 (5.41)	5 (2.15)	4.096	0.043

Table 6. The clinical manifestation observed in all 769 IBD patients

3.6 Medical treatment

At the moment, medical treatment of IBD mainly included four kinds of pharmaceuticals: 5-aminosalicylic acid (5-ASA) or sulfasalazine, corticoids, immunosuppressant (we use azathioprine in our hospital), and tumor necrosis factor monocolonal antibody.

5-ASA or sulfasalazine was a base-line agent wildly used in mild IBD patients or used for maintenance therapy. For those IBD patients of active stage, we prescripted 4g/day of this kind of medicine. And the maintenance dosage dropped to 2g/day. Short-term intravenous or oral corticosteroid treatment was used in moderate-to-severe IBD patients. Methylprednisolone given intravenously usually start from the dosage of 40-60mg/day, and 7-10 days later, we changed to corticoids via oral route. The whole treatment course with corticoids was usually tapered within 12-25 weeks. Azathioprine was used as a second-line agent for corticosteroid-dependent or corticosteroid-refractory individuals. It was also used as the replacement therapy during the course of corticosteroid tapering. As for Infliximab, it only began to be used in CD and UC since 2008 and 2009 respectively. Infliximab was listed in China in September 2007, and was mainly used in IBD patients suffered from fistula or in those with corticosteroid- and/or immunosuppressant-refractory.

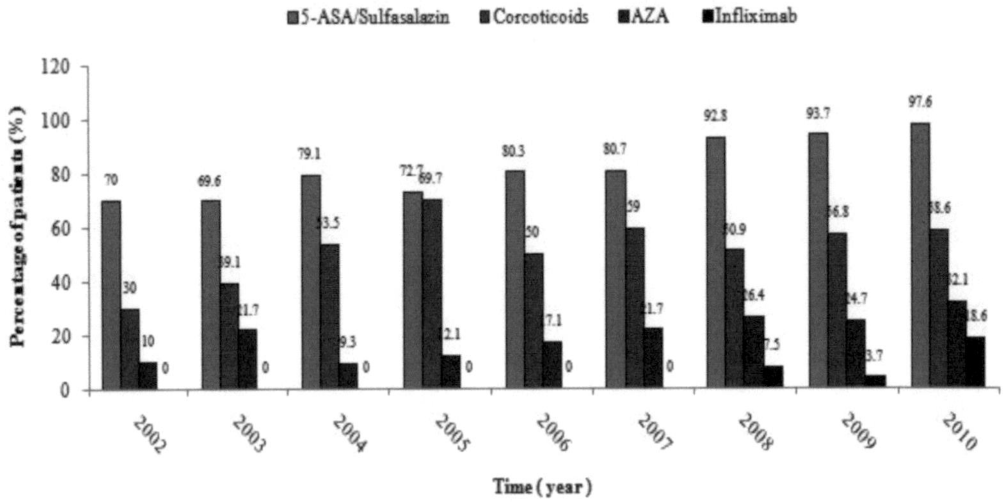

Fig. 3. Medical treatments for CD during 2002-2010

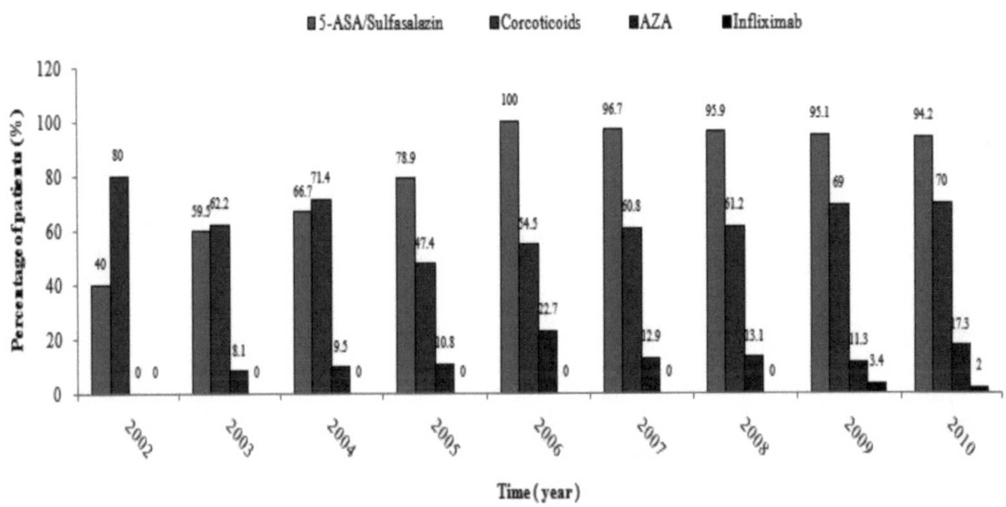

Fig. 4. Medical treatments for UC during 2002-2010

The overview situation of the usage of four pharmaceuticals stated above in CD patients from 2002 to 2010 was shown in Figure 3. As we could see, 5-ASA/ sulfasalazine was always a base-line agent used in most patients (range from 70% to 97.6%). The percentages of patients using corticoids became rather stable since the year of 2006, about half of the hospitalized CD patients had the records of using corticoids. The same trend of AZA could be observed since the year of 2007. And that of UC was listed in Figure 4. 5-ASA/sulfasalazine also played an important role in treating UC, 94.2% to 100% patients were given the agent during 2006-2010. Since 2006 to 2010, the corticoids were also applied to more than half of UC patients; the data was a little bit higher than that of CD patients (63.1% vs 55.06%). The application of AZA was a little bit lower than that in CD. In 2010,

Infliximab is more commonly used in CD patients (especially complicated with fistula) than in UC patients.
An interesting phenomenon could be observed was the change of corticoids using in both diseases. From the year of 2002 to 2005, the trends of corticoids application were just in the opposite directions in CD and UC. In CD, it turned out to be a raising curve; while in UC, the ratio dropped from 80% to 47.4%. But after that, since the year of 2006, in both diseases the use of corticoids became stable.

3.7 Repeated-hospitalization

Within all the 769 patients, 195 individuals had experiences of repeated-hospitalization (25.36%). 148 were CD and 47 were UC, accounted for the total number of each group 27.61% (148/536) and 20.17% (41/233), respectively. In CD cohort, 80 were male (54.1%) and 68 were female (45.9%). As for UC, 29 were male (61.7%) and 18 were female (38.3%).
The times of repeated-hospitalization ranged from 2 to 22. Detailed information was listed in Table 7. The reasons for repeated-hospitalization mainly included intestinal obstruction, severe GI bleeding, high temperature (>39°C) difficult to control, fistula, etc.

Times	2	3	4	5	>=6	Sum.
N	109	35	15	18	18*	195

* Within these 18 patients, 8 were hospitalized for 6 times, 3 for 7 times, 1 for 8 times, 2 for 9 times, 2 for 14 times, 1 for 15 times and 1 for 22 times.

Table 7. Overview of repeated-hospitalization

The interval between every 2 hospitalizations ranged from 0-94 months. And the mean interval of UC was longer than that of CD (Tab. 8).

	Mean interval (m)	Range (m)
CD (n=148)	6.29±10.71	0-92
UC (n=47)	10.04±15.39	0-94
Total (n=195)	6.94±12.13	0-94

Table 8. Overview of intervals between every 2 hospitalizations

4. Discussion

Significant changes have been observed in the epidemiology of IBD in the last two decades. Traditionally, the incidence of IBD was higher in the developed, industrialized countries; as for CD it ranged from $0.7/10^5$ to $11.6/10^5$ and for UC from $2.0/10^5$ to $14.3/10^5$. In contrast, nowadays it became more prevalent in the previously low incidence areas such as developing countries. In particular, the incidence and prevalence of IBD increased significantly in the Asia-Pacific region in recent years. Several recent studies confirmed that, in Asia, the prevalence of CD is $3.6/10^5$ to $7.7/10^5$, and of UC is $4.0/10^5$ to $44.3/10^5$; the morbidity of CD ranges from $0.5/10^5$ to $1/10^5$, of CD the data is between $1/10^5$ and $2/10^5$ (Leong et al., 2004; Al-Ghamdi et al., 2004). In China, it is inferred that the prevalence may be $1.4/10^5$ for CD, and $11.6/10^5$ for UC. The difference of clinical epidemiology, diagnosis and treatment between Asia-Pacific IBDs and that of western countries may be contributed to the diversities of environment, genetic background and medical systems. Lakatos et al reported , the incidence of UC in developing countries is similar to that observed in North America and Western Europe, while the incidence of CD is still relatively low, suggesting that the environmental factors may act faster or differently in UC than in CD (Lakatos L & Lakatos PL, 2007).

As stated before, Rui Jin Hospital affiliated to Shanghai Jiao Tong University is a tertiary level and first-class hospital, which is one of the largest public hospitals in China. This retrospective study enrolled all 769 hospitalized IBD patients from three departments in our hospital from May 2002 to December 2010. Thus, we can take it into granted that the current study, for the first time, systematically provide a relatively intact image of IBD patients in Shanghai during the past 9 years, which is also a valuable reference of the whole situation in China.

Grossly, our study revealed that the prevalence of IBD in Shanghai gradually increased during the observing 9 years. The potential explanations for the increasing trend may be at least partially contributed to the popularity of western life style and diet habits in recent years. As we can see, with the development of economic, literature, as well as tourism, international interactions are more frequent, therefore the gap of environment, diet habit, and life style becomes lessen. The phenomenon that changes of life style and diet habit paralleling with the change of IBD prevalence also indicates the importance of environment mechanism in IBD.

A second reason that may also contributed to the increasing of diagnostic yield of IBD is the improvement of inspection methods. As mentioned before, since 2003 when the DBE, MSCTE and CE became more and more popular in clinical application in our hospital, the diagnostic ratio of IBD also increased obviously. CE is a painless procedure that enables visualization of the entire small bowel and is highly acceptable to both doctors and patients. The disadvantages and limitations of this diagnostic modality include disability to control the direction, the random nature of the images, and the lack of a facility for sampling. The high cost of CE in China also precludes its use as a first-line diagnostic modality for small bowel disease. DBE was regarded as a revolutionary development for the diagnosis of small bowel diseases (Zhong et al., 2007). The entire small bowel could be visualized, usually with a combination of antegrade and retrograde approaches. DBE is used as a gold standard diagnostic modality for small bowel disease. MSCTE serves as a screening method now days in our hospital, when the relatively low cost of this modality taken into account. We failed to take enteroclysis into account, since we conducted it only in little amount of patients.

Nevertheless, differ from other previous studies; our team reported a significantly higher prevalence of CD than that of UC. Among the total of 769 IBD patients enrolled in this study, 536 (69.7%) were suffered from CD and 233 (30.3%) were suffered from UC. Mean age at diagnosis in UC patients was older than in CD, duration of each disease didn't show much difference. Male patients were more than female patients in both diseases in each time-stratifying group. The main reason could be that CD involved small bowel easily, and the three novel inspection techniques mentioned above largely developed the blind spots in small bowel. And that may also give a reasonable explanation why it was the diagnostic yield of CD not the UC rose significantly.

We chose several relatively special serologic targets in this retrospective study in IBD. The laboratory indexes observed included: the number of PLT, the level of CRP and ESR, tumor markers (CEA, CA-125, CA-199). In our study, there existed no obvious differences of the CRP and/or ESR between UC group and CD group. Both markers were higher in CD than in UC. As for tumor indicators, CA-125 and CA-199 seemed to have some abnormal tendency comparing with normal population. But further and detailed research is necessary before getting more convinced conclusions.

With the invention and development of immunomodulators and biologics, obvious changes have been introduced into IBD treatment in the past decade. Infliximab, a chimeric monoclonal antibody against tumor necrosis factor alpha, was first approved for the treatment of CD in 1998 (Hanauer et al., 2002; Sands et al., 2004; Targan et al., 1997); subsequently, three other biologic agents (Adalimumab, Certolizumab and Natalizumab) became available for induction and maintenance of remission in CD (Colombel et al., 2007; Feagan et al., 2008; Sandborn et al., 2007). Infliximab is the only biologic agent approved for the treatment of UC after demonstrating success in the ACT I and ACT II trials. In China, Infliximab was not listed until September 2007. We are now using it in more IBD patients in 2011, but since the clinical data of this year is not included within the current study, we have little to discuss here.

As for immunosuppressive agents (such as azathioprine, methotrexate, and 6-mercaptopurine), many studies during the last ten years have focused on their application in the treatment of both UC and CD (Ananthakrishnan et al., 2010; Cosnes et al., 2005). Azathioprine was used as a second-line agent for corticosteroid-dependent or corticosteroid-refractory individuals. And in our experience, it was more used as the replacement therapy during the course of corticosteroid tapering. Patient was usually asked to start using AZA two weeks before corticosteroid tapering at the dosage of 10 mg/day.

The goals of IBD therapies can be summarized as: inducing remission, preventing complications, improving life quality, and reducing hospitalization as well as surgical rates (Bai & Peng, 2010). Thus, predicting of disease outcome is of great importance. Chow and his team reported that thrombocytosis in IBD patients at diagnosis predicted corticosteroid-dependency, structuring phenotype of CD and presence of anaemia in UC predicted subsequent course of corticosteroid refractoriness (Chow et al., 2009). In the further research, we will convince the conclusion by collecting and analyzing the related data.

With regard to relapsing, for hospitalized IBD patients, repeated-hospitalization may be looked on as an indicator. In our current study, about 1/5 patients suffered relapse within a mean interval about 7 months. The patients hospitalized for more than 6 times were mostly for treatment with Inflixmab. As for the predictive factors of relapse, is the defect of this retrospective study. We will do more detailed work in our future research.

There are several limitations in our current study. First, we could not eliminate the possibility of referral bias. For the hospitalized IBD patients were in moderate-severe situations, which means patients suffer mild IBD may be cared by outpatient department. So the conclusion of this study maybe more reliable in reflecting the situation of moderate-severe patients. Second, the important marker of disease activity, CDAI, was not captured in this study, that would be the part included in our further study. Last but not least, data of some patients were not intact. The nutrition support, especially the enteral nutrition support, may induce illness ease, promote mucosal healings, and help maintaining the long-term stability of the disease. The lack of this part is also a pity. Nutrition therapy in patients with IBD is probably both undervalued and underused. Maybe we could try to make up for it in our future prospective study.

5. Conclusion

At present, large clinical material in IBD is still limited in Chinese population. This study, for the first time, systematically provided a relatively intact image of hospitalized IBD patients in Shanghai. The result is also a valuable reference of the whole situation in China.
In summary, in this 9-year retrospective study, an increasing prevalence of IBD in Shanghai was observed, which is synchronized with that in the western countries. The changes of life style and diet habits, the improvement of diagnostic modalities may play important role in it. We have more options, such as biologics, for IBD treatment besides the traditional medicine of 5-ASA, corticosteroids and immunosuppressants. The combination and adjustment of medicine are of great significance in inducing remission and maintaining the long-term stability of the disease. To choose appropriate diagnostic modality for patients, to establish effective surveillance indexes, and to develop individualized treatment program will contribute much to pharmacoeconomics.

6. References

Ananthakrishnan, AN.; McGinley, EL.; Binion, DG.& Saeian K.(2010). A novel risk score to stratify severity of Crohn's disease hospitalizations. The American Journal of Gastroenterology, Vol.105, No.8, pp. 1799-1807, ISSN 0002-9270

Al-Ghamdi, AS.;Al-Mofleh, IA.;Al-Rashed, RS.; Al-Amri, SM.; Aljebreen, AM.;Isnani, AC.& El-Badawi, R.(2004). Epidemiology and outcome of Crohn's disease in a teaching hospital in Riyadh. World Journal of Gastroenterology, Vol.10, No.9, pp. 1341-1344, ISSN 1007-9327

Baert, F.; Caprilli, R.& Angelucci, E.(2007). Medical therapy for Crohn's disease: top-down or step-up? Digestive diseases, Vol.25, No.3, pp. 260-266, ISSN 0257-2753

Bai, A.&Peng, Z.(2010). Biological therapies of inflammatory bowel disease. Immunotherapy, Vol.2, No.5, pp. 727-742, ISSN 1750-743X

Cosnes, J.; Nion-Larmurier, I.; Beaugerie, L.; Afchain, P.; Tiret, E.& Gendre, JP.(2005). Impact of the increasing use of immunosuppressants in Crohn's disease on the need for intestinal surgery. Gut, Vol.54, No.2, pp. 237-241, ISSN 0017-5749

Chow, DK.; Sung, JJ.; Tsoi, KK.; Wong, VW.; Wu, JC.; Leong, RW. & Chan, FK. (2009). Predictors of corticosteroid-dependent and corticosteroid-refractory inflammatory bowel disease: analysis of a Chinese cohort study. Alimentary pharmacology & therapeutics, Vol.29, No.8, pp. 843-854, ISSN 0269-2813

Colombel, JF.; Sandborn, WJ.; Rutgeerts, P.; Enns, R.; Hanauer, SB.; Panaccione, R.; Schreiber, S.; Byczkowski, D.; Li, J.; Kent, JD.& Pollack PF. (2007). Adalimumab for maintenance of clinical response and remission in patients with Crohn's disease: the CHARM trial. Gastroenterology, Vol.132, No.1, pp. 52-65, ISSN 0016-5085

Cao, Q.;Si, JM.; Gao, M.; Zhou, G.;Hu, WL.& Li JH.(2005). Clinical presentation of inflammatory bowel disease: a hospital based retrospective study of 379 patients in eastern China. Chinese medical journalJ (Engl), Vol.118, No.9, pp. 747-752, ISSN 0366-6999

Colombel, JF.;Vernier-Massouille, G.;Cortot, A.; Gower-Rousseau, C.&Salomez, JL.(2007). Epidemiology and risk factors of inflammatory bowel diseases. Bulletin de l'Académie nationale de médecine, Vol.191, No.6, pp. 1118-1123, ISSN 0001-4079

Domènech E. (2006). Inflammatory bowel disease: current therapeutic options. Digestion, Vol.73, No.1, pp. 67-76, ISSN 0012-2823

Edwards, CN.; Griffith, SG.; Hennis, AJ. & Hambleton, IR. (2008). Inflammatory bowel disease: incidence, prevalence, and disease characteristics in Barbados, West Indies. Inflammatory bowel diseases, Vol.14, No.10, pp. 1419-1424, ISSN 1078-0998

Feagan, BG.; Panaccione, R.; Sandborn, WJ.; D'Haens, GR.; Schreiber, S.; Rutgeerts, PJ.; Loftus EV, Jr.; Lomax, KG.; Yu, AP.; Wu, EQ.; Chao, J.& Mulani P. (2008). Effects of adalimumab therapy on incidence of hospitalization and surgery in Crohn's disease: results from the CHARM study. Gastroenterology, Vol.135, No.5, pp. 1493-1499, ISSN 0016-5085

Goh, K.&Xiao, SD. (2009) .Inflammatory bowel disease: a survey of the epidemiology in Asia. Journal of digestive disease, Vol.10, No.1, pp. 1-6, ISSN 1751-2972

Hanauer, SB.; Feagan, BG.; Lichtenstein, GR.; Mayer, LF.; Schreiber, S.; Colombel, JF.; Rachmilewitz, D.; Wolf, DC.; Olson, A.; Bao, W.; Rutgeerts, P.; & ACCENT I Study Group. (2002). Maintenance infliximab for Crohn's disease: the ACCENT I randomised trial. Lancet, Vol.359, No.9317, pp. 1541-1549, ISSN 0023-7507

Kappelman, MD.; Rifas-Shiman, SL.; Porter, CQ.; Ollendorf, DA.; Sandler, RS.; Galanko, JA.& Finkelstein, JA. (2008). Direct health care costs of Crohn's disease and ulcerative colitis in US children and adults. Gastroenterology, Vol.135, No.6, pp. 1907-1913, ISSN 0016-5085

Lennard-Jones, JE. (1989). Classification of inflammatory bowel disease. Scandinavian Journal of Gastroenterology Vol.170, pp. 2-6, ISSN 0085-5928

Lakatos, L.&Lakatos, PL. (2007). Changes in the epidemiology of inflammatory bowel diseases. Orvosi hetilap, Vol.148, No.5, pp. 223-228, ISSN 0030-6002

Leong, RW.; Lau, JY.& Sung，JJ. (2004). The epidemiology and phenotype of Crohn's disease in the Chinese population. Inflammation Bowel Disease, Vol.10, No.5, pp. 646-651, ISSN 1078-0998

Nguyen, GC.; Munsell, M. & Harris ML. (2008). Nationwide prevalence and prognostic significance of clinically diagnosable protein-calorie malnutrition in hospitalized inflammatory bowel disease patients. Inflammation Bowel Disease, Vol.14, No.8, pp. 1105-1111, ISSN 1078-0998

Sands, BE.; Anderson, FH.; Bernstein, CN.; Chey, WY.; Feagan, BG.; Fedorak, RN.; Kamm, MA.; Korzenik, JR.; Lashner, BA.; Onken, JE.; Rachmilewitz, D.; Rutgeerts, P.; Wild, G.; Wolf, DC.;Marsters, PA.; Travers, SB. Blank, MA. & van, Deventer SJ.(2004). Infliximab maintenance therapy for fistulizing Crohn's disease. The New England Journal of Medicine, Vol.350, No.9, pp. 876-885, ISSN 0028-4793

Sandborn, WJ.; Rutgeerts, P.; Enns, R.; Hanauer, SB.; Colombel, JF.; Panaccione, R.; D'Haens, G.; Li, J.; Rosenfeld, MR.; Kent, JD.& Pollack PF.(2007). Adalimumab induction therapy for Crohn disease previously treated with infliximab: a randomized trial. Annals of internal medicine, Vol.146, No.12, pp. 829-838, ISSN 0003-4819

Targan, SR.;Hanauer, SB.; van, Deventer SJ.; Mayer, L.; Present, DH.; Braakman, T.; DeWoody, KL.; Schaible, TF.& Rutgeerts PJ.(1997). A short-term study of chimeric monoclonal antibody cA2 to tumor necrosis factor alpha for Crohn's disease. Crohn's Disease cA2 Study Group. The New England Journal of Medicine, Vol.337, No.15, pp. 1029-1035, ISSN 0028-4793

Veluswamy, H.; Suryawala, K.; Sheth, A.; Wells, S.; Salvatierra, E.; Cromer, W.; Chaitanya,GV.; Painter, A.; Patel, M.; Manas, K.; Zwank, E.; Boktor, M.; Baig, K.; Datti, B.; Mathis, MJ.; Minagar, A.; Jordan, PA.& Alexander, JS.(2010). African-American inflammatory bowel disease in a Southern U.S. health center. The New England journal of medicine, Vol.10, pp. 104-112, ISSN 0028-4793

Zhong, J.; Ma, T.; Zhang, C.; Sun, B.; Chen, S.; Cao, Y. & Wu Y. (2007). A retrospective study of the application on double-balloon enteroscopy in 378 patients with suspected small-bowel diseases. Endoscopy, Vol.39, No.3, pp. 208-215, ISSN 0013-726X

Part 3

Management of Inflammatory Bowel Disease

14

The Role of Diet, Prebiotic and Probiotic in the Development and Management of Inflammatory Bowel Diseases (IBD)

Abdulamir, A.S.[1,2], Muhammad Zukhrufuz Zaman[3], Hafidh R.R.[1,4] and Abu Bakar F.[1,3]
[1]*Institute of Bioscience, University Putra Malaysia, Serdang, Selangor,*
[2]*Microbiology department, College of Medicine, Alnahrain University, Baghdad*
[3]*Faculty of Food Science and Technology, University Putra Malaysia, Serdang, Selangor*
[4]*Microbiology department, College of Medicine, Baghdad University*
[1,3]*Malaysia*
[2,4]*Iraq*

1. Introduction

Inflammatory bowel disease (IBD) refers to a chronic inflammation condition of the intestinal tract concerning both small and large intestine. The major types of IBD are Crohn's disease (CD) and ulcerative colitis (UC). Both are chronic, relapsing and remitting diseases. The etiology of these diseases is quite complicated that involves genetic and environmental factors including diets, geographical and socioeconomic status and microbial factors. This chapter provides and discusses information about diet, prebiotic and probiotic and their role in the development and management of IBD.

Diet has important role in the development of IBD or protection against IBD. The nutritional components contribute in the balance of intestinal microflora either positively or negatively depending on the diet itself. Foods have been previously considered by consumers barely in term of taste and immediate nutritional needs. Instead of those two aspects, many consumers consider the foods ability to provide specific benefits beyond their nutritional as stringent reasons for choosing foods as their daily diet. Thus, functional foods have become an important and rapidly growing segment of the food markets, especially for the prevention and mangemnt of bowel-related diseases such as IBD. On the other hand, Prebiotic components and probiotic bacteria have also been used in the prevention and treatment of IBD, and they exhibit proven efficacy in many clinical studies. Prebiotic such as inulin and fructooligosaccharides (FOS) are commercially available in the markets, as well as probiotic supplemented food such as yogurt and fermented milk. Further information regarding this both food products will be discussed later in this chapter.

This chapter reviews the role of diet and its different elements namely, fibers, proteins, fatty acids (saturated and unsaturated fatty acids), and carbohydrates in the development and management of inflammatory bowel diseases (IBD). In addition, the chapter will discuss the link between life style and nutritional status with the enteric microbiota, and the balance between harmful bacteria and the beneficial bacteria (prebiotic components and probiotic bacteria). Moreover, the mechanisms of such relationship between the enteric microbiota and diet will be discussed and explained. And the exact role of prebiotic and probiotic bacteria will be discussed thoroughly in the prevention, management and treatment of IBD along with the underlying mechanisms.

2. The healthy and unhealthy diet for intestine

Foods have a large impact on human digestive tract, particularly for those who have severe intestinal disorder such as constipation, inflammatory bowel disease, and colorectal cancer. Consumption of water, fiber containing food, prebiotic bacteria, probiotic bacteria, fruits and vegetables are thought to be beneficial for intestine, whereas specific red and processed meat are inconsistently exert detrimental effect to intestine. Prebotic and probiotic have been considered as healthy diet for the intestine. Water is required to keep foods and other substances move along more smoothly through the digestive tract as well as to make stools softer and easier to pass. In 117 patients with chronic functional constipation, a daily fiber intake of 25 g can increase the stools frequency and this effect was significantly enhanced by increasing water intake to 1.5-2.0 liters per day (Anti et al., 1998). In contrast, carbonated water improve dyspepsia, constipation and gallbladder emptying, however it decreases satiety in patients with functional dyspepsia and constipation (Cuomo et al., 2002). In early study, Lepkovsky et al. (1957) investigated the gastrointestinal regulation of water in rats fed with or without water. Rats fed without water ate less food than rats fed with water. However, the gastric contents (49% water) were similar within the both group, indicate close regulation of water in the gastric content. The authors suggested that diet without water resulted in decreasing appetite and food intake. Schoorlemmer and Evered (2002) revealed that a sensor located in the gastrointestinal tract or perhaps in the mesenteric veins, but not the hepatic portal vein or the liver mediated the inhibition of feeding during water deprivation. Therefore, water is considered as an important component that takes a part in maintaining the intestinal healthy.

Dietary fiber is an intrinsic substance of plants that are resistant to enzymatic digestion in the gastrointestinal track of human (Schneeman and Tietyen, 1994). It is usually differentiated into insoluble fiber (not dissolve in water) and soluble fiber (dissolve in water). Chemically, insoluble fiber consists of cellulose, hemicelluloses and lignin, while soluble fiber consists of pectin, gum and mucilage. Insoluble fiber enhances the movement of material through the digestive track and contributing bulk and moisture to the stool. Thus, it can be of benefit to those who suffer with constipation and irregular stools. Insoluble fiber is found in food such as whole grains, wheat bran and many vegetables. Soluble fiber absorbs water to form a gel-like material and can help lower blood cholesterol and glucose levels. Oat, peas, beans, nuts, some fruits and vegetables are good sources of soluble fiber. Consuming foods rich in fiber exert numerous benefits such as improved large bowel function, slowed digestion and absorption of carbohydrate and fat, and reduced risk for certain diseases (Schneeman and Tietyen, 1994). Average intake of dietary fiber in the United States is about 5 g/day. However, according to the American Dietetic Association, the recommended daily intake of fiber is 25-35 g (Slavin, 2008). Fiber should be increasingly consumed in certain time period rather than consumed promptly to achieve value of recommended daily intake, as it may cause stomach cramping and gas. In 2001, Bliss et al. revealed that dietary fiber may improve fecal incontinence. In their study, patients with fecal incontinence who are given dietary fiber as psylium or gum arabic showed significantly fewer incontinence stools than with placebo treatment.

Consumption of fruits and vegetables are believed to exert many beneficial effects to intestine, as they are sources of fiber. Chang et al. (2010) reported that consumption of kiwi fruit for 4 weeks be able to shorten colon transit time, increases defecation frequency, and improves bowel function in adults diagnosed with constipation. In another study with eight healthy volunteers, Shinohara et al. (2010) investigated the effect of apple intake on fecal microbiota in humans. They revealed that the number of bifidobacteria, *Lactobacillus* and *Streptococcus* in feces increase after the intake of 2 apples/day for 2 weeks. In contrast, the decreased numbers of *Clostridium perfringens, Enterobacteriaceae* and *Pseudomonas* was observed in the same groups. Their findings indicate that apple consumption improved intestinal environment and apple pectin was thought to be main component underlying this beneficial effect. In addition, Tamura et al. (2011) found that the occupation ratio of *Bacteroides* and *Clostridium* cluster IV were significantly higher in fecal flora of mice given Japanese apricot treatment compared to the control. The authors also suggested this Japanese apricot fiber possesses the fecal lipid excretion effects and feces bulking effects.

3. The kinds and nutritional status of diets and their role in the development of IBD

3.1 Sugar and refined carbohydrate

Many studies have been conducted to observe the role of sugar in the development of IBD. Martini and Brandes (1976) were among the earliest to reveal that intake of sugar and highly refined carbohydrate containing foods were higher in CD patients compared to the control. Mayberry et al. (1978) in UK observed the dietary breakfast on 100 CD patients and 100 controls, matched for age and sex. No significant difference was noted for the type of foods taken at breakfast, except for fruit and fruit juice, which were taken more often by control. Nevertheless, CD patients were observed to add significantly higher amount of sugar to their beverages and cereals compared to control. In later studies, a higher sugar intake in CD patients compared to control was eventually confirmed (Mayberry et al., 1980; Silkoff et al., 1980). Since then, numerous studies have confirmed the high level of sugar consumption noticed either in foods or beverages of CD patients (Jarnerot et al. 1983; Katschinski et al., 1988; Matsui et al., 1990, Reif et al., 1997).

Some debates have raised an issue on whether the increased sugar intake is a course or effect of the disease. However, the fact that increased sugar pattern has also been observed in new onset CD signifying that such pattern may contribute a role in the development of the disease. In a case controlled study, researchers used the odd ratio (OR) or relative risk (RR) as appropriate method for investigating the relationship between diet and disease. Persson et al. (1992) revealed that calculated RR of CD was increased for subjects who consume high amount of sucrose (>55 g/day) (RR= 2.6; 95% confidence interval (CI)= 1.4-5.0). Reif et al. (1997) found that a high sucrose intake was associated with the increase for IBD, with OR= 2.85 and 5.3 against population and clinic control, respectively. In addition, they found that lactose consumption exhibited no effect while fructose intake was negatively associated with risk of IBD. Sakamoto et al. (2005) used food frequency questionnaire (FFQ) to compare pre-illness diet in 108 CD and 126 UC patients with the diet of 211 controls in Japan. They found that high consumption of sugars and sweeteners (OR= 2.12; 95% CI= 1.08-4.17) and sweets (OR= 2.83; 95% CI= 1.38-5.83) were positively associated with CD risk. High intake of sweets was also observed to be positively associated with UC risk (OR= 2.86; 95% CI= 1.24-6.57).

3.2 Dietary fat

Dietary fat is suggested to be an important factor in the development of IBD. Hydrogenated fat such as margarine was found to contribute in the development of IBD. The causal relationship between margarine and IBD was previously proposed based on the association between the onsets of margarine consumption with the first report of ganulomatous ileitis (Geerling et al., 1999). Maconi et al. (2010) reported that moderate and high consumption on margarine (OR= 11.8 and OR= 21.37) was associated with UC.
An increase of fat consumption was observed in the pre-illness period of IBD, particularly of UC patients (Reif et al., 1997). The kind of fat observed in the study including animal fat, vegetable fat, saturated fat, monounsaturated fat, polyunsaturated fat and cholesterol, in which high intake of animal fat and cholesterol give high OR value of 4.09 and 4.57, respectively (Reif et al., 1997). Geerling et al. (2000) found in their study that high intake of monounsaturated fatty acids (MUFA) and polyunsaturated fatty acids (PUFA) were also associated with the development of UC. Similarly, Sakamoto et al. (2005) revealed that the intake of total fat, MUFA, and n-6 fatty acids was positively associated with CD risk, although they failed to found association with UC. An epidemiological study from Japan discovered that increasing incidence of CD (between 1966 and 1985) was in parallel increase with daily intake of animal protein, total fat and animal fat, particularly n-6 PUFA relative to n-3 PUFA (Shoda et al., 1996).

3.3 Dietary protein

Important source of protein such as meat, cheese, milk, eggs and fish are widely taken as dietary protein. Patients with CD and UC as well as ulcerative proctitis disorders exhibit higher protein intake compared to the control subject with other gastrointestinal disorders (Gee et al., 1985). Tragone et al. (1995) also found higher protein intake in UC but not CD patients compared to the control. On the other hand, Reif et al. (1997) failed to find the association between protein intake and the risk of IBD in their case control study. Shoda et al. (1996) who conducted an epidemiologic analysis of CD in Japan showed that increased incidence of CD was strongly correlated with increased dietary intake of animal protein (r= 0.908) and milk protein (r= 0.924). However, risk of CD is not correlated with fish protein (r= 0.055) and is inversely correlated with vegetable protein (r= -0.941). The study also suggests that the development of CD may be contributed by high intake of animal protein and n-6 PUFA with less n-3 PUFA. In recent study, Maconi et al. (2010) reported that high consumption of cheese was significantly associated (OR= 3.7; 95% CI= 1.14-12.01) with CD.
Allergy to milk protein was also proposed to be associated with the etiology of UC. Truelove et al. (1961) reported in earlier time that milk exclusion from the diet of patients led to clinical improvement, but an exacerbation of UC was observed when milk was re-added into the diet. Taylor and Truelove (1961) supported the theory with their discovery on raised circulating antibodies to cow's milk protein. Decades later, Glassman et al. (1990) reported a relationship between hypersensitivity to cow's milk during infancy and subsequent development of UC. Several studies investigated perinatal risk factor on the development of IBD found that the lack of breastfeeding is also an independent risk factor associated with development of CD (Koletzko et al., 1989; Thompson et al., 2000) and UC (Corrao et al., 1998) later in childhood. However, Koletzko et al. (1991) revealed that the association between breastfeeding and the increase risk of IBD remains obscure (Koletzko et al., 1991). Although discrepancies appear in many study, the relationship between protein intake and the development of IBD seems to be evidenced.

3.4 Other dietary components

Many dietary components either as whole foods or micronutrients have been examined for their risk in the development of IBD. Persson et al. (1992) found that consumption of fast food at least twice a weak associated with the increased relative risk of either CD (RR= 3.4; 95% CI= 1.3-9.3) or UC (RR= 3.9; 95% CI= 1.4-10.6). Reif et al. (1997) reported a positive association between retinol and the risk of IBD, while high intake of fluids, magnesium, vitamin C and fruits was negatively associated with the risk of IBD. In other study, a positive correlation was found between the intake of vitamin E (OR= 3.23; 95% CI= 1.45-717) and CD risk, whereas the intake of vitamin C (OR= 0.45; 95% CI= 0.21-0.99) was negatively related to UC risk (Sakamoto et al., 2005). A higher consumption of vitamin B_6 was observed in UC patients compared to the control (Geerling et al., 2000).

D'Souza et al. (2008) used the FFQ in a control case study to investigate the impact of dietary patterns in pediatric CD risk. They found that a characterized diet by meat, fatty food and dessert was positively associated with CD risk (OR= 4.7; 95% CI= 1.6-14.2). On the other hand, a diet characterized by fruits, vegetables, olive oil, fish, grains and nut was inversely associated with CD risk (OR= 0.2; 95% CI= 0.1-0.5). In other recent study, Maconi et al. (2010) evaluated the association between specific dietary pattern and IBD risk on adult. The dietary patterns were termed as refined (pasta, sweets, red and processed meat, butter and margarine), prudent (white meat, tuna fish, fish, eggs and potatoes) and healthy (bread, cheese, fruit and vegetables as well as olive oil). They observed that a "refine" pattern was associated with an increased risk of UC and CD. In contrast, the "prudent" diet was significantly associated with a decreased risk of UC and CD whiles the "healthy" pattern exhibited non significant association with increased risk of CD, and it was not consistently associated with UC. Although a meaningful conclusion cannot be drawn, these studies imply that specific dietary patterns has distinct role in the development of IBD either in children or adults.

4. Mechanisms underlying the association of diet with IBD

Diet is thought to play an important role in the development and treatment of IBD. However, the association between nutrition and IBD is complicated and involves several aspects such as nutritional support for malnourished patients, primary therapy for active disease and maintenance of remission, and nutrients risk factors involved in the etiology of IBD (Hartman et al., 2009). Malnutrition is commonly observed in patients with IBD, particularly CD (O'Sullivan et al., 2006; Razack and Seidner, 2007). Enteral nutrition has been applied as an adjunct therapy to correct or prevent malnutrition in CD patients in both adults and children (Dupont et al., 2008; Day et al., 2008; El-Matary, 2009). Enteral nutrition has also been considered to induce and maintain remission in CD (Tsujikawa et al., 2003; Griffiths, 2005; Smith, 2008). Nevertheless, mechanisms underlying the action of enteral nutrition are yet to be fully understood, although several mechanisms have been proposed by many researchers. These mechanisms include improvement of nutritional status (Beatti et al., 1994), down regulation of pro-inflammatory cytokines (de Jong et al., 2007), modification of gut flora (Leach, 2008), anti-inflammatory effects (Fell, 2005), promoting epithelial healing (Fell et al., 2000), decreased gut permeability (Guzy et al., 2009) and decreased antigenic load to the gut (Beatti et al., 1994).

The association between diet and IBD is likely to be determined by major components found in the foods. The ability of foods containing fiber in preventing the development of IBD is determined by the end products resulted from the fermentation of fiber in the gut. Fiber is metabolized by gastrointestinal bacteria to produce lactate, gas and short chain fatty acids (SCFA) such as acetate, propionate and butyrate. The most important SCFA is butyrate since it has anti-inflammatory effects by inhibiting NFκβ and thus preventing transcription of pro-inflammatory cytokines. Butyrate is also known to reduce colonic permeability by promoting activation of peroxisome proliferator activated receptor γ (PPAR-γ) (Venkatraman et al., 2003). In addition, N-3 PUFA, particularly eicosapentaenoic acid (EPA) and docosahexaenoic acid (DHA) have been associated with the prevention of IBD. These PUFA influence the inflammatory response through several mechanisms such as antagonizing the production of inflammatory eicosanoid mediators from arachidonic acid, suppress production of some inflammatory cytokines and downregulate the expression of a number of genes involved in inflammation (Gil, 2002).

5. The link among diet, prebiotic and enteric microbiota mainly probiotic bacteria

The human gastrointestinal tract that typically refers to stomach and intestine is colonized by an intricate community of microorganisms. The stomach is a home of typically 10^3 colony forming units (CFU)/g content (Gibson and Beaumont, 1996). The large intestine is the main colonization site of more than 500 indigenous microbial species which can reach up to 10^{12} CFU/g lumen contents (Conway, 1995; Gibson and Beaumont, 1996). A wide range of compounds that have both positive and negative effects on gut physiology is produced through fermentation process by predominantly strict anaerobe gut microflora. For instance, short-chain fatty acids (SCFA), mainly butyrate supplies energy metabolism for the large gut mucosa and colonic cell growth. This SCFA is the end fermentation products of complex carbohydrate and protein that usually present in human diet. In contrast, H_2S produced by sulfate-reducing bacteria is highly toxic and may induce ulcerative colitis (Gibson and Beaumont, 1996). From the host's perspective, the key function of gut microflora is to prevent colonization by potentially harmful microorganisms. The imbalanced gut microflora has been linked to the development of certain disorders such as gastroenteritis, colon cancer and inflammatory bowel disease (Gibson and Macfarlane, 1994). The composition of gut microflora is considered to be fairly stable over long periods. However, numerous factors such as competition for nutrients, metabolic interaction among bacteria, various host condition and individual dietary preferences may influence alteration of the pattern (Berg, 1981; Hill, 1986; Rowland and Tanaka, 1993). Therefore, it is of the foremost interest to manipulate the gut microflora composition toward an increased number of beneficial bacteria that provide health promising properties to the gut.

The groups of beneficial bacteria that help maintain health and treat disease is broadly known as probiotic. Several definitions of probiotic have been suggested for over the years. Fuller (1989) defined probiotic as a live microbial food supplements which have beneficial effects on the host by improving its intestinal microbial balance. A probiotic bacterium should fulfill certain criteria to be described as useful. These include acid and bile stability, adherence to intestinal cells, persistence for some time in the gut, ability to produce antimicrobial substances, antagonism against pathogenic bacteria, ability to modulate the immune response, being of human origin and having generally regarded as safe (GRAS) status (Dunne et al., 2001). In human, probiotic has been associated with lactobacilli (e.g. *Lactobacillus acidophilus, L. delbruekii* and *L. casei*) and bifidobacteria (e.g. *Bifidobacterium bifidum, B. adolescentis, B. infantis* and *B. longum*). Other known bacteria include streptococci (e.g. *Streptococcus lactis* and *S. salivarius* ss. thermophilus), nonpathogenic *E. coli* and *Saccharomyces boulardii* (Gibson and Roberfroid, 1995; Shanahan, 2001).

A practical approach in increasing the number and activities of probiotic is through dietary supplementation, particularly with intake of the so called prebiotic. Gibson and Roberfroid (1995) defined a prebiotic as 'a non digestible food ingredient that beneficially affects the host by selectively stimulating the growth and/or activity of one or a limited number of bacteria in the colon, and thus improves host health'. They revealed that food constituents can be categorized as prebiotic if meet the following requirements: 1) Resistant to hydrolysis and absorption in the upper part of gastrointestinal tract; 2) Act as selective substrate for one or a limited number of beneficial bacteria commensal to the colon; 3) Able to alter the colonic flora in favor to healthier composition; and 4) Induce luminal or systemic properties that are beneficial to the host health. Fructooligosaccharides (FOS), inulin, lactulose and galactooligosaccharides are commercially available prebiotic of proven efficacy. Inulin and FOS can be found in human breast milk and in food such as banana, asparagus, leeks, onion, garlic, wheat, chicory and tomatoes (Niness, 1999). Galactooligosaccharides (GOS), a mixture of oligosaccharides derived from lactose is frequently used as supplement in food and infant formula milk (Niness, 1999; Roberfroid, 2007). In their in vitro study, Wang and Gibson (1993) demonstrated that FOS and inulin are selectively fermented by most strains of bifidobacteria. The prebiotic effects of inulin and oligofructose in vivo have also been shown in many studies (Buddington et al., 1996; Kleesen et al., 1997). Moreover, the ability of these oligosaccharides in increasing the numbers of gut probiotic, particularly bifidobacteria has been shown in many human feeding studies. Breast milk is rich in human oligosaccharides and therefore the number of bifidobacteria in the gut microflora of breast-fed infants is higher than that in formula-fed infants (Gibson and Roberfroid, 1995; Harmsen et al., 2000). The predominance of bifidobacteria in breast-fed infants is usually associated with lower risk of intestinal infection. However, Moro et al. (2002) reported that after 28 days of feeding, the number of fecal bifidobacteria and lactobacilli in infant fed with a cow milk supplemented with FOS and GOS were significantly increased compared to the placebo group.

The link between prebiotic and probiotic has been pronounced to enhance the efficacy of the both agents in maintaining the health of intestine. Synbiotics have been defined as 'a mixture of probiotics and prebiotics that beneficially affects the host by improving the survival and implantation of live microbial dietary supplements in the gastrointestinal track, by selectively stimulating the growth and/or by activating the metabolism of one a limited number of health promoting bacteria, and thus improving host welfare' (Gibson and Roberfroid, 1995). There are only few studies carried out to investigate the efficacy of synbiotics in human. Bouhnik et al. (1996) investigated the effect of symbiotic containing *Bifidobacterium* spp. and inulin fermented milk in healthy people. The authors reported that intake of *Bifidobacterium* spp. significantly increased fecal bifidobacteria, but no extra numbers of that particular probiotic was observed merely due to the addition of inulin. However, 2 weeks after trials, the volunteers who received symbiotic product had significantly higher number of *Bifidobacterium* spp. compared to those receiving probiotic alone. In addition, it was found that the trend whereby *Bifidobacterium* spp population decreases in the gut microflora of eldery may be reversed by the consumption of inulin (Kleessen et al., 1997).

6. The role of prebiotic and probiotic bacteria in the prevention of IBD

The inflammatory bowel disease is of complicated etiology, wherein genetic factors, immunity system and environmental factors as well as the interaction among them are supposed to play a pivotal role in the development of these disease states. The convincing evidence for interaction of these factors has been exposed in experimental animal models of either CD or UC (Elson et al., 1995; Strober et al., 1998; Blumberg et al., 1999). The environment factors such as the composition and metabolic activity of the gastrointestinal microbiota are likely to be the most important aspect. Its relationship with the host is so specific, thus alteration in the balance of microorganisms might initiate the pathogenesis of IBD. Some of intestinal bacterial resident are considered harmful as they are involved in toxin production, mucosal invasion or activation of inflammatory responses. These bacteria include *Mycobacterium paratubercolusis, Listeria monocytogenes*, adherent *E. coli* and measles virus. The equilibrium between protective and harmful bacteria inside the gastrointestinal tract exists in healthy people. However, this equilibrium is broken in IBD people (termed as dysbiosis), resulting in chronic intestinal inflammation (Tamboli et al., 2004). Major modification in gastrointestinal microbiota in IBD patient includes increased numbers of coliforms, bacteroids and *E.coli*, as well as decreased numbers of lactic acid bacteria (Kennedy et al., 2000; Borruel et al., 2002). Distribution of lesions in this intestinal inflammation disorder is found greatest in areas with the highest numbers of luminal bacteria (Shanahan, 2000). The consumption of probiotic has been known to exert many beneficial effects. Probiotics facilitate host defense against infection through competitive metabolic interactions, production of antimicrobials, and inhibition of adherence or translocation of pathogen. In a view point of IBD, Shanahan (2000) revealed that anti-inflammatory effects of probiotic require signal with gastrointestinal epithelium and mucosal regulatory T cells or dendritic cells.

Many studies revealed that oral administration of probiotic in tandem with prebiotic promote the prevention of IBD. Prebiotic is growth substrates specifically directed toward indigenous beneficial bacteria in colon, thus amplify the probiotic effects in preventing IBD. Although there is no recommended daily dose of prebiotic, but Roberfroid et al. (1998) suggested that a minimum daily dose of 4 g of inulin or FOS would be sufficient to increase the numbers of bifidobacteria in the intestine. In people with IBD, intake of prebiotic is required to prevent the disease recurrence, since prebiotic served as substrate for probiotic to produce SCFAs particularly butyrate that exert protective effects to the gut. For instances, Videla et al. (1994) reported that prebiotic inulin increases colonic butyrate and reduces inflammation and disease severity in animal models of colitis. Germinated barley foodstuff (GBF) rich in fiber also alleviate the symptomatology in both animal models of UC and patients with UC (Bamba et al., 2002). GFB is efficiently increases luminal butyrate production by stimulating the growth of protective bacteria (Kanauchi et al., 2002, Kanauchi et al., 2003). Therefore, the prebiotic and probiotic are likely work synergistically in the prevention of IBD.

7. The role of prebiotic and probiotic in the management and treatment of IBD

Prebiotic and probiotic have been widely involved in the management and treatment of IBD. Many studies on the use of prebiotic in the management of IBD are presented in Table 1. Fernandez-Banares et al. (1999) shown that a diet with Plantago ovate seeds was as effective as mesalazine in maintenance of remission in inactive UC patients in a randomized controlled trial. Oral administration of GBF has been known to reduce clinical activity and prolonged remission time in UC patients (Kanauchi et al., 2002; Kanauchi et al., 2003; Hanai et al., 2004). In a recent study, Casellas et al. (2007) investigated the effect of oligofructose-enriched inulin in patients with active UC. They revealed that at day 7, an early significant reduction of fecal calprotectin was observed in patients who had taken oligofructose-enriched inulin, but not in placebo group. Fecal calprotectin has been used as an objective and quantitative marker of intestinal inflammation and its levels correlated significantly with histologic and endoscopic assessment of disease activity in UC (Roseth et al., 1997; Konikoff and Denson, 2006). Inulin has also been assayed in a placebo controlled clinical trial in patients with relapsing pouchitis (Welters et al., 2002). Dietary supplementation with inulin (24 g/day for 3 weeks) resulted in an increase of butyrate level, lower in pH, decreased numbers of *Bacteroides fragilis* and diminished level of secondary bile acids in feces. The authors further revealed that inulin was associated with reduction of endoscopic and histological scores of mucosal inflammation in the ileal reservoir. Nevertheless, more clinical trials are required to further validate the efficacy of dietary fiber as prebiotic in the management of IBD.

Prebiotic	Disease	Number of patients	Duration	Outcome Results	Reference
Inulin (24 g/day)	Pouchitis	20 adults	2.2 months	Reduction of inflammation of the mucosa of the ileal reservoir.	Welters et al. (2002)
Plantago ovata seed	UC	105 adults	12 months	Maintain remission as effective as mesalamine, Increased in fecal butyrate.	Fernandez-Banarez et al. (1999)
Synbiotic 2000 *	CD	30 adults	24 months	Fail to prevent postoperative recurrence.	Chermesh et al. (2007)
Synergy 1 (inulin and oligofructose) 6 g/day and *Bifidobacterium longum*	UC	18 adults	1 months	Reduction of β-defensins 2, 3, and 4, TNFα and Interleukin 1α.	Furrie et al. (2005)
Germinated barley foodstuff (30 g/day)	UC	10 adults	1 months	Reduction of clinical activity index scores and increase in stool butyrate concentrations.	Mitsuyama et al. (1998)

*: Synbiotic 2000 is combination of probiotic (Lactobacillus raffinolactis, L. paracasei, L. plantarum, Pediococcus pentosaceus) and prebiotic (2.5 g β-glucan, 2.5 g inulin, 2.5 g pectin and 2.5 g resistant starch).

Table 1. Studies of probiotics in the management of inflammatory bowel disease (IBD)

Many clinical studies have confirmed the efficacy of probiotic in the management and treatment of IBD (Table 2). In 1999, Venturi et al. reported the efficacy of VSL#3 (at 6 g/day) as maintenance treatment in patients with ulcerative colitis in remission and intolerance to 5-aminosalicylic acid (5-ASA). They observed that 75% of patients given VSL#3 remained in remission without any side effects throughout the 12 months period. VSL#3 is comprised of lyophilized viable cell of 4 strains of *Lactobacillus* (*L. casei, L. achidophilus, L. plantarum* and *L. bulgaricus*), 3 strains of *Bifidobacterium* (*B. longum, B. breve* and *B. infantis*) and 1 strain of *Streptococcus thermophilus*. In addition, the mixture of probiotic is found to be able to upregulate the intestinal mucosal alkaline sphingomyelinase and reduce the inflammation risk in UC patients (Soo et al., 2008). A non-patoghenic *E. coli*, Nissle 1917, also exhibits similar efficacy with mesalazine (the standard treatment) in the maintenance of UC (Rembacken et al., 1999; Kruis et al., 2004). In other study, the ability of *Saccharomyces boulardii* to induce the remission in 71% of patients with mild to moderate UC was reported (Guslandi et al., 2003).

There are only few controlled clinical studies using probiotic in CD and the results were somehow inconsistent. Malin et al. (1996) reported that intake of *Lactobacillus rhamnosus* GG ($2{\times}10^{10}$ CFU/day, for 10 days) in pediatric CD stimulates the gut IgA levels, which could promote the gut immune response. Furthermore, using the same probiotic strain and dose, Gupta et al. (2000) reported an improved clinical scores and intestinal permeability in an open-labeled pilot study with four children with CD. In contrast, Prantera et al. (2002) reported the ineffectivity of *Lactobacillus rhamnosus* GG in preventing post operative disease recurrence or reducing severity of recurrent lesion in patients with CD. In addition, *Lactobacillus johnsonii* La1 was also unable to prevent endoscopic recurrence in the 12 week period following ileo-caecal resection (Van Gossum et al., 2005). Chermesh et al. (2007) showed that post operative recurrence of CD patients was not prevented by Synbiotic 2000, a combination of 4 probiotic lactic acid bacteria (*Lactobacillus raffinolactis, L. paracasei, L. plantarum, Pediococcus pentosaceus*) and 4 prebiotic fermentable fibers (beta-glucans, inulin, pectin, resistant starch). However, combination treatment of antibiotic rifaximin and probiotic VSL#3 resulted in a significantly lower incidence of severe endoscopic recurrence compared with mesalazine treatment (Campieri et al., 2000). Combination of VSL#3 and *Saccharomyces boulardii* was also observed to give a therapeutic effect in patients with CD.

Gionchetti et al. (2000) investigated the efficacy of VSL#3 (at 6 g/day) oral administration in the maintenance of remission in chronic pouchities in the double blind controlled study. They found that 15% patients in the VSL#3 group had relapses, compared with 100% patients in the placebo group ($P<0.001$) over a nine month trial period. The mechanism of VSL#3's impressive effect has not been established. However, Gionchetti et al. (1999) have previously found that the intake of VSL#3 increases faecal concentration of lactobacilli, bifidobacteria and streptococci, as well as increases tissue levels of IL-10 in patients with chronic pouchitis. Since the efficacy disappears after stopping therapy, the efficacy of VSL#3 therapy was thought to be due to the ongoing presence of these factors. In contrast, Kuisma et al. (2003) showed that *Lactobacillus rhamnosus* GG was ineffective to prevent relapses in patients with chronic pouchitis in a placebo controlled trial. In an open-labeled study, combined *Lactobacillus rhamnosus* LGG and prebiotic fructooligosaccharide, when administered as adjuvant to antibiotic therapy, induce remission in patients with pouchitis (Friedman and Goerge, 2000).

Probiotic Strains and dose	Disease	Patients number and condition	Duration	Outcome Results	Reference
VSL#3 *	UC, in remission	20 adults (12 male, 8 female), intolerance to 5-ASA	12 months	75% patients remained in remission during study period, no side effects	Venturi et al. (1999)
Eschericia coli Nissle 1917 (1×10^{11}cfu/day)	UC, active	116 adult adults, treated with prednisolon + gentamicin plus either probiotic of mesalazine	3 months	Prebiotic induce remission as effective as mesalazine (standard treatment)	Rembacken et al. (1999)
Eschericia coli Nissle 1917 (1×10^{11} cfu/day)	UC, in remission	116 adult adults	12 months	Prebiotic shown equivalent efficacy with mesalazine in the maintenance of remission	Rembacken et al. (1999)
VSL#3	UC, active	30 adults	6 weeks	VSL#3 resulted in combined induction of remission/response rate of 70%, with no adverse effects	Bibiloni et al. (2005)
Saccharomyces boulardii	UC, in remission	25 adults, unsuitable for steroid therapy	1 months	71% patients remained in remission	Guslandi et al. (2003)
Yakult ** (1×10^{10} cfu/day)	UC	21 adults (11 male, 10 female)	12 months	73% patients treated with probiotic remained in remission, while only 10% placebo	Ishikawa et al. (2003)
Saccharomyces boulardii	CD, in remission	32 adults (20 male, 12 female)	6 months	Probiotic plus mesalamine reduced relapsing incindence compared to mesalamine alone	Guslandi et al. (2000)
Lactobacillus rhamnosus GG (2×10^{10} cfu/day)	CD	4 children	6 months	Improve gut barrier function, pediatric crohn's disease activity index (PCDAI) were 73% lower than baseline	Gupta et al. (2000)
Lactobacillus GG (1×10^{10} cfu/day)	CD	14 adults	10 days	Increase the IgA immune response, thus promote the gut immunological barrier	Malin et al. (1996)
VSL#3 (1.8×10^{12} cfu/day)	Pouchitis	40 adults	9 months	Reduced risk of relapse recurring, only 15% patient in probiotic group relapsed compared with 100% in placebo group	Gionchetti et al. (2000)
Cultura *** (5×10^{10} cfu/day)	Pouchits	10 adults	1 months	50% endoscopic improvement, but no histological improvement	Laake et al. (2003)
VSL#3 (1.8×10^{12} cfu/day)	Pouchitis	36 adults	12 months	Induced remission in 85% patients	Mimura et al. (2004)

*: VSL#3 (VSL Pharmaceuticals Inc., Fort Lauderdale, Florida, USA) contain 4 strains of Lactobacillus (L. casei, L. achidophilus, L. plantarum and L. bulgaricus), 3 strains of Bifidobacterium (B. longum, B. breve and B. infantis) and 1 strain of Streptococcus thermophilus.
**: Yakult (Yakult Honsha Co. Ltd., Tokyo, Japan) contain Bifidobacterium breve, B. bifidum and Lactobacillus acidhophilus.
***: Cultura® (TINE Dairies BA, Oslo, Norway) contain 1×1010 live Lactobacillus acidophilus and Bifidobacterium lactis per 100 g.

Table 2. Studies of probiotics in the management of inflammatory bowel disease (IBD)

8. The underlying mechanisms of the protective effects of probiotic bacteria

Many studies have been addressed to disentangle the mechanisms on how probiotic bacteria exert their beneficial effects on human health. Although not entirely understood, several mechanisms underlying the useful action of probiotic have been proposed by researchers. The mechanisms include production of inhibitory substances, competitive exclusion of microbial adherence or translocation, modulation of immune response and reinforcement of barrier function. These functions are likely interrelated in supporting the protective effect of probiotic. Furthermore, it should be emphasized that the action of probiotic is species and strains specific, thus, appropriate choice of microorganism is of particular attention to improve the efficacy of probiotic treatment.

8.1 Production of inhibitory substances

Probiotic bacteria produce various substances that perform as inhibitory agents to pathogenic bacteria. The inhibitory agents such as organic acids, hydrogen peroxide and bacteriocins are typically produced by probiotic. These compounds may reduce the number of viable cells as well as inhibit bacterial metabolism or toxin production (Rolfe, 2000). Several strains of Lactobacilli produce acetic, lactic and propionic acid that decrease the local pH thus inhibit the growth of many Gram-negative pathogenic bacteria. Some strains of Lactobacillus inhibit the growth of Salmonella enterotica merely by the production of lactic acid (Makras et al., 2006). The 2-component lantibiotics (lanthionine and methyllanthionine) are small microbial peptide bacteriocins produced by Gram positive bacteria such as Lactococcus lactis (Lawton et al., 2007). At nanomolar concentration, these peptides actively inhibit multidrug resistant pathogens by targeting the lipid II component of the bacterial cell wall (Morgan et al., 2005). Lactobacilli are also known to produce non-lanthione containing bacteriocins. A large group of bacteriocins with highly divergence sequences are produced by Lactobacillus strains including L. plantarum, L. sakei, L. acidophilus NCFM, and L. johnsonii NCC 533 (Makarova et al., 2006; Chaillou et al., 2005; Altermann et al., 2005; Pridmore et al., 2004). In addition, Collado et al. (2005) reported that several strains of human fecal Bifidobacteria produce bacteriocin like compounds that exert toxicity to both Gram-positive and negative bacteria.

8.2 Competitive exclusion of microbial adhesion or translocation

The adhesive properties of probiotic bacteria on epithelial cells enable the competitive inhibition of bacterial adhesion site, thus hampering colonization of pathogenic bacteria (He et al., 2001; Lee and Puong, 2002; Boudeau et al., 2003). Some probiotic have the ability to block the intestinal mucosal receptor, thus prevent adhesion of pathogenic bacteria. Several strains of Lactobacilli and Bifidobacteria are able to compete with many pathogenic bacteria such as Bacteroides vulgates, Enterobacter aerogene, Listeria monocytogenes, Staphylococcus aureus, Salmonella enterica, enterotoxigenic E. coli and enteropathogenic E. coli for intestinal epithelial cell binding (Collado et al., 2007; Candela et al., 2005; Roselli et al., 2006; Sherman et al., 2005). Displacement of pathogenic bacteria can also occur even if the pathogen have attached to intestinal epithelial cells prior to prebiotic treatment (Collado et al., 2007; Candela et al., 2005). Nevertheless, specific strains of probiotic or its combinations are required to inhibit or displace specific strains of pathogen (Collado et al., 2007).

8.3 Modulation of immune response

Probiotic bacteria play a key role in stimulating the immunity by increasing immunoglobulin A (IgA) production (Gewirtz et al., 2002). Bakker-Zierikzee et al. (2006) reported that fecal sIgA levels increase in infants fed with Bifidobacterium animalis enriched formula, and suggested that the use of probiotic may reinforce innate function. Interestingly, beside resulting in increased levels of fecal sIgA, spleen cells of mice treated with non viable LGG exhibited enhanced secretion of IL-6 which stimulate IgA antibody response at the mucosal surface (He et al., 2005). Moreover, probiotic protects the intestine from pathogen induced injury by modulating the balance of pro and anti-inflammatory cytokine production. Probiotic increase anti-inflammatory interleukin (IL)-10 and inhibited generation of inflammatory Th1 cells as well as decreases pro-inflammatory IL-12 (Hart et al., 2004). For instances, VSL#3 induces the production of IL-10 in human and murine dendritic cells (Drakes et al., 2004; Hart et al., 2004). Di Giancinto et al. (2005) reported that VSL#3 also stimulate IL-10 production in chemically induced IBD.

The ability of probiotic in suppressing pro-inflammatory cytokine production has been accounted for their efficacy in the treatment of IBD. Pena et al. (2005) said that LGG inhibit lipopolisaccharide (LPP) and Helicobacter pylori-stimulated tumor necrosis factor (TNF) production by murine macrophage. The authors further explained that substances derived from LGG decrease TNF production in macrophages in LGG conditioned cell culture media. In addition, Lactobacillus casei strain Shirota (LcS) inhibits the regulation of LPS-induced IL-6 and the production of IFN-γ by peripheral blood mononuclear cells isolated from normal and chronic colitis mice (Matsumoto et al., 2005). In colonic biopsies of inflamed mucosa from UC patients, Bifidobacterium longum was found to reduce the secretion of pro-inflammatory TNF-α and IL-8 (Bai et al., 2006). Moreover, Sturm et al. (2005) reported that E. coli Nissle 1917 inhibits peripheral bold T-cell cycle progression and expansion, increase IL-10 and decrease the liberation of TNF, IFN-γ and IL-2.

8.4 Reinforcement of barrier function

The defensive mechanisms of the intestinal epithelium are manifested by the intestinal barrier function which requires effective tight junctional complexes between the epithelial cells. The intestinal disintegrates are likely occur when the tight junctional structure or its function are disrupted, resulting in an increased ability of pathogenic bacteria to attach to the gut mucosa. Many studies revealed that the processes involved in mucosal barrier formation are possibly modulated by probiotic, as well as shown the function of probiotic in upregulating expression of defensins, mucins or other proteins associated with tight junction such as claudins and occludins. Therefore, the ability of probiotic in inducing barrier formation is considered as an important mode underlying their efficacy in the prevention and treatment of IBD. Zyrek et al. (2007) have shown that in vitro E.coli Nissle 1917 restored the disrupted epithelial barrier in the polarized T84 cell infected by enteropthogenic E. coli strains E2348/68. They found that E.coli Nissle 1917 increases expression and distribution of zonula occludens-2 (ZO-2) protein and of distinct protein kinase C isotopes to the cell surfaces to exert that protective function. Probiotic VSL#3 increased mucin gene expression and excretion in intestinal epithelial cells (Caballero-Franco et al., 2007). VSL#3 and Lactobacillus fermentum maintain the intestinal barrier function by upregulating the human β-defensin-2 (Schlee et al., 2008). β-defensin is an inducible antimicrobial peptide synthesized by the intestinal epithelial cells to prevent

bacterial adherence and invasion (Wehkamp et al.,2004). In rats with ethanol induced colitis, LGG increases the production of Muc6 and basal mucosal PGE2, resulting in an increased thickness of the mucosal mucus layer of the stomach (Lam et al., 2007). In addition to bacteria, Garcia Vilela et al. (2008) reported that yeast Saccharomyces boulardii induces the improvement but not normalization in leaky gut of CD patients.
The prevention of cytokine-induced epithelial damage by enhancing intestinal epithelial cell survival is another mechanism contributing the clinical efficacy of probiotic. Probiotic exhibit cytoprotective function by reducing intestinal epithelial apoptosis (Yan and Polk., 2002; Lin et al., 2008). Apoptosis is a major factor in the colonic inflammatory response and the pathogenesis of IBD (Sartor, 2002). LGG is found to prevents cytokine-induced apoptosis either in human or mouse intestinal epithelial cells by activating antiapoptotic Akt in a phosphatidylinositol-3-kinase (PI3K)-dependent manner, as well as preventing proapoptotic p38/MAPK activation (Yan and Polk, 2002).

9. Conclusion

Inflammatory bowel disease is a complex disorder in which both genetic and environmental factors involved in the pathogenesis of IBD. Most pivotal etiological factor for IBD is the alteration of gastrointestinal microbial flora to a larger proportion of harmful rather than beneficial bacteria. The alteration is likely to be strongly affected by the type of diet intake. Fibers containing foods are considered as good substances that may enhance the number of beneficial bacteria in the gut, thus maintaining the health of the gut. The end products of fiber fermentation by bacteria in the gut exert many beneficial impacts on either bacteria or host. For instance, short chain fatty acids, particularly butyrate that provides energy to the host and involved in regulating the anti-inflammatory constituents, was found to protect the gut. Efforts to manipulate the bacterial composition of the gut toward a more salutary regiment are of emerging interest today. The most prominent effort is by introducing probiotic (such as lactobacilli and bifidobacteria) and prebiotic (such as inulin and fructooligosaccharide) into the intestine. Probiotics and prebiotics have been used as altervative to current drug treatment in large number of studies of gastrointestinal disorder, particularly IBD. Several evidences support the efficacy of probiotic and prebiotic in the prevention and treatment of UC, CD or pouchitis. However, many trials have given conflicting results; thus large clinical trials using standardized methodology are required to reconfirm the evidences. In addition, more research should be better focused on mechanisms underlying the protective effects of probiotic and prebiotic; thus can be translated into meaningful clinical trial outcome.

10. References

Altermann, E., Russell, W.M., Azcarate-Peril, M.A., Barrangou, R., Buck, B.L., McAuliffe, O., Souther, N., Dobson, A., Duong, T., Callanan, M., Lick, S., Hamrick, A., Cano, R., Klaenhammer, T.R. (2005). Complete genome sequence of the probiotic lactic acid bacterium *Lactobacillus acidophilus* NCFM. *Proceeding of the National Academy of Sciences USA*, Vol. 102, pp. 3906-3912.

Anti, M., Lamazza, A., Pignataro, G., Pretaroli, A.R., Armuzzi, A., Pace, V., Valenti, A., Leo, P., Lascone, E., Castelli, A., Marmo, R., Gasbarrini, G. (1998). Water supplementation enhances the effect of high-fiber diet on stoolfrequency and laxative consumption in adult patients with functional constipation. *Hepato-Gastroenterology*, Vol. 45, pp. 728-732.

Bai, A.P., Ouyang, Q., Xiao, X.R., Li, S.F. (2006). Probiotics modulate inflammatory cytokine secretion from inflamed mucosa in active ulcerative colitis. *International Journal of Clinical Practice*, Vol. 60, pp. 284–288.

Bakker-Zierikzee, A.M., Van Tol, E.A.F, Kroes, H., Alles, M.S., Kok, F.J., Bindels, J.G. (2006). Faecal SIgA secretion in infants fed on pre- or probiotic infant formula. *Pediatric Allergy and Immunology*, Vol. 17, pp. 134 -140.

Bamba, T., Kanauchi, O., Andoh, A., Fujiyama, Y. (2002) A new prebiotic from germinated barley for nutraceutical treatment of ulcerative colitis. *Journal of Gastroenterology and Hepatology*. Vol. 17, pp. 818–824.

Beattie, R.M., Schiffrin, E.J., Donnet-Hughes, A., Huggett, A.C., Domizio, P., MacDonald, T.T., Walker-Smith, J.A. (1994). Polymeric nutrition as the primary therapy in children with small bowel Crohn's disease. *Alimentary and Pharmacology Therapeutic*, Vol. 8, pp. 609-615.

Berg, J. O. (1981). Cellular location of glycoside hydrolases in *Bacteroides fragilis*. *Current Microbiology*, Vol. 5, pp. 13-17.

Bibiloni, R., Fedorak, R.N., Tannock, G.W., Madsen, K.L., Gionchetti, P., Campieri, M., De Simone, C., Sartor, B. (2005). VSL#3 Probiotic-mixture induces remission in patients with active ulcerative colitis. *American Journal of Gastroenterology*, Vol. 100, pp. 1-8.

Bliss, D.Z., Jung, H.J., Savik, K., Lowry, A., Le-Moine, M., Jensen, L., Werner, C., Schaffer, K. (2001). Supplementation with dietary fiber improves fecal incontinence. *Nursing Research*, Vol. 50, pp. 203-213.

Blumberg, R.S., Saubermann, L.J., Strober, W. (1999). Animal models of mucosal inflammation and their relation to human inflammatory bowel disease. *Current Opinion in Immunology*, Vol. 11, pp. 648–656.

Boudeau, J., Glasser, A.L., Julien, S., Colombel, J.F., Darfeuille-Michaud, A. (2003). Inhibitory effect of probiotic *Escherichia coli* strain Nissle 1917 on adhesion to and invasion of intestinal epithelial cells by adherent-invasive *E. coli* strains isolated from patients with Crohn's disease. *Alimentary Pharmacology and Therapeutic*, Vol. 18, pp. 45–56.

Borruel, N., Carol, M., Casellas, F., Antolin, M., de Lara, F., Espin, E., Naval, J., Guarner, F., Malagelada, J.R. (2002). Increased mucosal tumour necrosis factor α production in Crohn's disease can be downregulated ex vivo by probiotic bacteria. *Gut*, Vol. 5, pp. 659–664.

Bouhnik, Y., Flourie, B., Andrieux, C., Bisetti, N., Briet, F., Rambaud, J.C. (1996). Effect of *Bifidobacterium* sp. fermented milk ingested with and without inulin on colonic bifidobacteria and enzymatic activities in healthy humans. *European Journal of Clinical Nutrition*. Vol. 50, pp. 269–273.

Buddington, R.K., Williams, C.H., Chen, S.C., Witherly, S.A. (1996). Dietary supplementation of neosugar alters the fecal flora and increases activities of some reductive enzymes in human subjects. *American Journal of Clinical Nutrition*, Vol. 63, pp. 709-716.

Caballero-Franco, C., Keller, K., De, S.C., Chadee, K. (2007). The VSL#3 probiotic formula induces mucin gene expression and secretion in colonic epithelial cells. *American Journal of Physiology Gastrointestinal and Liver Physiology*. Vol. 292, pp. G315–G322.

Campieri, M., Rizzello, F., Venturi, A., Gilberto, P., Ugolini, F., Helwig, U., Amadini, C., Romboli, E., Gionchetti, P. (2000). Combination of antibiotic and probiotic treatment is efficacious in prophylaxis of post-operative recurrence of Crohn's disease: A randomized controlled study vs mesalamine. *Gastroenterology*, Vol. 118, pp. G4179.

Candela, M., Seibold, G., Vitali, B., Lachenmaier, S., Eikmanns, B.J., Brigidi, P. (2005). Real-time PCR quantification of bacterial adhesion to Caco-2 cells: competition between bifidobacteria and enteropathogens. *Research in Microbiology*. Vol. 156, pp. 887- 895.

Casellas, F., Borruel, N., Torrejon, A., Varela, E., Antolin, M., Guarner, F., Malagelada, J.R. (2007). Oral oligofructose-enriched inulin supplementation in acute ulcerative colitis is well tolerated and associated with lowered fecal calprotectin. *Alimentary Pharmacology and Therapeutics*, Vol. 25, pp. 1061-1067.

Chaillou, S., Champomier-Verges, M.C., Cornet, M. Crutz-Le Coq, A.M., Dudez, A.M., Martin, V., Beaufils, S., DArbon-Rongere, E., Bossy, R., Loux, V., Zagorec, M. (2005). The complete genome sequence of the meat-borne lactic acid bacterium *Lactobacillus sakei* 23K. *Nature Biotechnology*, Vol. 23, pp. 1527-1533.

Chang, C.C., Lin, Y.T., Lu, Y.T., Liu, Y.S., Liu, J.F. (2010). Kiwifruit improves bowel function in patients with irritable bowel syndrome with constipation. *Asia Pacific Journal of Clinical Nutrition*, Vol. 19, pp. 451-457.

Chermesh, I., Tamir, A., Reshef, R., Chowers, Y,, Suissa, A., Katz, D., Gelber, M., Halpern, Z., Bengmark, S., Eliakim, R. (2007). Failure of synbiotic 2000 to prevent postoperative recurrence of Crohn's disease. *Digestive Diseases and Sciences*, Vol. 52, pp, 385–389.

Collado, M.C., Hernandez, M., Sanz, Y. (2005). Production of bacteriocin-like inhibitory compounds by human fecal Bifidobacterium strains. *Journal of Food Protection*, Vol. 68, pp. 1034 -1040.

Collado, M.C., Meriluoto, J., Salminen, S. (2007). Role of commercial probiotic strains against human pathogen adhesion to intestinal mucus. *Letters in Applied Microbiology*, Vol. 45, pp. 454–460.

Conway, P.L. (1995). Microbial ecology of the human large intestine. In: *Human Colonic Bacteria: Role in Nutrition, Physiology and Pathology*, Gibson, G.R., Macfarlane, G.T., pp. 1-1, CRC Press, Boca Raton.

Corrao, G., Tragnone, A., Caprilli, R., Caprilli, R., Trallori, G., Papi, C., Andreoli, A., Di Paolo, M., Riegler, G., Rigo, G.P., Ferrau, O., Mansi, C., Ingrosso, M., Valpiani, D., Coorperative Investigators of the Italian Group for the Study of the Colon and the Rectum. (1998). Risk of inflammatory bowel disease attributable to smoking, oral contraception and breastfeeding in Italy: a nationwide case-control study. International *Journal of Epidemiology*, Vol. 27, pp. 397–404.

Cuomo, R., Grasso, R., Sarnelli, G., Capuano, G., Nicolai, E., Nardone, G., Pomponi, D., Budillon, G., Ierardi, E. (2002). Effects of carbonated water on functional dyspepsia and constipation. *European Journal of Gastroenterology and Hepatology*, Vol. 12, pp. 991-999.

D'Souza, S., Levy, E., Mack, D., Israel, D., Lambrette, P., Ghadirian, P., Deslandres, C., Morgan, K., Seidman, E.G., Amre, D.K. (2008). Dietary Patterns and Risk for Crohn's Disease in Children. Inflammatory Bowel Disease, Vol. 14, pp. 367-373.

Day, A.S., Whitten, K.E., Sidler, M., Lemberg, D.A. (2008). Systematic review: nutritional therapy in paediatric Crohn's disease. *Alimentary Pharmacology Therapeutic*, Vol. 27, pp. 293–307.

de Jong, N.S., Leach, S.T., Day, A.S. (2007). Polymeric formula has direct anti-inflammatory effects on enterocytes in an in vitro model of intestinal inflammation. *Digestive Diseases and Sciences*, Vol. 52, pp. 2029-2036.

Di Giacinto, C., Marinaro, M., Sanchez, M., Strober, W., Boirivant, M. (2005). Probiotics ameliorate recurrent Th1-mediated murine colitis by inducing IL-10 and IL-10-dependent TGF-beta-bearing regulatory cells. *The Journal of Immunology*, Vol. 174, pp. 3237–3246.

Drakes, M., Blanchard, T., Czinn, S. (2004). Bacterial probiotic modulation of dendritic cells. *Infection and Immunity*, Vol. 72, pp. 3299-3309.

Dunne, C., O'Mahony, L., Murphy, L., Thornton, G., Morrissey, D., O'Halloran, S., Feeney, M., Flynn, S., Fitzgerald, G., Daly, C., Kiely, B., O'Sullivan, G.C., Shanahan, F, Collins, J.K. (2001). In vitro selection criteria for probiotic bacteria of human origin: correlation with in vivo findings. *American Journal of Clinical Nutrition*,Vol. 73, pp. 386s-392s.

Dupont, B., Dupont, C., Justum, A.M., Piquet, M.A, Reimund, JM. (2008). Enteral nutrition in adult Crohn's disease: present status and perspectives. *Molecular Nutrition and Food Research*, Vol. 52, pp. 875–884.

El-Matary, W. (2009). Enteral nutrition as a primary therapy of Crohn's disease: the pediatric perspective. *Nutrition in Clinical Practice*, Vol. 24, pp. 91–97.

Elson, C.O., Sartor, R.B., Tennyson, G.S., Riddell, R.H., (1995). Experimental models of inflammatory bowel disease. *Gastroenterology*, Vol. 109, pp. 1344–67.

Fell, J.M., Paintin, M., Arnaud-Battandier, F., Beattie, R.M., Hollis, A., Kitching, P., Donnet-Hughes, A., MacDonald, T.T., Walker-Smith, J.A. (2000). Mucosal healing and a fall in mucosal pro-inflammatory cytokine mRNA induced by a specific oral polymeric diet in paediatric Crohn's disease. *Alimentary and Pharmacology Theraputic*, Vol. 14, 281-289.

Fell, J.M. (2005). Control of systemic and local inflammation with transforming growth factor beta containing formulas. *JPEN Journal of Parenteral and Enteral Nutrition*, Vol. 29, pp. S126-S128; discussion S129-S133, S184-S188.

Fernandez-Banares, F., Hinojosa, J., Sanchez-Lombrana, J.L., Navarro, E., Martinez-Salmeron, J.F., Garcia-Puges, A., Gonzalez-Huix, F., Riera, J., Gonzalez-Lara, V., Dominguez-Abascal, F., Gine, J.J., Moles, J., Gomollon, F., Gassul, M.A., Spanish Group for the Study of Crohn's Disease and Ulcerative Colitis (GETECCU). (1999). Randomized clinical trial of Plantago ovata seeds (dietary fiber) as compared with mesalamine in maintaining remission in ulcerativecolitis. *The American Journal of Gastroenterology*, Vol. 94, pp. 427–433.

Fuller, R. (1989). Probiotics in man and animals. *Journal of Applied Bacteriology*, Vol. 66, pp. 365-378.

Furrie, E., Macfarlane, S., Kennedy, A., Cummings, J.H., Walsh, S.V., Macfarlane, G.T. (2005). Synbiotic therapy (*Bifidobacterium longum*/Synergy 1) initiates resolution of inflammation in patients with active ulcerative colitis: a randomised controlled pilot trial. *Gut*, Vol. 54, pp. 242-249.

Friedman, G., George, J. (2000). Treatment of refractory 'pouchitis' with probiotic and probiotic therapy. *Gastroenterology*, Vol. 118, pp. A4167.

Garcia Vilela, E., De Lourdes De Abreu Ferrari, M., Oswaldo Da Gama Torres, H., Guerra Pinto, A., Carolina Carneiro Aguirre, A., Paiva Martins, F., Marcos Andrade Goulart, E., Sales Da Cunha, A. (2008). Influence of Saccharomyces boulardii on the intestinal permeability of patients with Crohn's disease in remission. *Scandinavian Journal of Gastroenterology*, Vol. 43, pp. 842–848.

Gee, M.I., Grace, M.G.A., Wensel, R.H., Sherbaniuk, R.W., Thompson, A.B.R. (1985). Nutritional status of gastroenterology outpatients: comparison of inflammatory bowel disease with functional disorders. *Journal of the American Dietetic Association*, Vol. 85, pp. 1591–1599.

Gibson, G.R., MacFarlane, G.T. (1994). Intestinal bacteria and disease, In: human health: the contribution of microorganisms, Gibson, S.AW., pp. 53-62, Springer-Verlag, London.

Geerling, B.J., Stockbrugger, R.W., Brummer, R.J. (1999). Nutrition and inflammatory bowel disease: an update. *Scandinavian Journal of Gastroenterology*, Vol. 230, pp. 95–105.

Geerling, B.J., Dagnelie, P.C., Badart-Smook, A., Russel, M.G., Stockbrügger, R.W., Brummer, R.J. (2000). Diet as a risk factor for the development of ulcerative colitis. *American journal of Gastroenterology*, Vol. 95, pp. 1008-1013.

Gewirtz, A.T., Liu, Y., Sitaraman, S.V., Madara, J.L. (2002). Intestinal epithelial pathobiology: past, present and future. *Best Practice and Research Clinical Gastroenterology*, Vol. 16, pp. 851–867.

Gibson, G.R., Beaumont, A. (1996). An overview of human colonic bacteriology in health and disease. In: *Gut Flora and Health - Past, Present and Future*, Leeds, A.R., Rowland, I.R., pp. 3-11, The Royal Society of Medicine Press Ltd., London.

Gibson, G.R., Roberfroid, M.B. (1995). Dietary Modulation of the Colonic Microbiota: Introducing the Concept of Prebiotics. *The Journal of Nutrition*, Vol. 125, pp. 1401–1412.

Gil, A. (2002). Polyunsaturated fatty acids and inflammatory diseases. *Biomedicine and Pharmacotherapy*, Vol., 56, pp. 388–396.

Gionchetti, P., Rizzello, F., Venturi, A., Brigidi, P., Matteuzzi, D., Bazzocchi, G., Poggioli, G., Miglioli, M., Campieri, M. (2000). Oral bacteriotherapy as maintenance treatment in patients with chronic pouchitis: a double-blind, placebo-controlled trial. *Gastroenterology*, Vol. 119, pp. 305–309.

Gionchetti, P., Rizzello, F., Cifone, G., Venturi, A., D'Alo, S., Peruzzo, S., Bazzocchi, G., Miglioli, M., Campieri, M. (1999). In vivo effect of a highly concentrated probiotic on IL-10 pelvic pouch tissue levels(Abstract). *Gastroenterology*, Vol. 116, pp. A723.

Glassman, M.S., Newman, L.J., Berezin, S., Gryboski, J.D. (1990). Cow's milk protein sensitivity during infancy in patients with inflammatory bowel disease. *The American Journal of Gastroenterology*, Vol. 85, pp. 838–40.

Griffiths, A.M. (2005). Enteral nutrition in the management of Crohn's disease. *Journal Parenteral and Enteral Nutrition*, Vol. 29 (Suppl.4), pp. S108–12.

Gupta, P., Andrew, H., Kirschner, B.S., Guandalini, S. (2000). Is *Lactobacillus* GG helpful in children with crohn's disease? results of a preliminary, open-label study. *Journal of Pediatric Gastroenterology and Nutrition*, Vol. 31, pp. 453–457.

Guslandi, M., Mezzi, G., Sorghi, M., Testoni, P.A. (2000). Saccharomyces boulardii in maintenance treatment of crohn's disease. *Digestive Diseases and Sciences*, Vol. 45, pp. 1462–1464.

Guslandi, M., Giollo, P., Testoni, P.A. (2003). A pilot trial of *Saccharomyces boulardii* in ulcerative colitis. *European Journal of Gastroenterology and Hepatology*. Vol. 15, pp. 697–698.

Guzy, C., Schirbel, A., Paclik, D., Wiedenmann, B., Dignass, A., Sturm, A. (2009). Enteral and parenteral nutrition distinctively modulate intestinal permeability and T cell function in vitro. *European Journal of Nutrition*, Vol. 48, pp. 12-21.

Hanai, H., Kanauchi, O., Mitsuyama, K., Andoh, A., Takeuchi, K., Takayuki, I,. Araki, Y., Fujiyama, Y., Toyonaga, A., Sata, M., Kojima, A., Fukuda, M., Bamba, T. (2004). Germinated barley foodstuff prolongs remission in patients with ulcerative colitis. *International Journal of Molecular Medicine*, Vol. 13, pp. 643-647.

Harmsen, H.J.M., Wildeboer-Veloo, A.C.M., Raangs, G.C., Wagendorp, A.A., Klijn, N., Bindels, J.G., Welling, G.W. (2000) Analysis of intestinal flora development in breast-fed and formula-fed infants using molecular identification and detection methods. *Journal of Pediatric Gastroenterology and Nutrition*. Vol. 30, pp. 61–67.

Hart, A.L., Lammers, K., Brigidi, P., Vitali, B., Rizzello, F., Gionchetti, P., Campieri, M., Kamm, M.A., Knight, S.C., Stagg, A.J. (2004). Modulation of human dendritic cell phenotype and function by probiotic bacteria. *Gut*, Vol. 53, pp. 1602–1609.

Hartman, C., Eliakim, R., Shamir, R. (2009). Nutritional status and nutritional therapy in inflammatory bowel diseases. *World Journal of Gastroenterology*, Vol. 15, pp. 2570-2578.

He, F., Ouwehand, A.C., Isolauri, E., Hashimoto, H., Benno, Y., Salminen, S. (2001). Comparison of mucosal adhesion and species identification of bifidobacteria isolated from healthy and allergic infants. *FEMS Immunology and Medical Microbiology*, Vol. 30, pp. 43–47.

He, F., Morita, H., Kubota, A., Ouwehand, A.C., Hosoda, M., Hiramatsu, M., Kurisaki, J. (2005). Effect of orally administered non-viable Lactobacillus cells on murine humoral immune responses. *Microbiology and Immunology*, Vol. 49, pp. 993–997.

Hill, M.F. (1986). Factors affecting bacterial metabolism, In: *Microbial Metabolism in the Digestive Tract*, Hill, M.J., pp. 22-28, CRC Press, Boca Raton, FL.

Ishikawa, H., Akedo, I., Umesaki, Y., Tanaka, R., Imaoka, A, Otani, T. (2002). Randomized controlled trial of the effect of Bifidobacteria-fermented milk on ulcerative colitis. *Journal of the American College of Nutrition*, Vol. 22, pp. 56–63.

Jarnerot, G., Jarnmark, I., Nilsson, K. (1983). Consumption of refined sugar by patients with Crohn's disease, ulcerative colitis or irritable bowel syndrome. *Scandinavian Journal of Gastroenterology*, Vol. 18, pp. 999–1002.

Kanauchi, O., Suga, T., Tochihara, M., Hibi, T., Naganuma, M., Homma, T., Asakura, H., Nakano, H., Takahama, K., Fujiyama, Y., Andoh, A., Shimoyama, T., Hida, N., Haruma, K., Koga, H., Mitsuyama, K., Sata, M., Fukuda, M., Kojima, A., Bamba, T. (2002). Treatment of ulcerative colitis by feeding with germinated barley foodstuff: first report of a multicenter open control trial. *Journal of Gastroenterology*, Vol. 37 (Suppl.14), pp. 67–72.

Kanauchi, O., Mitsuyama, K., Homma, T., Takahama, K., Fujiyama, Y., Andoh, A., Araki, Y., Suga, T., Hibi, T., Naganuma, M., Asakura, H., Nakano, H., Shimoyama, T., Hida, N., Haruma, K., Koga, H., Sata, M., Tomiyasu, N., Toyonaga, A., Fukuda, M., Kojima, A., Bamba, T. (2003). Treatment of ulcerative colitis patients by long-term administration of germinated barley foodstuff: multi-center open trial. *International Journal of Molecular Medicine*, Vol. 12, No. 5, pp. 701-704.

Katschinski, B., Logan, R.F.A., Edmond, M., Langman, M.J.S. (1988). Smoking and sugar intake are separate but interactive risk factors in Crohn's disease. *Gut*, Vol. 29, pp. 1202–1206.

Kennedy, R.J., Kirk, S.J., Gardiner, K.R. (2000). Promotion for a favorable gut flora in inflammatory bowel disease. *JPEN Journal of Parenteral and Enteral Nutrition*, Vol. 24, pp. 189–95.

Kleessen, B., Sykura, B., Zunft, H.J., Blaut, M. (1997). Effects of inulin and lactose on fecal microflora, microbial cativity and bowel habit in eldery constipated persons. *American Journal of Clinical Nutrition*, Vol. 65, pp.1397-1402.

Koletzko, S., Sherman, P., Corey, M., Griffiths, A., Smith, C. (1989). Role of infant feeding practices in development of Crohn's disease in childhood. *British Medical Journal*, Vol. 298, pp.1617-1618.

Koletzko, S., Griffith, A., Corey, M. Smith, C., Sherman, P. (1991). Infant feeding practices and ulcerative colitis in childhood. *British Medical Journal*, Vol. 302, pp. 1580-1581.

Konikoff, M.R., Denson, L.A. (2006). Role of fecal calprotectin as a biomarker of intestinal inflammation in inflammatory bowel disease. *Inflammatory Bowel Disease*, Vol. 12, pp. 524–534.

Kruis, W., Fric, P., Potrotnieks, J., Lukas, M., Fixa, B., Kascak, M., Kamm, M.A., Weismueller, J., Beglinger, C., Stolte, M., Wolff, C., Schulze, J. (2004). Maintaining remission of ulcerative colitis with *Escherichia Coli* Nissle 1917 is as effective as with standard mesalazine", *Gut*, Vol. 53, pp. 1617–1623.

Kuisma, J., Mentula, S., Jarvinen, H., Kahri, A., Saxelin, M., Farkkila, M. (2003). Effect of *Lactobacillus rhamnosus* GG on ileal pouch inflammation and microbial flora. *Alimentary Pharmacology and Therapeutic*. Vol. 17, pp. 509–515.

Lam, E.K., Tai, E.K., Koo, M.W., Wong, H.P., Wu, W.K., Yu, L., So, W.H., Woo, P.C., Cho, C.H. (2007). Enhancement of gastric mucosal integrity by *Lactobacillus rhamnosus* GG. *Life Sciences*, Vol. 80, pp. 2128–2136.

Laake, K.O., Line, P.D., Aabakken, L., Lotveit, T., Bakka, A., Eide, J., Roseth, A., Grzyb, K., Bjorneklett, A., Vatn, M.H. (2003). Assessment of mucosal inflammation and circulation in response to probiotics in patients operated with ileal pouch anal anastomosis for ulcerative colitis. *Scandinavian Journal of Gastroenterology*, Vol.. 38, pp. 409-14.

Lawton, E.M., Ross, R.P., Hill, C., Cotter, P.D. (2007). Two-peptide lantibiotics: a medical perspective. *Mini Reviews in Medicinal Chemistry*, Vol. 7, pp. 236 -1247.

Leach, S.T., Mitchell, H.M., Eng, W.R., Zhang, L., Day, A.S. (2008). Sustained modulation of intestinal bacteria by exclusive enteral nutrition used to treat children with Crohn's disease. *Alimentary and Pharmacology Therapeutic*, Vol. 28, pp. 724-733.

Lee, Y.K., Puong, K.Y. (2002) Competition for adhesion between probiotics and human gastrointestinal pathogens in the presence of carbohydrate. *British Journal of Nutrition*, Vol. 88 (suppl 1), pp. S101-S108.

Lepkovsky, S., Lyman, R., Fleming, D., Nagumo, M., Dimick, M.M. (1957). Gastrointestinal Regulation of Water and Its Effect on Food Intake and Rate of Digestion. *American Journal of Physiology*, Vol. 188, pp. 327-331.

Lin, P.W., Nasr, T.R., Berardinelli, A.J., Kumar, A., Neish, A.S. (2008). The probiotic *Lactobacillus* GG may augment intestinal host defense by regulating apoptosis and promoting cytoprotective responses in the developing murine gut. *Pediatric Research*, Vol. 64, pp. 511–516.

Maconi, G., Ardizzone, S., Cucino, C., Bezzio, C., Russo, A.G., Porro, G.B. (2010). Pre-illnes changes in dietary habits and diets as a risk factor for inflammatory bowel disease: A case control study. *World Journal of Gastroenterology*, Vol. 16, pp. 4297-4304.

Makarova, K., Slesarev, A., Wolf, Y., Sorokin, A., Mirkin, B., Koonin, E., Pavlov, A., Pavlova, N., Karamychev, V., Polouchine, N., Shakhova, V., Grigoriev, I., Lou, Y., Rohksar, D., Lucas, S., Huang, K., Goodstein, D.M., Hawkins, T., Plengvidhya, V., Welker, D., Hughes, J., Goh, Y., Benson, A., Baldwin, K., Lee, J.H., Díaz-Muñiz, I., Dosti, B., Smeianov, V., Wechter, W., Barabote, R., Lorca, G., Altermann, E., Barrangou, R., Ganesan, B., Xie, Y., Rawsthorne, H., Tamir, D., Parker, C., Breidt, F., Broadbent, J., Hutkins, R., O'Sullivan, D., Steele, J., Unlu, G., Saier, M., Klaenhammer, T., Richardson, P., Kozyavkin, S., Weimer, B., Mills, D. (2006). Comparative genomics of the lactic acid bacteria. *Proceeding of the National Academy of Sciences USA*, Vol. 103, pp. 15611-15616.

Makras, L., Triantafyllou, V., Fayol-Messaoudi, D., Adriany, T., Zoumpopoulou, G., Tsakalidou, E., Servin, A., De Vuyst, L. (2006). Kinetic analysis of the antibacterial activity of probiotic lactobacilli towards *Salmonella enterica* serovar Typhimurium reveals a role for lactic acid and other inhibitory compounds. *Research in Microbiology*. Vol. 157, pp. 241-247.

Malin, M., Suomalainen, H., Saxelin, M., Isolauri, E. (1996). Promotion of IgA immune response in patients with Crohn's disease by oral bacteriotherapy with *Lactobacillus* GG. *Annals of Nutrition and Metabolism*, Vol. 40, pp. 137- 145.

Martini, G.A., Brandes, J.W. (1976). Increased consumption of refined carbohydrates in patients with Crohn's disease. *Klinische Wochenschrift*, Vol. 54, pp. 367–371.

Matsui, T., Iida, M., Fujishima, M., Imai, K., Yao, T. (1990). Increased sugar consumption in Japanese patients with Crohn's disease. *Gastroenterologia Japonica*, Vol. 25, pp. 271.

Matsumoto, S., Hara, T., Hori, T., Hori, T, Mitsuyama, K., Nagaoka, M., Tomiyasu, N., Suzuki, A., Sata, M. (2005). Probiotic Lactobacillus-induced improvement in murine chronic inflammatory bowel disease is associated with the down-regulation of pro-inflammatory cytokines in lamina propria mononuclear cells. *Clinical and Experimental Immunology*, Vol. 140, pp. 417– 426.

Mayberry, J.F., Rhodes, J., Newcombe, R.G. (1978). Breakfast and dietary aspects of Crohn's disease. *British Medical Journal*, Vol., pp. 1401.

Mayberry, J.F., Rhodes, J., Newcombe, R.G. (1980). Increased sugar consumption in Crohn's disease. *Digestion*, Vol. 20, pp. 323–326.

Mimura, T., Rizello, F., Helwig, U., Poggioli, G., Schreiber, S., Talbot, I.C., Nicholls, R.J., Ginonchetti, P., Campieri, M., Kamm, M.A. (2004). Once daily high dose probiotic therapy (VSL#3) for maintaining remission in recurrent or refractory pouchitis. *Gut*, Vol. 53, pp. 108-114.

Mitsuyama, K., Saiki, T., Kanauchi, O., Iwanaga, T., Tomiyasu, N., Nishiyama, T., Tateishi, H., Shirachi, A., Ide, M., Suzuki, A., Noguchi, K., Ikeda, H., Toyonaga, A., Sata, M. (1998). Treatment of ulcerative colitis with germinated barley foodstuff feeding: a pilot study. *Alimentary Pharmacology and Therapeutic*, Vol. 12, pp. 1225-1230.

Morgan, S.M., O'Connor, P.M., Cotter, P.D., Ross, R.P.,Hill, C. (2005). Sequential actions of the two component peptides of the lantibiotic lacticin 3147 explain its antimicrobial activity at nanomolar concentrations. *Antimicrobial Agents and Chemotherapy*, Vol. 49, pp. 2606 –2611.

Moro, G. Minoli, I., Mosca, M., Fanaro, S., Jelinek, J., Stahl, B., Boehm, G. (2002). Dosage-related bifidogenic effects of galactoand fructooligosaccharides in formula-fed term infants. Journal of Pediatric Gastroenterology and Nutrition, Vol. 34, pp. 291–295.

Niness, K.R.(1999). Inulin and oligofructose: what are they? *Journal of Nutrition*, Vol. 129, pp. 1402S-1406S.

O'Sullivan, M., O'Morain, C. (2006). Nutrition in inflammatory bowel disease. *Best Practice and Research Clinical Gastroenterology*, Vol. 20, pp. 561–573.

Pena, J.A., Rogers, A.B., Ge, Z., Ng, V., Li, S.Y., Fox, J.G., Versalovic, J. (2005). Probiotic *Lactobacillus* spp. diminish *Helicobacter hepaticus*-induced inflammatory bowel disease in interleukin-10-deficient mice. Infection and Immunity, Vol. 73, pp. 912–920.

Persson, P.G., Ahlbom, A., Hellers, G. (1992). Diet and inflammatory bowel diseases: a case control study. *Epidemiology*, Vol. 3, pp. 47-52.

Prantera, C., Scribano, M.L, Falasco, G., Andreoli, A., Luzi, C. (2002). Ineffectiveness of probiotics in preventing recurrence after curative resection for Crohn's disease: a randomised controlled trial with *Lactobacillus* GG. *Gut*, Vol. 51, pp. 405–409.

Pridmore, R.D., Berger, B., Desiere, F., Vilanova, D., Barretto, C., Pittet, A.C., Zwahlen, M.C., Rouvet, M., Altermann, E., Barrangou, R., Mollet, B., Mercenier, A., Klaenhammer, T., Arigoni, F., Schell, M.A. (2004). The genome sequence of the probiotic intestinal bacterium *Lactobacillus johnsonii* NCC 533. *Proceeding of the National Academy of Sciences USA*. Vol. 101, pp. 2512–2517.

Razack, R., Seidner, D.L. (2007). Nutrition in inflammatory bowel disease. *Current Opinion in Gastroenterology*, Vol. 23, 400–405.

Reif, S., Klein, I., Lubin, F., Farbstein, M., Hallak, A., Gilat, T. (1997). Pre-illness dietary factors in inflammatory bowel disease. *Gut*, Vol. 40, pp. 754–760.

Rembacken, B.J., Snelling, A.M., Hawkey, P.M., Chalmers, D.M., Axon, A.T. (1999). Non-pathogenic Escherichia coli versus mesalizine for the treatment of ulcerative colitis: a randomised trial. *Lancet*, Vol. 354, pp. 635–639.

Roberfroid, M. (2007). Prebiotics: the concept revisited. *Journal of Nutrition*, Vol. 137, pp. 830S-837S.

Roberfroid, M.B., Van Loo, J.A.E., Gibson, G.R. (1998). The bifidogenic nature of chicory inulin and its hydrolysis products. *Journal of Nutrition*, Vol. 128, pp. 11–19.

Rolfe R.D. (2000). The role of probiotic cultures in the control of gastrointestinal health. *Journal of Nutrition*, Vol. 130 (suppl), pp. 396–402.

Roselli, M., Finamore, A., Britti M.S., Mengheri, E. (2006). Probiotic bacteria *Bifidobacterium animalis* MB5 and *Lactobacillus rhamnosus* GG protect intestinal Caco-2 cells from the inflammation-associated response induced by enterotoxigenic *Escherichia coli* K88. *British Journal of Nutrition*, Vol. 95, pp. 1177–1184.

Roseth, A.G., Aadland, E., Jahnsen, J., Raknerud, N. (1997). Assessment of disease activity in ulcerative colitis by faecal calprotectin, a novel granulocyte marker protein. *Digestion*, Vol. 58, pp. 176–80

Rowland, I.R., Tanaka, R. (1993). The effects of transgalactosylated oligosaccharides on gut flora metabolism in rats associated with a human faecal microflora. *Journal of Applied Bacteriology*. Vol. 74, pp. 667-674.

Sakamoto, N., Kono, S., Wakai, K., Fukuda, Y., Satomi, M., Shimoyama, Inaba, Y., Miyake, Y., Sasaki, S., Okamoto, K., Kobashi, G., Washio, m., Yokoyama, T., Date, C, Tanaka, H., The Epidemiology Group of the Research Committee on Inflammatory Bowel Disease in Japan. (2005). Dietary Risk Factors for Inflammatory Bowel Disease, A Multicenter Case-Control Study in Japan. *Inflammatory Bowel Disease*, Vol. 11, pp. 154-163.

Sartor, R.B. (2002). Mucosal immunology and mechanisms of gastrointestinal inflammation. In: *Sleisenger & Fordtran's Gastrointestinal and Liver Disease: Gastrointestinal and Liver Disease: Pathophysiology, Diagnosis, Management* (7th edition), Feldman, M., Friedman, L.S., Sleisenger, M.H., pp. 21-51, W.B. Saunders, Philadelphia.

Schlee, M., Harder, J., Koten, B., Stange, E.F., Wehkamp, J., Fellermann, K. (2008). Probiotic lactobacilli and VSL#3 induce enterocyte beta-defensin 2. *Clinical and Experimental Immunology*, Vol. 151, pp. 528–535.

Schneeman, B. O., Tietyen, J. (1994). Dietary fiber. *In: Modern Nutrition in Health and Disease (8th edition)*, Shills, M. E., Olson, J. A., Shike, M., pp. 89–100. Lea and Febiger, Philadelphia.

Schoorlemmer, G.H.M., Evered, M.D. (2002). Reduced feeding during water deprivation depends on hydration of the gut. *American Journal of Physiology Regulatory Integrative and Comparative Physiology*. Vol. 283, pp. R1061-R1069.

Shanahan, F. (2000). Probiotics and Inflammatory bowel disease: is there a scientific rationale? *Inflammatory Bowel Disease*, Vol. 6, pp. 107–15.

Shanahan, F. (2001). Inflammatroy bowel disease: Immunodiagnostics, immunotherapeutics, and ecotherapies. *Gastroenterology*, Vol. 120, pp. 622–35.

Sherman, P.M., Johnson-Henry, K.C., Yeung, H.P., Ngo, P.S.C., Goulet, J., Tompkins, T.A. (2005). Probiotics reduce enterohemorrhagic *Escherichia coli* O157:H7- and enteropathogenic *E. coli* O127:H6-induced changes in polarized T84 epithelial cell monolayers by reducing bacterial adhesion and cytoskeletal rearrangements. *Infection and Immunity*, Vol. 73, pp. 5183–5188.

Shinohara, K., Ohashi, Y., Kawasumi, K., Terada, A., Fujisawa, T. (2010). Effect of apple intake on fecal microbiota nad metabolites in humans. *Anaerobe*, Vol. 16, pp. 510-515.

Shoda, R., Matsueda, K., Yamato, S., Umeda, N. (1996). Epidemiologic analysis of Crohn disease in Japan: increased dietary intake of n-6 polyunsaturated fatty acids and animal protein relates to the increased incidence of Crohn disease in Japan. *The American Journal of Clinical Nutrition*, Vol. 63, pp. 741-745.

Silkoff, K., Hallak, A., Yegena, L., Rozen, P., Mayberry, J.F., Rhodes, J., Newcombe, R.G. (1980). Consumption of refined carbohydrate by patients with Crohn's disease in Tel-Aviv-Yafo. *Postgraduate Medical Journal*, Vol. 56, pp. 842–846.

Slavin, J.L. (2008). Position of the American dietetic association: health implications of dietary fiber. *Journal of the American Dietetic Association*, Vol. 108, pp. 1716-1731.

Smith, P.A. (2008). Nutritional therapy for active Crohn's disease. *World Journal of Gastroenterology*, Vol. 14, pp. 4420–4423.

Soo, I., Madsen, K.L., Tejpar, Q., Sydora, B.C., Sherbaniuk, R., Cinque, B., Di Marzio, L., Cifone, M.G., Desimone, C., Fedorak, R.N. (2008). VSL#3 probiotic upregulates intestinal mucosal alkaline sphingomyelinase and reduces inflammation. *Canadian Journal of Gastroenterology*, Vol. 22, pp. 237–242.

Strober, W., Fuss, I.J., Ehrhardt, R.O., Neurath, M., Boirivant, M., Ludviksson, B. (1998). Mucosal immunoregulation and inflammatory bowel disease: new insights from murine models of inflammation. *Scandinavian Journal of Immunology*, Vol. 48, pp. 453–458.

Sturm, A., Rilling, K., Baumgart, D.C., Gargas, K., Abou-Ghazalie, T., Raupach, B., Eckert, J., Schumann, R.R., Enders, C., Sonnenborn, U., Wiedenmann, B., Dignas, A.U. (2005). *Escherichia coli* Nissle 1917 distinctively modulates T-cell cycling and expansion via toll-like receptor 2 signaling. *Infection and Immunity*, Vol. 73, pp. 1452–1465.

Tamboli, C.P., Neut, C., Desreumaux, P., Colombel, J.F. (2004). Dysbiosis in inflammatory bowel disease. *Gut*, Vol. 53, pp. 1-4.

Tamura, M. Ohnishi, Y., Kotani, T., Gato, N. (2011). Effects of new dietary fiber from Japanese apricot (Prunus mume Sieb. et Zucc.) on gut function and intestinal microflora in adult mice. *International Journal of Molecular Sciences*, Vol. 12, pp. 2088-2099.

Taylor, K.B., Truelove, S.C. (1961). Circulating antibodies to milk proteins in ulcerative colitis. *British Medical Journal*, Vol. 2, pp. 924–929.

Thompson, N.P., Montgomery, S.M., Wadsworth, M.E., Pounder, R.E., Wakefield, A.J. (2000). Early determinants of inflammatory bowel disease: use of two national longitudinal birth cohorts. *European Journal of Gastroenterology Hepatology*, Vol. 12, pp. 25–30.

Truelove, S.C. (1961). Ulcerative colitis provoked by milk. *British Medical Journal*, Vol. 1, pp. 154–160.

Tsujikawa, T., Andoh, A., Fujiyama, Y. (2003). Enteral and parenteral nutrition therapy for Crohn's disease. *Current Pharmceutical Design*, Vol. 9, pp. 323–332.

Van Gossum, A., Dewit, O., Geboes, K., Baert, F., De Vos, M., Louis, E., Enslen, M., Paintin, M., Franchimont, D. (2005). A randomized placebo-controlled clinical trial of probiotics (*L. johnsonii*, La1®) on early endoscopic recurrence of Crohn's disease (CD) after ileo-caecal resection (Abstract). *Gastroenterology*, Vol. 128 (Suppl. 2), pp. A98.

Venkatraman, A., Ramakrishna, B.S., Shaji, R.V., Nanda Kumar, N.S. Pulimoof, A., Patra, S. (2003). Amelioration of dextran sulfate colitis by butyrate: role of heat shock protein 70 and NF-kappaB. *American Journal of Physiology Gastrointestinal and Liver Physiology*. Vol. 285, pp. G177–G184.

Venturi, A., Gionchetti, P., Rizzello, F., Johansson, R., Zucconi, E., Brigidi, P., Matteuzzi, D., Campieri, M. (1999). Impact on the composition of the faecal flora by a new probiotic preparation: preliminary data on maintenance treatment of patients with ulcerative colitis. *Alimentary Pharmacology and Therapeutic*, Vol. 13, pp. 1103-1108.

Videla, S., Vilaseca, J., Guarner, F., Salas, A., Treserra, F., Crespo, E., Antolin, M., Malagelada, J.R. (1994). Role of intestinal microbiota in chronic inflammation and ulceration of the rat colon. *Gut*, Vol. 35, pp. 1090–1097.

Wang, X., Gibson, G.R. (1993). Effects of in vitro fermentation of oligofructose and inulin by bacteria growing in the human large intestine. *Journal of Applied Bacteriology*, Vol. 75, pp. 373-380.

Wehkamp, J., Harder, J., Wehkamp, K., Wehkamp-von Meissner, B., Schlee, M., Enders, C., Sonnenborn, U., Nuding, S., Bengmark, S, Fellermannm K., Schroder, J.M. Stange, F. (2004). NF-κB- and AP-1-mediated induction of human beta defensin-2 in intestinal epithelial cells by *Escherichia coli* Nissle 1917: a novel effect of a probiotic bacterium. *Infection and Immunity*, Vol. 72, pp. 5750 –5758.

Welters, C.F., Heineman, E., Thunnissen, F.B., Van der Bogaard, A.E., Soeters, P.B., Baeten, C.G. (2002). Effect of dietary inulin supplementation on inflammation of pouch mucosa in patients with an ileal pouchanal anastomosis. *Diseases of the Colon and Rectum*, Vol. 45, pp. 621–627.

Yan, F., Polk, D.B. (2002). Probiotic bacterium prevents cytokine-induced apoptosis in intestinal epithelial cells. *The Journal of Biological Chemistry*, Vol. 277, pp. 50959-50965.

Zyrek, A.A., Cichon, C., Helms, S., Enders, C., Sonnenborn, U., Schmidt, M.A. (2007). Molecular mechanisms underlying the probiotic effects of Escherichia coli Nissle 1917 involve ZO-2 and PKC zeta redistribution resulting in tight junction and epithelial barrier repair. *Cellular Microbiology*, Vol. 9, pp. 804–816.

15

The Use of Pomegranate (*Punica granatum* L.) Phenolic Compounds as Potential Natural Prevention Against IBDs

Sylvie Hollebeeck, Yvan Larondelle,
Yves-Jacques Schneider and Alexandrine During
Institut des Sciences de la Vie, UCLouvain, Louvain-la-Neuve
Belgium

1. Introduction

Phenolic compounds (PCs) are plant secondary metabolites that are integral part of the "normal" human diet. The daily intake of PCs depends on the diet but is commonly evaluated at *ca.* 1g/day for people who eat several fruits and vegetables per day (Scalbert & Williamson, 2000). PCs may be interesting to prevent the development of inflammatory diseases, more particularly in the gastrointestinal tract, where their concentration may reach levels of up to several hundred µM (Scalbert & Williamson, 2000). Many studies have indeed reported on anti-inflammatory properties of different PCs (see (Calixto *et al.*, 2004; Rahman *et al.*, 2006; Romier *et al.*, 2009; Shapiro *et al.*, 2009), for reviews).

Pomegranate *(Punica granatum L.)* belongs to the *Punicaceae* family, which includes only two species. More than 500 cultivars of *Punica granatum* exist with specific characteristics such as fruit size, exocarp and aril color, etc. Originating from the Middle East, pomegranate is now widely cultivated throughout the world, and also widely consumed. Pomegranate has been used for centuries in the folk medicine of many cultures. As described in the review of Lansky *et al.* (2007), the bark and the roots are believed to have anthelmintic and vermifuge properties, the fruit peel has been used as a cure for diarrhea, oral aphthae, and as a powerful astringent, the juice as a blood tonic, and the flowers as a cure for *diabetes mellitus.*

Numerous investigations have highlighted the anti-inflammatory potential of the PCs found in this fruit, and more especially of hydrolysable tannins called ellagitannins (ETs), which are mainly located in pomegranate peels. These ETs are extracted into the juice upon commercial processing of the whole fruit (Gil *et al.*, 2000).

This chapter first describes the PCs found in pomegranate fruit, then focuses on ETs in relation to their metabolic fate after ingestion as well as to their anti-inflammatory properties on the intestine, and finally discusses gut microflora modifications following pomegranate ingestion and their impact on intestinal inflammation.

2. Phenolic compounds identified in the pomegranate fruit

The pomegranate fruit is a berry of 5 to 12 cm diameter with a leathery, deep red peel (husk, rind, and pericarp are synonyms). The fruit's interior is separated by membranous walls into compartments containing arils filled with pulp. Each aril contains one angular seed. PCs are present in different parts of pomegranate plants; they are found in seeds, arils, fruit peels, leaves, flowers, tree bark, and roots (Lansky & Newman, 2007). Here, we will be focusing on the PCs of the pomegranate fruit since the commercial processing of the whole fruit is largely used in the juice industry. Different classes of PCs are found in the pomegranate fruit. The amounts of each PC are largely affected by the raw material, e.g. pomegranate cultivars and climatic conditions during fruit maturation and ripening (Borochov-Neori *et al.*, 2009), but also by the post-harvest storage, and the technological treatments leading to juice production and distribution (Tomás-Barberan *et al.*, 2000).

One important component of pomegranate PCs is ellagic acid (EA) (**Figure 1**). EA can be found in its free form (aglycone form), in a conjugated form with a glycoside moiety or more commonly complexed in the form of ETs. The occurrence of the free form in the nature is however quite uncommon (Clifford & Scalbert, 2000).

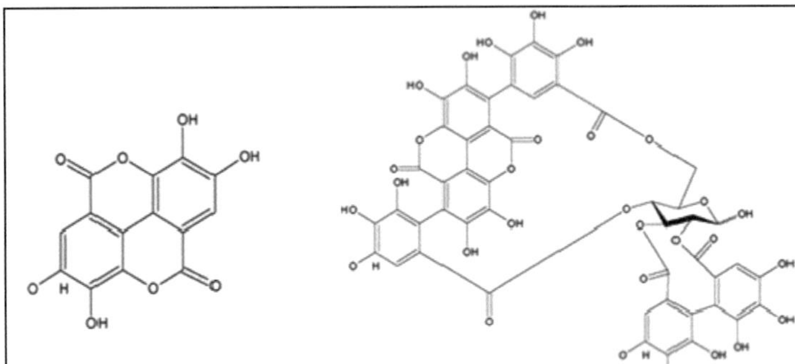

1 2

Fig. 1. Chemical structures of EA (1) and punicalagin (2) (Lansky & Newman, 2007).

Regarding pomegranate juice production, the phenolic profile has been reported to be very different if made from isolated arils only or from the whole fruit (Gil *et al.*, 2000). In the same study, commercial pomegranate juices, made by pressing the whole fruit, were reported to show an antioxidant activity three times higher than red wine and green tea infusion, while hand-pressed pomegranate juice showed a lower antioxidant activity. This difference was attributed to the elevated amount of pomegranate peel ETs that are transferred into the juice during whole fruit pressing. Numerous studies have highlighted that commercial pomegranate juices present a very high antioxidant activity, mainly attributed to their high content in ETs and more particularly in punicalagin (**Figure 1**), which offers more than 50% of the total antioxidant activity (Gil *et al.*, 2000; Li *et al.*, 2006; Schubert *et al.*, 1999; Seeram *et al.*, 2005a; Tzulker *et al.*, 2007).

Given the wide difference in antioxidant activity observed with the two methods of juicing, it is useful to distinguish PCs found in juice made from the arils only, from those identified in the peel. Hydroxybenzoic acids were mainly found in the arils, except for gallic acid that was present at a higher level in the peel (Amakura *et al.*, 2000; Fischer *et al.*, 2011). Hydroxycinnamic acids are identified only in the arils, except for free caffeic acid and chlorogenic acid that were reported to be present only in the fruit peels (Amakura *et al.*, 2000; Fischer *et al.*, 2011; Lansky & Newman, 2007). Among the flavonoids, luteolin and luteolin 7-O-glucoside (flavones), as well as naringenin 7-O-rutinoside (flavanones), catechin, epicatechin and epigallocatechin 3-gallate (flavanols), and quercetin, kaempferol, rutin, kaempferol 3-O-glucoside and kaempferol 3-O-rhamnoglycoside (flavonols), were also exclusively identified in the fruit peel (Lansky & Newman, 2007; de Pascual-Teresa *et al.*, 2000), whereas the flavonol dihydrokaempferol-hexoside was identified in the arils, but not in the peel (Fischer *et al.*, 2011). Still in the class of flavonoids, the pomegranate fruit contains a collection of different anthocyanins (delphinidin 3,5-diglucoside, delphinidin 3-glucoside, cyanidin 3-glucoside, cyanidin-pentoside-hexoside, cyaniding 3-rutinoside, cyaniding 3-pentoside, cyanidin 3-hexoside, cyanidin 3,5-diglucoside, pelargonidin 3-glucoside, pelargonidin 3,5-diglucoside), which are present in both arils and peels in similar concentrations (Fischer *et al.*, 2011). Pomegranate fruits are very rich in hydrolysable tannins, including gallotannins and ETs, essentially present in the peel with about 44g/kg of dry matter of that material (Fischer *et al.*, 2011). Gallotannins represent less than 0.01% and less than 2% of total hydrolysable tannins, respectively in the peel and in the juice made from arils only. ETs are predominantly found in the peel, with about 20 components identified (Fischer *et al.*, 2011). As indicated before, the most abundant ET is punicalagin with a concentration of about 10.5 g/kg of dry matter of pomegranate peel, and its levels can be superior to 2g/L in industrial juice (Amakura *et al.*, 2000; Borges *et al.*, 2010; Fischer *et al.*, 2011; Lansky & Newman, 2007; Martin *et al.*, 2009, Seeram *et al.*, 2005b).

3. Metabolic fate of pomegranate ellagitannins

In order to evaluate the health effects of ETs, it is critical to understand their oral bioaccessibility from the pomegranate matrix as well as their bioavailability.

3.1 Bioaccessibility and intestinal absorption

After ingestion, PCs may undergo changes until they reach the site where they could have an impact. In the gastro-intestinal tract, PCs are submitted, on one hand, to abiotic physico-chemical changes and enzymatic attacks, accompanying the digestion in the upper part of the tract, and, on the other hand, to biotic changes with the participation of the gut microflora found in the lower part of the tract, and especially in the colon.

Concerning the abiotic changes, an *in vitro* simulated gastric digestion showed that ETs are quite stable under acidic conditions and are not hydrolyzed by stomach enzymes, while an important increase of free EA was observed in the duodenal digestion conditions (Gil-Izquierdo *et al.*, 2002). Similarly, in the duodenal conditions, a significant release of EA from the standard punicalagin was also reported by Larrosa *et al.* (2006b) and it was assumed to be due to a spontaneous hydrolysis of punicalagin in the neutral pH conditions. When pomegranate juice was submitted to both *in vitro* gastric and duodenal digestions, no significant differences in total soluble phenolic contents (determined by the Folin-Ciocalteu) were noticed before and after gastric digestion, while, after duodenal digestion, 29% of the total initial phenolic content in a soluble form were available for absorption (Perez-Vicente *et al.*, 2002). These results confirm that pomegranate PCs undergo modifications under duodenal conditions. To our knowledge, no other data are available on the fate of ETs or EA with reference to abiotic changes, related to enzymatic attacks and pH variations, encountered in the gastro-intestinal tract. In the lower part of the gastro-intestinal tract, ETs seem to be transformed by the gut microflora (*i.e.* biotic changes). An *in vivo* study conducted on pigs showed that EA, resulting from ET hydrolysis, is metabolized by the gut microflora that is already active in the jejunum and much more concentrated in the colon. This progressive metabolic processing is illustrated in **Figure 2**. Urolithins D, C, A and B are sequentially produced, by successive losses of hydroxyl groups, resulting in an increased lipophilicity as well as in an increased intestinal absorption rate (Espín *et al.*, 2007). When rats fed with punicalagin at a daily rate ranging from 0.6 to 1.2 g for 37 days, their feces showed an increased presence of punicalagin and its hydrolysis products (punicalin, gallagic acid, and EA) up to day 18. Afterwards, a decrease of punicalagin and punicalin amounts was observed concomitantly with an increase in urolithin acompounds (Cerdá *et al.*, 2003b). Human fecal samples from 6 healthy volunteers were incubated with EA, punicalagin and an extract of walnut (rich in ETs) to search for the occurrence of urolithin A. Samples were analyzed at 5, 24, 48, and 72h of incubation. Urolithin A in its aglycone form was identified in all the samples collected, but not urolithin A conjugates, suggesting that the aglycones should first be absorbed before being metabolized in the conjugated forms by the intestinal cells and/or liver (Cerdá *et al.*, 2005). In another study, the occurrence of the different urolithins (**Figure 2**) in their aglycone form was analyzed after incubation of pomegranate by-products with human fecal samples obtained from three healthy volunteers. The four urolithins D, C, A and B were identified (Bialonska *et al.*, 2010).

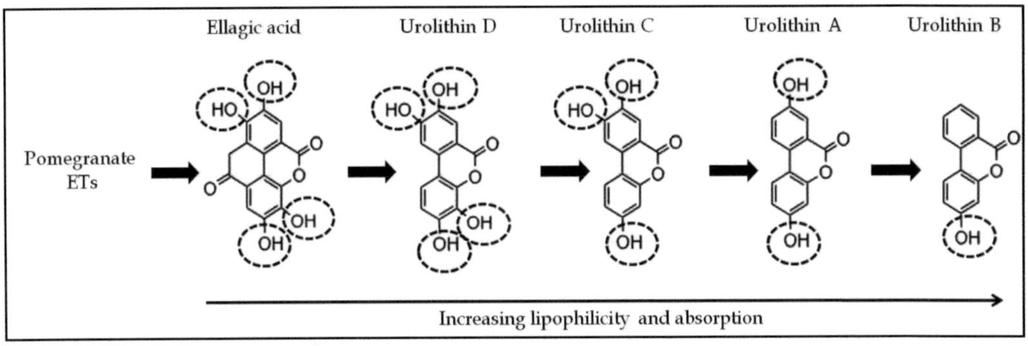

Fig. 2. Metabolism of pomegranate ETs by the human intestinal microflora (adapted from Espín *et al.* (2007)).

Concerning the intestinal absorption, EA was shown to enter into the intestinal cells and to be further metabolized in dimethyl EA conjugates (e.g. dimethyl EA glucuronides and dimethyl EA sulphates) in an *in vitro* study using proliferating Caco-2 cells, suggesting the involvement of phase II enzymes (methylation, glucuronidation and sulphation) (Larrosa *et al.*, 2006b). In another *in vitro* study (Whitley *et al.*, 2003), with differentiated Caco-2 cells in a bicameral system, labeled standard EA was incubated in the apical compartment to evaluate its trans- or para-cellular transport. Cellular uptake seemed very extensive and probably governed by passive diffusion at the apical side. However, the passage across the epithelial cell monolayer appeared very limited since the quantity of EA found in the basolateral compartment was very low in this model. In accordance with this observation, a preferential apical efflux of EA was observed even though the multidrug resistance-associated protein 2 (MRP2) and the P-glycoprotein, two apical efflux transporters expressed in Caco-2 cells, were not involved. In addition, intracellular binding processes were shown to decrease EA passage. Once in the intestinal cells, EA appeared indeed to bind irreversibly to DNA and proteins (Whitley *et al.*, 2003), as it was already demonstrated for the flavonoid quercetin (Walle *et al.*, 2003). The high irreversible binding ability of EA to DNA did not require prior oxidation and may be due to its great ability to intercalate DNA (Dixit & Gold, 1986; Teel *et al.*, 1987; Thulstrup *et al.*, 1999). In contrast, the covalent binding ability of EA to proteins may require its prior oxidation by reactive oxygen species that could be abolished by glutathione (Whitley *et al.*, 2003). In the *in vivo* study on pigs mentioned above (Espín *et al.*, 2007), ET metabolites were shown to be absorbed in the intestinal tissues. The metabolites detected in the pig jejunum tissues were, in increasing amounts, urolithin D, urolithin C, urolithin A, urolithin A glucuronide, and urolithin C methyl ether, following the increase degree of lipophilicity. By contrast, EA conjugates were not detected in the intestinal tissues but were present in bile and in urines, suggesting EA absorption in the stomach. The colon tissues were also analyzed and only small amounts of urolithins A and B were detected. The results of these *in vitro* and *in vivo* studies indicate that the resulting products of microbial transformation, namely the urolithins, are absorbed along with EA and further metabolized in the enterocytes by phase II (methylation, glucuronidation and sulphation) enzymes.

3.2 Blood circulation, distribution and excretion

Except for the studies of Cerdá *et al.* (2003a & 2003b) reporting trace amounts of punicalagin in rat plasma after a high daily consumption of 0.9 g punicalagin for 37 days, many *in vivo* animal studies indicate that ETs are not found as such in the blood circulation (Borges *et al.*, 2007; Cerdá *et al.*, 2004a & 2004b; Espín *et al.*, 2007; González-Barrio *et al.*, 2010; Mertens-Talcott *et al.*, 2006; Seeram *et al.*, 2006). In their pig study, Espín *et al.* (2007) reported that animals fed with acorns rich in ETs and EA (single feeding) showed the occurrence of urolithin A and B as aglycone and conjugates in their plasma 24h, but not 3h, after ingestion. The same ET metabolites were also detected in trace amounts in the 24h urines. These observations indicate that pigs are able to produce rapidly the microflora metabolites (24h after a single ingestion), in contrast with rats that needed several days (Cerdá *et al.*, 2003b). In pigs regularly fed with acorns and after a 24h fasting period, urolithins A and B as aglycone and as conjugates and EA conjugates were detected in both plasma and urines as well. The bile content of these animals, after gall bladder removal, showed a wide range of urolithins (urolithin A, C and D) conjugates, mainly the glucuronides, as well as EA conjugates, while no urolithin B aglycone and/or conjugates were found. The metabolites found in the bile coincide with those found in the lumen, except for the aglycone EA that was not detected in the bile. The presence of a wide range of ET metabolites in the bile and the very low clearance of these compounds in urines suggested an important enterohepatic circulation (Espín *et al.*, 2007). Interestingly enough, the study of Cerdá *et al.* (2003b) on rats fed with punicalagin for 37 days did not only report on fecal analyses (see section 3.1), but also on plasma and urine levels of ET metabolites. They showed that, during a first period of about 20 days, the main metabolites detected in plasma and urines were derived only from punicalagin hydrolysis through conjugation in methyl ether or glucuronide forms, whereas, after 20 days, urolithins and their glucuronides were detected, which may be due, as for the fecal observations, to a modification of the gut microflora composition. After mice ingested a single dose (0.8 mg per animal) of an ET-enriched pomegranate peel extract, standardized to 37% ETs and 3.5% EA, plasma samples were collected over 24h. EA was detected in the plasma 30 min after pomegranate extract ingestion and was cleared after 2h, while neither urolithin A nor urolithin A conjugates were detected during the 24h (Seeram *et al.*, 2007). The pharmacokinetics of EA was evaluated after oral administration of a pomegranate leaf extract to rats. A rapid increase of EA was observed in the plasma with a maximum concentration reached 0.54h after ingestion and a plasma half-life of 5h (Lei *et al.*, 2003).

Human studies on healthy volunteers seem to confirm the results obtained in animal studies. A first trial was conducted on one subject who ingested 180 mL of pomegranate juice containing 25 mg of EA and 318 mg of ETs. In order to evaluate EA bioavailability, blood samples were collected until 6h after consumption. A maximum concentration was detected 1h post-ingestion and EA was cleared after 4h (Seeram *et al.*, 2004). On the basis of that preliminary study, another study was performed on 18 healthy human volunteers who consumed 180 mL of pomegranate juice containing 1561 mg/L of punicalagin, 121 mg/L of EA, and 417 mg/L of other ETs. Blood samples were analyzed during the 6h following ingestion and urines were collected in 12h batches the day before, the day of, and the day after ingestion. Again, no ETs were detected as intact form in plasma. By contrast, EA could be detected. It peaked at 0.98±0.06 h post-ingestion (T_{max}), with a maximum concentration (C_{max}) of 0.06±0.01 µmol/L (18.64 ng/mL), and an elimination half-life ($T_{1/2}$) of 0.71±0.08 h. It was cleared within 5h. The area under the curve (AUC) was 0.17±0.02 (µmol*h)*L^{-1} (50.07 ng*h/mL). Interestingly, urolithin A and B as aglycone and as conjugates began already to appear in blood collected 0.5h after ingestion and higher concentrations were found in 6h plasma samples. EA and dimethyl EA glucuronide were detected in urines of the day of juice consumption, respectively for 5 and 15 of the 18 subjects, but not of the following day. Urolithin A and B glucuronides appeared in the urines collected the second 12h of the day of the study, and in the urines collected the day after (Seeram *et al.*, 2006). After 6 healthy volunteers ingested 1 L of pomegranate juice per day for 5 days, the occurrence of metabolites in plasma and urines was examined (Cerdá *et al.*, 2004a). Neither punicalagin nor EA, in free or in conjugated form, was found in plasma samples, whereas urolithins conjugates were detected (urolithin A glucuronide, an unidentified aglycone metabolite and urolithin B glucuronide). The urines revealed the presence of 3 additional microflora metabolites (urolithin A, urolithin B, and an unidentified aglycone metabolite). The metabolites found in plasma and urines presented high inter-individual variability (Cerdá *et al.*, 2004a). Another study conducted on 40 healthy volunteers investigated the metabolic fate of ETs from 4 different sources of ET-rich foodstuffs, *i.e.* strawberries, red raspberries, walnuts, and oak-aged red wine. Each group of 10 volunteers received a single dose of ET-containing foodstuff and the urines were collected in 5 fractions, at 8, 16, 32, 40, and 56h after food intake (Cerdá *et al.*, 2004b). As previously observed with pomegranate juice consumption (Cerdá *et al.*, 2004a), neither ETs nor EA were detected in none of the urine fractions collected. Whatever the foodstuff ingested, urolithin B glucuronide was detected in all the urines from 32h to 56h following ingestion, and urolithin B in some of them (Cerdá *et al.*, 2004b). In another human study, 2 capsules corresponding to 800 mg of pomegranate extract (330.4 mg of punicalagin and 21.6 mg of EA), were administered to 11 healthy volunteers. No punicalagin was found in human plasma, while EA appeared in plasma with similar pharmacokinetic parameters as previously observed: T_{max}=1h, C_{max}=33.8±12.7 ng/mL, $T_{1/2}$=0.94h and AUC=118.01 ng*h/mL. The microflora metabolites were detected as well (e.g. urolithin A, hydroxyl urolithin A, urolithin A glucuronide, urolithin B and dimethyl urolithin B glucuronide). Again, these different metabolites were not present in all the subjects tested, which could be explained by the difference in microflora composition responsible for ET degradation (Mertens-Talcott *et al.*, 2006). A single intake of raspberry containing ETs was given to 10 healthy humans and 4 humans with ileostomy. Blood was collected during 24h and urines were collected at 4, 7, 24 and 48h post-ingestion. Urolithins were detected in the plasma of the healthy volunteers, but not in the plasma of the patients with ileostomy, confirming that urolithins are formed in the large intestine. No ETs in an intact or conjugated form were detected in the plasma of any subjects during 24h after raspberry intake. Small amounts of EA and EA glucuronide were detected in the urines from both groups. However, urolithin A and B glucuronides were only identified in the urines of healthy subjects collected at 7 to 48h post-ingestion (González-Barrio *et al.*, 2010). In sum, these human studies indicate that there is no absorption of the ETs in an intact form. Concerning the distribution in non-intestinal tissues, an *in vitro* study reported that urolithins A and B entered into the human breast cancer MCF-7 cells and were metabolized in urolithin sulphate and glucuronide conjugates (Larrosa *et al.*, 2006a). In the mice study of Seeram *et al.* (2007), prostate, liver, kidney, lung and brain tissues were analyzed 24h after pomegranate extract ingestion. Neither EA, nor ETs, nor urolithin A in free or conjugated form was detected in any tissues when pomegranate was orally administrated. In the pig study performed by Espín *et al.* (2007), liver, kidney, heart, lung, brain, and muscle tissues were analyzed after a 117 day-ET rich diet, and again no ET metabolites were detected. Nevertheless, in the rat study performed by Cerdá *et al.* (2003a), 5 punicalagin metabolites (two EA conjugates, gallagic acid, urolithin A glucuronide, and urolithin C glucuronide) were detected in the two organs investigated, namely liver and kidney.

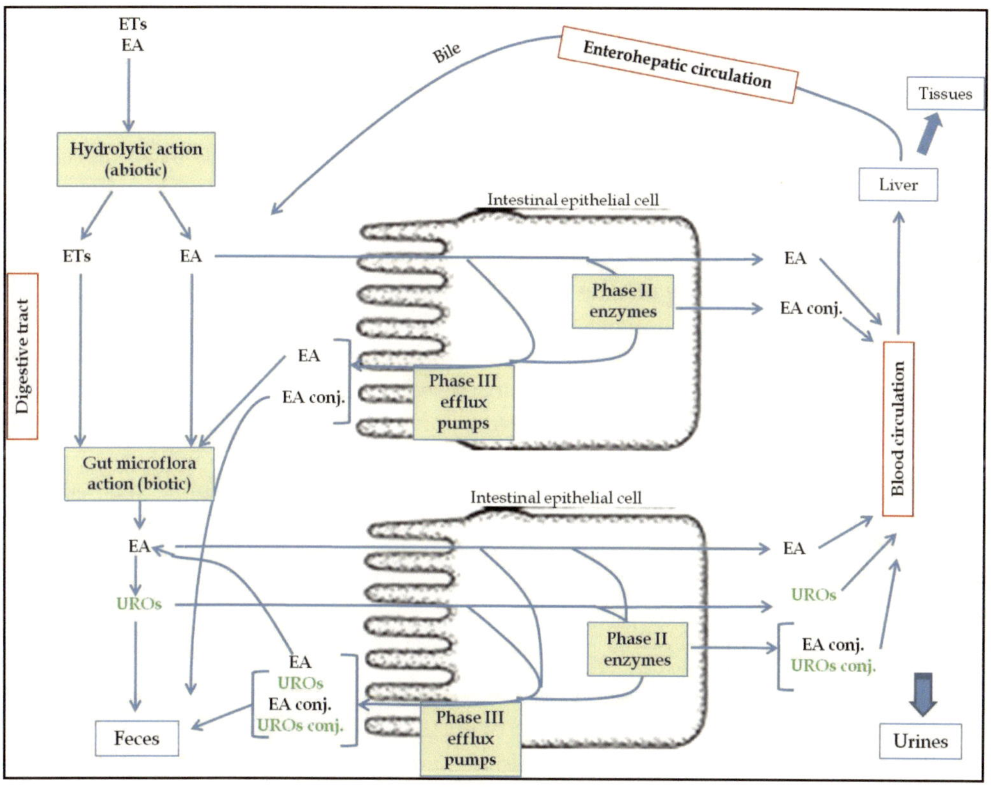

Abbreviations: conj., conjugates ; EA, ellagic acid; ETs, ellagitannins; UROs, urolithins.
The compounds in green result from a microbial action on EA.

Fig. 3. Model of the metabolic fate of ellagitannins and ellagic acid in the human intestine.

As summarized in **Figure 3**, upon ingestion of pomegranate, ETs seem to be partially hydrolyzed in the upper part of the gastrointestinal tract to release EA that is further metabolized by the colon microflora to form the bioavailable urolithins. Free EA found in pomegranate could already be absorbed in the small intestine epithelial cells, while intact ETs need to reach the large intestine where they are shown to be extensively transformed in urolithins by the intestinal microflora before being absorbed. Once urolithins and EA are absorbed, they are conjugated to give methyl ether, glucuronide or sulphate conjugates by phases II enzymes. These conjugates can be found in the plasma, as well as in the intestinal lumen, directly after conjugation in the intestinal cell, or via the enterohepatic circulation. Part of them is not absorbed and is excreted in the feces. The urolithins and EA, either conjugated or in their free form, can temporarily accumulate in the intestinal tissues before being liberated in the plasma.

4. Effects of pomegranate phenolic compounds on the intestinal inflammatory response in IBD-related models

Since the last years, anti-inflammatory effects related to pomegranate consumption were reported in intestinal *in vitro* and in *vivo* studies, suggesting a role for pomegranate-derived products in IBD prevention. Causes of IBDs are not well known but two main hypotheses are put forward. The first hypothesis suggests that a deregulation of the mucosal immune system provokes excessive immunologic responses against the normal gut microflora, while the second one proposes that changes in the composition of the gut microflora associated with a disrupted epithelial barrier lead to an abnormal inflammatory response from the intestinal mucosa (Stecher & Hardt, 2008). In this section, *in vitro* and *in vivo* studies highlighting the anti-inflammatory properties of pomegranate PCs will be reviewed.

4.1 *In vitro* anti-inflammatory effects of pomegranate phenolic compounds

Anti-cancer effects of pomegranate have been described in *in vitro* studies on cell proliferation and apoptosis using human colon cancer cells (Larrosa *et al.*, 2006b; Seeram *et al.*, 2005b). Even if IBDs are associated with increased risk for colorectal cancer and if there are similarities in the biology of IBD-associated colon cancer and sporadic cancer (Rhodes & Campbell, 2002), these highlighted effects are not, strictly speaking, related to the intestinal inflammation response developed by IBD patients, and therefore, will not be detailed in this section. Among *in vitro* studies on intestinal epithelial cells, only three studies investigated the intestinal anti-inflammatory potential of pomegranate extracts, pomegranate juice or pomegranate PCs. They were carried out on human colon epithelial cells: Caco-2 cells (Romier-Crouzet *et al.*, 2009; Sergent *et al.*, 2010) and HT-29 cells (Adams *et al.*, 2006). In these studies, intestinal inflammation was induced either by IL-1β (Romier-Crouzet *et al.*, 2009), or TNF-α (Adams *et al.*, 2006) or by a mixture of pro-inflammatory molecules, *i.e.* IL-1β, IFN-γ, TNF-α and LPS (Romier-Crouzet *et al.*, 2009; Sergent *et al.*, 2010). Additional *in vitro* studies have evaluated the potential role of pomegranate for preventing IBDs by using other types of cells involved in the intestinal immune response, such as murine splenic lymphocytes CD4+ T cells (S.I. Lee *et al.*, 2008), RAW 264.7 murine macrophages (C.J. Lee *et al.*, 2010; Panichayupakaranant *et al.*, 2010), or the human basophilic cell line KU812 (Rasheed *et al.*, 2009). In these studies, inflammation was induced either by LPS (C.J. Lee *et al.*, 2010; Panichayupakaranant *et al.*, 2010) or by phorbol-12-myristate 13-acetate plus calcium ionophore A23187 (PMACI) (Rasheed *et al.*, 2009).

4.1.1 *In vitro* effects on inflamed intestinal cells

Ellagic acid. Anti-inflammatory effects of EA were evaluated by measuring inflammatory-related cytokine (the pro-inflammatory cytokines IL-6, IL-8, MCP-1 and the anti-inflammatory IL-10) secretion and mRNA expression in differentiated Caco-2 cells stimulated with the pro-inflammatory cocktail (IL-1β, IFN-γ, TNF-α and LPS) (Sergent *et al.*, 2010). For the experiments, cells were seeded on a microporous membrane in bicameral inserts. Two-day treatments were started at day-19 by adding EA (50 μM final concentration) to the apical side of the cells, while the cocktail of pro-inflammatory stimuli was concomitantly introduced to the basolateral side. The amounts of pro-inflammatory cytokines were quantified with ELISA assays after pooling the media from both compartments. EA decreased MCP-1 and IL-8 secretion but not significantly, and had no effect on IL-6 and IL-10 secretions, while mRNA expression of the four cytokines was not affected. Nevertheless, in that study, EA down-regulated the transcription of three genes involved in the intestinal inflammation: CD14 (Cluster of differentiation 14 gene) encoding a protein acting as LPS receptor, IL1R1 (Interleukin 1 receptor type 1 gene), and PLA2G2A (phospholipase A2 gene). EA also significantly down-regulated the transcription factor STAT3 (signal transducer and activator of transcription 3) involved in the persistent activation of NF-κB (the nuclear factor-kappa B), an inducible nuclear transcriptional factor associated with the intestinal inflammatory response (Yu *et al.*, 2009) and the gene CYP1A1 (Cytochrome P450, family 1, subfamily A, polypeptide 1) (Sergent *et al.*, 2010).

Pomegranate peel extract. A pomegranate peel extract, used at the concentration of 50 μM gallic acid equivalent (GAE), was reported to inhibit NF-κB activity in confluent Caco-2 cells temporarily transfected with a NF-κB-luciferase construct and under IL-1β stimulation. The same extract tested on Il-1β-stimulated and non-transfected confluent Caco-2 cells was also found to inhibit slightly Erk1/2 phosphorylation, but had no effect on JNK phosphorylation (2 major members of the mitogen-activated-protein kinase (MAPK) cascades involved in the intestinal inflammatory response). In addition, it significantly decreased IL-8 secretion as well as cyclooxygenase-2 (COX-2) activity, as measured by the synthesis of prostaglandin-E2 (PGE2) upon incubation of the cells with arachidonic acid (Romier-Crouzet *et al.*, 2009).

Pomegranate juice, tannins and punicalagin. Effects of pomegranate juice, total pomegranate tannins and punicalagin on inflammatory proteins involved in cell signaling cascades were evaluated using HT-29 colon cancer cells stimulated with TNFα. The juice was commercially available (POM Wonderful LLC, Los Angeles, CA) and was used in a concentrated form containing 1.74 g/L punicalagin, while purified punicalagin as well as total pomegranate tannins were isolated from the fruit peel and normalized at equivalent concentrations of those found in the juice. The induced COX-2 protein expression was decreased with all the three preparations, in a dose dependent manner. In addition, the pomegranate juice was shown to significantly inhibit the protein kinase B (AKT) activity, which is known for increasing COX-2 expression (Adams *et al.*, 2006).

4.1.2 *In vitro* effects on immune cells

Other pomegranate anti-inflammatory properties have been highlighted not directly on the intestinal epithelial cells but also on immune cells since both cell types are interacting during the intestinal inflammatory response.

Macrophage cells. In inflammatory events, macrophage cells, stimulated by the pro-inflammatory cytokines secreted by the activated T cells, produce in turn a large amount of pro-inflammatory mediators (e.g. TNFα, interleukins, and reactive oxygen species (ROS)). RAW 264.7 murine macrophages were used to study the anti-inflammatory properties of 4 ETs isolated from pomegranate peels, namely punicalagin, punicalin, strictinin A, and granatin B (C.J. Lee *et al.*, 2010). Inflammation was induced by 24h pre-incubation with LPS (1 μg/mL), leading to a high secretion of NO and PGE2 as well as to an up-regulation of iNOS and COX-2 protein expression. Inhibitory effects on NO production were observed for the 4 isolated ETs (at 100 μM) with the following decreasing order of intensity: granatin B > strictinin A > punicalagin > punicalin. That NO inhibition was neither due to NO-scavenging activity, nor to iNOS activity inhibition, but was the consequence of a decrease in iNOS protein expression with the strongest effect attributed to granatin B. Only granatin B significantly reduced PGE2 production and COX-2 expression in a dose dependent manner after 8h of treatment, while granatin B showed no effect on COX-2 expression after 18h exposure (C.J. Lee *et al.*, 2010). An inhibition of NO production was also found with a standardized pomegranate peel extract containing 13% w/w EA, in LPS-induced (100 μg/mL) RAW 264.7 cells. This peel extract revealed marked anti-NO effects, equivalent to that of L-nitroarginine, a NO synthase inhibitor, with an IC_{50} (concentration at which 50% of the inhibitory effect is observed) of 10.7 μg/mL. Standard EA was also tested and revealed even higher anti-NO effects with an IC_{50} value of 1.9 μg/mL (Panichayupakaranant *et al.*, 2010).

Mast cells. Mast cells are other key players in the inflammation that release, upon activation, numerous mediators by discharging their granules and/or by synthesizing them. These mediators play a role by recruiting leucocytes to the inflammation site, and by activating many of them to produce their own mediators of inflammation. The anti-inflammatory potential of a standardized pomegranate fruit extract (POMx, POM Wonderful brand) has been evaluated on KU812 cells, a model of human mast cells, which were stimulated with 40 nM of phorbol 12-myristate 13-acetate (PMA) plus 1 μM of calcium ionophore (CI) (Rasheed *et al.*, 2009). The cells were pre-treated with POMx (20-100 μg/mL) for 1h prior to stimulation with PMA-CI for 4h. POMx significantly inhibited IL-6 and IL-8 secretions and decreased the corresponding gene expressions in a dose-dependent manner. Furthermore, POMx attenuated JNKp54/p46 and ERKp44/p42 phosphorylation, but had no effect on p38-MAPK phosphorylation in PMA-CI-induced mast cells. POMx inhibited the PMA-CI-induced degradation of IκBα and nuclear translocation of p65 NF-κB. Finally, POMx significantly inhibited the NF-κB DNA binding activity in KU812 cells transfected with a NF-κB-luciferase construct and exposed to PMA-CI (Rasheed *et al.*, 2009).

T cells. Naïve T cells (Th0) activation initiates an adaptive immune response, and then, plays a central role in the development of autoimmune diseases. In IBDs, effector T cells (Th1, Th2 and Th17) predominate over regulatory T cells (Th3, Tr). These activated T cells secrete pro-inflammatory cytokines (IL-4, IL-5, IL-12, IL-13, IL-17, INFγ, etc.) that stimulate macrophages. Punicalagin was identified as a potent immune suppressant in activated murine splenic CD4+ T cells. Indeed, a 24h exposure of these cells to punicalagin (5 μM) decreased the secretion of IL-2, a protein stimulating growth and differentiation of T cells. A reduction of IL-2 mRNA levels was also observed with 5 μM punicalagin (S.I. Lee *et al.*, 2008). Furthermore, after 6h incubation, punicalagin (2.5-40 μM) significantly inhibited the activation of the nuclear factor activated T cells (NFAT), a transcription factor for IL-2 expression after T cell activation, in a dose-dependent way, in NFAT-Jurkat cells stimulated with PMA (10 ng/mL) and CI (1 μM) (S.I. Lee *et al.*, 2008).

4.2 *Ex vivo* intestinal anti-inflammatory effects of pomegranate PCs

A single dose (34 mg/kg body weight (bw)) of pomegranate fruit extract (POMx, POM Wonderful brand) was orally administrated to experimental rabbits. After 2h, blood samples of the experimental and the control groups were collected in order to test the inhibitory effects of plasma samples on the activities of COXs *ex vivo* by using purified enzyme preparations. Both COX-1 and COX-2 activities were reduced *ex vivo* in presence of the experimental plasma (2h post-supplementation with POMx) *versus* the control plasma (prior supplementation), with a higher effect on COX-2 activity. These results suggested that pomegranate fruit extract component and/or metabolites may inhibit the activity of eicosanoid generating enzymes, and then exert anti-inflammatory effects *ex vivo* (Shukla *et al., 2008).*

4.3 *In vivo* intestinal anti-inflammatory effects of pomegranate phenolic compounds

Although all the *in vitro* studies seem to show anti-inflammatory effects of the pomegranate fruit in intestinal inflammation, its biological activity should be proven *in vivo*.

Among the *in vivo* studies on the effects of pomegranate PCs on intestinal inflammation related to IBDs, four studies conducted on murine models were reported in the literature: three with rats (Larrosa *et al.*, 2010; Ogawa *et al.*, 2002; Rosillo *et al.*, 2011) and one with mice (Singh *et al.*, 2009). Experimental models of IBD were induced by a daily oral administration of dextran sulphate sodium (DSS) at 2-5% (v/v) in drinking water or by intra-colonic administration of trinitrobenzene sulfonic acid (TNBS).

4.3.1 Rat studies

Ellagic acid. To evaluate the prophylactic effects of EA in the treatment of IBDs (Ogawa *et al.*, 2002), EA was administered to rats, as such or in an encapsulated form. The microsphere capsules allowed EA to reach the terminal ileum and colon where microcapsules dissolved. Encapsulated or not, EA was administrated orally twice daily for the last 6 days during the 7 day treatment with DSS to one group of rats. Another DSS-induced colitis rat group received superoxide dismutase (SOD), a well-known anti-oxidative agent, intra-rectally twice daily for the last 6 days. Colonic mucosa of DSS-treated animals showed typical inflammatory changes such as erosions, ulcerations, and infiltration of immune cells. The administration of encapsulated EA (1-10 mg/kg bw) prevented the development of DSS-induced colitis with an effective dose on 50% of rats (ED_{50}) of 2.3 mg/kg bw. The same effects were observed with non-encapsulated EA, but at higher concentrations (ED_{50} 32.9 mg/kg bw). Treatments with EA also prevented the decrease in colon length due to DSS treatment, and again a higher effect was observed with the encapsulated EA. Lipid peroxidation in the colonic mucosa, determined by the thiobarbituric acid-reactive substance (TBARS) assay, was significantly decreased by the encapsulated EA treatment, but was not affected by free EA. Similar effects were observed after SOD administration, supporting the idea that EA prevents the colitis development by radical scavenging or other anti-oxidative actions (Ogawa *et al.*, 2002). EA was orally administrated to rats at both doses (10 and 20 mg/kg bw) 48, 24 and 1h before TNBS intra-colonic administration and 24h after. Both doses of EA significantly decreased the extent and severity of the colonic damage and the leukocyte infiltration, and increased the mucus production by goblet cells. EA decreased COX-2 and iNOS protein expressions induced by TNBS. EA also inhibited both MAPK (ERK, JNK, and p38) pathways by preventing their phosphorylation and NF-κB pathway by preventing the IκBα degradation and the nuclear translocation of p65 in the intestinal epithelial cells from inflamed rat colon (Rosillo *et al.*, 2011).

Pomegranate polyphenolic extract and urolithin A. A DSS-induced colitis rat model was used to study the anti-inflammatory effects of a commercial pomegranate extract ("Nutragranate from Nutracitrus S.L., Elche, Spain), and of urolithin A (see section 3). Rats received a standard diet for 25 days with 5% DSS for the last 5 days. The test groups received the standard diet supplemented either with pomegranate extract (250 mg/kg bw/day) or with urolithin A (15 mg/kg bw/day) (Larrosa *et al.*, 2010). Typical histological changes of inflammation were observed in the colon of DSS-induced colitis rats, together with increases in the prostaglandin E synthase (PTGES) and COX-2 protein levels and in their catalysis product, namely PGE_2, and with an up-regulation of iNOS mRNA expression associated with higher levels of NO in the colon mucosa. Urolithin A supplementation significantly attenuated the histological changes induced by DSS in colon mucosa, while the pomegranate extract showed non-significant attenuations. Both supplementations decreased the PTGES and COX-2 protein levels, and lowered PGE_2 production in the colon mucosa with more efficient effects in the case of the pomegranate extract. In addition, both supplementations allowed to significantly decrease NO levels in colon mucosa (Larrosa *et al.*, 2010).

4.3.2 Mice studies

Pomegranate flower extract and EA-rich fraction. The potential beneficial properties of a pomegranate flower extract and of its EA-rich fraction were evaluated in mice with ulcerative colitis induced by a daily administration of DSS (2%) in drinking water for 7 days (Singh *et al.*, 2009). Treatments were administrated concomitantly with DSS and during a period of 48h before. Colonic tissues were harvested on the day 8 after DSS treatment for macroscopic and biochemical analyses. As expected, DSS administration induced mucosal injuries and reduced colon length. Administration of the pomegranate extract and its EA-rich fraction significantly attenuated most of the DSS-induced macroscopic changes. Body weight loss, stool consistency, and bleeding, were also improved by both treatments, as well as the histopathological changes induced by DSS in the colon. DSS administration was also associated with an increase in myeloperoxidase (MPO) activity from an intense infiltration of neutrophils in the colon in association with an acute inflammation. A decrease of MPO activity in colonic tissues was also observed with both treatments. In addition, both treatments decreased histamine levels in colonic tissues, suggesting a prevention of histamine release. Finally, they also decreased the oxidative stress, measured by the TBARS assay, and the superoxide anion generation, which were significantly increased in DSS-treated mice (Singh *et al.*, 2009).

4.3.3 Human studies

To our knowledge, no human study has yet been conducted to evaluate anti-inflammatory properties of pomegranate in subjects suffering from IBDs. There is a serious need for this kind of studies to validate the purported beneficial effects of pomegranate-derived products. Nevertheless, a study conducted on healthy human subjects showed an increase by 6% of serum antioxidant status, 2h after consumption of a commercial pomegranate juice (POM Wonderful LLC, Los Angeles, CA), and by 11% after a daily consumption of 250 mL of that juice for 1 week (Rosenblat *et al.*, 2010). The increment of antioxidant status and reduction of oxidative damage after pomegranate juice consumption were also observed in another study conducted on healthy elderly subjects who consumed daily 250 mL of juice for 4 weeks (Guo *et al.*, 2008). In physiological inflammation, ROS are scavenged by substances naturally found in our organism. However, in IBDs, the chronic pathological inflammatory response is characterized by an overproduction of ROS leading to persistent oxidative stress and to functional alterations in DNA, proteins and lipids (Bartsch & Nair, 2006; Kapoor *et al.*, 2005). It can thus be speculated that oxidative status improvements offered by the consumption of pomegranate products can attenuate IBD severity.

5. Effects of pomegranate phenolic compounds on the gut microflora associated to IBD pathogenesis

The human gut microflora is estimated to contain 10^{18} of microorganisms (Davis & Milner, 2009) with about 10^{14} bacteria classified within 4 bacterial phyla, namely Firmicutes, Bacteroidetes, Actinobacteria, and Proteobacteria (Seksik, 2010). Gut microflora is composed of beneficial bacteria (like *Bifidobacterium* spp. from the Actinobacteria phylum, and *Lactobacillus* spp. from the Firmicutes phylum), but also comprises deleterious bacteria (like certain members of *Clostridium* spp. or *Staphylococcus* spp. from the Firmicutes phylum). Archae, fungi and protozoa also make up the human gut microflora but little is known about their activities. The gut microflora is a critical component in the development and prevention/treatment of IBDs and its composition differs in IBD patients compared to healthy patients (Swidsinski *et al.*, 2002). Nutrients, such as PCs, may influence that composition by enhancing or depleting the growth of beneficial bacteria, and by increasing or decreasing deleterious bacteria (Laparra & Sanz, 2010). Changes of gut microflora composition after consumption of pomegranate PCs have thus been investigated in different ways. Several studies have highlighted the antimicrobial effects of pomegranate extracts or PCs on isolated bacteria or fungi. A pomegranate peel extract showed antimicrobial effects (evaluated by measuring the zone of inhibition (IZ)) against different multi-drug resistant pathogenic organisms according to the following decreasing order: *Staphylococcus aureus, Salmonella paratyphi, Shigella dysenteriae* > *Candida albicans* > *Bacillus subtilis, Escherichia coli* (Ahmad & Beg, 2001). EA, gallagic acid, punicalin, and punicalagin, which were isolated from a pomegranate peel extract, were also evaluated for their antimicrobial activities against pathogenic fungi (*C. albicans, Cryptococcus neoformans,* and *Aspergillus fumigatus*), a non-pathogenic strain of *E. coli,* and pathogenic bacteria (*Pseudomonas aeruginosa* and *Mycobacterium intracellulare*). EA and punicalin did not show any antimicrobial activity at the highest concentration tested (20 µg/ml). However, gallagic acid and punicalagin inhibited the growth of *E. coli, P. aeruginosa,* and *C. neoformans* with IC_{50} values lower than 15 µg/mL (Reddy *et al.*, 2007). Another study also highlighted the inhibitory effects of a pomegranate peel extract against antibiotic-resistant pathogenic bacteria and fungi. Significant inhibitory effects were observed against a pathogenic strain of *E. coli,* and the pathogenic *S. aureus, B. subtilis, Listeria monocytogenes, P. aeruginosa* and *Yersinia enterocolitica.* An antifungal activity was also observed against *Candida utilis, Saccharomyces cerevisae,* and *Aspergillus niger* (Al-Zoreky, 2009). The effects of the standardized commercial pomegranate peel extract POMx and of pure punicalagin, punicalin, EA, and gallic acid were evaluated on the growth of intestinal bacteria in liquid cultures. POMx and punicalagin inhibited the growth of *S. aureus* and of *Clostridium* spp.. Interestingly enough, the growths of the probiotic *Lactobacillus* spp. and *Bifidobacteria* spp. were relatively unaffected neither by the extract POMx nor by the pure polyphenols, except for the growths of the probiotics *Bifidobacterium breve* and *Bifidobacterium infantis,* which were significantly enhanced by POMx. In this study, POMx application resulted in a decrease of pH media that could partially explain its inhibition towards pathogenic bacteria that are more susceptible to low pH than probiotic bacteria (Bialonska *et al.*, 2009). Another pomegranate peel extract was evaluated for its antibacterial activity towards *Propionibacterium acnes, S. aureus, Staphylococcus epidermidis, E. coli, Salmonella typhimurium, Salmonella typhi* and *Shigella sonnei*. After exposure to pomegranate peel extract (200 mg/mL), inhibitory effects were observed against the deleterious gram-positive bacteria *P. acnes, S. aureus* and *S. epidermidis*, while no inhibitory effect was seen on the non-pathogenic gram-negative bacteria *E. coli,* and on the pathogenic gram-negative *S. typhimurium, S. typhi* , and *S. sonnei* (Panichayupakaranant *et al.*, 2010). Normal human gut microflora also contains harmless saprophyte yeasts, like *Candida* spp., in a normal gastrointestinal tract. However, if the immune defenses are compromised, these yeasts can cause infections. In a recent study, *Candida* spp. were incubated with punicalagin or a pomegranate peel extract (Endo *et al.*, 2010).

Punicalagin showed strong antifungal activities against *C. albicans* and *Candida parapsilosis*, while the pomegranate peel extract did not show any antifungal activity. In the same study, the pomegranate peel extract was also tested against *E. coli, P. aeruginosa, B. subtilis,* and *S. aureus* and showed inhibitory effects only against *S. aureus*. The antimicrobial and antifungal activities of pomegranate PCs are summarized in **Table 1.**

The antimicrobial potential of pomegranated-derived products has also been tested in feces, which represent a more complex model than isolated bacteria or fungi. Bialonska *et al.* (2010) investigated the potential antibacterial activities of POMx and punicalagin on bacteria present in fecal samples obtained from 3 healthy human subjects without any gastrointestinal disease history. The samples were used to inoculate batch-culture vessels and both POMx and punicalagin were added under anaerobic conditions. Bacterial enumeration was assessed by a fluorescence *in situ* hybridization technique (FISH) using ribosomal RNA-targeted oligonucleotide probes for *Bifidobacterium* spp., *Lactobacillus-Enterococcus* group, *Clostridium coccoides-Eubacterium rectale* group, *Clostridium histolyticum* group, as well as for the totality of bacteria. POMx significantly increased the number of *Bifidobacterium* spp., as well as the *Lactobacillus-Enterococcus* group and the total number of bacteria. By contrast, it did not change the growth of the commensal *Clostridium coccoides-Eubacterium rectale* group and *C. histolyticum* group. Punicalagin had no significant effect on any bacteria (Bialonska *et al.*, 2010). Another study (Larrosa *et al.*, 2010) investigated the effects of Nutragranate and urolithin A (see section 3) on the gut microflora composition in DSS-induced colitis rats *vs.* control rats. Both supplementations for 10 days resulted in an increase of *Bifidobacterium* spp, *Lactobacillus* spp. and *Clostridium* spp. in the control rats. After DSS administration for 5 days, the increases of *Bifidobacterium* spp, *Lactobacillus* spp. and *Clostridium* spp were maintained in rats fed with urolithin A, but were reduced in rats eating the pomegranate extract. In addition, significant increases of *E. coli,* of the whole *Enterobacteriaceae* family and of total aerobic bacteria were observed in the DSS-induced colitis model (without any supplementation). These increases were significantly lower in the groups supplemented with the pomegranate extract or urolithin A. The inflammatory status induced by DSS generated differences in the metabolism of pomegranate PCs. As such, in the healthy rats eating the pomegranate extract, the expected metabolite urolithin A was significantly recovered in feces (190 µg/g), but not ETs or EA. In the DSS-treated rats eating the pomegranate extract, EA was predominant in feces, while urolithin A was detected in much lower quantities (8 µg/g). These differences can be put in parallel with the microbial effects observed and suggest that urolithin A formation in the gut lumen is an important

	Antimicrobial activity of pomegranate-derived products								
Pomegrenate-derived products	**PPE[1]**	**PPE[2]**	**PPE[3]**	**PPE[4]**	**POMx[5]**	**Gallic acid[5]**	**EA[5]**	**Punicalin[5]**	**Punicalagin[5]**
Dose tested	8 mg/mL	150 mg/mL	200 mg/mL		0.01% (v/v)	0.05% (v/v)	0.05% (v/v)	0.05% (v/v)	0.05% (v/v)
Microbia (CFU)	10^6	10^4	10^8	10^6	10^8	10^8	10^8	10^8	10^8
BACTERIA									
Firmicutes									
Staphylococcus aureus	IZ: 13 mm MIC: 2 mg/ml	IZ: 31-40 mm	IZ: 16-19 mm MIC: 7.8 µg/ml	MIC: 125 µg/ml	-3%[a] *	97% [a]	75% [a]	86% [a]	-27% [a] *
Staphylococcus epidermidis			IZ: 19 mm MIC: 15.6 µg/ml						
Bacillus subtilis	IZ: 17 mm MIC: 0.5 mg/ml	IZ: 10-20 mm							
Listeria monocytogenes	IZ: 20 mm								
Lactobacillus acidophilus					83% [a] *	126% [a]	66% [a] *	131% [a]	95% [a]
Lactobacillus casei ssp. casei					81% [a]	102% [a]	67% [a] *	101% [a]	70% [a]
Lactobacillus paracasei ssp. paracasei					90% [a]	110% [a]	79% [a] *	107% [a]	81% [a]

Lactobacillus pentosus		88% [a] *	107% [a]	77% [a] *	109% [a]	86% [a]
Lactobacillus rhamnosus		79% [a] *	105% [a]	74% [a] *	108% [a]	82% [a]
Bifidobacterium breve		275% [a] *	112% [a]	81% [a]	121% [a]	130% [a] *
Bifidobacterium infantis		241% [a] *	99% [a]	122% [a]	106% [a]	106% [a]
Bifidobacterium longum		99% [a]	96% [a]	93% [a]	121% [a]	68% [a]
Bifidobacterium bifidum		83% [a] *	83% [a] *	114% [a]	96% [a]	86% [a]
Bifidobacterium animalis ssp. lactis		112% [a]	109% [a]	52% [a] *	78% [a] *	78% [a] *
Clostridium perfringens		-13% [a] *	46% [a]	0% [a] *	90% [a]	-26% [a] *
Clostridium clostriidoforme		58% [a]	114% [a]	0% [a] *	103% [a]	0% [a] *
Clostridium ramosum		0% [a] *	70% [a]	26% [a] *	65% [a]	-16% [a] *
Bacteroidetes						
Bacteroides fragilis		73% [a]	107% [a]	24% [a] *	117% [a]	83% [a]
Actinobacteria						
Propionibacterium acnes	IZ: 22 ± 2 mm MIC: 15.6 µg/ml					

Pomegrenate-derived products	**PPE[1]**	**PPE[2]**	**PPE[3]**	**PPE[4]**	**POMx[5]**	**Gallagic acid[6]**	**EA[6]**	**Punicalin[6]**	**Punicalagin[6]**
Dose tested	8 mg/mL	150 mg/mL	200 mg/mL		0.01% (v/v)	20 µg/ml	20 µg/ml	20 µg/ml	20 µg/ml
Microbia (CFU)	10^6	10^4	10^8	10^6	n.d.	n.d.	n.d.	n.d.	n.d.
Actinobacteria									
Mycobacterium intracellulare						/	/	/	/
Proteobacteria									
Salmonella paratyphi		IZ: 31-40 mm							
Salmonella enteritidis	MIC : 4 mg/ml								
Salmonella typhimurium			/						
Salmonella typhi			/						
Shigella dysenteriae		IZ: 31-40 mm							
Shigella sonnei			/						
Escherichia coli	IZ: 16 mm MIC : 1 mg/ml	IZ: 10-20 mm	/			IC_{50}: 15 µg/ml	/	/	IC_{50}: 10 µg/ml
Pseudomonas aeruginosa	IZ: 18 mm					IC_{50}: 6.0 µg/ml	/	/	IC_{50}: 3.5 µg/ml

Yersinia enterocolitica	IZ: 19 mm MIC : 0.25 mg/ml						
FUNGI							
Candida albicans		IZ: 21-30 mm	MIC: 3.9 μg/ml	/	/	/	/
Candida parapsilosis			MIC: 3.9 μg/ml				
Candida utilis	IZ: 18 mm						
Cryptococcus neoformans				IC_{50}: 10 μg/ml MIC: 20 μg/ml	/	/	IC_{50}: 7 μg/ml MIC: 20 μg/ml
Aspergillus fumigatus				/	/	/	/
Aspergillus niger	IZ: 12 mm						
Saccharomyces cerevisae	IZ: 14 mm						

Abbreviations: CFU, colony forming unit; IZ, inhibitory zone; MIC, minimum inhibitory concentration; n.d., no data; POMx, a pomegranate fruit extract (POM Wonderful brand); PPE, pomegranate peel extract.

[a] Means of human gut bacteria growth (with PCs) compared to means of control growth (significant differences are indicated by an asterisk ($p \leq 0.05$))

/ : No inhibitory activity

[1] Al-Zoreky, 2009; [2] Ahmad & Beg, 2001; [3] Panichayupakaranant *et al.*, 2010; [4] Endo *et al.*, 2010; [5] Bialonska *et al.*, 2009; [6] Reddy *et al.*, 2007.

Table 1. Antimicrobial effects of pomegranate or PCs on isolated microorganisms.

step for the pomegranate extract to affect the gut microflora composition (Larrosa *et al.*, 2010). The effect of pomegranate extracts or of their derived PCs on the gut microbiota can occur at different levels and could partially explain their beneficial role in IBDs. First, tannins are known to complex enzymes, in particular those secreted by the gut microbiota, leading to changes in their structural conformation and thereby inhibiting their enzymatic activities. Furthermore, tannins might form complexes with proteins of cell walls, and by that way, could result in the decrease of both cell permeability and substrate transport into cells. Tannins may also form stable complexes with metal ions (*e.g.*, Fe and Cu), resulting in the decrease of their availability to bacteria and therefore affecting the activity of their metalloenzymes. Finally, as already mentioned, another effect of pomegranate extracts could be the decrease of pH within the intestinal lumen. Most of the time, a low pH favors probiotic bacteria, while deleterious bacteria would be more affected by acidic conditions (Puupponen-Pimia *et al.*, 2005).

6. Conclusion

Plant-derived secondary metabolites are the basis for many drugs or food supplements currently used to treat or prevent pathologic conditions. Since recent research works have shown that the repeated oral administration of high doses of pomegranate to rats and mice was not toxic (Cerdá *et al.*, 2003a, Patel *et al.*, 2008), it is expected that pomegranate peel polyphenolic extracts do not show any severe toxicity in humans. However, further investigations are needed to confirm its safety in humans. The pomegranate peel is a by-product of the pomegranate juice industry that contains high amounts of ETs. When the pomegranate is ingested, these ETs are metabolized mainly in active urolithins by the gut microflora but a lower metabolization occurred in inflamed conditions. In addition to its high antioxidant activity, pomegranate presents anti-inflammatory properties potentially interesting against IBDs by acting on several mechanisms involved in the intestinal inflammatory response. These mechanisms include the interaction with the NF-κB and MAPK cascade pathways, the reduction of the mRNA expression and protein secretion of various pro-inflammatory cytokines, the decrease of the inducible isoforms of iNOS and COX-2 and their resulting products NO and PGE2, known to participate in an increase of the inflammatory status. It also improves the luminal microbiota composition. These different effects were mainly observed in *in vitro* models of intestinal epithelial and immune cells. Results generated *in vivo* go in the same direction, *i.e.* pomegranate PCs can decrease the inflammatory status of animals with induced-inflammation. However, the number of animal studies remains quite limited and to our knowledge, no one human study has been published yet in a peer-reviewed journal. Therefore, since increasing evidence *in vitro* and *in vivo* converge to indicate beneficial effects of pomegranate PCs on intestinal inflammation, further *in vivo* studies are necessary and trials on human subjects should be designed to investigate the pomegranate potential and especially that of pomegranate peel extracts on IBDs.

7. References

Adams, L. S.; Seeram, N. P., Aggarwal, B. B., Takada, Y., Sand, D. & Heber, D. (2006). Pomegranate juice, total pomegranate ellagitannins, and punicalagin suppress inflammatory cell signaling in colon cancer cells. *Journal of Agricultural & Food Chemistry,* Vol.54, No.3, pp.980-985, ISSN 0021-8561.

Ahmad, I. & Beg, A. Z. (2001). Antimicrobial and phytochemical studies on 45 indian medicinal plants against multi-drug resistant human pathogens. *Journal of Ethnopharmacology,* Vol.74, No.2, pp.113-123, ISSN 0378-8741.

Al-Zoreky, N. S. (2009) Antimicrobial activity of pomegranate (punica granatum l.) fruit peels. *International Journal of Food Microbiology,* Vol.134, No.3, pp.244-248, ISSN 0168-1605.

Amakura, Y.; Okada, M., Tsuji, S. & Tonogai, Y. (2000). Determination of phenolic acids in fruit juices by isocratic column liquid chromatography. *Journal of Chromatography A,* Vol.891, No.1, pp.183-188, ISSN 0021-9673.

Bartsch, H. & Nair, J. (2006). Chronic inflammation and oxidative stress in the genesis and perpetuation of cancer: Role of lipid peroxidation, DNA damage, and repair. *Langenbeck's Archives of Surgery,* Vol.391, No.5, pp.499-510, ISSN 1435-2443.

Bialonska, D., Kasimsetty, S. G., Schrader, K. K. & Ferreira, D. (2009). The effect of pomegranate (punica granatum L.) byproducts and ellagitannins on the growth of human gut bacteria. *Journal of Agricultural & Food Chemistry,* Vol.57, No.18, pp.8344-8349, ISSN 0021-8561.

Bialonska, D.; Ramnani, P., Kasimsetty, S. G., Muntha, K. R., Gibson, G. R. & Ferreira, D. (2010). The influence of pomegranate by-product and punicalagins on selected groups of human intestinal microbiota. *International Journal of Food Microbiology,* Vol.140, No.2-3, pp.175-182, ISSN 0168-1605.

Borges, G.; Roowi, S., Rouanet, J. M., Duthie, G. G., Lean, M. E. & Crozier, A. (2007). The bioavailability of raspberry anthocyanins and ellagitannins in rats. *Molecular Nutrition & Food Research,* Vol.51, No.6, pp.714-25, ISSN 1613-4125.

Borges, G.; Mullen, W. & Crozier, A. (2010). Comparison of the polyphenolic composition and antioxidant activity of european commercial fruit juices. *Food & Function,* Vol.1, No.1., pp.73-83, ISSN 2042-6496.

Borochov-Neori, H.; Judeinstein, S., Tripler, E., Harari, M., Greenberg, A., Shomer, I. & Holland, D. (2009). Seasonal and cultivar variations in antioxidant and sensory quality of pomegranate (punica granatum L.) fruit. *Journal of Food Composition & Analysis,* Vol.22, No.3, pp.189-195, ISSN 0889-1575.

Calixto, J. O. B.; Campos, M. M., Otuki, M. F. & Santos, A. R. S. (2004). Anti-inflammatory compounds of plant origin. Part II. Modulation of pro-inflammatory cytokines, chemokines and adhesion molecules. *Planta Medica,* Vol.70, No.2, pp.93-103, ISSN 0032-0943.

Cerdá, B.; Cerón, J. J., Tomás-Barberán, F. A. & Espín, J. C. (2003a). Repeated oral administration of high doses of the pomegranate ellagitannin punicalagin to rats for 37 days is not toxic. *Journal of Agricultural & Food Chemistry,* Vol.51, No.11, pp.3493-3501, ISSN 0021-8561.

Cerdá, B.; Llorach, R., Cerón, J. J., Espín, J. C. & Tomás-Barberán, F. A. (2003b). Evaluation of the bioavailability and metabolism in the rat of punicalagin, an antioxidant polyphenol from pomegranate juice. *European Journal of Nutrition,* Vol.42, No.1, pp.18, ISSN 1436-6207.

Cerdá, B.; Espín, J. C., Parra, S., Martínez, P. & Tomás-Barberán, F. A. (2004a). The potent *in vitro* antioxidant ellagitannins from pomegranate juice are metabolised into bioavailable but poor antioxidant hydroxy–6H–dibenzopyran–6– one derivatives by the colonic microflora of healthy humans. *European Journal of Nutrition,* Vol.43, No.4, pp.205-220, ISSN 1436-6207.

Cerdá, B.; Tomas-Barberan, F. A. & Espin, J. C. (2004b). Metabolism of antioxidant and chemopreventive ellagitannins from strawberries, raspberries, walnuts, and oak-aged wine in humans: Identification of biomarkers and individual variability. *Journal of Agricultural & Food Chemistry,* Vol.53, No.2, pp.227-235, ISSN 0021-8561.

Cerdá, B.; Periago, P., Espín, J. C. & Tomás-Barberán, F. A. (2005). Identification of urolithin A as a metabolite produced by human colon microflora from ellagic acid and related compounds. *J Agric Food Chem,* Vol.53, No.14, pp.5571-5576, ISSN 0021-8561.

Clifford, M. N. & Scalbert, A. (2000). Ellagitannins-nature, occurrence and dietary burden. *Journal of the science of food & agriculture,* Vol.80, No.7, pp.1118-1125, ISSN 0022-5142.

Davis, C. D. & Milner, J. A. (2009). Gastrointestinal microflora, food components and colon cancer prevention. *The Journal of Nutritional Biochemistry,* Vol.20, No.10, pp.743-752, ISSN 0955-2863.

De Pascual-Teresa, S.; Santos-Buelga, C. & Rivas-Gonzalo, J. C. (2000). Quantitative analysis of flavan-3-ols in spanish foodstuffs and beverages. *Journal of Agricultural & Food Chemistry,* Vol.48, pp.5331-5337, ISSN 0021-8561.

Dixit, R. & Gold, B. (1986). Inhibition of N-methyl-N-nitrosourea-induced mutagenicity and DNA methylation by ellagic acid. *Proceedings of the National Academy of Sciences of the United States of America,* Vol.83, No.21, pp.8039-8043, ISSN 0027-8424.

Endo, E. H.; Garcia Cortez, D. A., Ueda-Nakamura, T., Nakamura, C. V. & Dias Filho, B. P. (2010). Potent antifungal activity of extracts and pure compound isolated from pomegranate peels and synergism with fluconazole against candida albicans. *Research in Microbiology,* Vol.161, No.7, pp.534-540, ISSN 0923-2508.

Espín, J. C.; González-Barrio, R., Cerdá, B., López-Bote, C., Rey, A. I. & Tomás-Barberán, F. A. (2007). Iberian pig as a model to clarify obscure points in the bioavailability and metabolism of ellagitannins in humans. *Journal of Agricultural & Food Chemistry,* Vol.55, No.25, pp.10476-10485, ISSN 0021-8561.

Fischer, U. A.; Carle, R. & Kammerer, D. R. (2011). Identification and quantification of phenolic compounds from pomegranate (punica granatum L.) peel, mesocarp, aril and differently produced juices by HPLC-DAD-ESI/MS^n. *Food Chemistry,* Vol.127, No.2, pp.807-821, ISSN 0308-8146.

Gil, M. I.; Tomas-Barberan, F. A., Hess-Pierce, B., Holcroft, D. M. & Kader, A. A. (2000). Antioxidant activity of pomegranate juice and its relationship with phenolic composition and processing. *Journal of Agricultural & Food Chemistry,* Vol.48, No.10, pp.4581-4589, ISSN 0021-8561.

Gil-Izquierdo, A.; Zafrilla, P. & Tomas-Barberan, F. A. (2002). An *in vitro* method to simulate phenolic compound release from the food matrix in the gastrointestinal tract. *European Food Research & Technology,* Vol.214, No.2, pp.155-159, ISSN 1438-2377.

González-Barrio, R.; Borges, G., Mullen, W. & Crozier, A. (2010). Bioavailability of anthocyanins and ellagitannins following consumption of raspberries by healthy humans and subjects with an ileostomy. *Journal of Agricultural & Food Chemistry,*Vol.58, No.7, pp.3933-3939, ISSN 1520-5118.

Guo, C.; Wei, J., Yang, J., Xu, J., Pang, W. & Jiang, Y. (2008). Pomegranate juice is potentially better than apple juice in improving antioxidant function in elderly subjects. *Nutrition Research,* Vol.28, No.2, pp.72-77, ISSN 0271-5317.

Kapoor, M.; Clarkson, A. N., Sutherland, B. A. & Appleton, I. (2005). The role of antioxidants in models of inflammation: Emphasis on L-arginine and arachidonic acid metabolism. *Inflammopharmacology,* Vol.12, No.5-6, pp.505-519, ISSN 0925-4692.

Lansky, E. P. & Newman, R. A. (2007). Punica granatum (pomegranate) and its potential for prevention and treatment of inflammation and cancer. *Journal of Ethnopharmacology,* Vol.109, No.2, pp.177-206, ISSN 0378-8741.

Laparra, J. M. & Sanz, Y. (2010). Interactions of gut microbiota with functional food components and nutraceuticals. *Pharmacological Research,* Vol.61, No.3, pp.219-225, ISSN 1043-6618.

Larrosa, M.; González-Sarrías, A., García-Conesa, M. T., Tomás-Barberán, F. A. & Espín, J. C. (2006a). Urolithins, ellagic acid-derived metabolites produced by human colonic microflora, exhibit estrogenic and antiestrogenic activities. *Journal of Agricultural and Food Chemistry,* Vol.54, No.5, pp.1611-1620, ISSN 0021-8561.

Larrosa, M.; Tomás-Barberán, F. A. & Espín, J. C. (2006b). The dietary hydrolysable tannin punicalagin releases ellagic acid that induces apoptosis in human colon adenocarcinoma Caco-2 cells by using the mitochondrial pathway. *The Journal of Nutritional Biochemistry,* Vol.17, No.9, pp.611-625, ISSN 0955-2863.

Larrosa, M.; González-Sarrías, A., Yáñez-Gascón, M. J., Selma, M. V., Azorín-Ortuño, M., Toti, S., Tomás-Barberán, F., Dolara, P. & Espín, J. C. (2010). Anti-inflammatory properties of a pomegranate extract and its metabolite urolithin-A in a colitis rat model and the effect of colon inflammation on phenolic metabolism. *The Journal of Nutritional Biochemistry,* Vol.21, No.8, pp.717-725, ISSN 0955-2863.

Lee, C.-J.; Chen, L.-G., Liang, W.-L. & Wang, C.-C. (2010). Anti-inflammatory effects of punica granatum Linne *in vitro* and *in vivo*. *Food Chemistry,* Vol.118, No.2, pp.315-322, ISSN 0308-8146.

Lee, S.-I.; Kim, B.-S., Kim, K.-S., Lee, S., Shin, K.-S. & Lim, J.-S. (2008). Immune-suppressive activity of punicalagin via inhibition of NFAT activation. *Biochemical and Biophysical Research Communications,* Vol.371, No.4, pp.799-803, ISSN 0006-291X.

Lei, F.; Xing, D.-M., Xiang, L., Zhao, Y.-N., Wang, W., Zhang, L.-J. & Du, L.-J. (2003). Pharmacokinetic study of ellagic acid in rat after oral administration of pomegranate leaf extract. *Journal of Chromatography B,* Vol.796, No.1, pp.189-194, ISSN1570-0232.

Li, Y.; Guo, C., Yang, J., Wei, J., Xu, J. & Cheng, S. (2006). Evaluation of antioxidant properties of pomegranate peel extract in comparison with pomegranate pulp extract. *Food Chemistry,* Vol.96, No.2, pp.254-260, ISSN 0308-8146.

Martin, K. R.; Krueger, C. G., Rodriquez, G., Dreher, M. & Reed, J. D. (2009). Development of a novel pomegranate standard and new method for the quantitative measurement of pomegranate polyphenols. *Journal of the Science of Food & Agriculture,* Vol.89, No.1, pp.157-162, ISSN 0022-5142.

Mertens-Talcott, S. U.; Jilma-Stohlawetz, P., Rios, J., Hingorani, L. & Derendorf, H. (2006). Absorption, metabolism, and antioxidant effects of pomegranate (punica granatum L.) polyphenols after ingestion of a standardized extract in healthy human volunteers. *Journal of Agricultural & Food Chemistry,* Vol.54, No.23, pp.8956-8961, ISSN 0021-8561.

Ogawa, Y.; Kanatsu, K., Iino, T., Kato, S., Jeong, Y. I., Shibata, N., Takada, K. & Takeuchi, K. (2002). Protection against dextran sulfate sodium-induced colitis by microspheres of ellagic acid in rats. *Life Sciences,* Vol.71, No.7, pp.827-839, ISSN 0024-3205.

Panichayupakaranant, P.; Tewtrakul, S. & Yuenyongsawad, S. (2010). Antibacterial, anti-inflammatory and anti-allergic activities of standardised pomegranate rind extract. *Food Chemistry,* Vol.123, No.2, pp.400-403, ISSN 0308-8146.

Patel, C.; Dadhaniya, P., Hingorani, L. & Soni, M. G. (2008). Safety assessment of pomegranate fruit extract: Acute and subchronic toxicity studies. *Food & Chemical Toxicology,* Vol.46, No.8, pp.2728-2735, ISSN 0278-6915.

Perez-Vicente, A.; Gil-Izquierdo, A. & Garcia-Viguera, C. (2002). *In vitro* gastrointestinal digestion study of pomegranate juice phenolic compounds, anthocyanins, and vitamin C. *Journal of Agricultural & Food Chemistry,* Vol.50, No.8, pp.2308-2312, ISSN 0021-8561.

Puupponen-Pimia, R.; Nohynek, L., Hartmann-Schmidlin, S., Kahkonen, M., Heinonen, M., Maatta-Riihinen, K. & Oksman-Caldentey, K. M. (2005). Berry phenolics selectively inhibit the growth of intestinal pathogens. *Journal of Applied Microbiolology,* Vol.98, No.4, pp.991-1000, ISSN 1364-5072.

Rahman, I.; Biswas, S. K. & Kirkham, P. A. (2006). Regulation of inflammation and redox signaling by dietary polyphenols. *Biochemical Pharmacology,* Vol.72, No.11, pp.1439-1452, ISSN 0006-2952.

Rasheed, Z.; Akhtar, N., Anbazhagan, A. N., Ramamurthy, S., Shukla, M. & Haqqi, T. M. (2009). Polyphenol-rich pomegranate fruit extract (POMx) suppresses PMACI-induced expression of pro-inflammatory cytokines by inhibiting the activation of MAP kinases and NF-κB in human KU812 cells. *Journal of Inflammation London England,* Vol.6, No.1, pp.1-12, ISSN 1476-9255.

Reddy, M. K.; Gupta, S. K., Jacob, M. R., Khan, S. I. & Ferreira, D. (2007). Antioxidant, antimalarial and antimicrobial activities of tannin-rich fractions, ellagitannins and phenolic acids from punica granatum L.. *Planta Medica,* Vol.73, No.5, pp.461-467, ISSN 0032-0943.

Rhodes, J. M. & Campbell, B. J. (2002). Inflammation and colorectal cancer: IBD-associated and sporadic cancer compared. *Trends in Molecular Medicine,* Vol.8, No.1, pp.10-16, ISSN 1471-4914.

Romier, B.; Schneider, Y. J., Larondelle, Y. & During, A. (2009). Dietary polyphenols can modulate the intestinal inflammatory response. *Nutrition Reviews,* Vol.67, No.7, pp.363-378, ISSN 0029-6643.

Romier-Crouzet, B.; Van De Walle, J., During, A., Joly, A., Rousseau, C., Henry, O., Larondelle, Y. & Schneider, Y. J. (2009). Inhibition of inflammatory mediators by polyphenolic plant extracts in human intestinal Caco-2 cells. *Food & Chemical Toxicology,* Vol.47, No.6, pp.1221-1230, ISSN 0278-6915.

Rosenblat, M.; Volkova, N., Attias, J., Mahamid, R. & Aviram, M. (2010). Consumption of polyphenolic-rich beverages (mostly pomegranate and black currant juices) by healthy subjects for a short term increased serum antioxidant status, and the serum's ability to attenuate macrophage cholesterol accumulation. *Food & Function,* Vol.1, No.1, pp.99-109, ISSN 2042-6496.

Rosillo, M.A.; Sanchez-Hidalgo, Cárdeno, M A. & Alarcón de la Lastra, C. (2011). Protective effect of ellagic acid, a natural polyphenolic compound, in a murine model of Crohn's disease. *Biochemical Pharmacology.* In Press, Accepted Manuscript, Available online 7 July 2011

Scalbert, A. & Williamson, G. (2000). Dietary intake and bioavailability of polyphenols. *Journal of Nutrition,* Vol.130, No.8, pp.2073S-2085S, ISSN 0022-3166.

Schubert, S. Y.; Lansky, E. P. & Neeman, I. (1999). Antioxidant and eicosanoid enzyme inhibition properties of pomegranate seed oil and fermented juice flavonoids. *Journal of Ethnopharmacology,* Vol.66, No.1, pp.11-17, ISSN 0378-8741.

Seeram, N. P.; Lee, R. & Heber, D. (2004). Bioavailability of ellagic acid in human plasma after consumption of ellagitannins from pomegranate (punica granatum L.) juice. *Clinica Chimica Acta,* Vol.348, No.1-2, pp.63-68, ISSN 0009-8981.

Seeram, N. P.; Adams, L. S.; Henning, S. M.; Niu, Y., Zhang, Y.; Nair, M. G. & Heber, D. (2005a). *In vitro* antiproliferative, apoptotic and antioxidant activities of punicalagin, ellagic acid and a total pomegranate tannin extract are enhanced in combination with other polyphenols as found in pomegranate juice. *The Journal of Nutritional Biochemistry,* Vol.16, No.6, pp.360-367, ISSN 0955-2863.

Seeram, N.; Lee, R., Hardy, M. & Heber, D. (2005b). Rapid large scale purification of ellagitannins from pomegranate husk, a by-product of the commercial juice industry. *Separation & Purification Technology,* Vol.41, No.1, pp.49-55, ISSN 1383-5866.

Seeram, N. P.; Henning, S. M., Zhang, Y., Suchard, M., Li, Z. & Heber, D. (2006). Pomegranate juice ellagitannin metabolites are present in human plasma and some persist in urine for up to 48 hours. *Journal of Nutrition,* Vol.136, No.10, pp.2481-2485, ISSN 0022-3166.

Seeram, N. P.; Aronson, W. J., Zhang, Y., Henning, S. M., Moro, A., Lee, R. P., Sartippour, M., Harris, D. M., Rettig, M., Suchard, M. A., Pantuck, A. J., Belldegrun, A. & Heber, D. (2007). Pomegranate ellagitannin-derived metabolites inhibit prostate cancer growth and localize to the mouse prostate gland. *Journal of Agricultural & Food Chemistry*, Vol.55, No.19, pp.7732-7737, ISSN 0021-8561

Seksik, P. (2010). Gut microbiota and IBD. *Gastroentérologie Clinique et Biologique,* Vol.34, Supplement 1, pp.S44-S51, ISSN 0399-8320.

Sergent, T.; Piront, N., Meurice, J., Toussaint, O. & Schneider, Y.-J. (2010). Anti-inflammatory effects of dietary phenolic compounds in an *in vitro* model of inflamed human intestinal epithelium. *Chemico-Biological Interactions,* Vol.188, No.3, pp.659-667, ISSN 0009-2797.

Shapiro, H.; Lev, S., Cohen, J. & Singer, P. (2009). Polyphenols in the prevention and treatment of sepsis syndromes: Rationale and pre-clinical evidence. *Nutrition,* Vol.25, No.10, pp.981-997, ISSN 0899-9007.

Shukla, M.; Gupta, K., Rasheed, Z., Khan, K. A. & Haqqi, T. M. (2008). Bioavailable constituents/metabolites of pomegranate (*Punica granatum* L) preferentially inhibit COX2 activity *ex vivo* and IL-1beta-induced PGE_2 production in human chondrocytes *in vitro. Journal of Inflammation,* No.5, pp.9-19, ISSN 1476-9255.

Singh, K.; Jaggi, A. S. & Singh, N. (2009). Exploring the ameliorative potential of punica granatum in dextran sulfate sodium induced ulcerative colitis in mice. *Phytotherapy Research,* Vol.23, No.11, pp.1565-1574, ISSN 0951-418X.

Stecher, B. & Hardt, W.-D. (2008). The role of microbiota in infectious disease. *Trends in Microbiology,* Vol.16, No.3, pp.107-114, ISSN 0966-842X.

Swidsinski, A.; Ladhoff, A., Pernthaler, A., Swidsinski, S., Loening-Baucke, V., Ortner, M., Weber, J., Hoffmann, U., Schreiber, S., Dietel, M. & Lochs, H. (2002). Mucosal flora in inflammatory bowel disease. *Gastroenterology,* Vol.122, No.1, pp.44-54, ISSN 0016-5085.

Teel, R. W.; Martin, R. M. & Allahyari, R. (1987). Ellagic acid metabolism and binding to DNA in organ explant cultures of the rat. *Cancer Lett,* Vol.36, No.2, pp.203-11, ISSN 0304-3835.

Thulstrup, P. W.; Thormann, T., Spanget-Larsen, J. & Bisgaard, H. C. (1999). Interaction between ellagic acid and calf thymus DNA studied with flow linear dichroism UV-Vis spectroscopy. *Biochemical & Biophysical Research Communications,* Vol.265, No.2, pp.416-421, ISSN 0006-291X.

Tomás-Barberan, F. A.; Ferreres, F. & Gil, M. I. (2000). Antioxidant phenolic metabolites from fruit and vegetables and changes during postharvest storage and processing, In: *Studies in natural products chemistry,* Atta ur, Rahman, pp.739-795, Elsevier, Retrieved from < http://www.sciencedirect.com/science/article/B8H3X-4P29JR8-N/2/d48b0692d1551a20bfa8ad48816421d5>.

Tzulker, R.; Glazer, I., Bar-Ilan, I., Holland, D., Aviram, M. & Amir, R. (2007). Antioxidant activity, polyphenol content, and related compounds in different fruit juices and homogenates prepared from 29 different pomegranate accessions. *Journal of Agricultural & Food Chemistry,* Vol.55, No.23, pp.9559-9570, ISSN 0021-8561.

Walle, T.; Vincent, T. S. & Walle, U. K. (2003). Evidence of covalent binding of the dietary flavonoid quercetin to DNA and protein in human intestinal and hepatic cells. *Biochemical Pharmacology,* Vol.65, No.10, pp.1603-1610, ISSN 0006-2952.

Whitley, A. C.; Stoner, G. D., Darby, M. V. & Walle, T. (2003). Intestinal epithelial cell accumulation of the cancer preventive polyphenol ellagic acid extensive binding to protein and DNA. *Biochemical Pharmacology,* Vol.66, No.6, pp.907-915, ISSN 0006-2952.

Yu, H.; Pardoll, D. & Jove, R. (2009). STATs in cancer inflammation and immunity: A leading role for stat3. *Nature Reviews Cancer,* Vol.9, No.11, pp.798-809, ISSN 1474-175X.

16

Drug Targeting in IBD Treatment – Existing and New Approaches

Katerina Goracinova, Marija Glavas-Dodov,
Maja Simonoska-Crcarevska and Nikola Geskovski
Institute of Pharmaceutical technology, Faculty of Pharmacy
University Ss. Cyril and Methodius, Skopje
Macedonia

1. Introduction

Recent advances in understanding of inflammatory bowel diseases (IBD) pathogenesis, despite the questions remaining still unanswered, have led to improved approaches in ulcerative colitis (UC) and Crohn`s disease (CD) treatment. In depth investigation of immunopathology of IBD and mucosal inflammation enabled the identification of new strategies for drug targeting, new points of therapeutic attack, cytokine based therapies and new therapeutic agents. Further understanding of the genetic background of this disease will enable discovery of potential gene therapy target molecules related to chronic intestinal inflammation, like new therapeutic targets in IBD.

There is a vast body of information and research associated with current medical treatments, their undesirable effects and limited efficacy. Different drug delivery strategies were employed to overcome limited performance of conventional IBD therapy and many more will be designed to enable safe and efficacious delivery of newly developed therapeutic agents. Both diseases, UC and CD involve different parts of the gastrointestinal (GI) system. CD may involve any part of the GI tract, although most commonly the terminal ileum and colon, while UC usually involves only the colon and always extends proximally from the rectum. T helper 1 (Th1) stimulated immune dysregulation is characteristic for CD while T helper 2 (Th2) stimulated immune dysregulation causes inflammatory mediatory imbalance characteristic for UC (Bouma & Strober, 2003; Hedley, 2000; Sands, 2007; Sellin, 2005). Treatment of UC and CD varies depending on subtype and severity, but significant overlap is seen. The most common therapeutic agents for IBD, aminosalycilates and corticosteroids, have been incorporated into different dosage forms and drug delivery systems (DDS) in order to accomplish successful topical delivery of these agents at the site of inflammation (in CD - terminal ileum, or colon, the site of inflammation for both subtypes) (Green et al., 2002; Haddish-Berhane et al., 2007; Sands, 2007). The most critical step in the development of a reliable DDS for IBD treatment is to achieve improved localization and controlled release of the active substance at the site of inflammation, minimizing the premature release and subsequent absorption in the blood stream. However, the main disadvantage of today's therapy and DDS for management of IBD is the inability to target the drug directly to the site of action (inflammation) and/or to maintain high local concentration. In addition to poor localization extensive metabolism at the level of the epithelial cells of the intestinal wall (ex. hydroxylation of budesonide by cytochrome P450 isoenzyme CYP3A4 in hepatocytes and epithelial cells) might further impair local concentration required for improved drug efficacy (Fedorak & Bistritz, 2005; Klotz & Schwab, 2005).

2. Conventional design strategies for GI targeting

The efficacy of the treatment of IBD depends on the functionality of the strategy for the delivery of therapeutic concentrations of the drug substance at the site of inflammation. In addition, minimizing the intestinal absorption using different formulation design approaches will improve the safety and reduce the adverse effects of the treatments. Various chemical modifications and formulation technologies based on the intestinal physiology (motility, intraluminal pH, and intestinal transit times) as well as distribution of IBD in the GI tract have been developed in order to improve the efficacy and precision of drug release to the affected areas.

These conventional approaches are mainly focused to targeting a particular site in the GI tract and delivery of prodrugs, colonic microflora activated systems, pH dependent and time dependent systems in a form of single or multiunit dosage forms (Gazzaniga et al., 2006; Ishibashi et al., 1998). Delivery strategies and release mechanisms employed in these dosage forms rely on the enzymatic activity of the GI microflora, pH difference between different parts of the GI tract, GI transit time and increased luminal pressure in the colon due to strong peristaltic waves (Leopold, 2001). The conditions in the complex and dynamic GI tract environment are the source of variability of drug release, absorption and patient response even if healthy individuals are concerned. Moreover, due to the pathological changes in response to the IBD, factors like GI tract pH, motility, transit time and microflora activity will become the source of increased variability in the response and effectiveness of different formulations for treatment of the GI diseases. Before mentioned factors and variables suggest that these design approaches might suffer from limited efficacy in concentrating the active substance at the site of inflammation, preventing drug absorption and systemic exposure to these agents. Moreover, if single unit dosage forms are used, their residence time in GI tract will be under constant threat of persistent diarrhea in IBD patients (Bourgeois, 2005; Chourasia & Jain, 2003; Roy & Shahiwala, 2009).

Today it is widely accepted that the delivery of the active substance influences clinical efficacy of the drug product. Based upon this view, clinical studies for the efficacy and safety of different conventional marketed DDS describing the site of drug release, drug release rate, subsequent absorption from the GI tract, systemic absorption and local concentration of the anti-inflammatory agents are the baseline for rational approach in prescribing different doses and dosage forms for IBD, once the location and the type of the disease are known. Due to the clinical efficacy studies valuable information for the usefulness of different dosage forms for the treatment of mild or moderate disease, induction or maintaining remission etc. related to the disease pattern and drug disposition are available (Clemett & Markham, 2000; Prakash, 1999). Moreover, there is increasing number of papers trying to investigate and explain variation in luminal pH in UC and CD patients, mucosal flora profiles for UC and CD which will further improve the understanding of the effect of these variables on the drug release pattern and disposition as well as clinical efficacy of different drug products, but will also help the profiling of different phenotypes of IBD (Friend, 2005; Haddish-Berhane et al., 2007; Nugent et al., 2001).

2.1 Prodrug approach

The rationale behind the utilization of a prodrug approach for drug targeting in IBD is multilateral. Nevertheless, the first 5-ASA prodrug was developed to deliver sulfonamide specifically to the colon, later it was realized that sulfasalazine (sulfapyridyne-azo linkage-5ASA) is efficient for UC treatment as it can successfully perform colon specific delivery of 5-ASA after oral administration, at the same time it can reduce the absorption in the upper intestines due to increased hydrophylicity and/or molecular size (Friend, 2005; Sands, 2007). Azo prodrug approach for colon targeting will improve local concentration of the active substance at the site of therapeutic action, resulting with increased efficacy and fewer side effects of the therapy (Bourgeois, 2005; Oz & Ebersole, 2008; Sands, 2000) . These cannot be linearly applied to all azo conjugates as the side effects may originate from the carrier molecule or degradation products also released during the azo bond cleavage.

The trigger that releases the active substances from their azo-prodrugs is the colon micoflora enzymatic activity. Contrary to the small intestine (10^4 CFU/ml mainly gram positive facultative bacteria), colonic flora is of much higher order (10^{11}–10^{12} CFU/ml) and is mainly consisted of an anaerobic bacteria (Mcconnell et al., 2008; Sinha & Kumria, 2001). For the fermentation of undigested substrates in the small intestine like disaccharides, polysaccharides, mucopolysaccharides, and fulfillment of microflora energy demands, these commensal bacteria produce different types of enzymes like azoreductase, β-galactosidase, β-xylosidase, nitroreductase, glycosidase, deaminase etc. (Bourgeois, 2005; Han & Amidon, 2000; Oz & Ebersole, 2008; Yang, 2008). Most of these anaerobic bacteria are capable of reducing azo linkages, thus releasing the active drug from the azo product. Beside azo prodrugs based on azo linkage of the drug with different carriers, other systems for colon drug targeting based on colonic microflora activity are also developed. The rationale behind glucuronide conjugates development as colon targeting systems is based on the β-glucuronidase activity in the lower GI tract; cyclodextrin (CyD) conjugates are based on poor digestion of the complex through the GI tract except in the colon by the colonic microflora; the drug is released from dextran-drug conjugates due to dextranase activity in the region of caecum and colon; amino acid conjugates are probably hydrolyzed by the microbial flora activity at the location of the caecum and colon, etc. (Bourgeois, 2005; Chourasia & Jain, 2003). Examples of the prodrug products available on the market and of the prodrug systems still under research are presented in Table 1.

The functionality of these delivery systems is directly influenced by i). the stability of the conjugate in the upper GI tract, ii). colon specific complex degradation and iii). toxicity of the carrier or the cleavage products. Their capacity when applied for targeting in IBD treatment is to release and increase localization and concentration of the drug substance at the specific site in GI tract (site specific delivery). Commercially available 5-ASA conjugates are not able to completely prevent prodrug hydrolysis and 5-ASA absorption in the upper GI tract. Although the approaches presented in the literature using different polymer carriers might probably overcome this weakness, apparently creating a balance among the resilience against hydrolysis in the upper GI tract and required drug release rate in colon is not an easy task.

Conjugates	Drug	Carrier molecule	Release mechanism	Source
Azo prodrugs				
Sulfasalazine	5-ASA	Sulfapyridine	Enzymatic cleavage (azoreduction) of the azo-bond by azo-reductases in the colon	Marketed product
Balsalazide	5-ASA	4-aminobenzoyl-β-alanine		Marketed product
Olsalazine (disodium azodisalicylate)	5-ASA	One molecule of 5-ASA is used as a carrier for the other		Marketed product
Non-absorbable polymer-drug azo conjugate	5-ASA	Sulphanilamidoethyl-ene polymer		(Brown et al., 1983)
Water soluble polymer-drug azo conjugate	5-ASA	*N*-(-hydroxypropyl) methacrylamide copolymer		(Kopecek, 1990)
Bioadhesive polymer-drug azo conjugate	5-ASA	*N*-(2-hydroxypropyl) methacrylamide copolymers with bioadhesive moiety (fucosylamine)		(Kopecek et al., 1992)
Amino-acid conjugates				
Drug-amino acid conjugate	5-ASA	Glycine	Enzymatic hydrolysis of the amide bond by the GI microorganisms in the caecum and colon	(Jung et al., 1998)
Glycoside and glucuronide conjugates				
Drug-glycoside conjugate (coupling through β–glycosidic bond)	Prednisolone or Dexametha-sone	β-D-glucoside	Enzymatic hydrolysis - cleavage of the polar moiety by bacterial glycosidases in the colon	(Friend & Chang, 1985)
Drug-glycoronide conjugate	Budesonide	β-D-glucuronide	Enzymatic hydrolysis - Deglucuronidation of the drug - glucuronic acid prodrug by the β –glucuronidase secreted by GI bacteria in the colon	(Friend, 1991; Nolen et al., 1995)

Cyclodextrin (CyD) conjugates				
Prednisolone Succinate-CyD Ester Conjugate	Prednisolone	α-CyD	Enzymatic hydrolysis - Bacterial enzymatic degradation of CyD rings to small saccharides followed by ester hydrolysis in the lower parts of GI tract	(Yano et al., 2001)
Polysaccharide conjugates				
Dextran conjugate	5-ASA	Oxidised dextran (dialdehyde dextran) coupled to alpha NH_2 groups from 5-ASA to form imine bonds which are further reduced to secondary amine bonds to improve stability in water	Enzymatic hydrolysis of the amine complex by deaminases and the dextrane glycoside bonds in the distal ileum and proximal colon by dextranases to oligomers which are further split by colonic esterases	(Ahmad et al., 2006)
Dendrimer conjugates				
Hydrophylic polyamidoamine dendrimer (PAMAM)	5-ASA	PAMAM (drug is bound to the polymer *via* spacers containing azo bonds: p-aminobenzoic acid spacer and p-aminohippuric acid spacer)	Enzymatic cleavage of the azo-bond by colonic azo-reductases	(Wiwattana patapee et al., 2003)

Table 1. Conjugates for colon drug targeting

2.2 pH, time and microbiologically dependent systems for colon targeting

Drug delivery approaches for pH and time dependent systems currently on the market are based on polymer coating or matrix technology for single or multiple unit dosage forms. Eudragit S coated 5-ASA tablets (Asacol®) and Eudragit L coated 5-ASA tablets (Salofalk®, Claversal®, Mesazal®, Calitoflak®) represent purely pH dependent delayed release systems which release the active substance upon the dissolution of the polymer coating, generally at pH 7 or pH 6 for Eudragit S and Eudragit L coating, respectively (Klotz & Schwab, 2005; Leopold, 2001; Wilding et al., 2000). Entocort® is designed as Eudragit L100-55 coated budesonide/ethylcellulose beads in gelatin capsule in order to delay the release of the active substance till pH 5.5 and further sustain the drug release through GI tract due to the presence of ethylcellulose (Fedorak & Bistritz, 2005; Friend, 2005; Klotz & Schwab, 2005). The coating of combined Eudragit enterosoluble and swelling polymers (Eudragit L/S/RL an RS) in Budenofalk microgranules is supposed to delay the release until pH 6.4. It is assumed that multiunit coated beads will provide more uniform transit and distribution through the GI tract and accordingly more uniform drug release as they are less subjected to the differences in the transit time due to the environmental changes. Accordingly, the exposition of the dosage forms to an acidic environment due to the differences in the gastric emptying process for pellets and tablets might be different. Pellets are continuously emptied from the stomach (unless settled at the greater curvature or float because of the high or low density, respectively) during the digestive period, and non-desintegrating tablets, like enteric coated tablets, are emptied during the interdigestive period. The description of the drug release site according to the solubility of the enterosolvent coating is a valuable orientation point, but at the same time very general as it can be only applied in ideal circumstances and is subjected to number of inter-, intra-individual variables as well as different disease factors. However, it might be expected that patients with UC will have the greatest benefit as by design pH dependent dosage forms will deliver most of the dose in the distal ileum and colon. Latest published research data on small bowel pH in patients with ileal CD (3 patients with ileal CD, 8 patients with operated ileal CD and 4 normal controls) point that small bowel pH was similar to the control group and sufficiently high to allow the dissolution of enterosolvent delayed release dosage forms coated with polymer that requires pH less than 7 to be dissolved (ex. Eudragit L) (Nugent et al., 2000). As these systems usually need at least 30 minutes (max. 1 hour) to complete the dissolution in vitro it seems that the drug will be released during the transit through the small bowel towards the colon. Another study that measured the luminal pH and mean transit time in patients with mild to moderate UC clearly state that more than 50% of examined patients (10 males, 4 with extensive and 6 with distal colitis) failed to achieve the sustained pH level needed for dissolution of some delayed release 5-ASA preparations (proximal, distal small bowel pH as well as right and left colon pH were measured). A different study confirmed that colonic pH is lower in patients with mild to moderate UC compared to the control group, but small bowel pH was not significantly changed compared to the controls (Friend, 2005; Oliveira, L. & Cohen, 2011). Opposite findings, from confirmed efficacy to incomplete drug release, are also found through the reports from clinical studies in the literature. As pH dependent systems are widely used in today's practice careful and individual approach in prescribing of the delayed release systems for IBD would benefit the patient.

Time based delivery systems release the drug in a sustained manner as they pass down the GI tract. Pentasa® is based on ethylcellulose coated beads that release 5-ASA slowly and continuously throughout the small bowel and colon in a time-dependent manner (Klotz & Schwab, 2005; Larouche, 1995; Wilding et al., 2000). Scintigraphic evaluation of the disposition, dispersion and movement of the Pentasa® microgranules through the GI tract (app. 1 mm in diameter) point that the particles showed fluid like properties in a fasted stomach, rapid exponential emptying in a progressive manner over 30-60 min period with no signs of delay. Colon arrival was observed within 4-6 hours on average followed by subsequent wide distribution of the beads through the colon. Accumulation of time controlled system in the ileo-caecal junction might present serious problem and should be carefully avoided by stimulating the colonic activity and gastrocolonic responce with a carefully scheduled light meal (Adkin et al., 1993; Price et al., 1993; Wilding et al., 2000). If the release of 5-ASA is successfully postponed or minimized by the presence of a ethylcellulose polymeric membrane till reaching the lower parts of the GI tract, this type of dosage form due to its wide multiunit distribution at the site of inflammation would be beneficial as the release is expected in a sustained manner through the entire colon.

Compared to pH dependent single unit dosage forms that release the drug in a short period after the dissolution of the coating, multiple dose units spread all over the region of interest and release the drug in a sustained manner at the site of action.

pH and time dependent systems were developed in order to combine delayed dissolution and sustained diffusion through swellable or non-swellable coatings or matrices. Apriso® is formulated as enteric coated microgranules with delayed release starting at pH 6.0 and polymer matrix core which will provide extended release of the active substance and deliver the drug continuously from the small bowel through the colon (Brunner et al., 2003; Oliveira, L. & Cohen, 2011; Sandborn et al., 2010).

Time dependent delivery systems like TIME CLOCK™ and Pulsincap™ are developed as colon drug delivery systems based on the observation that the small intestinal transit time doesn't exceed a mean of 3-4 hours (Bourgeois, 2005; Chourasia & Jain, 2003; Gazzaniga et al., 2008). These systems usually show burst drug release after the lag time, mainly due to the superdisintegrants and highly swellable agents which act upon the dissolution and permeability of the protective coating. TIME-CLOCK™ system, proposed by Pozzi et al. (Pozzi et al., 1994) is composed of tablet core containing the drug and bulking agents like lactose, polyvinyl pyrrolidone, corn starch and lubricant magnesium stearate, coated with hydrophobic dispersion of carnauba wax, bees' wax, polyoxyethylene sorbitan monooleate and hydroxypropyl methylcellulose in water. Drug release is not dependent to normal physiological conditions, pH, digestive state and anatomical position. The lag time can be modulated by altering the thickness of the coating. Pulsincap™ system consists of water insoluble capsule containing the formulation closed at the open end with a swellable hydrogel plug. Lag time is controlled by the type, dimensions and position of the plug and rapid drug release at particular site in GI tract is ensured by incorporation of disintegrants or effervescent agents. Pulsatile pH and time dependent multiple unit dosage forms composed of enterosolvent outer layer and a second membrane of water insoluble and enteric polymers are also suitable for colon drug targeting. OROS-CT™ system can be a single osmotic unit or may incorporate as many as 5-6 push-pull units, each 4 mm in diameter, encapsulated within a hard gelatin capsule (Leopold, 2001; Verma et al., 2000, 2002). Because of its drug-impermeable enteric coating, the release from each push-pull unit is prevented and delayed until higher pH values. When the acid resistant coating dissolves, water enters the unit, causing the osmotic push compartment to swell. Drug gel is forced out through the orifice due to the swelling effect and increased osmotic pressure in the push compartment at a rate precisely controlled by the rate of water transport through the semipermeable membrane. For treating ulcerative colitis, each push pull unit is designed with a 3-4 hours post gastric delay to prevent drug delivery in the small intestine. OROS-CT™ units can maintain a constant release rate for up to 24 hours in the colon or can deliver drug over a period as short as four hours.

Except the previously presented examples, approaches based on modification and combination of two or more conventional designs in order to improve the delivery and site specificity in the GI tract are presented through literature. Sinha and Kumria developed conventional enteric/coated time dependent single unit dosage form for colon specific delivery of water insoluble drugs or slightly soluble drugs (Sinha & Kumria, 2002). Time dependent delivery was achieved using xanthan gum, guar gum, chitosan and Eudragit E as binders. The most successful in sustaining the drug release in the upper GI tract was chitosan. Moreover, application of chitosan for site specific targeting of less soluble substances was favorable as the release was retarded only till microbial degradation or polymer solubilization took place in the colon. Another variation of pH and time dependent

single unit system for colonic delivery was published by Ishibashi et al (Ishibashi et al., 1998). Drug release from the capsule in the upper parts of the GI tract was postponed by the acidoresistant layer at the capsule surface. To prevent the contact among the outer anionic layer and inner cationic (Eudragit E) polymer, an intermediate water soluble layer was introduced. After gastric empting both layers dissolve quickly, exposing the cationic layer to the intestinal environment. The cationic layer delayed the release till its complete dissolution due to the presence of the organic acid in the inner capsule body together with the drug.
Microgranular system coated with outer layer of enterosolvent Eudragit FS (dissolves at pH higher than 6.8) and inner layer composed of combination of pH independent cationic polymers Eudragit RL and Eudragit RS demonstrated the potential for delayed release till pH 6.5 and sustained release through the colon for approximately 12 hours (Gupta et al., 2000 as cited in Gupta et al., 2001). Different enzymatically cleavable polymers are also reported to be synthesized for application in colonic microflora activated systems. First biodegradable enzymatically cleavable polymers for colon drug targeting are the azo polymers composed of hydrophobic and hydrophilic moiety connected by an azo segment. Their microbial degradation and consequently drug release rate from the coated drug dosage forms depends upon their hydrophilicity. Careful adjustment among the hydrophilic and hydrophobic part is a necessity for maintaining gastric resistance and sustained release in the lower GI tract. However, reduction of the azo compound is usually very slow which might lead to incomplete release of the drug substance. Major drawback of these compounds is coming from the toxicity of the primary aromatic amines resulting from the microbial reduction of the more hydrophilic azo compounds and with more hydrophobic polymers reduction will be stopped at the hydrazo compounds instead of leading to the amines which will influence the drug release rate and mechanism. Azo crosslinked co-polymers of styrene and hydroxyethylmethacrylate and methyl methacrylate polymers crosslinked through bifunctional azo aromatic compounds, azo aromatic group containing polyurethanes and pH sensitive terpolymers containing hydroxyethylmethacrylate, methyl methacrylate and methacrylic acid were also investigated as sustained release coatings and water insoluble hydrogels for colon targeting (Bourgeois, 2005; Leopold, 2001). More examples of technologies and combined formulation approaches for pH, time, microbiologically and pressure dependent single and multiple unit drug delivery systems for colon targeting are presented in Table 2.

3. Disease oriented strategies for drug targeting in IBD

During the past fifteen years vast body of research has been done on CD and UC complex cascade of immunologically driven interactions by inflammatory substances and cytokines. Detailed knowledge of different stages of these pathways (Rivkin, 2009; Rutgeerts et al., 2004; Van Deventer, 1999; Wong et al., 2008) is very useful for identifying new therapeutic targets for IBD therapy as well as clarification of the mechanisms of action of current therapeutic agents. Improved understanding of the mechanisms of disease and mechanism of action of the active substances at the molecular levels brought new ideas and models for rational drug targeting and drug delivery at the site of action (organ, tissue, and cell) at the same time reducing the concentration at the non-targeted sites. It has been proven that development of rational delivery approaches for old therapeutic agents might improve the efficacy, decrease the side effects of the therapy, and even improve therapeutic potential of the drug substance.

On the other hand, advances in the understanding of the pathophysiology of IBD led to a great interest in the evaluation of new therapeutic agents with novel and improved therapeutic actions and new therapeutic targets. Biological therapy came about as a consequence of improved understanding of the mechanism and pathophysiology of the disease and it was the most important addition to the IBD therapy in 50 years. Development of sophisticated drug targeting carriers for per oral delivery of new protein and peptide therapeutic agents for the treatment of IBD is by no means essential not only to provide stability, efficacy and improved targeting at the site of inflammation but to decrease the serious side effect of the biological therapeutics when administered through conventional parenteral dosage forms. The underlying mechanism of the novel disease oriented experimental strategies for drug targeting is based on complete understanding of the mechanisms of the disease and drug action.

In order to cover the basic principles of the disease oriented strategies for GI targeting based on micro- and nano-sized carriers and to emphasize the advantages and disadvantages of this design approach, short summary of the disease ethyology and pathogenesis will be given. Common working hypothesis for explanation and understanding of etiology and pathogenesis of IBD is that IBD results from inappropriate and exaggerated mucosal immune response of the innate and adaptive immune system to normal constituents of the mucosal microflora that is in part determined by the genetic factor. Immunopathogenesis results from secretion of toxic peroxide anions, proteases, and oxygen/nitrogen radicals by activated macrophages and T-cells that kill the invading bacteria. But, these substances, except destroying the antigen, will also cause indiscriminate damage to the surrounding tissue. In healthy GI tract the inflammation ceases once the antigen is eliminated and the immune cells are no longer directly stimulated. But in IBD the immune cells are stimulated from commensal bacteria or GI tract bacterial microflora which is a trigger for continuous inflammation, mounting and accumulating inflammatory mediators and inflammatory substances with increasing potential for inflammation induced damage to the epithelial barrier. Inflammation induced damage will allow increased permeability and infiltration of bacteria into the lamina propria causing further stimulation of the immune cells, magnifying the inflammatory response and creating a vicious circle of continuous tissue damage. Increased permeability of the epithelial barrier, accompanied with increase of M-cell number as well as increased uptake activity of the immunoregulatory cells at the site of inflammation are the main disease related factors resulting with increased interaction with the physical systems like micro- and nano-particles (MPs and NPs) and increased concentration of these polymeric carriers loaded with drug substance at the site of action (Babbs, 1992; Beckman & Ames, 1997; Cuvelier et al., 1994; Grisham & Granger, 1988; Ina et al., 1999; Nikolaus et al., 1998; Oz & Ebersole, 2008; Uguccioni et al., 1999). During inflammation the particles will be concentrated in an increased manner in the lamina propria and in the follicle region not only through the usual gateway like antigen sampling microfold cells (M-cells) overlying the lymphoid follicles of Payer's patches in the small intestines and colonic mucosal lymphoid organs in the colon but through the leaky inflamed epithelium as well (Fujimura et al., 1992; Van Assche & Rutgeerts, 2002; Yeh et al., 1998). Further, the interaction of the physical systems with the aberrantly present enormously active immunorelated cells (macrophages, dendritic cells) at the site of inflammation will increase the concentration of the active substance in the inflammation related elements which actually represent therapeutic targets for the anti-inflammatory agents.

Polymer	Design approach	Sources
Eudragit E 100 Cationic copolymer soluble in water (<pH 5) **Eudragit L 100** Anionic copolymer dissolves at pH≥6.0 **Eudragit S 100** Anyonic copolymer dissolves at pH≥7.0 **Eudragit RL 100** **Eudragit RS 100** Neutral copolymers insoluble in water with pH independent swelling **Eudragit FS 30D Anionic copolymer dissolves at pH above 7.0**	CODES™ - colon specific drug delivery technology for single unit (tablets) and multiple unit (pellets) dosage forms - developed as a combination of pH, time and microbiological approach Composition: Enteric coating polymer/s (delayed release): Eudragit L, HPMCP Inner acid soluble coating (sustained release): Eudragit E Polysacharide containing core	(Katsuma et al., 2004, Omar et al., 2007)
	pH dependent reservoir system pH dependent polymers (delayed release): Eudragit L100 and Eudragit S100	(Khan et al., 2000)
	Combined pH and time dependent reservoir system pH dependent polymer (delayed release): Eudragit S, Eudragit L Time dependent polymers (sustained release): Eudragit RL and Eudragit RS	(Akhgari et al., 2006; Patel, 2010)
	pH dependent reservoir systems with or without disintegrants acting upon the increased permeability or dissolution of the acid resistant layer	(Bott et al., 2004; Ibekwe et al., 2006; Kshirsagar, 2009)
Ethylcellulose Insoluble in water	pH and time dependent system Time dependent polymer matrix: ethylcellulose/hydroxyethylcellulose Enterosolvent polymer coat: Eudragit S 100	(Alvarez-Fuentes et al., 2004)
	Time and microbiologically dependent multi-reservoir drug delivery system Time dependent coating was composed of ethylcellulose combined with microbiologically degradable pectin	(Wei et al., 2008)
Hydroxypropyl methylcellulose phthalate (HPMCP) **HP50; HP 55** Soluble in: water (pH>5.0; pH > 5.5)	Pressure controlled system: disintegrates due to the colon luminal inner pressure composed of HPMCP enterosolvent coating over ethylcellulose coating	(Jeong et al., 2001)
	pH and microbiologically controlled multiparticulated system composed of HPMCP, pectin and chitosan	(Oliveira, G.F., 2010)

Table 2. Conventional approaches for colon targeting

This phenomenon is equable to epithelial EPR effect (enhanced permeability and retention due to increased tumor capillary endothelial permeability) employed for drug targeting in solid tumors, as the potential strategy for targeting the inflamed tissue in GI tract is based on quite similar principles of increased permeability and retention by the endothelial tissue (Lamprecht, 2010; Pastorelli et al., 2008). Compared to conventional GI site targeting using pH, time dependent, pressure or microbiologically dependent systems, this approach is a an improvement in the principle of accumulation as it targets directly the site of inflammation. The fact that often the exact location of the site of inflammation is not known is not an issue for this design approach as drug delivery systems accumulate at the site of inflammation due to the increased permeability of the inflamed mucosa as well as particle uptake due to the interaction with aberrantly present macrophages and dendritic cells at the site of inflammation (Nakase et al., 2000; Tabata et al., 1996). The DDS designed by this targeting approach have to be fabricated with specific physicochemical properties and to be able to overcome the barriers including steep pH gradient, premature binding to the mucus layer, premature uptake or absorption and premature clearance, in order to reach the site of inflammation and accumulate according to the epithelial EPR effect in the GI tract.

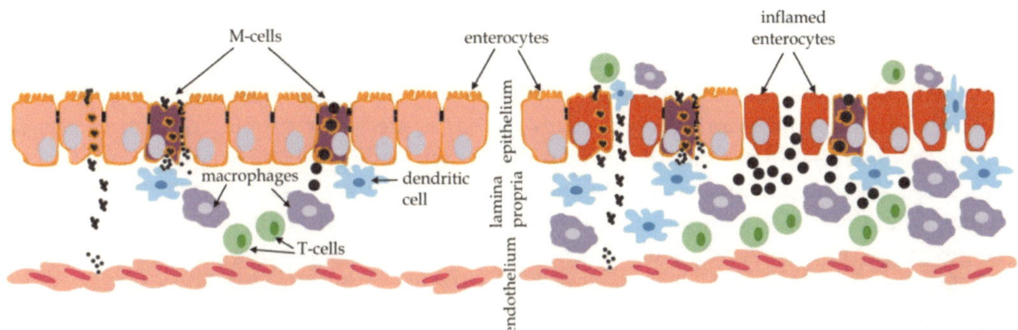

Fig. 1. Translocation of the particles through GI tract epithelium - mechanistic approach (the sieving effect and partitioning between mucus/glycocalyx and GI tract epithelium is not presented), 1. Un-inflamed mucosa: endocytotic uptake and/or transcytosis through enterocytes (particles size<500 nm); lymphatic uptake - particles adsorbed by M-cells of the Peyer's patches (particle size <5 μm) and enhanced adhesion of the MPs and NPs to the intestinal epithelium elicited by the adequate muco/bioadhesive coating 2. Inflamed mucosa: increased particle uptake due to cytokine induced disruption and leaky epithelium; presence of large intercellular pores due to the lower expression of tight junction proteins; improved lymphatic uptake due to the increased M-cell population and large population of macrophages, dendritic cells and natural killer cells in lamina propria and in the mucus layer.

Sophisticated manipulation of the physicochemical properties during the fabrication of the targeted DDS will provide functionality of the proposed targeting mechanism. Among them in addition to particle size and particle size distribution are the stability in GI tract, zeta potential, hydrophylicity, hydrophobicity, swelling properties, muco/bioadhesivity, surface active groups, density, porosity, etc.

3.1 Physicochemical properties affecting the efficacy of the DDS

Targeting IBD using disease oriented strategy requires particle stability and inertness in the upper GI tract, increased retention time in the lower parts of the GI tract, specific interaction of the particles with the inflamed mucosal tissue and immunoregulatory elements as well as controlled release at the site of action. Improved concentration of the DDS and controlled release of the drug substance at the site of therapeutic action will contribute to improved efficacy as well as decreased systemic exposure and side effects from the therapy. The importance and tailoring of the physicochemical properties of the DDS according to selected targeting mechanism as well as physiological and patophysiological conditions at the therapeutic site of action will be discussed through design, production and physicochemical characterization of budesonide loaded chitosan-Ca-alginate MPs intended for targeting and treatment of IBD.

Particle size: Very well known fact about the particle size of the DDS is that accelerated elimination and premature clearance due to the diarrhea, a major symptom of IBD, will be circumvented by size reduction effect and formulation of MPs or NPs for inflammation targeting (Lamprecht et al., 2005; Nakase et al., 2000; Nakase et al., 2001). In order to achieve improved localization and prolonged residence time due to increased epithelial permeability and enormous immunoregulatory cells activity at the site of inflammation, the beads should have an optimal particle size, probably between 4 and 15 μm (Coppi et al., 2001, 2002; Lamprecht et al., 2001, 2001a). Carrier systems in that size range are able to attach more efficiently to the mucus layer and accumulate in the inflamed region even without the need for macrophage uptake. NPs have also shown potential for specific accumulation in the areas with inflamed tissue increasing the selectivity of local drug delivery. When particles of different sizes are compared one simple conclusion can be drawn; that increased retention of particles of all sizes bellow 10 μm is noticed in inflamed tissue and with further size reduction the retention effect is maximized and the clearance minimized at the size of approximately 100 nm (Lamprecht et al., 2001, 2001a).

The mucus gel layer covering the intestinal/colonic mucosa is the first barrier to overcome in order to achieve increased localization in the Payer patches, intestinal lymphoid tissue and lamina propria. It is well known that UC and, to a lesser extent, CD is associated with an alteration and reduction of the protective mucus layer in the large intestine. In active UC there was a trend for the mucus layer to become progressively thinner and significantly more discontinuous as disease severity increases. The number of goblet cells in UC, which synthesize both mucin and intestinal trefoil factor, is reduced in active disease and the gel layer is consequently thinner. Mucin quality is also affected by the depletion or decreased sulfation and by increased quantity of sialic acid residues (Fujimura et al., 1992; Nakase et al., 2001; Yeh et al., 1998). Recently, data developed mainly through the investigation of most common UC induced model, dextran sulphate model, were published, pointing that the defects in the inner mucus layer may allow massive bacterial penetration into the normal sterile crypts and trigger the inflammation. Probably this pathology of the outer and inner compact and protective mucus layer contributes to the effect of increased permeability of the intestinal mucosa and improved localization of the particulate systems during inflammation. CD, unlike UC, is deep seated, therefore cytokines may initially stimulate mucus secretion, and increase thickness, but as the inflammation becomes more extensive it might begin to impair mucus production by the epithelium (Dieleman et al., 1998; Kojouharoff et al., 1997; Ni et al., 1996).

Translocation of the particles across the enterocytes/colonocytes and M cells after diffusion through mucus/glycocalyx layer as a diffusional and enzymatic barrier for healthy intestinal tissue is also affected by size and surface chemistry. Plausible mechanistic explanation for size dependent disposition and translocation of MP and NP-DDS in healthy

GI tract includes the following processes i). endocytotic uptake - particles absorbed by intestinal enterocytes through endocytosis (particles size<500 nm); ii). lymphatic uptake - particles adsorbed by M cells of the Peyer's patches (particle size <5 μm) and iii). an enhanced adhesion of the microparticles and nanoparticles to the intestinal epithelium elicited by the adequate muco/bioadhesive coating, resulting, overall in a marked improvement of the absorption into the intestinal cells due to the ability of creating favorable concentration gradient for absorption or escaping from the multi-drug resistance pump proteins. But usually, because of the low endocytic activity of the enterocytes and the presence of tight junctions, translocation is mainly performed across the M-cells. Macrophages in M-cells invaginate the basolateral membrane to an extent that they come very close to the apical membrane, sometimes even protruding into the lumen. Literature data point that further biological fate after internalization depends on the size and chemistry as well. It is reported that internalized particles between 2 - 5 μm will remain longer in the Payer's patches, consequently showing very small systemic distribution compared to smaller nano sized particles. Particles bellow 2 μm migrated from the patches to mesenteric lymph nodes. Altered mucus layer during IBD, leaky epithelium and increased activity of the immunoregulatory cells in the inflamed mucosa are additional variables contributing to the improved localization of MPs and NPs at the site of inflammation but at the same time they assist the translocation and biological fate of the MP/NP-DDS to be even less predictable (Lamprecht, 2010; Nixon et al., 1996; Reece et al., 2001).
Implementing previously stated targeting principles we have designed microparticulated polyelectrolyte muco/bioadhesive DDS for inflammation targeting using the enhanced permeability effect as targeting strategy (Crcarevska et al., 2009; Glavas Dodov et al., 2009; Mladenovska et al., 2007; Mladenovska et al., 2007; Simonoska Crcarevska et al., 2008). We hypothesized that polyelectrolyte particles with a size from 1-5 μm, narrow particle distribution, positive surface charge, pH and crosslinking dependent swelling/bioadhesion and release might be suitable DDS for interaction and increased accumulation in the inflamed tissue. However, the distribution is not only size related property, but a complex interrelationship among size, shape, density, hydrophylicity/ hydrophobicity, swelling properties, surface active groups, surface charge of the drug carrier etc. Consequently, only complex combination of different attributes of the DDS might result with efficacious targeting and performance.
Surface active groups, zeta potential and muco/bioadhesion: Number of polymers with muco/bioadhesive properties are cited in literature. Anionic polymers (polyacrylates and cellulose derivatives) and cationic polymers (chitosan) interact with mucus layer through non-covalent interactions (hydrophobic interactions, hydrogen binding, van der Waals interactions, electrostatic interactions) modulated by pH and ionic strength of the environment. Alginate (anionic polymer) is also citied among polymers with mucoadhesive properties involving hydrogen bonding of alginate carboxylic groups with mucus layer as a mechanism of mucoadhesive interaction (Chickering, 1995; Deacon et al., 2000; Fiebrig, 1994; 1995; Gombotz & Wee, 1998; Hejazi & Amiji, 2003; Wittaya-Areekul et al., 2006). Thiolated polymers of polyacrylates and cellulose derivatives as well as chitosan thiolated polymers exibit cationic covalent bonding building strong covalent disulfide bonds with the cysteine domains of mucins (Bernkop-Schnurch et al., 1999). Other synthetic polymers used in bioadhesive formulations are: polyvinyl alcohol, polyamides, polycarbonates, polyalkylene glycols, polyvinyl ethers, esters and halides, polymethacrylic acid, polymethyl methacrylic acid, methylcellulose, ethyl cellulose, hydroxypropyl cellulose, hydroxypropyl

methylcellulose, sodium carboxymethylcellulose and various biodegradable polymers like poly(lactides), poly(glycolides), poly(lactide-co-glycolides), polycaprolactones, polyalkyl cyanoacrylates, polyorthoesters etc.

Having in mind bio/mucoadhesive properties of natural biopolymers, cationic chitosan and anionic alginate were selected for formulation of the budesonide loaded microparticulated DDS with a potential for IBD targeting. Sodium alginate LF 10/60 which consists of 65–75% of guluronic acid (G) and 25–35% of manuronic acid (M) was used for particle preparation because MG types compared with MM and GG types of sodium alginate have better flexibility (Smidsrød, 1973), and polymer gels formed from alginate with high percentage of guluronic acid (>70%) have highest mechanical strength and stability towards monovalent ions (Martinsen, 1991). Chitosan with low viscosity, highly deacetylated was chosen for polyelectrolyte complexation with sodium alginate. The fact that the deacetylated chains are fully stretched by the electrostatic repulsion among the -NH3+ groups (and the acetylated blocks are micelle-like agglomerates because of the hydrophobic forces), leads to a conclusion that higher degree of deacetylation might contribute to more efficient process of coating. Additional physicochemical stability of the alginate-chitosan polyelectrolyte complex was provided by crosslinking with inorganic calcium chloride. The method of preparation was simple and highly reproducible one step spray-drying procedure (Goracinova, 2005) carried out through concomitant spraying of core (budesonide containing alginate solution) and coating solutions (chitosan/calcium chloride solution) through adopted two fluid-nozzle. Processes of ionotropic gelation/polyelectrolite complexation are simultaneously performed during the short contact of the core and coating solution at the tip of the nozzle followed by drying in a spray drying chamber. Theoretically, during one-step procedure (Fig. 2.A) both chitosan molecules and calcium ions are competing with each other at the same time for the negatively charged groups of the alginate molecules and this competition may result in slightly bound chitosan molecules at the particle surface, hence keeping their flexibility when the particles are suspended in aqueous milieu. As a result, they are able to interact with the mucin chains and show good mucoadhesivity. Zeta potential of the particles is positive and in a magnitude of 30 – 45 mV (buffer solutions from pH 2.0 till pH 6.8) providing good stability against agglomeration. Considering, that chitosan–Ca–alginate MPs showed a positive value of the zeta potential at all pH media an assumption for the presence of chitosan at the surface of the particles can be made (Borges et al., 2005). 14C sodium acetate was used for quantitative determination of amino groups at the MPs surface and 14C glycine ethyl ester was used for carboxyl group quantification. Although amino groups were prevalent at the surface, also carboxyl groups were present at the surface of the carrier. Compared to the one step procedure, when two step spray drying procedure was applied for MPs production (preparation of alginate particles by spray drying with subsequent crosslinking in a solution of calcium chloride and chitosan) particle's zeta potential was negative, pointing that most of the chitosan amino groups are crosslinked with the carboxyl alginate groups or that the chitosan is deeply infiltrated within the pores of the microspheres without forming a continuous coating layer at the surface (Fig. 2.B). Surface properties of prepared beads are essential for efficacy of the DDS, since positive charge originating from chitosan is crucial for the interaction with negatively charged mucus and cell membranes. During the inflammation these surfaces are becoming even more negative due to the increased production of sialic acid and sialic acid residues during inflammation (Martinac et al., 2005). Considering the expecting performance of the DDS under development and the benefit of increase residence time at the site of inflammation, it is obvious that by utilization of one step spray drying procedure expected mucoadhesivity of prepared MPs will be obtained.

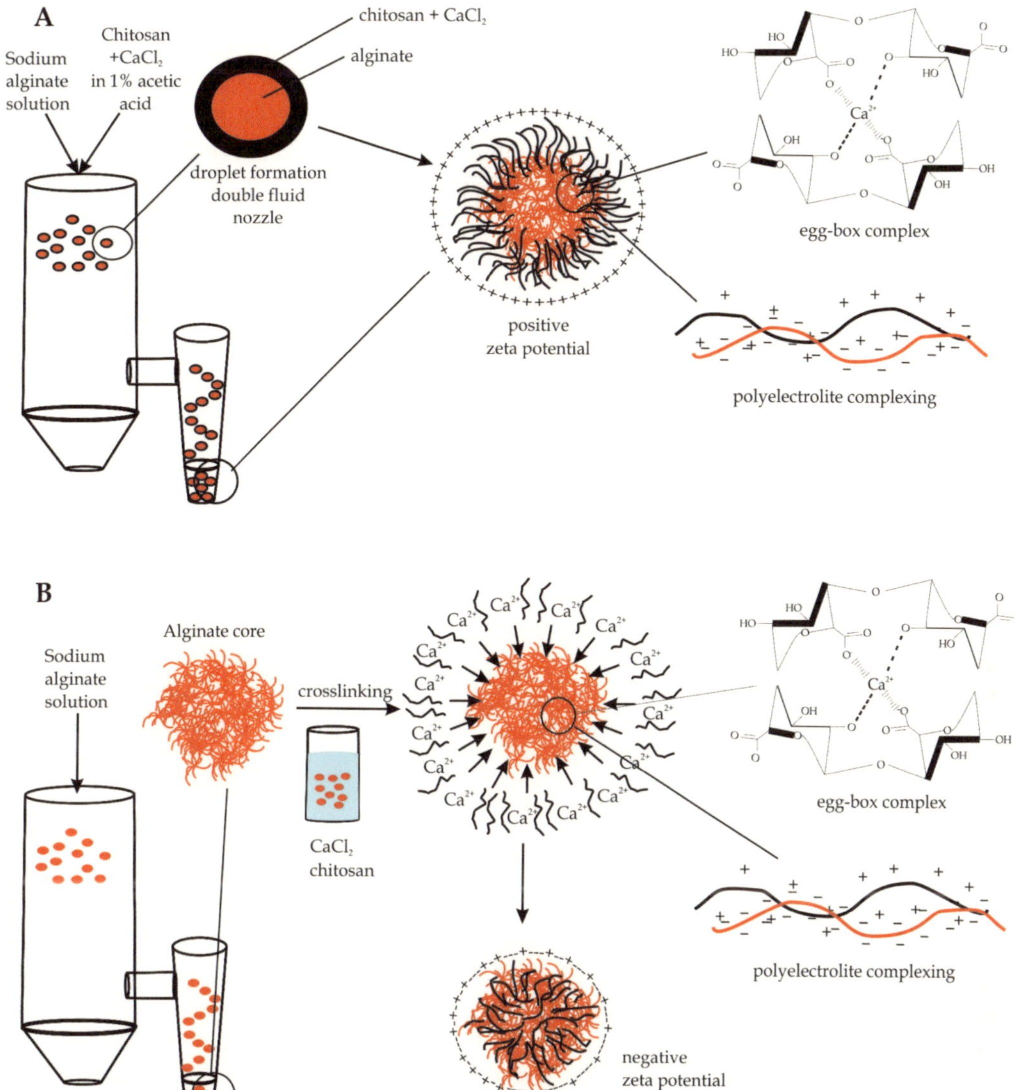

Fig. 2. Different structural and surface properties of chitosan-Ca-alginate MPs prepared by: A. one step spray-drying procedure; B. two step spray-drying procedure

As crosslinked polyelectrolyte matrices posses different properties compared to the starting polymers, physicochemical stability in the bio-environment of the upper GI tract, at the same time increased site-specificity and interaction with the bio-environment in the lower parts of GI tract (swelling, muco/bioadhession and controlled drug release) were adjusted through the degree of crosslinking during the production process. As mucoadhesiveness of the polymers and physicochemical stability of the chitosan-Ca-alginate MPs depend on their solubility, flexibility of the polymer backbone and its polar functional groups, it is obvious that it can be modified during the cross-linking procedure (Huang et al., 2000; Wittaya-Areekul et al., 2006). By controlling the degree of crosslinking, through optimization of the process conditions, concentration of polymer and calcium chloride solutions, the polyelectrolyte bio-matrices were tailored to be inert in the bio-environment of the upper parts of GI tract, showing relatively low degree of swelling and high physicochemical stability. This slightly swollen matrices travel freely through the GI tract until reaching biological fluids with higher pH values and composition which will favor de-crosslinking of the matrix, inducing swelling and controlled drug release of the active substance.

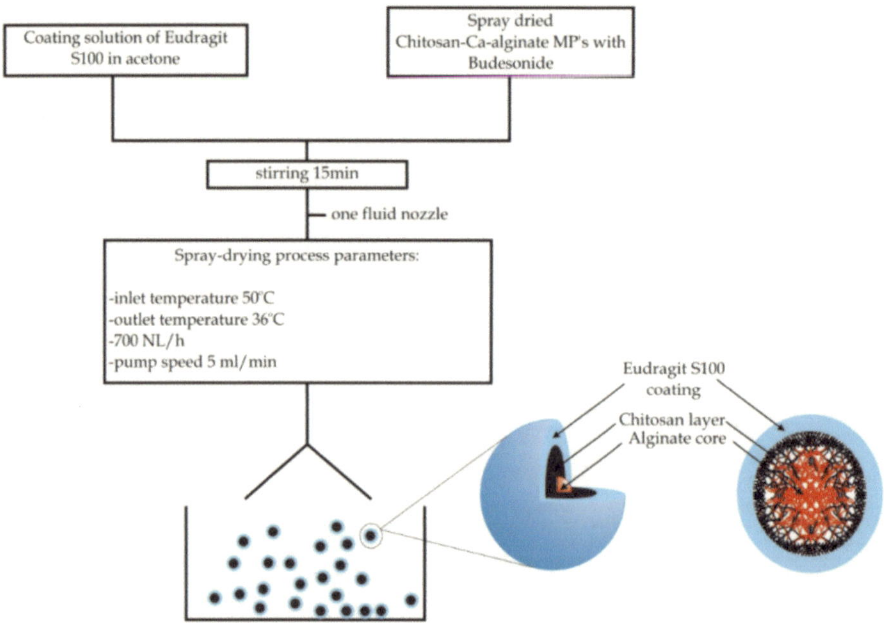

Fig. 3. Schematic presentation of coating procedure of budesonide loaded chitosan–Ca-alginate MPs (EMPB)

Physicochemical changes in the hydrogel environment induce relaxation of the polymer network which initiates mucus layer interaction as a result of pH, ion exchange and microbiologically induced swelling of the polymer (chitosan enzymatic degradation in colon) network. Prolonged residence time of the bioresponsive matrices at the site of action will further improve targeting of the inflammation facilitating and improving the contact with the mucosal tissue, providing better conditions for particle uptake by the inflamed tissue or improved absorption. Increased localization and uptake as well as controlled drug release at the site of action will provide significant improvement of the therapeutic efficacy. In order to avoid any undesirable erroneous performance in the upper GI tract, the chitosan-Ca-alginate MPs loaded with budesonide (MPB) were additionally coated with enterosolvent polymer (EMPB), as a second control barrier to the drug release at pH range from 2.0 to 6.8 (Fig. 3).

In order to test the suitability of prepared particles for efficient treatment of IBD *in vivo,* studies on rat model of TNBS induced colitis were performed. GI tract time distribution study indicated that complete gastric emptying was reached within 2 hours, while after 6th hour most of the MPs were located in the colon where the radioactive material deposits remained detectable even after 24 hours. When correlated with GI time distribution studies the *in vitro* swelling behavior, mucoadhesion and *in vitro* drug release correlated with the expected performance *in vivo* (Fig. 4A, B).

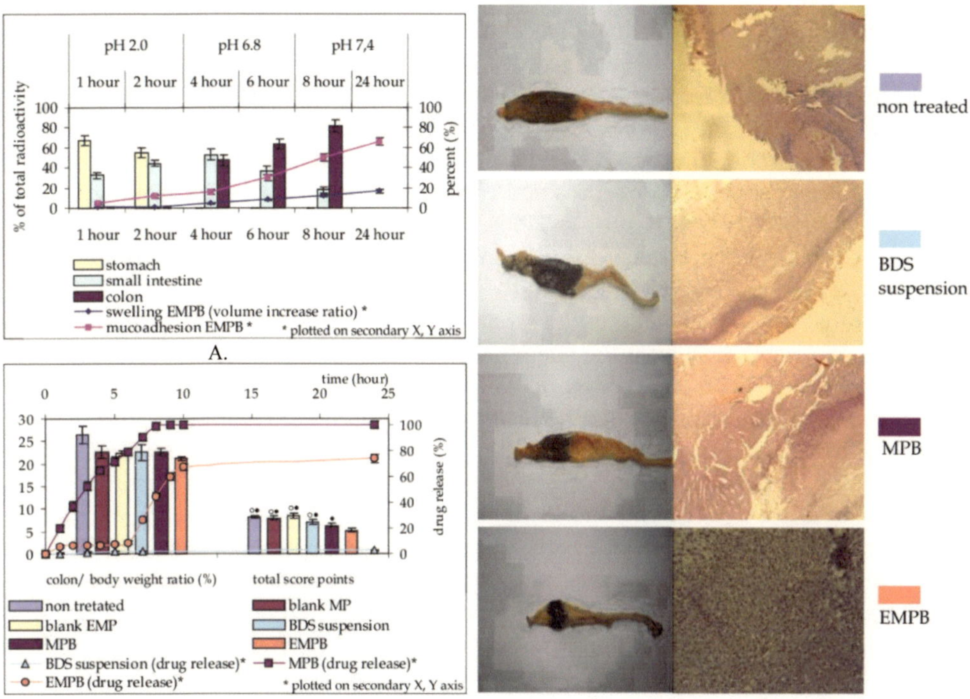

B. C.

Fig. 4. **A.** GI tract distribution of ^{99m}Tc labeled MPs after peroral administration to Wistar rats with TNBS induced colitis (mean ± SD, n=12), swelling and mucoadhesive properties of EMPB (mean ± SD, n=3). **B.** *In vitro* release profiles of BDS suspension, MPB and EMPB (2 hours at pH 2.0; additional 4 hours at pH 6.8 and up to 24 hours at pH 7.4) (mean ± SD, n=3); Colon/body weight ratio and total score points after the treatment with EMPB, MPB, BDS suspension, blank uncoated and Eudragit coated MPs (MP and EMP), as well as non treated animals sacrificed 6th day after colitis induction, (mean ± SD; n=5), ○ statistically significant difference (P<0.05) compared to MPB, • statistically significant difference (P<0.05) compared to EMPB.
C. Photographs and histology of a representative colon specimens of animals with TNBS induced colitis: non treated group-severe inflammation with complete destruction of mucosa structure followed by loss of epithelium; treated with BDS suspension - focal ulcerations, necrosis with demarcation, loss of the necrotic epithelium, and formation of granulation tissue; treated with MPB - lower degree of necrosis with distinct boundary of necrotic lesions, focal erosive changes, but also, formation of granulation tissue, regeneration and parts with normal proliferating mucosa; treated with EMPB - focal ulcerative lesions, necrosis with focal character and distinct boundary from the normal tissue, lower parts of mucosa with large granulation tissue. Regeneration tendency could be observed easily.

Efficacy of prepared MPs (selected uncoated and Eudragit coated formulations, $CaCl_2$:alginate=1:0.625) was evaluated on male Wistar rats using experimentally TNBS induced colitis (Crcarevska et al., 2009). For comparison, adequate blank MPs, as well as budesonide (BDS) suspension were used. After 5 days of daily administration by oral gavage of prepared formulations, the rats were sacrificed and colon/body weight ratio, gross morphological and histological evaluation, and clinical activity score as inflammatory indices were determined. Individual clinical and histological evaluation showed that colitis severity was suppressed in following order BDS suspension < MPB < EMPB (Fig. 4C). Clinical activity score decreased in the same order (Fig. 4B). Statistical analysis of total score points indicated that the incorporation of budesonide into MPs showed significant differences in favor of efficacy of the DDS with expected accumulation at the site of inflammation, mucoadhesive properties and controlled release at the site of action (one-way ANOVA, $P<0.05$) (Crcarevska et al., 2009). Fig. 4B comparatively presents the drug dissolution profiles of the tested formulations to the efficacy of designed systems in the treatment of TNBS induced colitis.

It is obvious that the system showing postponed release until colon and controlled release during colon residence time or at the site of action demonstrated highest *in vivo* efficacy. In fact this is most likely due to the unique combination of bio/mucoadhesive properties of designed system along with physicochemical and biopharmaceutical properties, hence, by its design providing improved localization in the inflamed tissue and/or prolonged residence time in colon. Namely, carrier system with such properties possess ability to attach more efficiently to the mucus layer in the lower GI tract and accumulate in the inflamed region even without need for macrophage uptake, although the particles were designed to be taken up by macrophages easily as well. The system is inert in the upper GI tract, showing minimal adhesion and swelling but, anyway, second line defense was added with Eudragit coating in order to prevent any nonspecific adherence in the upper GI tract and provide increased drug control release through GI tract. Thus, budesonide is effectively delivered in a controlled manner to the colon due to the increased accumulation effect in the inflamed tissue of the MPs itself and controlled release at the site of action. Controlled drug release allows pharmacological effects to be extended due to the prolonged residence time of the carrier system at the targeted inflamed area. In fact, enteric coated MPs are specific complex system different from uncoated MPs, by their *in vitro* and hence *in vivo* performance. Although both systems show improved *in vivo* efficacy, the Eudragit coated one outperformed non coated MPs during the *in vivo* studies.

4. Specific colon targeting

Theoretically, the selectivity of inflammation targeting in GI tract can be improved by attachment of various ligands at the surface of the carriers. Specific interactions with the receptors uniformly present at large areas or only in a specialized areas in the GI tract will improve bioadhesion and absorption, capacity for endocytosis and cell localization. Number of ligands and ligand-receptor pairs are discovered and examined for targeting the healthy and diseased tissue. Among them are receptor-recognizable ligands, such as lectins, toxins, viral haemagglutinins, invasins, transferrin, and vitamins (Vitamin B12, folate, riboflavin and biotin), which may improve the specificity of the delivery systems for the target cells (Brayden et al., 2005; Clark et al., 1998; De Boer, 2007; Foster & Hirst, 2005; Leamon & Low, 2001; Lee et al., 2005; Ota et al., 2002; Roth-Walter et al., 2004, 2005; Russell-Jones et al., 1999;

Vinogradov et al., 1999). The most exploited ligands for GI targeting are different types of lectins due to their specificity for the membrane associated carbohydrate rich material mainly composed of olligosacharides conjugated with membrane lipids, proteins or peptide glycans. When conjugated to DDS and macromolecular drugs, depending on the lectin structure and sugar specificity, lectins may adhere and bind to the cellular surface or induce cellular uptake and internalization routing of the DDS. However, there are two distinct layers present in the intestinal mucosa, mucus layer and the glycocalix that are reach with oligosaccharides. Carbohydrate domains of glycolipids and glycoproteins protrude outwards the cell membrane to create, together with the acidic mucopolysaccharides, a thick meshwork or glycocalyx. Adhesion of the lectinised DDS at the mucus layer will produce effect similar to non-specific mucoadhesives, prolonging the residence time at the site of absorption, and dependent on the physicochemical properties of the carrier as well as the type and intensity of mucoadhesive interaction increased concentration gradient between the lumen and enterocytes and facilitated absorption might be also provided (Gao et al., 2007; Gupta, 2009; Irache et al., 2008; Smart, 2004). Anyway, this highly viscous mucus layer is also a barrier to the diffusion of the DDS towards transmembrane mucin associated oligosaccharides into the glycocalyx contributing to low accessibility and low predictability of cytoadhesion and/or cytoinvasion with lectin mediated DDS. If the physicochemical properties of the carrier (particle size, polymer properties, surface charge, surface active groups as well as the nature of attached ligand) promote mucus diffusion, partitioning of the formulation to the cell surface is possible due to the reversibility of the lectin-mucin interaction, even if the similar oligosaccharides in the mucus layer and glycocalyx are the targeted one. Interaction with the specific carbohydrates of the glycocalyx is also possible and it will induce cytoadhesion increasing the concentration gradient and improving absorption. Apart from this interaction, lectins might interact with carbohydrate domains of glycolipids and glycoproteins protruding outwards the cell membrane into the glycocalyx (glycosylated cell receptor interaction). Lectins interacting wih the glycocalix of certain region or certain cell types in GI tract are so called "bioadhesives of second generation" (Lehr, 2000; Tao et al., 2003). Direct adhesion to the cell wall will certainly overcome the limitation of mucoadhesion contact time improvement limited to few hours, extending the residence time and the interaction time to several days. However, glycocalyx sieve function is again important for the receptor accessibility and the interaction with glycosylated receptors at the cell membrane which for some lectines as wheat germ agglutinin (WGA) for epidermal growth factor (EGF)-receptor might induce receptor mediated endocytosys and internalization of nano-scaled carrier systems into acidic endosomal compartments, releasing the drug into the cytoplasm or part of the nano-carriers can also follow transcytotic patway (Lochner et al., 2003).

The features of different sites and cell types as well as characteristics of the overlying mucus layer and glycocalyx (thickness and glycosylation pattern) are well documented through literature. Folicle associated epithelium covering the Payer patches with its M-cells specialized in transcytosis; weak mucus production, unique ultrastructure of the glycocalyx and glycosylation pattern, number of infiltrated B cells, T cells, macrophages and dendritic cells, lack of subepithelial myofibroblast sheat and its basal lamina much more porous compared to regular epithelia are characteristics that support different translocation pattern and membrane receptor accessibility (Gabor et al., 2004; Gupta, 2009). Also, although M-cells highly express diverse terminaly glycosylated glycoconjugates which may be exploited as receptors, the uptake of particles by M-cells is not entirely dependent on specific ligand binding, since adherence to M-cells by any mechanism leads to endocytosis, phagocytosis, pinocytosis, and macropinocytosis or any other mechanism used for the ingestion of the extracellular material. Colonic mucosa doesn't contain Payer's patches but it contains large lymphoid follicles of a dome-type configuration, extended as far as the lamina propria of the mucosa and associated with massive lymphoid aggregations spreading beyond the muscularis mucosa from the submucosa. The epithelium covering these follicles, is associated with a few goblet cells, contains M-cells and many migrating lymphocytes crossing through discontinuities of the basal lamina in the vicinity of the M-cells, and is specialized, differing from the surrounding mucosa (Fujimura et al., 1992).

In order to integrate this concepts of glycotargeting into the inflammation targeting the influence of mucus production impairment and reduction of the protective mucus layer in the intestines during inflammation, increased epithelial permeability, characteristic increased immunoregullatory cells activity in the inflamed tissue (section 3), presence of occasional erosions for ex. at the apical surface of the colonic lymphoid follicles in a size range of 2–6 µm in CD, revealing the naked surface of the dome beneath the epithelium and alteration of the glycolation pattern during the inflammation, have to be considered as additional factors influencing the design of the DDS. Additional decoration of the micro- and nano-carriers for inflammation targeting designed for increased accumulation due to the epithelial EPR effect might further improve the concentration of the active substance in the targeted cells due to the effect of cytoadhesion and cytoinvasion. E. coli K99 fimbriae adhesin was used to target 6-methyl prednisolone to the inflamed tissue in GI tract of the Chron's patients. Peptide, protein and DNA therapeutics delivery to the sites of therapeutic action will be also possible through the design of these specialized decorated cytoadhesive and cytoinvasive nanocarriers (section 5). Targeting the lectine molecules expressed at the mammalian cell surface, like galectins which are β-galactoside binding proteins, or direct lectine targeting, is also used for normal and diseased colon targeting.

Alteration of glycolylation pattern is seen during inflammation and neoplastic colonic disease. Abnormality in epithelial cell glycoconjugates is commonly present in both UC and CD and it may reflect abnormality in mucus glycoprotein synthesis in IBD. As a result altered lectin binding by colonic epithelial glycoconjugates in UC and CD can be seen. Up to date only limited data are available on the "sugar code" of the GI tract inflammation (Gabius, 2000). It is well known that the enterocytes, follicle-associated epithelial cells, M-cells, immunoregulatory elements and colonocites differ by their glycosylation pattern, but the data on the abnormality, differences and characteristics of epithelial glycoconjugates during UC and CD are very scarce (Yeh et al., 1998). Even less data can be found about the type of interaction mediated by certain oligosaccharide sequence and possible homing of the carrier payload into the cell or cell routing triggered by receptor ligand linking.

Histochemical studies are useful for understanding the altered lectin binding and changes in the glycosylation map during cancer and inflammation. In the study of Rhodes et al. high proportion of binding of the lectins of peanut agglutinin (PNA), Ulex europeus I (UEAI) and Griffonia simplicifolia II (GSII) to UC and CD mucosal samples was shown (Kiss et al., 1997; Rhodes et al., 1986, 1988, 2008). It was shown that PNA exhibited specificity for inflamed biopsies without binding to the mucosa or free mucus of the normal biopsies. PNA positivity, when present, was most marked in the surface epithelium, particularly in the supranuclear region of the epithelial cells. PNA identifies Gal(β1,3)GalNAc which is normally obscured by the terminal sialic acid that is added to mucus sialoglycoprotein in the Golgi apparatus as the final step in mucin synthesis. The finding of UEAI (fucose binding) positivity in a small proportion of UC and CD rectal biopsies, but not in normal rectal mucosa, may be due to reduced sialylation or increased fucosylation. Other lectins used in this study like wheat germ agglutinin (WGA), soy bean (SBA), grifonia seed (GSI) showed similar affinity to normal, UC and CD biopsies.

In the study of Melo-Junior et al. (Melo-Junior et al., 2004), it was found that WGA presented recognition pattern for diseased tissue. The authors claim that N-acetylglucosamine was absent or not accessible for lectin recognition in normal tissues, as well as mannosides and galactose. L-fucose was found in the intestinal crypts of normal glands and UC intestinal biopsies showed intense WGA binding in the gland cells of intestinal crypts, indicating high expression of N-acetylglucosamine in these cells in UC. Also, fucose binding Lotus tetragonolobus agglutinin was highly bound to UC gland epithelium pointing to increased L-fucose levels.

5. Biological and gene therapies for inflammatory bowel diseases

Although investigations of IBD pathogenesis did not clear up all misunderstandings of this disease and causes of IBD are still unknown, in depth studies of immunopathology of IBD and mechanism driving the uncontrolled inflammation enabled the development of design strategies for improvement of the efficacy of the conventional therapeutic agents as well as identification of new therapeutic targets and novel therapeutic active agents. Genetic factors and defects in innate and adaptive immune pathways have been identified, and biological therapies that target specific pathophysiological mechanisms of IBD selectively blocking the inflammatory mechanisms have been designed.

The fundamentals of biological treatment strategies involve neutralization of pro-inflammatory cytokines that plays central role in pathogenesis of CD and UC, use of anti-inflammatory cytokines and inhibition of neutrophil adhesion or T-cell signaling. Since the discovery of the central role of the proinflammatory cytokine TNF α in the inflammatory cascade of UC and CD, based on large randomized clinical trials, anti-TNF-α agents have substantially extended the therapeutic armamentarium in IBD. A variety of biological agents have been used to inhibit TNF-α in patients with IBD, including the mouse/human chimeric monoclonal antibody (infliximab), the humanized monoclonal antibody CDP571, the human soluble TNF-α p55 receptor (onercept), the human monoclonal antibody D2E7 (adalimumab), the p75 soluble TNF receptor fusion protein (etanercept), and the polyethylene glycol (PEG)ylated anti-TNF-α antibody fragment CDP-870. Among these, infliximab (formerly cA2) and CDP571 have shown the most promise, particularly in CD. However, up to date with few isolated approaches for local administration (Worledge et al., 2000; AVX-470 in preclinical studies) most of these agents are administered through conventional parenteral dosage forms resulting with lower concentration at the site of inflammation as well as direct intrusion in the human immune system, number of contraindications and serious adverse effects. In addition to these agents that directly antagonize and block the activity of TNF-α, alternative pathways for improved therapeutic approach are investigated. First of all, gene delivery that will provide sustained production of anti-inflammatory proteins has significant promise for local treatment of IBD. Also, transcription factors that regulate the synthesis of TNF-α and other proinflammatory cytokines are identified like new therapeutic targets. Among them the key transcription factor of lymphocytes and macrophages, NF-κB that plays a major role in regulating more than hundred proinflammatory cytokines, including TNF-α, is becoming an attractive

target for therapeutic intervention in IBD. A NF-κB decoy therapeutic system using a synthetic double stranded oligonucleotide to competitively inhibit binding and interaction of NF-κB to their target genoms and prevent the gene induction, transcription and production of the proinflammatory cytokines, is already presented in the literature as promising therapy for IBD and other inflammatory diseases. Successful intracellular and intranuclear delivery of the stable NF-κB decoy to the site of inflammation and action in GI tract is a field yet to be explored (Tahara et al., 2011). Finaly, RNA interference therapy utilizing short interfering (siRNA), usually composed of 20-25 nucleotides targeted to cytosol will trigger gene silencing mechanism through RNA interference where siRNA can block the expression of a specific gene (TNF-α or different proinflammatory gene expression in IBD) and proinflammatory protein synthesis, thus providing for successful therapeutic approach in IBD (Kriegel & Amiji, 2011).
Gene therapy can be delivered to local sites in GI tract, produce and concentrate a therapeutic protein in intestinal tissue, and release negligible amounts into the circulation (Kriegel & Amiji, 2011). Examples presented through literature for design approaches for gene, peptide and protein targeting in IBD relay on the previous experience with nano- and micro-carriers for inflammation and vaccine non specific or specific targeting. Higher concentration of the carrier in the inflamed tissue due to enhanced permeability of GI tract epithelium as well as increased activity of immune regulatory cells during UC and CD, increased residence time and improved carrier/cell non-specific or specific interaction are processes assisting the uptake and endosomal release in cytosol or different trafficking pathways after triggering internalization. Non-viral nano-sized vectors based on natural and/or synthetic polymers for tissue and cell specific delivery with encapsulated DNA, siRNA or oligonucleotide payload have shown promising stability, intracellular uptake, further trafficking (endosomal/lysosomal escape) and successful transfection efficacy. NiMOS (nanoparticles in microspheres system) is based on 200 nm non-condensing type B gelatin NPs encapsulated into pH and enzyme attack protective 1-5 μm poly(epsilon-caprolactone) (PCL) microspheres (Xu et al., 2011). As PCL is degraded by lipases in the small and large intestine it is expected that plasmid DNA loaded NPs might be internalized by the enterocytes or other cells in GI tract for transfection of the encoded protein. These particles loaded with anti-inflammatory murine IL-10 expressing plasmid DNA were evaluated for efficacy of transfection, through measurement of the mRNA and anti-inflammatory protein levels in TNBS induced colitis in Balb/c mice's. Concomitant effect of reduction of pro-inflammatory cytokines and chemokines together with increased messenger RNA (mRNA) and antiinflamatory IL-10 levels were reported by the authors (Bhavsar & Amiji, 2007). It is well known that successful delivery of siRNAs in the cytoplasm, will initiate a process that cleaves the complementary mRNA to prevent its processing and translation, blocking the expression of a specific gene eg. those expressed in a disease (Plevy & Targan, 2011). NiMOS was also used for oral TNF-α specific siRNA delivery (Kriegel & Amiji, 2011) and the system was evaluated for the efficacy of oral TNF-α gene silencing using Balb/c mice's TNBS induced colitis model. It was pointed that the system is promising and that lower expression of TNF-α due to silencing preceded the downregulation of other inflammatory cytokines and within time showed similar effect on the chemokine production. The concept of gene therapy for oral delivery and treatment of IBD has received significant attention, while the GI tract offers an ideal target due to large surface area and access to the luminal site of inflammation after oral administration. As the research in this field is growing day by day successful local gene delivery will probably

offer tailor made control of immune responses and inflammatory reactions for an individual patient, contributing to the overall success of the anti-inflammatory therapy during IBD.

6. Acknowledgments

For the experimental work presented the authors would like to acknowledge the support of NATO Science for Peace program: grant No. 978023

7. References

Adkin, D.A., Davis, S.S., Sparrow, R.A. & Wilding, I.R. (1993). Colonic transit of different sized tablets in healthy subjects. *Journal of Controlled Release,* Vol. 23, No. 2, (February 2003), pp. 147-156, ISSN 0168-3659

Ahmad, S., Tester, R.F., Corbett, A. & Karkalas, J. (2006). Dextran and 5-aminosalicylic acid (5-asa) conjugates: Synthesis, characterisation and enzymic hydrolysis. *Carbohydrate Research,* Vol. 341, No. 16, (November 2006), pp. 2694-2701, ISSN 0008-6215

Akhgari, A., Sadeghi, F. & Garekani, H.A. (2006). Combination of time-dependent and ph-dependent polymethacrylates as a single coating formulation for colonic delivery of indomethacin pellets. *International Journal of Pharmaceutics,* Vol. 320, No. 1-2, (August 2006), pp. 137-142, ISSN 0378-5173

Alvarez-Fuentes, J., Fernandez-Arevalo, M., Gonzalez-Rodriguez, M.L., Cirri, M. & Mura, P. (2004). Development of enteric-coated timed-release matrix tablets for colon targeting. *Journal of Drug Targeting,* Vol. 12, No. 9-10, (December 2004), pp. 607-612, ISSN 1061-186X

Babbs, C.F. (1992). Oxygen radicals in ulcerative colitis. *Free Radical Biology and Medicine,* Vol. 13, No. 2, (August 1992), pp. 169-181, ISSN 0891-5849

Beckman, K.B. & Ames, B.N. (1997). Oxidative decay of DNA. *Journal of Biological Chemistry,* Vol. 272, No. 32, (August 1997), pp. 19633-19636, ISSN 0021-9258

Bernkop-Schnurch, A., Schwarz, V. & Steininger, S. (1999). Polymers with thiol groups: A new generation of mucoadhesive polymers? *Pharmaceutical Research,* Vol. 16, No. 6, (June 1999), pp. 876-881, ISSN 0724-8741

Bhavsar, M. D. & Amiji, M. M. (2007). Gastrointestinal distribution and in vivo gene transfection studies with nanoparticles-in-microsphere oral system (NiMOS). *Journal of controlled release,*Vol. 119, No. 3, (June 2007), pp. 339-348, ISSN 0168-3659

Borges, O., Borchard, G., Verhoef, J.C., De Sousa, A. & Junginger, H.E. (2005). Preparation of coated nanoparticles for a new mucosal vaccine delivery system. *International Journal of Pharmaceutics,* Vol. 299, No. 1-2, (August 2005), pp. 155-166, ISSN 0378-5173

Bott, C., Rudolph, M.W., Schneider, A.R., Schirrmacher, S., Skalsky, B., Petereit, H.U., Langguth, P., Dressman, J.B. & Stein, J. (2004). In vivo evaluation of a novel ph- and time-based multiunit colonic drug delivery system. *Alimentary Pharmacology & Therapeutics,* Vol. 20, No. 3, (August 2004), pp. 347-353, ISSN 0269-2813

Bouma, G. & Strober, W. (2003). The immunological and genetic basis of inflammatory bowel disease. *Nature Reviews Immunology,* Vol. 3, No. 7, (October 2003), pp. 521-533, ISSN 14741733

Bourgeois, S. (2005). Polymer colon drug delivery systems and their application to peptides, proteins, and nucleic acids. *American journal of drug delivery,* Vol. 3, No. 3, (n.d.), pp. 171-204, ISSN 1175-9038

Brayden, D.J., Jepson, M.A. & Baird, A.W. (2005). Keynote review: Intestinal peyer's patch m cells and oral vaccine targeting. *Drug Discovery Today,* Vol. 10, No. 17, (September 2005), pp. 1145-1157, ISSN 1359-6446

Brown, J.P., Mcgarraugh, G.V., Parkinson, T.M., Wingard, R.E., Jr. & Onderdonk, A.B. (1983). A polymeric drug for treatment of inflammatory bowel disease. *Jornal of Medicinal Chemistry,* Vol. 26, No. 9, (September 1983), pp. 1300-1307, ISSN 0022-2623

Brunner, M. , Greinwald, R. , Kletter, K., Kvaternik, H., Corrado, M. E., Eichler, H. G. & Müller, M. (2003). Gastrointestinal transit and release of 5-aminosalicylic acid from 153Sm-labelled mesalazine pellets vs. Tablets in male healthy volunteers. *Alimentary pharmacology & therapeutics,* Vol. 17, No. 9, (May 2003), pp. 1163-1169, ISSN 0269-2813

Chickering, D.E. (1995). Bioadhesive microspheres: I. A novel electrobalance-based method to study adhesive interactions between individual microspheres and intestinal mucosa. *Journal of controlled release,* Vol. 34, No. 3, (June 1995), pp. 251-261, ISSN 0168-3659

Chourasia, M.K. & Jain, S.K. (2003). Pharmaceutical approaches to colon targeted drug delivery systems. *Journal of. Pharmacy & Pharmaceutical Sciences,* Vol. 6, No. 1, (January-April 2003), pp. 33-66, ISSN 1482-1826

Clark, M.A., Hirst, B.H. & Jepson, M.A. (1998). M-cell surface beta1 integrin expression and invasin-mediated targeting of yersinia pseudotuberculosis to mouse peyer's patch m cells. *Infection and Immunity,* Vol. 66, No. 3, (March 1998), pp. 1237-1243, ISSN 0019-9567

Clemett, D. & Markham, A. (2000). Prolonged-release mesalazine: A review of its therapeutic potential in ulcerative colitis and crohn's disease. *Drugs,* Vol. 59, No. 4, (April 2000), pp. 929-956, ISSN 0012-6667

Coppi, G., Iannuccelli, V., Bernabei, M. & Cameroni, R. (2002). Alginate microparticles for enzyme peroral administration. *International Journal of Pharmaceutics,* Vol. 242, No. 1-2, (August 2002), pp. 263-266, ISSN 0378-5173

Coppi, G., Iannuccelli, V., Leo, E., Bernabei, M.T. & Cameroni, R. (2001). Chitosan-alginate microparticles as a protein carrier. *Drug Development and Industrial Pharmacy,* Vol. 27, No. 5, (May 2001), pp. 393-400, ISSN 0363-9045

Crcarevska, M.S., Dodov, M.G., Petrusevska, G., Gjorgoski, I. & Goracinova, K. (2009). Bioefficacy of budesonide loaded crosslinked polyelectrolyte microparticles in rat model of induced colitis. *Journal of Drug Targeting,* Vol. 17, No. 10, (December 2009), pp. 788-802, ISSN 1029-2330

Cuvelier, C. A., Quatacker, J., Mielants, H., De Vos, M., Veys, E. & Roels, H. J. (1994). M-cells are damaged and increased in number in inflamed human ileal mucosa. *Histopathology,*Vol. 24, No. 5, (May 1994), pp. 417-426, ISSN 0309-0167

De Boer, A.G. (2007). Drug targeting to the brain. *Annual review of pharmacology and toxicology,* Vol. 47, No. 1, (February 2007), pp. 323-355, ISSN 0362-1642

Deacon, M.P., Mcgurk, S., Roberts, C.J., Williams, P.M., Tendler, S.J., Davies, M.C., Davis, S.S. & Harding, S.E. (2000). Atomic force microscopy of gastric mucin and chitosan mucoadhesive systems. *Biochemical Journal,* Vol. 348, No.3 (June 2000), pp. 557-563, ISSN 0264-6021

Dieleman, L.A., Palmen, M.J., Akol, H., Bloemena, E., Pena, A.S., Meuwissen, S.G. & Van Rees, E.P. (1998). Chronic experimental colitis induced by dextran sulphate sodium (dss) is characterized by th1 and th2 cytokines. *Clinical & Experimental Immunology,* Vol. 114, No. 3, (December 1998), pp. 385-391, ISSN 0009-9104

Fedorak, R.N. & Bistritz, L. (2005). Targeted delivery, safety, and efficacy of oral enteric-coated formulations of budesonide. *Advanced Drug Delivery Review,* Vol. 57, No. 2, (January 2005), pp. 303-316, ISSN 0169-409X

Fiebrig, I. (1994). Sedimentation analysis of potential interactions between mucins and a putative bioadhesive polymer. *Progress in colloid & polymer science,* Vol. 94, No. (n.d.), pp. 66-73, ISSN 0340-255X

Fiebrig, I. (1995). Transmission electron microscopy studies on pig gastric mucin and its interactions with chitosan. *Carbohydrate polymers,* Vol. 28, No. 3, (December 1995), pp. 239-244, ISSN 0144-8617

Foster, N. & Hirst, B.H. (2005). Exploiting receptor biology for oral vaccination with biodegradable particulates. *Advanced Drug Delivery Review,* Vol. 57, No. 3, (January 2005), pp. 431-450, ISSN 0169-409X

Friend, D.R. (1991). Colon-specific drug delivery. *Advanced drug delivery reviews,* Vol. 7, No. 1, (July-August 1991), pp. 149-199, ISSN 0169-409X

Friend, D.R. (2005). New oral delivery systems for treatment of inflammatory bowel disease. *Advanced Drug Delivery Review,* Vol. 57, No. 2, (January 2005), pp. 247-265, ISSN 0169-409X

Friend, D.R. (2005). New oral delivery systems for treatment of inflammatory bowel disease. *Advanced drug delivery reviews,* Vol. 57, No. 2, (January 2005), pp. 247-265, ISSN 0169409X

Friend, D.R. & Chang, G.W. (1985). Drug glycosides: Potential prodrugs for colon-specific drug delivery. *Journal of Medicinal Chemistry,* Vol. 28, No. 1, (January 1985), pp. 51-57, ISSN 0022-2623

Fujimura, Y., Hosobe, M. & Kihara, T. (1992). Ultrastructural study of m cells from colonic lymphoid nodules obtained by colonoscopic biopsy. *Digestive diseases and sciences,* Vol. 37, No. 7, (July 1992), pp. 1089-1098, ISSN 0163-2116

Gabius, H.J. (2000). Biological information transfer beyond the genetic code: The sugar code. *Naturwissenschaften,* Vol. 87, No. 3, (March 2000), pp. 108-121, ISSN 0028-1042

Gabor, F., Bogner, E., Weissenboeck, A. & Wirth, M. (2004). The lectin-cell interaction and its implications to intestinal lectin-mediated drug delivery. *Advanced Drug Delivery Review,* Vol. 56, No. 4, (March 2004), pp. 459-480, ISSN 0169-409X

Gao, X., Chen, J., Tao, W., Zhu, J., Zhang, Q., Chen, H. & Jiang, X. (2007). Uea i-bearing nanoparticles for brain delivery following intranasal administration. *International Journakl of Pharmaceutics,* Vol. 340, No. 1-2, (August 2007), pp. 207-215, ISSN 0378-5173

Gazzaniga, A., Maroni, A., Sangalli, M.E. & Zema, L. (2006). Time-controlled oral delivery systems for colon targeting. *Expert Opinion on Drug Delivery,* Vol. 3, No. 5, (September 2006), pp. 583-597, ISSN 1742-5247

Gazzaniga, A., Palugan, L., Foppoli, A. & Sangalli, M.E. (2008). Oral pulsatile delivery systems based on swellable hydrophilic polymers. *European Journal of Pharmaceutics and Biopharmaceutics,* Vol. 68, No. 1, (January 2008), pp. 11-18, ISSN 0939-6411

Glavas Dodov, M., Calis, S., Crcarevska, M.S., Geskovski, N., Petrovska, V. & Goracinova, K. (2009). Wheat germ agglutinin-conjugated chitosan-ca-alginate microparticles for local colon delivery of 5-fu: Development and in vitro characterization. *International Journal of Pharmaceutics,* Vol. 381, No. 2, (November 2009), pp. 166-175, ISSN 1873-3476

Gombotz, W.R. & Wee, S. (1998). Protein release from alginate matrices. *Advanced drug delivery reviews,* Vol. 31, No. 3, (May 1998), pp. 267-285, ISSN 0169-409X

Goracinova, K. Formulation and preparation of spray-dried alginate–Ca microparticles. Patent No. MP/MK/05/01/FF/BE/01/IP, 2005

Green, J.R., Mansfield, J.C., Gibson, J.A., Kerr, G.D. & Thornton, P.C. (2002). A double-blind comparison of balsalazide, 6.75 g daily, and sulfasalazine, 3 g daily, in patients with newly diagnosed or relapsed active ulcerative colitis. *Alimentary Pharmacology and Therapeutics,* Vol. 16, No. 1, (January 2002), pp. 61-68, ISSN 0269-2813

Grisham, M.B. & Granger, D.N. (1988). Neutrophil-mediated mucosal injury. Role of reactive oxygen metabolites. *Digestive diseases and sciences,* Vol. 33, No. 3 Suppl, (March 1988), pp. 6S-15S, ISSN 0163-2116

Gupta, V. K., Beckert, T. E. & Price, J. C. (2001). A novel ph- and time-based multi-unit potential colonic drug delivery system. I. Development. *International Journal of Pharmaceutics,* Vol. 213, No. 1-2, (February 2001), pp. 83-91, ISSN 0378-5173

Gupta, A. (2009). Targeting cells for drug and gene delivery: Emerging applications of mannans and mannan binding lectins. *Journal of scientific & industrial research (New Delhi, India: 1963),* Vol. 68, No. 6, (June 2009), pp. 465-483, ISSN 0022-4456

Haddish-Berhane, N., Farhadi, A., Nyquist, C., Haghighi, K. & Keshavarzian, A. (2007). Biological variability and targeted delivery of therapeutics for inflammatory bowel diseases: An in silico approach. *Inflammation & Allergy-Drug Targets,* Vol. 6, No. 1, (March 2007), pp. 47-55, ISSN 1871-5281

Han, H.K. & Amidon, G.L. (2000). Targeted prodrug design to optimize drug delivery. *AAPS PharmSci,* Vol. 2, No. 1, (March 2000), pp. E6, ISSN 1522-1059

Hedley, M.L. (2000). Gene therapy of chronic inflammatory disease. *Advanced Drug Delivery Review,* Vol. 44, No. 2-3, (November 2000), pp. 195-207, ISSN 0169-409X

Hejazi, R. & Amiji, M. (2003). Chitosan-based gastrointestinal delivery systems. *Journal of Controlled Release,* Vol. 89, No. 2, (April 2003), pp. 151-165, ISSN 0168-3659

Huang, Y., Leobandung, W., Foss, A. & Peppas, N.A. (2000). Molecular aspects of muco- and bioadhesion: Tethered structures and site-specific surfaces. *Journal of Controlled Release,* Vol. 65, No. 1-2, (March 2000), pp. 63-71, ISSN 0168-3659

Ibekwe, V.C., Liu, F., Fadda, H.M., Khela, M.K., Evans, D.F., Parsons, G.E. & Basit, A.W. (2006). An investigation into the in vivo performance variability of ph responsive polymers for ileo-colonic drug delivery using gamma scintigraphy in humans. *Jornal of Pharmaceutical Science,* Vol. 95, No. 12, (December 2006), pp. 2760-2766, ISSN 0022-3549

Ina, K., Kusugami, K., Hosokawa, T., Imada, A., Shimizu, T., Yamaguchi, T., Ohsuga, M., Kyokane, K., Sakai, T., Nishio, Y., Yokoyama, Y. & Ando, T. (1999). Increased mucosal production of granulocyte colony-stimulating factor is related to a delay in neutrophil apoptosis in inflammatory bowel disease. *Journal of Gastroenterology and Hepatology,* Vol. 14, No. 1, (January 1999), pp. 46-53, ISSN 0815-9319

Irache, J.M., Salman, H.H., Gamazo, C. & Espuelas, S. (2008). Mannose-targeted systems for the delivery of therapeutics. *Expert Opinion on Drug Delivery,* Vol. 5, No. 6, (June 2008), pp. 703-724, ISSN 1742-5247

Ishibashi, T., Hatano, H., Kobayashi, M., Mizobe, M. & Yoshino, H. (1998). Design and evaluation of a new capsule-type dosage form for colon-targeted delivery of drugs.

International Journal of Pharmaceutics, Vol. 168, No. 1, (June 1998), pp. 31-40, ISSN 0378-5173

Jeong, Y.I., Ohno, T., Hu, Z., Yoshikawa, Y., Shibata, N., Nagata, S. & Takada, K. (2001). Evaluation of an intestinal pressure-controlled colon delivery capsules prepared by a dipping method. *Jornal of Controlled Release,* Vol. 71, No. 2, (April 2001), pp. 175-182, ISSN 0168-3659

Jung, Y.J., Lee, J.S., Kim, H.H., Kim, Y.M. & Han, S.K. (1998). Synthesis and evaluation of 5-aminosalicyl-glycine as a potential colon-specific prodrug of 5-aminosalicylic acid. *Archives of pharmacal research,* Vol. 21, No. 2, (April 1998), pp. 174-178, ISSN 0253-6269

Katsuma, M., Watanabe, S., Takemura, S., Sako, K., Sawada, T., Masuda, Y., Nakamura, K., Fukui, M., Connor, A.L. & Wilding, I.R. (2004). Scintigraphic evaluation of a novel colon-targeted delivery system (codes) in healthy volunteers. *Journal of Pharmaceutical Science,* Vol. 93, No. 5, (May 2004), pp. 1287-1299, ISSN 0022-3549

Khan, M.Z., Stedul, H.P. & Kurjakovic, N. (2000). A ph-dependent colon-targeted oral drug delivery system using methacrylic acid copolymers. Ii. Manipulation of drug release using eudragit l100 and eudragit s100 combinations. *Drug Development and Industrial Pharmacy,* Vol. 26, No. 5, (May 2000), pp. 549-554, ISSN 0363-9045

Kiss, R., Camby, I., Duckworth, C., De Decker, R., Salmon, I., Pasteels, J.L., Danguy, A. & Yeaton, P. (1997). In vitro influence of phaseolus vulgaris, griffonia simplicifolia, concanavalin a, wheat germ, and peanut agglutinins on hct-15, lovo, and sw837 human colorectal cancer cell growth. *Gut,* Vol. 40, No. 2, (February 1997), pp. 253-261, ISSN 0017-5749

Klotz, U. & Schwab, M. (2005). Topical delivery of therapeutic agents in the treatment of inflammatory bowel disease. *Advanced Drug Delivery Review,* Vol. 57, No. 2, (January 2005), pp. 267-279, ISSN 0169-409X

Kojouharoff, G., Hans, W., Obermeier, F., Mannel, D.N., Andus, T., Scholmerich, J., Gross, V. & Falk, W. (1997). Neutralization of tumour necrosis factor (tnf) but not of il-1 reduces inflammation in chronic dextran sulphate sodium-induced colitis in mice. *Clinical & Experimental Immunology,* Vol. 107, No. 2, (February 1997), pp. 353-358, ISSN 0009-9104

Kopecek, J. (1990). The potential of water-soluble polymeric carriers in targeted and site-specific drug delivery. *Journal of Controlled Release,* Vol. 11, No. 1-3, (January 1990), pp. 279-290, ISSN 0168-3659

Kopecek, J., Kopecková, P., Brøndsted, H., Rathi, R., Ríhová, B., Yeh, P.Y. & Ikesue, K. (1992). Polymers for colon-specific drug delivery. *Journal of Controlled Release,* Vol. 19, No. 1-3, (March 1992), pp. 121-130, ISSN 0168-3659

Kriegel, C. & Amiji, M. (2011). Oral tnf-α gene silencing using a polymeric microsphere-based delivery system for the treatment of inflammatory bowel disease. *Journal of controlled release,*Vol. 150, No. 1, (February 2011), pp. 77-86, ISSN 01683659

Kshirsagar, S.J. (2009). In vitro in vivo comparison of two ph sensitive eudragit polymers for colon specific drug delivery. *Journal of pharmaceutical sciences and research,* Vol. 1, No. 4, (December 2009), pp. 61-70, ISSN 0975-1459

Lamprecht, A. (2010). Ibd: Selective nanoparticle adhesion can enhance colitis therapy. *Nature Reviews Gastroenterology and Hepatology,* Vol. 7, No. 6, (June 2010), pp. 311-312, ISSN 1759-5053

Lamprecht, A., Schafer, U. & Lehr, C.M. (2001). Size-dependent bioadhesion of micro- and nanoparticulate carriers to the inflamed colonic mucosa. *Pharmaceutical Research,* Vol. 18, No. 6, (June 2001), pp. 788-793, ISSN 0724-8741

Lamprecht, A., Ubrich, N., Yamamoto, H., Schafer, U., Takeuchi, H., Maincent, P., Kawashima, Y. & Lehr, C.M. (2001). Biodegradable nanoparticles for targeted drug delivery in treatment of inflammatory bowel disease. *Journal of Pharmacology and Experimental Therapeutics,* Vol. 299, No. 2, (November 2001), pp. 775-781, ISSN 0022-3565

Lamprecht, A., Yamamoto, H., Takeuchi, H. & Kawashima, Y. (2005). Nanoparticles enhance therapeutic efficiency by selectively increased local drug dose in experimental colitis in rats. *Journal of Pharmacology and Experimental Therapeutics,* Vol. 315, No. 1, (October 2005), pp. 196-202, ISSN 0022-3565

Larouche, J. (1995). Release of 5-asa from pentasa in patients with crohn's disease of the small intestine. *Alimentary pharmacology & therapeutics,* Vol. 9, No. 3, (June 1995), pp. 315-320, ISSN 0269-2813

Leamon, C.P. & Low, P.S. (2001). Folate-mediated targeting: From diagnostics to drug and gene delivery. *Drug Discovery Today,* Vol. 6, No. 1, (January 2001), pp. 44-51, ISSN 1878-5832

Lee, E.S., Na, K. & Bae, Y.H. (2005). Super ph-sensitive multifunctional polymeric micelle. *Nano Letters,* Vol. 5, No. 2, (February 2005), pp. 325-329, ISSN 1530-6984

Lehr, C.M. (2000). Lectin-mediated drug delivery: The second generation of bioadhesives. *J Control Release,* Vol. 65, No. 1-2, (March 2000), pp. 19-29, ISSN 0168-3659

Leopold, C.S. (2001). A practical approach in the design of colon-specific drug delivery systems, In:Book *Drug targeting* pp. (157-170), Wiley-VCH Verlag GmbH, ISBN 9783527600069

Lochner, N., Pittner, F., Wirth, M. & Gabor, F. (2003). Wheat germ agglutinin binds to the epidermal growth factor receptor of artificial caco-2 membranes as detected by silver nanoparticle enhanced fluorescence. Pharmaceutical Research,Vol. 20, No. 5, (May 2003), pp. 833-839, ISSN 0724-8741

Martinac, A., Filipovic-Grcic, J., Voinovich, D., Perissutti, B. & Franceschinis, E. (2005). Development and bioadhesive properties of chitosan-ethylcellulose microspheres for nasal delivery. *International Journal of Pharmaceutics,* Vol. 291, No. 1-2, (March 2005), pp. 69-77, ISSN 0378-5173

Martinsen, A. (1991). Comparison of different methods for determination of molecular weight and molecular weight distribution of alginates. *Carbohydrate polymers,* Vol. 15, No. 2, (n.d.), pp. 171-193, ISSN 0144-8617

Mcconnell, E.L., Short, M.D. & Basit, A.W. (2008). An in vivo comparison of intestinal ph and bacteria as physiological trigger mechanisms for colonic targeting in man. *Jornal of Controlled Release,* Vol. 130, No. 2, (September 2008), pp. 154-160, ISSN 1873-4995

Melo-Junior, M. R.; Lelles, A. M. S. & Albuquerque, F E. B. (2004). Altered lectin-binding sites in normal colon and ulcerative colitis. *Jornal Brasileiro de Patologia e Medicina Laboratorial,* (April 2004), Vol. 40, No. 2, pp. 123-125, ISSN 1676-2444

Mladenovska, K., Cruaud, O., Richomme, P., Belamie, E., Raicki, R.S., Venier-Julienne, M.C., Popovski, E., Benoit, J.P. & Goracinova, K. (2007). 5-asa loaded chitosan-ca-alginate microparticles: Preparation and physicochemical characterization. *International Journal of Pharmaceutics,* Vol. 345, No. 1-2, (December 2007), pp. 59-69, ISSN 0378-5173

Mladenovska, K., Raicki, R.S., Janevik, E.I., Ristoski, T., Pavlova, M.J., Kavrakovski, Z., Dodov, M.G. & Goracinova, K. (2007). Colon-specific delivery of 5-aminosalicylic acid from chitosan-ca-alginate microparticles. *International Journal of Pharmaceutics,* Vol. 342, No. 1-2, (September 2007), pp. 124-136, ISSN 0378-5173

Nakase, H., Okazaki, K., Tabata, Y., Uose, S., Ohana, M., Uchida, K., Matsushima, Y., Kawanami, C., Oshima, C., Ikada, Y. & Chiba, T. (2000). Development of an oral drug delivery system targeting immune-regulating cells in experimental inflammatory bowel disease: A new therapeutic strategy. *Journal of Pharmacology and Experimental Therapeutics,* Vol. 292, No. 1, (January 2000), pp. 15-21, ISSN 0022-3565

Nakase, H., Okazaki, K., Tabata, Y., Uose, S., Ohana, M., Uchida, K., Nishi, T., Debreceni, A., Itoh, T., Kawanami, C., Iwano, M., Ikada, Y. & Chiba, T. (2001). An oral drug delivery system targeting immune-regulating cells ameliorates mucosal injury in trinitrobenzene sulfonic acid-induced colitis. *Journal of Pharmacology and Experimental Therapeutics,* Vol. 297, No. 3, (June 2001), pp. 1122-1128, ISSN 0022-3565

Ni, J., Chen, S.F. & Hollander, D. (1996). Effects of dextran sulphate sodium on intestinal epithelial cells and intestinal lymphocytes. *Gut,* Vol. 39, No. 2, (August 1996), pp. 234-241, ISSN 0017-5749

Nikolaus, S., Bauditz, J., Gionchetti, P., Witt, C., Lochs, H. & Schreiber, S. (1998). Increased secretion of pro-inflammatory cytokines by circulating polymorphonuclear neutrophils and regulation by interleukin 10 during intestinal inflammation. *Gut,* Vol. 42, No. 4, (April 1998), pp. 470-476, ISSN 0017-5749

Nixon, D.F., Hioe, C., Chen, P.D., Bian, Z., Kuebler, P., Li, M.L., Qiu, H., Li, X.M., Singh, M., Richardson, J., Mcgee, P., Zamb, T., Koff, W., Wang, C.Y. & O'hagan, D. (1996). Synthetic peptides entrapped in microparticles can elicit cytotoxic t cell activity. *Vaccine,* Vol. 14, No. 16, (November 1996), pp. 1523-1530, ISSN 0264-410X

Nolen, H., 3rd, Fedorak, R.N. & Friend, D.R. (1995). Budesonide-beta-d-glucuronide: A potential prodrug for treatment of ulcerative colitis. *Journal of Pharmaceutical Science,* Vol. 84, No. 6, (June 1995), pp. 677-681, ISSN 0022-3549

Nugent, S.G., Kumar, D., Rampton, D.S. & Evans, D.F. (2001). Intestinal luminal ph in inflammatory bowel disease: Possible determinants and implications for therapy with aminosalicylates and other drugs. *Gut,* Vol. 48, No. 4, (April 2001), pp. 571-577, ISSN 0017-5749

Nugent, S.G., Kumar, D., Yazaki, E.T., Evans, D.F. & Rampton, D.S. (2000). Small intestinal luminal ph in crohn's disease: Implications for release of antiinflammatory drugs from ph-dependent capsules. *Gastroenterology,* Vol. 118, No. 4, Part 1, (April 2000), pp. A780-A780, ISSN 0016-5085

Oliveira, G.F. (2010). Chitosan–pectin multiparticulate systems associated with enteric polymers for colonic drug delivery. *Carbohydrate polymers,* Vol. 82, No. 3, (October 2010), pp. 1004-1009, ISSN 0144-8617

Oliveira, L. & Cohen, R.D. (2011). Maintaining remission in ulcerative colitis--role of once daily extended-release mesalamine. *Drug Design, Development and Therapy,* Vol. 5, (n.d.), pp. 111-116, ISSN 1177-8881

Omar, S., Aldosari, B., Refai, H. & Gohary, O.A. (2007). Colon-specific drug delivery for mebeverine hydrochloride. *Journal of Drug Targeting,* Vol. 15, No. 10, (December 2007), pp. 691-700, ISSN 1061-186X

Ota, T., Maeda, M. & Tatsuka, M. (2002). Cationic liposomes with plasmid DNA influence cancer metastatic capability. *Anticancer Research,* Vol. 22, No. 6C, (November-December 2002), pp. 4049-4052, ISSN 0250-7005

Oz, H.S. & Ebersole, J.L. (2008). Application of prodrugs to inflammatory diseases of the gut. *Molecules,* Vol. 13, No. 2, (February 2008), pp. 452-474, ISSN 1420-3049 \

Pastorelli, L., Saibeni, S., Spina, L., Signorelli, C., Celasco, G., De Franchis, R. & Vecchi, M. (2008). Oral, colonic-release low-molecular-weight heparin: An initial open study of parnaparin-mmx for the treatment of mild-to-moderate left-sided ulcerative colitis. *Alimentary Pharmacology & Therapeutics,* Vol. 28, No. 5, (September 2008), pp. 581-588, ISSN 1365-2036

Patel, J.M. (2010). Colon targeted oral delivery of ornidazole using combination of ph and time dependent drug delivery system. *International Journal of Pharmaceutical Research,* Vol. 2, No. 1, (January-March 2010), pp. 28-35, ISSN 1674-0440

Plevy, S. E. & Targan, S. R. (2011). Future therapeutic approaches for inflammatory bowel diseases. *Gastroenterology,*Vol. 140, No. 6, (May 2011), pp. 1838-1846, ISSN 0016-5085

Pozzi, F., Furlani, P., Gazzaniga, A., Davis, S.S. & Wilding, I.R. (1994). The time clock system: A new oral dosage form for fast and complete release of drug after a predetermined lag time. *Journal of Controlled Release,* Vol. 31, No. 1, (April 1994), pp. 99-108, ISSN 0168-3659

Prakash, A. (1999). Oral delayed-release mesalazine a review of its use in ulcerative colitis and Crohn`s disease. *Drugs (New York, N.Y.),* Vol. 57, No. 3, (March 1999), pp. 383-408, ISSN 0012-6667

Price, J.M., Davis, S.S., Sparrow, R.A. & Wilding, I.R. (1993). The effect of meal composition on the gastrocolonic response: Implications for drug delivery to the colon. *Pharmaceutical Research,* Vol. 10, No. 5, (May 1993), pp. 722-726, ISSN 0724-8741

Reece, J.C., Vardaxis, N.J., Marshall, J.A., Crowe, S.M. & Cameron, P.U. (2001). Uptake of hiv and latex particles by fresh and cultured dendritic cells and monocytes. *Immunology & Cell Biology,* Vol. 79, No. 3, (June 2001), pp. 255-263, ISSN 0818-9641

Rhodes, J. M., Black, R. R. & Savage, A. (1986). Glycoprotein abnormalities in colonic carcinomata, adenomata, and hyperplastic polyps shown by lectin peroxidase histochemistry. *Journal of Clinical Pathology,*Vol. 39, No. 12, (December 1986), pp. 1331-1334, ISSN 0021-9746

Rhodes, J. M., Black, R. R. & Savage, A. (1988). Altered lectin binding by colonic epithelial glycoconjugates in ulcerative colitis and crohn's disease. *Digestive Diseases and Sciences,*Vol. 33, No. 11, (November 1988) pp. 1359-1363, ISSN 0163-2116

Rhodes, J. M., Campbell, B. J. & Yu, L. G. (2008). Lectin-epithelial interactions in the human colon. *Biochemical Society Transactions,*Vol. 36, No. Pt 6, (December 2008), pp. 1482-1486, ISSN 1470-8752

Rivkin, A. (2009). Certolizumab pegol for the management of crohn's disease in adults. *Clinical Therapeutics,* Vol. 31, No. 6, (June 2009), pp. 1158-1176, ISSN 1879-114X

Roth-Walter, F., Bohle, B., Scholl, I., Untersmayr, E., Scheiner, O., Boltz-Nitulescu, G., Gabor, F., Brayden, D.J. & Jensen-Jarolim, E. (2005). Targeting antigens to murine and human m-cells with aleuria aurantia lectin-functionalized microparticles. *Immunology Letters,* Vol. 100, No. 2, (September 2005), pp. 182-188, ISSN 0165-2478

Roth-Walter, F., Scholl, I., Untersmayr, E., Fuchs, R., Boltz-Nitulescu, G., Weissenbock, A., Scheiner, O., Gabor, F. & Jensen-Jarolim, E. (2004). M cell targeting with aleuria aurantia lectin as a novel approach for oral allergen immunotherapy. *Journal of Allergy and Clinical Immunology,* Vol. 114, No. 6, (December 2004), pp. 1362-1368, ISSN 0091-6749

Roy, P. & Shahiwala, A. (2009). Multiparticulate formulation approach to pulsatile drug delivery: Current perspectives. *Journal of Controlled Release,* Vol. 134, No. 2, (March 2009), pp. 74-80, ISSN 1873-4995

Russell-Jones, G.J., Arthur, L. & Walker, H. (1999). Vitamin b12-mediated transport of nanoparticles across caco-2 cells. *International Journal of Pharmaceutics,* Vol. 179, No. 2, (March 1999), pp. 247-255, ISSN 0378-5173

Rutgeerts, P., Van Assche, G. & Vermeire, S. (2004). Optimizing anti-tnf treatment in inflammatory bowel disease. *Gastroenterology,* Vol. 126, No. 6, (May 2004), pp. 1593-1610, ISSN 0016-5085

Sandborn, W.J., Korzenik, J., Lashner, B., Leighton, J.A., Mahadevan, U., Marion, J.F., Safdi, M., Sninsky, C.A., Patel, R.M., Friedenberg, K.A., Dunnmon, P., Ramsey, D. & Kane, S. (2010). Once-daily dosing of delayed-release oral mesalamine (400-mg tablet) is as effective as twice-daily dosing for maintenance of remission of ulcerative colitis. *Gastroenterology,* Vol. 138, No. 4, (April 2010), pp. 1286-1296.e1283, ISSN 0016-5085

Sands, B.E. (2000). Therapy of inflammatory bowel disease. *Gastroenterology,* Vol. 118, No. 2 Suppl 1, (February 2000), pp. S68-82, ISSN 0016-5085

Sands, B.E. (2007). Inflammatory bowel disease: Past, present, and future. *Journal of Gastroenterology,* Vol. 42, No. 1, (January 2007), pp. 16-25, ISSN 0944-1174

Sellin, J. (2005). Treatment targets in inflammatory bowel disease. *Advanced Drug Delivery Review,* Vol. 57, No. 2, (January 2005), pp. 217-218, ISSN 0169-409X

Simonoska Crcarevska, M., Glavas Dodov, M. & Goracinova, K. (2008). Chitosan coated ca-alginate microparticles loaded with budesonide for delivery to the inflamed colonic mucosa. *European Journal of Pharmaceutics and Biopharmaceutics,* Vol. 68, No. 3, (March 2008), pp. 565-578, ISSN 0939-6411

Sinha, V.R. & Kumria, R. (2001). Colonic drug delivery: Prodrug approach. *Pharmaceutical Research,* Vol. 18, No. 5, (May 2001), pp. 557-564, ISSN 0724-8741

Sinha, V.R. & Kumria, R. (2002). Binders for colon specific drug delivery: An in vitro evaluation. *International Journal of Pharmaceutics,* Vol. 249, No. 1-2, (December 2002), pp. 23-31, ISSN 0378-5173

Smart, J.D. (2004). Lectin-mediated drug delivery in the oral cavity. *Advanced Drug Delivery Review,* Vol. 56, No. 4, (March 2004), pp. 481-489, ISSN 0169-409X

Smidsrød, O. (1973). The relative extension of alginates having different chemical composition. *Carbohydrate research,* Vol. 27, No. 1, (March 1973), pp. 107-118, ISSN 0008-6215

Tabata, Y., Inoue, Y. & Ikada, Y. (1996). Size effect on systemic and mucosal immune responses induced by oral administration of biodegradable microspheres. *Vaccine,* Vol. 14, No. 17-18, (December 1996), pp. 1677-1685, ISSN 0264-410X

Tahara, K., Samura, S., Tsuji, K., Yamamoto, H., Tsukada, Y., Bando, Y., Tsujimoto, H., Morishita, R. & Kawashima, Y. (2011). Oral nuclear factor-[kappa]b decoy oligonucleotides delivery system with chitosan modified poly(d,l-lactide-co-glycolide) nanospheres for inflammatory bowel disease. *Biomaterials,*Vol. 32, No. 3, (January 2011), pp. 870-878, ISSN 0142-9612

Tao, S.L., Lubeley, M.W. & Desai, T.A. (2003). Bioadhesive poly(methyl methacrylate) microdevices for controlled drug delivery. *Journal of Controlled Release,* Vol. 88, No. 2, (March 2003), pp. 215-228, ISSN 0168-3659

Uguccioni, M., Gionchetti, P., Robbiani, D.F., Rizzello, F., Peruzzo, S., Campieri, M. & Baggiolini, M. (1999). Increased expression of ip-10, il-8, mcp-1, and mcp-3 in ulcerative colitis. The *American Journal of Pathology,* Vol. 155, No. 2, (August 1999), pp. 331-336, ISSN 0002-9440

Van Assche, G. & Rutgeerts, P. (2002). Antiadhesion molecule therapy in inflammatory bowel disease. *Inflammatory Bowel Disease,* Vol. 8, No. 4, (July 2002), pp. 291-300, ISSN 1078-0998

Van Deventer, S.J. (1999). Anti-tnf antibody treatment of crohn's disease. *Annals of the Rheumatic Diseases,* Vol. 58, No. Suppl 1 (November 1999), pp. I114-120, ISSN 0003-4967

Verma, R.K., Krishna, D.M. & Garg, S. (2002). Formulation aspects in the development of osmotically controlled oral drug delivery systems. *Jornal of Controlled Release,* Vol. 79, No. 1-3, (Feb 2002), pp. 7-27, ISSN 0168-3659

Verma, R.K., Mishra, B. & Garg, S. (2000). Osmotically controlled oral drug delivery. *Drug Development and Industrial Pharmacy,* Vol. 26, No. 7, (July 2000), pp. 695-708, ISSN 0363-9045

Vinogradov, S., Batrakova, E., Li, S. & Kabanov, A. (1999). Polyion complex micelles with protein-modified corona for receptor-mediated delivery of oligonucleotides into cells. *Bioconjugate Chemistry,* Vol. 10, No. 5, (September-October 1999), pp. 851-860, ISSN 1043-1802

Wei, H., Qing, D., De-Ying, C., Bai, X. & Li-Fang, F. (2008). In-vitro and in-vivo studies of pectin/ethylcellulosefilm-coated pellets of 5-fluorouracil for colonic targeting. *Journal Pharmacy and Pharmacology,* Vol. 60, No. 1, (January 2008), pp. 35-44, ISSN 0022-3573

Wilding, I.R., Kenyon, C.J. & Hooper, G. (2000). Gastrointestinal spread of oral prolonged-release mesalazine microgranules (pentasa) dosed as either tablets or sachet. *Alimentary Pharmacology & Therapeutics,* Vol. 14, No. 2, (February 2000), pp. 163-169, ISSN 0269-2813

Wittaya-Areekul, S., Kruenate, J. & Prahsarn, C. (2006). Preparation and in vitro evaluation of mucoadhesive properties of alginate/chitosan microparticles containing prednisolone. *International Journal of Pharmaceutics,* Vol. 312, No. 1-2, (April 2006), pp. 113-118, ISSN 0378-5173

Wiwattanapatapee, R., Lomlim, L. & Saramunee, K. (2003). Dendrimers conjugates for colonic delivery of 5-aminosalicylic acid. *Journal of Controlled Release,* Vol. 88, No. 1, (February 2003), pp. 1-9, ISSN 0168-3659

Wong, M., Ziring, D., Korin, Y., Desai, S., Kim, S., Lin, J., Gjertson, D., Braun, J., Reed, E. & Singh, R.R. (2008). Tnfalpha blockade in human diseases: Mechanisms and future directions. *Clinical Immunology,* Vol. 126, No. 2, (February 2008), pp. 121-136, ISSN 1521-6616

Worledge, K. L., Godiska, R., Barrett, T. A. & Kink, J. A. (2000). Oral administration of avian tumor necrosis factor antibodies effectively treats experimental colitis in rats. *Digestive Diseases and Sciences,*Vol. 45, No. 12, pp. 2298-2305, ISSN 0163-2116

Xu, J., Ganesh, S. & Amiji, M. Non-condensing polymeric nanoparticles for targeted gene and sirna delivery. *International Journal of Pharmaceutics,* DOI: 10.1016/j.ijpharm. 2011.05.036, ISSN 0378-5173

Yang, L. (2008). Biorelevant dissolution testing of colon-specific delivery systems activated by colonic microflora. *Journal of Controlled Release,* Vol. 125, No. 2, (January 2008), pp. 77-86, ISSN 1873-4995

Yano, H., Hirayama, F., Arima, H. & Uekama, K. (2001). Prednisolone-appended alpha-cyclodextrin: Alleviation of systemic adverse effect of prednisolone after intracolonic administration in 2,4,6-trinitrobenzenesulfonic acid-induced colitis rats. *Journal of Pharmaceutical Science,* Vol. 90, No. 12, (December 2001), pp. 2103-2112, ISSN 0022-3549

Yeh, P., Ellens, H. & Smith, P.L. (1998). Physiological considerations in the design of particulate dosage forms for oral vaccine delivery. *Advanced Drug Delivery Review,* Vol. 34, No. 2-3, (December 1998), pp. 123-133, ISSN 1872-8294